Essence of
Office
Pediatrics

ESSENCE OF
OFFICE
PEDIATRICS

James A. Stockman III, M.D.
President
American Board of Pediatrics
Chapel Hill, North Carolina

Jacob A. Lohr, M.D.
Professor and Vice Chair
Department of Pediatrics
University of North Carolina School of Medicine
Pediatrician-in-Chief
North Carolina Children's Hospital
Chapel Hill, North Carolina

W.B. SAUNDERS COMPANY
A Harcourt Health Sciences Company
Philadelphia • London • New York • St. Louis • Sydney • Toronto

W.B. SAUNDERS COMPANY
A Harcourt Health Sciences Company

The Curtis Center
Independence Square West
Philadelphia, Pennsylvania 19106

Library of Congress Cataloging-in-Publication Data

Essence of pediatrics / [edited by] James A. Stockman III, Jacob A. Lohr
— 1st ed.

p. cm.

ISBN 0-7216-5845-8

1. Pediatrics.   2. Children—Diseases.   I. Stockman, James, A.
II. Lohr, Jacob A.
[DNLM: 1. Pediatrics. WS 200 E78 2001

RJ45 .E815 2001

618.92—dc21   99-050226

Essence of Office Pediatrics   ISBN 0–7216–5845–8

Printed in the United States of America

Last digit is the print number: 9   8   7   6   5   4   3   2   1

DEDICATION

To Missy, Jason, Lara, Jonathan, Brice,
Lee, Meredith, Samantha, Jamie, and Jennifer

Brojendra N. Agarwala, M.D.
Professor of Clinical Pediatrics, University of Chicago; Pediatric Cardiologist, University of Chicago Children's Hospital, Chicago, Illinois
Heart Block, Complete

Elizabeth M. Alderman, M.D.
Associate Professor of Clinical Pediatrics, Albert Einstein College of Medicine; Associate Attending Director of Adolescent Ambulatory Services, Montefiore Medical Center, Bronx, New York
Amenorrhea, Primary
Amenorrhea, Secondary

Kenneth Alexander, M.D., Ph.D.
Assistant Professor of Pediatrics and Microbiology, Duke University Medical Center, Durham, North Carolina
Coxsackie Virus A Infections
Coxsackie Virus B Infections

Judith F. Allanson, MBChB, FRCP, FRCP (C), DABMG, FCCMG
Professor of Pediatrics, University of Ottawa; Head, Clinical Section, Genetics Section, Genetics Patient Service Unit, Children's Hospital of Eastern Ontario, Ottawa, Ontario, Canada
Noonan Syndrome

Hugh D. Allen, M.D.
Professor of Pediatrics and Internal Medicine; Chief, Division of Pediatric Cardiology and Director, Cardiology Fellowship Program, The Ohio State University, Columbus Children's Hospital; Physician-in-Chief, Columbus Children's Hospital, Columbus, Ohio
Rheumatic Fever

Mary G. Ampola, M.D.
Professor of Pediatrics, Tufts University School of Medicine; Chief, Division of Metabolism, Department of Pediatrics and Director, Pediatric Amino Acid Laboratory, New England Medical Center, Boston, Massachusetts
Phenylketonuria

Marsha S. Anderson, M.D.
Assistant Professor, Pediatrics, Division of Pediatric Infectious Diseases, University of Colorado Health Sciences Center, Denver, Colorado; Director of Inpatient Medicine, The Children's Hospital, Denver, Colorado
Meningococcemia

Joel M. Andres, M.D.
Chief, Pediatric Gastroenterology, Arnold Palmer Children's Hospital and Nemours Children's Clinic, Orlando, Florida
Polyps and Polyposis, Juvenile

Anthony L. Anker, M.D.
Attending Physician, Emergency Department, Rogue Valley Medical Center, Medford, Oregon
Acetaminophen Poisoning
Aspirin Poisoning

Alia Y. Antoon, M.D.
Assistant Clinical Professor of Pediatrics, Harvard Medical School; Chief of Pediatrics, Shriners Hospitals for Children, Shriners Burns Hospital, Boston, Massachusetts
Burns, Outpatient

Leonard Apt, M.D.
Professor of Ophthalmology, Director Emeritus and Founder of Division of Pediatric Ophthalmology, University of California–Los Angeles School of Medicine; Jules Stein Eye Institute, Los Angeles, California
Hyphema

Steven Arkin, M.D.
Clinical Associate Professor of Pediatrics, Division of Pediatric Hematology/Oncology, Mount Sinai School of Medicine; Assistant Attending in Pediatrics, The Mount Sinai Hospital, New York, New York
Iron-Deficiency Anemia

Kenneth A. Arndt, M.D.
Professor of Dermatology, Harvard Medical School; Beth Israel Deaconess Medical Center, Boston, Massachusetts
Piebaldism, Waardenburg Syndrome, and Tuberous Sclerosis
Vitiligo and Pityriasis Alba

Stephen S. Arnon, M.D.
Chief, Infant Botulism Treatment and Prevention Program, Division of Communicable Disease Control, California Department of Health Services, Berkeley, California
Botulism, Infant

Stephen C. Aronoff, M.D.
Professor and Chairman, Department of Pediatrics, Temple University School of Medicine; Chief Medical Officer, Temple University Children's Medical Center, Philadelphia, Pennsylvania
Bites, Dog and Cat
Histiocytoses, Childhood

Andrew V. Atton, M.D.
Clinical Instructor, Yale University School of Medicine; Yale-New Haven Hospital, New Haven, Connecticut
Dermoid Cyst

Gilbert P. August, M.D.
Professor of Pediatrics, George Washington University; Department of Endocrinology, Children's National Medical Center, Washington, DC
Short Stature, Diagnosis

K. Scott Baker, M.D.
Assistant Professor of Pediatrics, University of Minnesota; Pediatric Hematology/Oncology and Blood and Marrow Transplant, Fairview–University Medical Center, Minneapolis, Minnesota
Rhabdomyosarcoma

J. Williamson Balfe, M.D., FRCP (C)
Professor of Pediatrics, University of Toronto; Pediatric Nephrologist and Director of Peritoneal Dialysis, Hospital for Sick Children, Toronto, Ontario, Canada
Hypertension, Management

John P. Barletta, M.D.
Staff Ophthalmologist, St. Joseph Mercy Hospital, Ann Arbor, Michigan
Cataracts

L. Jarrett Barnhill, M.D.
Associate Professor, Department of Psychiatry, University of North Carolina School of Medicine; Director, Developmental Neuropharmacology Clinic, University of North Carolina School of Medicine, Chapel Hill, North Carolina
Tourette Syndrome (TS) and Related Disorders

Robert A. Bashford, M.D.
Associate Professor, Departments of Ob-Gyn and Psychiatry, University of North Carolina School of Medicine and North Carolina Memorial Hospital, Chapel Hill, North Carolina
Conversion Disorder

Melisse Sloas Baylor, M.D.
Medical Officer, Division of Antiviral Drug Products, Food and Drug Administration, Rockville, Maryland
Cryptococcal Infections

Roberta K. Beach, M.D., MPH
Professor of Pediatrics and Adolescent Medicine, University of Colorado School of Medicine; Director, Pediatric and Adolescent Services, Westside Family Health Center, Denver Health Authority, Denver, Colorado
Rape Management

James H. Beaty, M.D.
Professor and Staff Physician, University of Tennessee, Department of Orthopaedic Surgery, Campbell Clinic, Memphis, Tennessee
Fractures, Hip (Apophysitis / Hip Pointer), Femoral Neck, and Femur

David S. Bell, M.D., FAAD
Chief, Department of Pediatrics, Medina Memorial Hospital, Medina, New York
Chronic Fatigue Syndrome

Jennifer J. Bell, M.D.
Senior Lecturer, Columbia University, College of Physicians and Surgeons, New York, New York
Precocious Puberty

Louis M. Bell, M.D.
Associate Professor of Pediatrics, University of Pennsylvania School of Medicine; Attending Physician, Section of Infectious Diseases and Division of Emergency Medicine, The Children's Hospital of Philadelphia, Philadelphia, Pennsylvania
Rubeola, Measles

Tom Belhorn, M.D., Ph.D.
Assistant Professor of Pediatrics, Division of Infectious Diseases, University of North Carolina at Chapel Hill, Chapel Hill, North Carolina
Echoviruses
Toxocariasis

James T. Bennett, M.D.
Professor of Orthopaedics, Chief Section of Pediatric Orthopaedics, Tulane University School of Medicine, New Orleans, Louisiana
Tibial Torsion, Internal

Pedro K. Beredjiklian, M.D.
Assistant Professor of Orthopaedic Surgery, University of Pennsylvania School of Medicine, Philadelphia, Pennsylvania
Sprengle Deformity

Jerry M. Bergstein, M.D.
Professor, Department of Pediatrics, Indiana University School of Medicine; Director, Section of Nephrology, James Whitcomb Riley Hospital for Children, Indianapolis, Indiana
Hemolytic-Uremic Syndrome

Matthew R. Biebel, M.D., FAAP
Children's Hospital of Wisconsin, Milwaukee, Wisconsin; Waukesha Memorial Hospital, Waukesha, Wisconsin
Brachial Plexus Palsy

Audrey H. Birnbaum, M.D.
Assistant Professor, Mount Sinai School of Medicine; Assistant Attending, Mount Sinai Hospital, New York, New York
Pancreatitis

James A. Blackman, M.D., MPH
Professor of Pediatrics, University of Virginia; Director of Research, Kluge Children's Rehabilitation Center, Charlottesville, Virginia
Cerebral Palsy

R. Dale Blasier, M.D.
Professor of Orthopaedic Surgery, Division of Pediatric Orthopaedics, University of Arkansas for Medical Sciences, Arkansas Children's Hospital, Little Rock, Arkansas
Fractures, Knee

Kenneth E. Bloom, M.D.
Clinical Associate Professor, Department of Dermatology and Pediatrics, University of Minnesota; Director, Dermatology Center for Children and Young Adults, Minneapolis, Minnesota
Pyogenic Granuloma (Lobular Capillary Hemangioma)

W. Clayton Bordley, M.D., MPH
Assistant Professor of Pediatrics, Clinical Assistant Professor of Emergency Medicine, University of North Carolina School of Medicine, Chapel Hill, North Carolina
Lead Toxicity

F. William Bora, M.D.
Professor of Orthopaedic Surgery, University of Pennsylvania School of Medicine, Philadelphia, Pennsylvania
Sprengel Deformity

Robert Bortolussi, M.D., FRCPC
Professor of Pediatrics and Microbiology, Dalhousie University; IWK Grace Health Centre, Halifax, Nova Scotia, Canada
Listeriosis

Gary D. Bos, M.D.
Associate Professor, Department of Orthopedic Surgery, University of North Carolina School of Medicine; Lineberger Comprehensive Cancer Center, University of North Carolina at Chapel Hill, Chapel Hill, North Carolina
Bone Tumors and Cysts (Benign)

Nancy E. Braverman, M.D.
Assistant Professor, Institute for Genetic Medicine, Johns Hopkins Hospital, Baltimore, Maryland
Maple Syrup Urine Disease

Timothy J. Brei, M.D.
Clinical Professor of Pediatrics, Section on Developmental Pediatrics, Medical Director, Myelomeningocele and Cerebral Palsy Programs; Attending Physician, James Whitcomb Riley Hospital for Children, Indianapolis, Indiana
Myelomeningocele

Philip P. Breitfeld, M.D.
Klingler Professor of Pediatrics, Indiana University School of Medicine, Indianapolis, Indiana
Leukemia, Acute Lymphocytic

Lela W. Brink, M.D.
Penn State Geisinger Health System, Pediatric Clinic, State College, Pennsylvania
Pneumothorax and Pneumomediastinum

John W. Brock III, M.D.
Associate Professor, Department of Urologic Surgery; Associate Professor, Department of Pediatrics; Director, Division of Pediatric Urology, Vanderbilt University Medical Center, Nashville, Tennessee
Penile Disorders, Micellaneous: Balanitis, Phimosis, Paraphimosis, and Meatal Stenosis
Epididymitis and Orchitis
Testis, Torsion of

Richard R. Brookman, M.D.
Professor and Chairman, Division of Adolescent Medicine, Department of Pediatrics, Virginia Commonwealth University, Richmond, Virginia
Suicide

Amy R. Brooks-Kayal, M.D.
Assistant Professor, Neurology and Pediatrics, University of Pennsylvania, Children's Hospital of Philadelphia, Philadelphia, Pennsylvania
Seizures, Complex Partial (Psychomotor, Limbic)

Ben H. Brouhard, M.D.
Professor of Pediatrics, Case Western Reserve University School of Medicine; Chairman, Department of Pediatrics, Metro Health Medical Center, Cleveland, Ohio
Hypertension, Evaluation and Management
Nephrotic Syndrome

Melissa R. Brown, M.D.
Clinical Instructor, Urology, Boston University, Boston, Massachusetts
Cryptorchidism and Undescended Testicles

George R. Buchanan, M.D.
Professor of Pediatrics, University of Texas Southwestern Medical Center, Dallas, Texas
Diamond-Blackfan Anemia

Robert A. Buckmire, M.D.
Instructor, Division of Otolaryngology, Head and Neck Surgery, University of North Carolina School of Medicine, Chapel Hill, North Carolina
Retropharyngeal and Peritonsillar Abscess

Charles A. Bullaboy, M.D., FAAP, FACC, FCCP
Professor of Pediatrics, Eastern Virginia Medical School; Pediatric Cardiologist, Children's Specialty Group, Children's Hospital of the King's Daughters, Norfolk, Virginia
Mitral Valve Prolapse
Pericarditis, Acute

Jacqueline M. Calkin, M.D.
Fellow, Department of Dermatology, University of California, San Francisco, San Francisco, California
Hypopigmented Lesions
Pigmented Lesions
Vascular Lesions

Robert M. Campbell, Jr., M.D.
Associate Professor, University of Texas Health Science Center, San Antonio, Texas; Staff Physician, Principle Investigator for Titanium Rib Project, Pediatric Orthopaedics, Christus Santa Rosa Children's Hospital, San Antonio, Texas
Fractures, Elbow

Edmund R. Campion, M.D.
Associate Professor of Orthopaedic Surgery, Residency Program Director, University of North Carolina School of Medicine, Chapel Hill, North Carolina
Kyphosis
Slipped Capital Femoral Epiphysis

S. Terry Canale, M.D.
Professor and Chief of Staff, University of Tennessee, Campbell Clinic, Department of Orthopaedic Surgery, Memphis, Tennessee
Fractures, Hip (Apophysitis/ Hip Pointer), Femoral Neck, and Femur

Charles E. Canter, M.D.
Associate Professor of Pediatrics, Washington University School of Medicine; Medical Director, Pediatric Cardiac Transplantation, St. Louis Children's Hospital, St. Louis, Missouri
Cardiomyopathy

Paul A. Carbonaro, M.D.
Chief Resident in Dermatology, University of Massachusetts Medical School, Worcester, Massachusetts
Bites, Insect, and Stings

Thomas O. Carpenter, M.D.
Associate Professor, Department of Pediatrics (Endocrine Section), Yale University School of Medicine; Attending Physician, Yale-New Haven Hospital, New Haven, Connecticut
Rickets

Bruce T. Carter, M.D.
Clinical Assistant Professor, Department of Ophthalmology, Clinical Associate Professor, Department of Pediatrics, University of Virginia School of Medicine, Charlottesville, Virginia
Corneal Abrasion

James T. Cassidy, M.D.
Professor of Child Health, Chief, Division of Pediatric Rheumatology, University of Missouri Health Sciences Center, Columbia, Missouri
Juvenile Rheumatoid Arthritis (JRA)

Sarah L. Chamlin, M.D.
Pediatric Dermatology Fellow, University of California School of Medicine, San Francisco, California
Cystic Hygroma
Papillomavirus Infection, Nongenital

Sam S. Chang, M.D.
Department of Urology, Vanderbilt University Medical Center, Nashville, Tennessee
Penile Disorders, Micellaneous: Balanitis, Phimosis, Paraphimos, and Meatal Stenosis
Epididymitis and Orchitis
Testis, Torsion of

David R. Chavez, M.D.
Fellow in Pediatric Urology, Duke University Medical Center, Durham, North Carolina; Clinical Research Fellow in Endocrinology, Beth Israel Hospital-Harvard Medical School, Boston, Massachusetts
Hydronephrosis, Fetal Obstructive Uropathy

Cindy W. Christian, M.D.
Assistant Professor of Pediatrics, University of Pennsylvania School of Medicine; Director, Child Abuse Services, The Children's Hospital of Philadelphia, Philadelphia, Pennsylvania
Child Abuse and Child Neglect

Esther K. Chung, M.D., MPH
Assistant Clinical Professor of General Pediatrics, University of California at San Francisco, San Francisco, California
Syphilis, Neonatal

Mary Williams Clark, M.D.
Professor, Orthopedic Surgery, Chief, Division of Pediatric Orthopedics, Medical College of Ohio; Mercy Children's Hospital, Toledo, Ohio
Talus, Congenital Vertical

Bernard A. Cohen, M.D.
Associate Professor of Pediatrics and Dermatology, Johns Hopkins University School of Medicine; Director of Pediatric Dermatology, Johns Hopkins Children's Center, Baltimore, Maryland
Acne Vulgaris
Hemangioma
Milia
Sunburn

Mitchell B. Cohen, M.D.
Professor of Pediatrics, University of Cincinnati; Attending Physician, Children's Hospital Medical Center, Cincinnati, Ohio
Gastroenteritis, Bacterial

Rebecca S. Coker, M.D.
Associate Clinical Professor, Pediatrics, East Carolina University, School of Medicine; Medical Director, TEDI BEAR Children's Advocacy Center, Greenville, North Carolina
Fetal Drug Exposure: Alcohol, Cocaine, Heroin

Barbara R. Cole, M.D.
Associate Professor of Pediatrics, Washington University; Director, Division of Pediatric Nephrology, St. Louis Children's Hospital, St. Louis, Missouri
Renal Dysplasia and Cystic Disease

Francisco Colon-Fontanez, M.D.
Fellow, Division of Pediatric Dermatology, Children's Hospital and Health Science Center, San Diego, California
Cutaneous Vascular Malformations (Port-Wine Stains)

W. Carl Cooley, M.D.
Associate Professor of Pediatrics, Dartmouth Medical School, Hanover, New Hampshire; Medical Director, Crotched Mountain Rehabilitation Center, Greenfield, New Hampshire
Down Syndrome

James Coplan, M.D.
Clinical Associate Professor of Pediatrics, University of Pennsylvania School of Medicine; Director of Training, Children's Seashore House of the Children's Hospital of Philadelphia, Philadelphia, Pennsylvania
Speech Disorders Other Than Stuttering

Enrique Criado, M.D.
Associate Professor of Surgery, Division of Vascular Surgery, University of North Carolina School of Medicine, Chapel Hill, North Carolina; Chief Vascular Surgery Unit, Fundación Hospital de Alcorcón, Madrid, Spain
Thrombosis, Deep Vein

Allen C. Crocker, M.D.
Associate Professor of Pediatrics, Harvard Medical School; Associate Professor of Maternal and Child Health, Harvard School of Public Health; Senior Associate in Medicine, Children's Hospital, Boston, Massachusetts
Mental Retardation

Gary L. Darmstadt, M.D.
Assistant Professor, Divisions of Dermatology and Infectious Disease, Department of Pediatrics, Children's Hospital and Regional Medical Center; Division of Dermatology, Department of Medicine, University of Washington School of Medicine, Seattle, Washington; Division of Community Health and Health Systems Department of Community Health, School of Hygiene and Public Health, Johns Hopkins Medical Institutions, Baltimore, Maryland
Drug Eruptions
Folliculitis
Furunculosis and Carbunculosis
Impetigo

Marsha L. Davenport, M.D.
Associate Professor of Pediatrics, University of North Carolina at Chapel Hill, Chapel Hill, North Carolina
Turner Syndrome

H. Dele Davies, M.D., MSc
Associate Professor, University of Calgary, Departments of Pediatrics, Microbiology and Infectious Diseases and Community Health, University of Calgary; Director, Child Health Research Unit, Alberta Children's Hospital, Calgary, Alberta, Canada
Pneumonia, Afebrile of Infancy

Pedro A. de Alarcon, M.D.
Professor of Pediatrics, Division Head, Pediatric Hematology/Oncology, University of Virginia Health System, Charlottesville, Virginia
Spherocytosis

Richard J. Deckelbaum, M.D., CM, FRCP (C)
Professor of Pediatrics, Robert R. Williams Professor of Nutrition, Director, Division of Gastroenterology and Nutrition, Department of Pediatrics, Director, Institute of Human Nutrition, Columbia University College of Physicians and Surgeons, New York, New York
Gastroenteritis, Parasitic

Gail J. Demmler, M.D.
Associate Professor, Pediatrics and Pathology, Baylor College of Medicine; Director Diagnostic Virology Laboratory and Attending Physician, Texas Children's Hospital, Houston, Texas
Cytomegalovirus Infections

Floyd W. Denny, Jr., M.D.
Professor Emeritus of Pediatrics, University of North Carolina School of Medicine, and University of North Carolina Hospitals, Chapel Hill, North Carolina
Pharyngitis/Tonsillitis
Scarlet Fever

John M. DeVaro, M.D.
Pediatric Ophthalmology, Memorial Health University Medical Center, Georgia Eye Institute, Savannah, Georgia
Amblyopia
Refractive Errors (Nearsightedness/Farsightedness/Astigmatism)

Frederick R. Dietz, M.D.
Professor of Orthopaedic Surgery, University of Iowa, Iowa City, Iowa
Clubfoot, Idiopathic (Talipes Equinovarus)

James G. Dinulos, M.D.
Acting Instructor, Division of Dermatology, Department of Pediatrics, Children's Hospital and Medical Center; Division of Dermatology, Department of Medicine, University of Washington School of Medicine, Seattle, Washington
Drug Eruptions

Theresa L. Dise, M.D.
Assistant Professor of Pediatrics, Tulane Medical School, New Orleans, Louisiana
Flatfeet (Flexible Pes Planovalgus)

Cynthia A. Doerr, M.D.
Epidemiologist, Pediatric Infectious Disease Consultant, Methodist Children's Hospital of South Texas, San Antonio, Texas
Endocarditis

Stephen E. Dolgin, M.D.
Chief, Pediatric Surgery and Associate Professor of Surgery, Pediatrics, Anatomy and Cell Biology, Mount Sinai School of Medicine, New York, New York
Hydrocele

John P. Dormans, M.D.
Associate Professor of Orthopaedic Surgery, The University of Pennsylvania School of Medicine; Chief of Orthopaedic Surgery, The Children's Hospital of Philadelphia, Philadelphia, Pennsylvania
Osteochondritis Dissecans (Knee and Elbow)

Amelia F. Drake, M.D.
Professor, University of
North Carolina School of Medicine,
Chapel Hill, North Carolina
*Foreign Bodies of the Ear, Nose,
and Esophagus*

Noam Z. Drazin, M.D.
Chief Resident Internal Medicine,
Cedars-Sinai Medical Center,
Los Angeles, California
Tapeworm Infestations

Fritz Dreifuss, M.D.†
Seizures, Absence (Petit Mal)
*Seizures, Generalized Tonic-Clonic
(Grand Mal)*
Seizures, Infantile Spasms
Seizures, Status Epilepticus

James C. Drennan, M.D.
Professor, Department of
Orthopaedics and Pediatrics,
University of New Mexico School of
Medicine; Medical Director/
Administrator, Carrie Tingley
Hospital, University of New Mexico
Health Sciences Center,
Albuquerque, New Mexico
Cavovarus Foot
Charcot-Marie Tooth Disease

Robert P. Drucker, M.D.
Director, Pediatric Student
Education, Duke University Medical
Center; Assistant Clinical Professor,
Duke University Medical Center,
Durham, North Carolina
Lung Abscess

Barbara S. Dudley, MSN, RN
Instructor in Pediatrics, Virginia
Commonwealth University's Medical
College of Virginia, Richmond,
Virginia
Lactose Intolerance

Robert M. Ehrlich, M.D., FRCPC
Professor Emeritus, Department of
Pediatrics, University of Toronto,
Toronto, Ontario; Consultant
Endocrinologist, Markham
Stouffville Hospital, Markham,
Ontario, Canada
Thyrotoxicosis

Lawrence F. Eichenfield, M.D.
Associate Professor of Pediatrics and
Medicine, University of California,
San Diego, School of Medicine;
Director, Pediatric and Adolescent
Dermatology, Children's Hospital,
San Diego, and UCSD School of
Medicine, San Diego, California
*Cutaneous Vascular Malformations
(Port-Wine Stains)*

S. Jean Emans, M.D.
Associate Professor of Pediatrics,
Harvard Medical School; Chief,
Division of Adolescent/Young Adult
Medicine, Children's Hospital,
Boston, Massachusetts
Uterine Bleeding, Irregular
*Vulvovaginitis in the Prepubertal
Child*

Owen B. Evans, M.D.
Professor and Chairman,
Department of Pediatrics, University
of Mississippi School
of Medicine, Jackson, Mississippi
Myositis

Karen D. Fairchild, M.D.
Assistant Professor of Pediatrics,
Division of Neonatology, University
of Maryland School of Medicine,
Baltimore, Maryland
Tracheoesophageal Fistula

Fuad S. Farah, M.D.
Professor of Medicine (Dermatology),
Upstate Medical University,
Syracuse, New York
*Ancylostomiasis and
Strongyloidiasis*
Ascariasis and Enterobiasis
*Filariasis: Onchocerciasis, Loiasis,
Lymphatic Filariasis*
Roundworm Infestations
*Streptocerciasis, Cutaneous Larva
Migrans, Visceral Larva Migrans*
*Trichinosis, Gnathostomiasis,
Angiostrongyliasis, Dracunculosis*

Mark A. Farber, M.D.
Assistant Professor, Vascular
Surgery, University of North
Carolina, Chapel Hill, North
Carolina
Thrombosis, Deep Vein

Heidi M. Feldman, M.D.
Associate Professor, Department of
Pediatrics, University of Pittsburgh
School of Medicine; Director,
Division of General Academic
Pediatrics, Children's Hospital of
Pittsburgh, Pittsburgh,
Pennsylvania
Stuttering

Gerald W. Fernald, M.D.
Professor Emeritus, Department
of Pediatrics, University of
North Carolina School of Medicine,
Chapel Hill, North Carolina
Cystic Fibrosis
Pneumonia, Mycoplasma

Gerald W. Fischer, M.D.
Professor of Pediatrics, Uniformed
Services University of the Health
Sciences, Bethesda, Maryland;
President and CEO, Biosynexus,
Inc., Rockville, Maryland
Intervertebral Disk Infections

Coy D. Fitch, M.D.
Professor and Chairman,
Department of Internal Medicine, St.
Louis University School of Medicine;
Chief of Medical Service, St. Louis
University Hospital, St. Louis,
Missouri
Malaria

Robert D. Fitch, M.D.
Associate Professor of Surgery,
Duke University Medical Center,
Durham, North Carolina
Tibial Bowing

Joseph F. Fitzgerald, M.D.
Professor of Pediatrics,
Director, Division of Pediatric
Gastroenterology, Hepatology
and Nutrition, James Whitcomb
Riley Hospital for Children,
Indiana University School of
Medicine, Indianapolis, Indiana
Peritonitis

John W. Foreman, M.D.
Professor of Pediatrics, Duke
University Medical Center; Chief,
Division of Pediatric Nephrology,
Department of Pediatrics, Duke
University Medical Center, Durham,
North Carolina
Renal Tubular Acidosis (RTA)

William S. Foshee, M.D.
Associate Professor of Pediatrics,
Medical College of Georgia;
Education Coordinator, University
Hospital, Augusta, Georgia
Sporotrichosis, Cutaneous

Carol M. Foster, M.D.
Professor, Department of Pediatrics,
Division of Endocrinology,
University of Michigan, Ann Arbor,
Michigan
Dysmenorrhea

Sandra L. Fowler, M.D.
Clinical Associate Professor of
Pediatrics, Division of Infectious
Diseases and Clinical Immunology,
Medical University of South
Carolina, Charleston, South
Carolina
Pneumonia, Viral

Elman G. Frantz, M.D.
Associate Professor, Pediatrics (Cardiology), University of North Carolina School of Medicine; Associate Director, C.V. Richardson Cardiac Catheterization Laboratory for Pediatric Services, University of North Carolina Hospitals, Chapel Hill, North Carolina
Coarctation of the Aorta
Transposition of the Great Arteries

Dianne M. Frazier, MPH, Ph.D.
Clinical Associate Professor, Department of Pediatrics, University of North Carolina at Chapel Hill, Chapel Hill, North Carolina
Galactosemia

Sharon F. Freedman, M.D.
Associate Professor of Ophthalmology, Assistant Professor of Pediatrics, Duke University Medical Center, Durham, North Carolina
Dacryostenosis, Dacryocystitis, and Related Obstructions
Strabismus

Andrew A. Freiberg, M.D.
Assistant Professor of Orthopaedic Surgery and Chief, Adult Reconstruction Service, University of Michigan Hospitals, Ann Arbor, Michigan
Freiberg Disease

Alison G. Freifeld, M.D.
Clinical Associate Professor, Infectious Diseases, University of Nebraska Medical Center, Omaha, Nebraska
Fever and Neutropenia

Ilona J. Frieden, M.D.
Clinical Professor Dermatology and Pediatrics, University of California School of Medicine, San Francisco, California
Cystic Hygroma
Human Papillomavirus Infections, Nongenital

Sheila Fallon Friedlander, M.D.
Associate Clinical Professor, UCSD School of Medicine and Children's Hospital, San Diego, California
Papular Urticaria

Henry S. Friedman, M.D.
James B. Powell, Jr. Professor of Neuro-Oncology, Duke University Medical Center, Durham, North Carolina
Brain Tumors: Medulloblastoma

Keith R. Gabriel, M.D.
Associate Professor, St. Louis University; Department Director, Cardinal Glennon Children's Hospital, St. Louis, Missouri
Growing Pains

John P. Gearhart, M.D.
Professor of Pediatric Urology, Professor of Pediatrics, Johns Hopkins School of Medicine; Director of Pediatric Urology, Johns Hopkins Hospital, Baltimore, Maryland
Hypospadias/Epispadias

John W. Georgitis, M.D.
Professor of Pediatrics and Chief, Section of Allergy, Immunology and Pulmonology, Wake Forest University School of Medicine, Winston-Salem, North Carolina
Angioedema
Urticaria

Anne A. Gershon, M.D.
Professor of Pediatrics, Director of Pediatric Infectious Diseases, Columbia University College of Physicians and Surgeons, New York, New York
Varicella-Zoster Virus Infections

Gerald S. Gilchrist, M.D.
Helen C. Levitt Professor, Department of Pediatric and Adolescent Medicine, Director, Mayo Clinic Comprehensive Hemophilia Center, Mayo Clinic and Foundation and Mayo Medical School; Consultant in Pediatric Hematology and Oncology, Mayo Eugenio Litta Children's Hospital, Rochester, Minnesota
Hemophilia A
Hemophilia B

Roger H. Giller, M.D.
Associate Professor of Pediatrics, University of Colorado School of Medicine; Director, Pediatric Bone Marrow Transplant Program, University of Colorado School of Medicine; Director, Pediatric Bone Marrow Transplant Program, The Children's Hospital, Denver, Colorado
Teratomas and Other Germ Cell Tumors (GCTs)

Charles M. Ginsburg, M.D.
Professor and Chairman, Marilyn R. Corrigan Distinguished Chair in Pediatric Research, University of Texas Southwestern Medical Center; Chief of Staff, Children's Medical Center, Dallas, Texas
Bites, Human

Jill P. Ginsberg, M.D.
Assistant Professor of Pediatrics, Baylor College of Medicine, Texas Children's Cancer Center, Houston, Texas
Ewing Sarcoma Family of Tumors

Laurie J. Glader, M.D.
Instructor in Pediatrics, Harvard Medical School; Assistant in Medicine, Children's Hospital, Boston, Massachusetts
Encopresis

Stuart Goldman, M.D.
Assistant Professor of Psychiatry, Harvard Medical School; Director of Psychiatric Education, Children's Hospital, Boston, Massachusetts
Conduct Disorders

Manuel R. Gomez, M.D.
Emeritus Professor of Pediatric Neurology, Mayo Medical School and St. Mary's Hospital, Rochester, Minnesota
Tuberous Sclerosis Complex (TSC)

Jerome L. Gorski, M.D.
Professor of Pediatrics and Communicable Diseases, Professor of Human Genetics, Director, Division of Pediatric Genetics, University of Michigan Medical School; Professor of Pediatrics and Communicable Diseases, Director, Division of Pediatric Genetics, C. S. Mott Children's Hospital, Ann Arbor, Michigan
Incontinentia Pigmenti

William D. Graf, M.D.
Assistant Professor, University of Washington School of Medicine; Attending Physician, Children's Hospital and Regional Medical Center, Seattle, Washington
Drowning

John M. Graham, Jr, M.D., ScD
Director of Clinical Genetics and Dysmorphology, Cedars-Sinai Medical Center; Professor of Pediatrics, UCLA School of Medicine, Los Angeles, California
Down Syndrome

Jane M. Grant-Kels, M.D.
Professor and Chairperson, University of Connecticut Health Center and John Dempsey Hospital, Farmington, Connecticut
Ichthyosis

Daniel M. Green, M.D.
Professor of Pediatrics, School of Medicine and Biomedical Sciences, University of Buffalo, State University of New York; Roswell Park Cancer Institute, Buffalo, New York
Wilms Tumor

Michael Green, M.D., MPH
Associate Professor of Pediatrics and Surgery, University of Pittsburgh School of Medicine; Division of Allergy, Immunology, and Infectious Diseases, Children's Hospital of Pittsburgh, Pittsburgh, Pennsylvania
Leptospirosis

Walter B. Greene, M.D.
Professor and Chairman, Department of Orthopedic Surgery, University of Missouri, Columbia, Missouri
Calcaneal Apophysitis (Sever Disease)
Knee, Anterior Pain
Patellar Dislocations and Fractures

Robert S. Greenwood, M.D.
Professor of Neurology and Pediatrics, University of North Carolina School of Medicine; Professor of Neurology and Pediatrics, Attending Physician, University of North Carolina Hospitals, Chapel Hill, North Carolina
Neurofibromatosis

Andrew J. Griffith, M.D., Ph.D.
Senior Staff Fellow, Neuro-Otology Branch and Laboratory of Molecular Genetics, National Institute on Deafness and Other Communication Disorders, National Institutes of Health, Bethesda, Maryland
Nerve Deafness: Congenital

Dennis P. Grogan, M.D.
Clinical Professor, Division of Orthopaedic Surgery, University of South Florida, College of Medicine; Chief of Staff, Shriners Hospital for Children, Tampa, Florida
Köhler Disease
Navicular, Accessory

Moses Grossman, M.D.
Professor Emeritus, Department of Pediatrics, University of California, San Francisco; Attending Physician, San Francisco General Hospital, San Francisco, California
Brucellosis

Steven K. Gudeman, M.D.
Private practice, Gastonia, North Carolina
Concussion
Craniosynostosis
Scalp Swelling, Post-Traumatic
Subdural and Epidural Hematomas

Joseph J. Gugenheim, Jr., M.D.
Clinical Associate Professor, Department of Orthopedic Surgery, Baylor College of Medicine; Member, Fondren Orthopedic Group, Texas Orthopedic Hospital, Houston, Texas
Ganglia (Hand and Foot) and Cysts (Popliteal)

Mary Anne Guggenheim, M.D.
Clinical Professor, University of Colorado School of Medicine, Denver Colorado; Adjunct Professor, WAMI Program, University, University of Washington School of Medicine, Bozeman, Montana; St. Peters Community Hospital, Helena, Montana
Seizures, Febrile

Ann P. Guillot, M.D.
Associate Professor, Department of Pediatrics, University of Vermont College of Medicine, Burlington, Vermont
Renal Vein Thrombosis

Alan R. Gurd, M.D., Mch, FRCS
Head, Pediatric Orthopaedic Surgery, Cleveland Clinic, Cleveland, Ohio
Femoral Torsion (Anteversion/Retroversion)

Cynthia Guzzo, M.D.
Adjunct Clinical Associate Professor, Department of Dermatology, University of Pennsylvania, Philadelphia, Pennsylvania; Director, Worldwide OTC Development, Merck Research Laboratories, Merck & Co., Inc., Blue Bell, Pennsylvania
Atopic Dermatitis

Colin D. Hall, MBChB
Professor and Interim Chair, Department of Neurology, University of North Carolina School of Medicine, Chapel Hill, North Carolina
Muscular Dystrophies

Margaret R. Hammerschlag, M.D.
Professor of Pediatrics and Medicine, SUNY Health Sciences Center at Brooklyn; Director, Division of Pediatric Infectious Diseases, University Hospital of Brooklyn, Kings County Hospital Center, Brooklyn, New York
Pneumonia, Chlamydial

Gregory W. Hammond, M.D., FRCP (C)
Professor, University of Manitoba; Director, Public Health Branch, Manitoba Health, Winnipeg, Manitoba, Canada
Rabies

Harvey J. Hamrick, M.D.
Professor of Pediatrics, Department of Pediatrics, University of North Carolina Hospitals, University of North Carolina at Chapel Hill, Chapel Hill, North Carolina
Cellulitis

John E. Handelsman, M.D., M Ch Orth, FRCS
Professor of Orthopaedics and Pediatrics, Albert Einstein College of Medicine, Bronx, New York; Chief, Pediatric Orthopaedic Surgery, Schneider Children's Hospital of Long Island Jewish Medical Center, New Hyde Park, New York
Hip Dysplasia, Developmental

Sonali G. Hanson, M.D.
Private practice; Consulting, St. Luke's Episcopal Hospital, The Methodist Hospital, Houston, Texas
Mastocytosis: Urticaria Pigmentosa
Neurocutaneous Melanosis
Scabies

Dennis C. Harper, Ph.D.
Professor of Pediatrics and Graduate Studies in Rehabilitation, University of Iowa College of Medicine, Iowa City, Iowa
Psychosomatic Illness
School Behavior Problems

Christopher J. Harrison, M.D.
Professor of Pediatrics and Microbiology and Immunology, Creighton University School of Medicine; Co-Director of Medical Education, Children's Hospital, Omaha, Nebraska
Otitis Media

William E. Hathaway, M.D.
Professor Emeritus of Pediatrics, University of Colorado School of Medicine, Denver, Colorado
von Willebrand Disease

Morey W. Haymond, M.D.
Professor of Pediatrics, Baylor College of Medicine, Houston, Texas
Diabetes Mellitus, Insulin Dependent
Diabetic Ketoacidosis

David M. Heilbronner, M.D.
Clinical Assistant Professor of Orthopaedics, Clinical Assistant Professor of Nursing, University of Virginia School of Medicine; Staff Physician, Martha Jefferson Hospital, Charlottesville, Virginia
Fractures, Tibial (Toddler's)

Jonathan D. Heiliczer, M.D.
Associate Professor of Pediatrics, University of Illinois College of Medicine; Director, Children's Kidney Center of Illinois, UIC Medical Center, Chicago, Illinois
Renal Failure, Acute, Management

Val G. Hemming, M.D.
Dean, School of Medicine, and Professor of Pediatrics, F. Edward Hebert School of Medicine, Uniformed Services University of the Health Sciences, Bethesda, Maryland
Pneumonia, Bacterial (Community Acquired)

Frederick W. Henderson, M.D.
Professor of Pediatrics, Pediatric Infectious Diseases, University of North Carolina School of Medicine; Attending Physician, University of North Carolina Children's Hospital, Chapel Hill, North Carolina
Laryngotracheobronchitis (Croup)
Toxic Shock Syndromes, Staphylococcal and Streptococcal

Richard C. Henderson, M.D., Ph.D.
Professor of Orthopaedics and Pediatrics, University of North Carolina at Chapel Hill, Chapel Hill, North Carolina
Tibia Vara (TV), Infantile and Adolescent (Late Onset Blount Disease)

J. Owen Hendley, M.D.
Professor of Pediatrics, University of Virginia Medical Center and University of Virginia Health System, Charlottesville, Virginia
Common Cold

Martin J. Herman, M.D.
Clinical Instructor Orthopedic Surgery, UMDNJ–Robert Wood Johnson Medical School, New Brunswick, New Jersey
Compartment Syndrome, Acute and Chronic

William A. Herndon, M.D.
Clinical Professor, Orthopaedic Surgery, University of Oklahoma College of Medicine, Oklahoma City, Oklahoma
Little League Elbow

John T. Herrin, MBBS, FRACP
Associate Clinical Professor Pediatrics, Harvard Medical School; Director Clinical Services, Division of Nephrology, Children's Hospital, Boston, Massachusetts
Tetany

John A. Herring, M.D.
Professor of Orthopaedic Surgery, University of Texas Southwestern Medical School Dallas; Chief of Staff, Texas Scottish Rite Hospital for Children, Dallas, Texas
Legg-Calvé-Perthes Disease

Seth V. Hetherington, M.D.
Clinical Associate Professor, Department of Pediatrics, Division of Pediatric Infectious Diseases, University of North Carolina Hospital School of Medicine; Senior Clinical Program Head, HIV/Opportunistic Infection Clinical Development, Glaxo Wellcome, Research Triangle Park, North Carolina
Aspergillosis

Peter Heydemann, M.D.
Associate Professor of Pediatrics and Neurology, Rush Medical College; Director, Pediatric Neurology, Co-Director, Muscular Dystrophy Association Clinic, Rush Medical Center, Chicago, Illinois
Myopathy

Raymond L. Hintz, M.D.
Professor of Pediatrics, Stanford University School of Medicine; Lucile Salter Packard Children's Hospital at Stanford, Stanford, California
Growth Hormone Deficiency

Jay A. Hochman, M.D.
Pediatric Gastroenterologist, Children's Center for Digestive Health Care, Atlanta Georgia
Gastroenteritis, Bacterial

David Edward E. Holck, M.D.
Assistant Professor of Surgery, Uniformed Services University of the Health Sciences (USUHS), School of Medicine, Bethesda, Maryland; Assistant Clinical Professor, Department of Ophthalmology, University of Texas Health Sciences Center; Director, Oculoplastics, Orbit and Ocular Oncology Services, Wilford Hall Medical Center, San Antonio, Texas
Epiphora (Tearing)
Eye Problems, Pediatric Blepharoptosis

Julie E. Hoover, M.D.
Fellow, Institute of Genetic Medicine, Johns Hopkins Hospital, Baltimore, Maryland
Maple Syrup Urine Disease

Marc E. Horowitz, M.D.
Professor of Pediatrics, Baylor College of Medicine, Texas Children's Cancer Center, Houston, Texas
Ewing Sarcoma Family of Tumors

Sharon L. Hostler, M.D.
McLemore Birdsong Professor of Pediatrics; Chief, Division of Developmental Pediatrics, Associate Chair for Medical Affairs, Medical Director, Kluge Children's Rehabilitation Center, University of Virginia School of Medicine, Charlottesville, Virginia
Anorexia Nervosa
Bulimia Nervosa

James F. Howard, Jr., M.D.
Professor of Neurology, Chief, Neuromuscular Disorders Section, Department of Neurology, The University of North Carolina School of Medicine; University of North Carolina Hospital, Chapel Hill, North Carolina
Myasthenia Gravis

Michelle S. Howenstine, M.D.
Clinical Associate Professor, Department of Pediatrics, Indiana University School of Medicine; Pediatric Pulmonologist, Riley Hospital for Children, Indianapolis, Indiana
Foreign Bodies of the Lung

John D. Hsu, M.D., CM, FACS
Clinical Professor, Department of Orthopedics, University of Southern California School of Medicine, Los Angeles; Chief, Department of Surgery, Chief of Orthopedics, Rancho Los Amigos National Rehabilitation Center, Downey, California
Fractures, Clavicle

Walter T. Hughes, M.D.
Professor of Pediatrics and Preventive Medicine, University of Tennessee College of Medicine; Emeritus Member, St. Jude's Children's Research Hospital, Memphis, Tennessee
Pneumonia, Pneumocystis Carinii

Gregory F. Hulka, M.D.
Assistant Professor, Duke University Medical Center, Durham, North Carolina
Brachial Cleft Cysts

Walter W. Huurman, M.D.
Professor, Orthopaedic Surgery, Director Children's Orthopaedics, University of Nebraska Medical Center, Omaha, Nebraska
Radial Head Subluxation (Nursemaid's Elbow) and Congenital Dislocations

David L. Ingram, M.D.
Professor of Pediatrics, University of North Carolina School of Medicine, Chapel Hill, North Carolina; Director of Pediatrics, CARElina Medical Associates, Raleigh, North Carolina
Gonorrhea
Syphilis, Noncongenital
Trichomonas vaginalis Infections

Sherwin J. Isenberg, M.D.
Professor of Ophthalmology, Departments of Ophthalmology and Pediatrics, University of California–Los Angeles School of Medicine; Jules Stein Eye Institute, Harbor–UCLA Medical Center, Los Angeles, California
Hyphema

Richard F. Jacobs, M.D., FAAP
Horace C. Cabe Professor of Pediatrics, University of Arkansas for Medical Sciences; Chief, Pediatric Infectious Diseases, Arkansas Children's Hospital, Little Rock, Arkansas
Tuberculosis, Background / Diagnosis
Tuberculosis, Treatment
Tularemia

Camila K. Janniger, M.D.
Clinical Associate Professor of Dermatology and Pediatrics and Chief, Pediatric Dermatology, New Jersey Medical School, Newark, New Jersey
Bites, Insect, and Stings
Molluscum Contagiosum

David Jardine, M.D.
Associate Professor of Anesthesiology, Adjunct Associate Professor of Pediatrics, Children's Hospital and Medical Center, University of Washington School of Medicine; Attending Staff, Department of Anesthesiology, Children's Hospital and Regional Medical Center, Seattle, Washington
Heat Stroke and Hemorrhagic Shock and Encephalopathy Syndrome (HSES)

Bernett L. Johnson, Jr., M.D.
Herman Beerman Professor of Dermatology, University of Pennsylvania School of Medicine; Senior Medical Director, Hospital of the University of Pennsylvania, Philadelphia, Pennsylvania
Melanocytic Nevus, Congenital

Wendi Johnson, M.D.
Medical Director/Supervisor, University Health and Counseling Services, University of Wisconsin - Whitewater, Whitewater, Wisconsin
Osgood-Schlatter Disease and Sinding-Larsen-Johansson Disease

Helen S. Johnstone, M.D.
Associate Professor of Pediatrics, University of Illinois at Chicago; Attending Physician, University of Illinois Hospital, Chicago, Illinois
Thalassemia, Major and Minor

Joseph L. Jorizzo, M.D.
Professor and Chair, Department of Dermatology, Wake Forest University School of Medicine, Winston-Salem, North Carolina
Urticaria

Natalie Pierre Joseph, M.D., MPH
University of Massachusetts Medical Center; Leominster Hospital; Adolescent/Pediatric Attending Physician, Fallon Clinic, Worcester, Massachusetts
Uterine Bleeding, Irregular

Jessica A. Kahn, M.D., MPH
Assistant Professor of Clinical Pediatrics, University of Cincinnati College of Medicine; Assistant Professor of Pediatrics, Children's Hospital Medical Center, Cincinnati, Ohio
Vulvovaginitis in the Prepubertal Child

Vicki Kalen, M.D.
Assistant Clinical Professor, University of Maryland School of Medicine, Baltimore, Maryland
Fractures, Proximal Humerus

Richard A. Kaplan, M.D., Ph.D.
Director, Pediatric Nephrology and Hypertension, Lutheran General Hospital, Park Ridge, Illinois
Renal Failure, Chronic, Management

Sheldon L. Kaplan, M.D.
Professor and Vice-Chairman for Clinical Affairs, Department of Pediatrics, Baylor College of Medicine; Chief, Infectious Diseases Service, Texas Children's Hospital, Houston, Texas
Osteomyelitis
Septic Arthritis

Michael Katz, M.D.
Reuben S. Carpentier Professor Emeritus of Pediatrics, Columbia University College of Physicians and Surgeons; Consultant Emeritus, New York-Presbyterian Hospital, New York, New York; Vice President for Research, March of Dimes, Birth Defects Foundation, White Plains, New York
Pinworm Infection (Enterobiasis)
Visceral Larva Migrans

Samuel L. Katz, M.D., DSC
Wilburt C. Davison Professor and Chairman Emeritus, Department of Pediatrics, Duke University; Duke University Medical Center, Durham, North Carolina
Poliomyelitis

Frank G. Keller, M.D.
Assistant Professor, Department of Pediatrics, West Virginia University School of Medicine, Morgantown, West Virginia
Histiocytoses, Childhood

Jay S. Keystone, M.D., MSC (CTM), FRCPC
Professor of Medicine, University of Toronto; Staff Physician, Centre for Travel and Tropical Medicine, Toronto General Hospital, Toronto, Ontario, Canada
Cysticercosis

Lowell R. King, M.D., FACS, FAAP
Professor of Urology, Division of Urology, Department of Surgery, University of New Mexico School of Medicine, Albuquerque, New Mexico; Emeritus Professor of Surgery, Duke University Medical Center, Durham, North Carolina
Hydronephrosis, Fetal Obstructive Uropathy

H. Neil Kirkman, M.D.
Professor Emeritus, Department of Pediatrics, University of North Carolina at Chapel Hill, Chapel Hill, North Carolina
Galactosemia

Ronald E. Kleinman, M.D.
Professor of Pediatrics, Harvard Medical School; Chief, Pediatric Gastroenterology and Nutrition, Massachusetts General Hospital, Boston, Massachusetts
Diarrhea, Chronic Nonspecific (CNSD) or Toddler's Diarrhea

Robert M. Kliegman, M.D.
Professor and Chair, Department of Pediatrics, Medical College of Wisconsin; Pediatrician-in-Chief, Children's Hospital of Wisconsin, Milwaukee, Wisconsin
Brachial Plexus Palsy

Mark W. Kline, M.D.
Professor of Pediatrics, Baylor College of Medicine, Houston, Texas
Fever without a Source (>2 Mos of Age)

Nancy E. Kline, Ph.D., CPNP
Assistant Professor of Pediatrics, Baylor College of Medicine; Pediatric Nurse Practitioner, Texas Children's Cancer Center, Texas Children's Hospital, Houston, Texas
Fever without a Source (>2 Mos of Age)

William C. Koch, M.D.
Associate Professor of Pediatrics, Department of Pediatrics, Division of Infectious Diseases, Medical College of Virginia, Virginia Commonwealth University; Attending Physician, Department of Pediatrics, Medical College of Virginia Hospitals, Richmond, Virginia
Fifth Disease (Erythema Infectiosum) and Other Parvovirus Infections

Patricia K. Kokotailo, M.D., MPH
Associate Professor of Pediatrics, Director, Pediatric Medical Education, Department of Pediatrics, University of Wisconsin, Madison, Wisconsin
Alcohol Use
Marijuana Use

David N. Korones, M.D.
Division of Pediatric Hematology and Oncology, Department of Pediatrics, Children's Hospital at Strong Memorial Hospital, Rochester, New York
Folic Acid Deficiency

Karen L. Kotloff, M.D.
Professor of Pediatrics and Medicine, University of Maryland School of Medicine, Baltimore, Maryland
Hepatitis A Virus
Hepatitis B Virus
Hepatitis C Virus
Salmonella and Salmonella Typhi

Stephen O. Kovacs, M.D.
Assistant Professor of Surgery, Hahnemann Hospital, Medical College of Pennsylvania, Philadelphia, Pennsylvania
Contact Dermatitis (Allergic and Irritant)

Bernice R. Krafchik, MB, ChB, FRCPC
Professor, Departments of Paediatrics and Medicine, University of Toronto; Head, Section of Dermatology, Division of Paediatric Medicine, Hospital for Sick Children, Toronto, Canada
Psoriasis

Richard M. Kravitz, M.D.
Assistant Professor of Pediatrics, Duke University School of Medicine; Assistant Professor of Pediatrics, Director, Pediatric Sleep Laboratory, Duke University Medical Center, Durham, North Carolina
Tracheomalacia

Leonard Kristal, M.D.
Clinical Assistant Professor of Dermatology and Pediatrics, State University of New York at Stony Brook, Stony Brook, New York
Intertrigol / Intertriginous Eruptions
Pityriasis Rosea

Daniel P. Krowchuk, M.D.
Professor of Pediatrics and Dermatology, Wake Forest University School of Medicine, Winston-Salem, North Carolina
Angioedema
Urticaria

David A. Kube, M.D.
Assistant Professor of Pediatrics, University of Tennessee; Assistant Professor of Pediatrics, Boling Center for Developmental Disabilities, Memphis, Tennessee
Dyslexia (Reading Disorder)

Stephen La Franchi, M.D.
Professor, Department of Pediatrics and Head, Pediatric Endocrinology, Oregon Health Sciences University, Portland, Oregon
Hypothyroidism

Elise E. Labbé, Ph.D.
Professor of Psychology, Department of Psychology, University of South Alabama, Mobile, Alabama
Headache, Other Than Migraine, Management

Gregory L. Landry, M.D.
Professor of Pediatrics, University of Wisconsin Hospital; Head Medical Team Physician, University of Wisconsin Athletic Teams, Madison, Wisconsin
Osgood-Schlatter Disease and Sinding-Larson-Johansson Disease

Beverly J. Lange, M.D.
Professor of Pediatrics, University of Pennsylvania School of Medicine; Professor of Clinical Oncology, The Children's Hospital of Philadelphia, Philadelphia, Pennsylvania
Hodgkin Disease
Leukemia, Acute Myelogenous

Craig B. Langman, M.D.
Professor of Pediatrics, Northwestern University, Evanston, Illinois; Head, Nephrology and Mineral Metabolism, Children's Memorial Medical Center, Chicago, Illinois
Rickets, X-Linked Hypophosphatemic (Vitamin D Resistant Rickets)

Ronald M. Laxer, M.D., FRCPC
Professor of Pediatrics and Medicine, Vice-Chairman, Department of Pediatrics, University of Toronto; Associate Pediatrician-in-Chief, Pediatric Rheumatologist, The Hospital for Sick Children, Toronto, Ontario, Canada
Ankylosing Spondylitis, Juvenile and Other Sero-Negative Arthritides

Howard M. Lederman, M.D., Ph.D.
Associate Professor of Pediatrics, Division of Pediatric Allergy and Immunology, Johns Hopkins University School of Medicine; Director, Immunodeficiency Clinic, Johns Hopkins Hospital, Baltimore, Maryland
Immunodeficiency Disorders

Bong S. Lee, M.D.
Associate Clinical Professor of Orthopedic Surgery, University of Pennsylvania School of Medicine; Director, Pediatric Hand Surgery, Children's Hospital of Philadelphia, Philadelphia, Pennsylvania
Finger and Nail Injuries

Peter A. Lee, M.D., Ph.D.
Professor of Pediatrics, Penn State University College of Medicine; Attending Physician, Milton S. Hershey Medical Center, Department of Pediatrics, Hershey, Pennsylvania
Sex Chromosome Abnormalities (Other Than Turner Syndrome)

Margaret W. Leigh, M.D.
Professor of Pediatrics, Chief, Division of Pulmonary Medicine and Allergy, University of North Carolina at Chapel Hill; Attending Physician, University of North Carolina Hospitals, Chapel Hill, North Carolina
Bronchopulmonary Dysplasia

Neal S. LeLeiko, M.D., Ph.D.
Vice Chair, Department of Pediatrics, Professor and Chief, Division of Pediatric Gastroenterology, Nutrition and Liver Diseases, The Mount Sinai School of Medicine, New York, New York
Pancreatitis

Amy A. Levine, M.D.
Clinical Assistant Professor, Pediatrics and Nutrition, University of North Carolina at Chapel Hill, Chapel Hill, North Carolina
Obesity

Moise L. Levy, M.D.
Professor of Dermatology and Pediatrics, Baylor College of Medicine; Chief, Dermatology Service, Texas Children's Hospital, Houston, Texas
Mastocytosis: Urticaria Pigmentosa
Neurocutaneous Melanosis
Scabies

Alan B. Lewis, M.D.
Professor of Pediatrics, Keck School of Medicine, University of Southern California; Associate Head, Division of Cardiology, Children's Hospital of Los Angeles, Los Angeles, California
Myocarditis

James P. Loehr, M.D.
Assistant Professor, Department of Pediatrics, University of North Carolina at Chapel Hill, Chapel Hill, North Carolina
Supraventricular Tachycardia

Jacob A. Lohr, M.D.
Professor and Vice Chair, Department of Pediatrics, University of North Carolina School of Medicine; Pediatrician-in-Chief, North Carolina Children's Hospital, Chapel Hill, North Carolina
Conjunctivitis (Acute Benign Infectious Conjunctivitis)

Sarah S. Long, M.D.
Professor of Pediatrics, MCP Hahnemann University School of Medicine; Chief, Infectious Diseases, St. Christopher's Hospital for Children, Philadelphia, Pennsylvania
Pertussis

Gerald M. Loughlin, M.D.
Professor of Pediatrics and Director, Eudowood Division of Pediatric Respiratory Sciences, Johns Hopkins University School of Medicine; Senior Vice President for Medical Affairs, Mt. Washington Pediatric Hospital, Baltimore, Maryland
Bronchiolitis
Obstructive Sleep Apnea

Stephen Ludwig, M.D.
Professor of Pediatrics, University of Pennsylvania School of Medicine; Associate Physician-in-Chief, Children's Hospital of Philadelphia, Philadelphia, Pennsylvania
Hypothermia

Susan Lurie, M.D.
Assistant Professor of Psychiatry, University of Colorado Health Sciences Center; Medical Director, Psychiatric Day Treatment Program, The Children's Hospital, Denver, Colorado
Anxiety Disorders

Sudesh P. Makker, M.D.
Professor of Pediatrics, Chief, Division of Nephrology, University of California–Davis, School of Medicine and University of California - Davis, Medical Center, Sacramento, California
Glomerulonephritides

J. Jeffrey Malatack, M.D.
Professor of Pediatrics, MCP Hahnemann School of Medicine; Director, Diagnostic Referral Service, St. Christopher's Hospital for Children, Philadelphia, Pennsylvania
Cat Scratch Disease

Susan B. Mallory, M.D.
Professor of Dermatology and Pediatrics, Washington University School of Medicine; Director, Pediatric Dermatology, St. Louis Children's Hospital, St. Louis, Missouri
Contact Dermatitis (Allergic and Irritant)
Neonatal Papules: Acne Neonatorum, Erythema Toxicum, and Milia

Kathleen A. Mammel, M.D.
Clinical Assistant Professor, Department of Pediatrics, Wayne State University School of Medicine, Detroit, Michigan; Director, Adolescent Pediatrics, William Beaumont Hospital, Royal Oak, Michigan
Breast Abscess

Caroline M. Mann, M.D.
Dermatology Outpatient Center, Barnes Clinic, St. Louis, Missouri
Neonatal Papules: Acne Neonatorum, Erythema Toxicum, and Milia

John Douglas Mann, M.D.
Professor of Neurology, University of North Carolina School of Medicine; Professor of Neurology, University of North Carolina Hospitals, Chapel Hill, North Carolina
Cerebral Edema

Paris T. Mansmann, M.D., FAAP, FACP, FACAAI
Associate Professor of Medicine, West Virginia University School of Medicine, Morgantown, West Virginia; Director of Allergy and Clinical Immunovirology, Director of Paul E. Keener Immunovirology Laboratory, Ruby Memorial Hospital of Robert C. Byrd Health Sciences Center, Morgantown, West Virginia
Acrodermatitis Enteropathica

S. Michael Marcy, M.D.
Clinical Professor of Pediatrics, University of Southern California and University of California at Los Angeles Schools of Medicine, Los Angeles, California; Staff Pediatrician, Kaiser Foundation Hospital, Panorama City, California
Mumps

Bruce J. Masek, Ph.D.
Associate Professor of Psychiatry, Harvard Medical School; Director, Behavioral Medicine, Department of Psychiatry, Children's Hospital and Massachusetts General Hospital, Boston, Massachusetts
Enuresis

Eric E. Mast, M.D., MPH
Chief, Hepatitis Surveillance Unit, Hepatitis Branch, National Center for Infectious Diseases, Centers for Disease Control and Prevention, Atlanta, Georgia
Hepatitis E and Non A-E Hepatitis

Ranjiv Mathews, M.D.
Assistant Professor, Pediatric Urology, The Johns Hopkins Hospital-Brady Urological Institute, Baltimore, Maryland
Hypospadias/Epispadias

David O. Matson, M.D., Ph.D.
Professor of Pediatrics, Eastern Virginia Medical School; Head, Infectious Diseases Section, Associate Director, Center for Pediatric Research, Norfolk, Virginia
Rotavirus Infections

Harold M. Maurer, M.D.
Chancellor, University of Nebraska Medical College of Medicine, Omaha, Nebraska
Rhabdomyosarcoma

Jay H. Mayefsky, M.D., MPH
Associate Professor of Pediatrics, Finch University of Health Sciences, The Chicago Medical School, North Chicago, Illinois; Director, Comprehensive Care Clinic, Cook County Children's Hospital, Chicago, Illinois
Roseola (Exanthem Subitum) and Other Human Herpesvirus 6/7 Infections

Mary Anne S. Mayo, M.D.
Assistant Professor, University of North Carolina Department of Pediatrics, University of North Carolina at Chapel Hill, Chapel Hill, North Carolina
Bites, Snake

Joseph Maytal, M.D.
Associate Professor of Pediatrics and Neurology, Albert Einstein College of Medicine, Bronx, New York; Chief, Pediatric Neurology, North Shore-Long Island Jewish Health System, Schneider Children's Hospital, New Hyde Park, New York
Seizures, Generalized, Myoclonic

Carol A. McCarthy, M.D.
Associate Professor of Pediatrics, University of Vermont College of Medicine, Burlington, Vermont; Director, Pediatric Infectious Disease, Maine Medical Center, Portland, Maine
Fever without a Source (<2 Mos of Age)

Kenneth L. McClain, M.D., Ph.D.
Associate Professor of Pediatrics, Texas Children's Cancer Center and Hematology Service, Baylor College of Medicine, Houston, Texas
Autoimmune Anemia

Elizabeth J. McFarland, M.D.
Assistant Professor of Pediatrics, University of Colorado Health Sciences Center; Director, Children's Hospital Immunodeficiency Program, The Children's Hospital, Denver, Colorado
Acquired Immune Deficiency Syndrome (AIDS)

Eugene D. McGahren III, M.D.
Associate Professor of Pediatric Surgery and Pediatrics, University of Virginia Health System, Department of Surgery, Charlottesville, Virginia
Cholecystitis
Choledochal Cyst
Pyloric Stenosis
Volvulus

Judeth K. McGann, M.D.
Adjunct Faculty, Tufts University School of Medicine; Director, Pediatric Hematology and Oncology Clinic, Eastern Maine Medical Center, Bangor, Maine
Folic Acid Deficiency

Sara C. McIntire, M.D.
Associate Professor of Pediatrics, University of Pittsburgh School of Medicine; Physician, Diagnostic Referral Service, Children's Hospital of Pittsburgh, Pittsburgh, Pennsylvania
Hallux Valgus

David M. McKalip, M.D.
Assistant Professor, Department of Neurological Surgery, University of California, San Francisco, San Francisco, California
Concussion
Craniosynostosis
Scalp Swelling, Post-Traumatic
Subdural and Epidural Hematomas

Julia A. McMillan, M.D.
Associate Professor of Pediatrics, Vice Chair for Education, Residency Program Director, Johns Hopkins University School of Medicine, Baltimore, Maryland
Meningoencephalitis, Viral

Dan G. McNamara, M.D.†
Pulmonary Valve Stenosis

Chapman T. McQueen, M.D.
Assistant Professor Pediatric Otolaryngology, University of North Carolina School of Medicine, Chapel Hill, North Carolina
Myringitis, Bullous
Otitis Externa

Paulette Mehta, M.D.
Professor and Medical Director, Pediatric Hematology/Oncology, University of Florida College of Medicine, Professor and Medical Director, Shands Teaching Hospital, Gainesville, Florida
Bone Marrow Transplantation: Care of the Child Post-Transplantation
Transient Erythroblastopenia of Childhood

Gregory A. Mencio, M.D.
Associate Professor, Department of Orthopaedics and Rehabilitation, Vanderbilt University School of Medicine, Nashville, Tennessee
Genu Varum and Genu Valgum

Mark J. Mendelsohn, M.D.
Associate Professor of Clinical Pediatrics, University of Virginia Health Sciences Center, Charlottesville, Virginia
Epistaxis, Management

Marian G. Michaels, M.D., MPH
Associate Professor of Pediatrics and Surgery, University of Pittsburgh School of Medicine; Pediatric Infectious Diseases, Children's Hospital of Pittsburgh, Pittsburgh, Pennsylvania
Toxoplasmosis

Richard J. Mier, M.D.
Professor of Pediatrics, University of Kentucky; Director of Pediatric Services, Shriners Hospital for Children, Lexington, Kentucky
Torticollis

Joseph G. Morelli, M.D.
Associate Professor of Dermatology and Pediatrics, University of Colorado School of Medicine, Denver, Colorado
Miliaria Rubra and Crystallina

Anna-Barbara Moscicki, M.D.
Professor of Pediatrics, Director of Clinics, Division of Adolescent Medicine, University of California–San Francisco School of Medicine, San Francisco, California
Human Papillomavirus Infections in Adolescents and Children, Genital

Kevin M. Mulhern, M.D.
Associate Professor of Medicine, University of Iowa College of Medicine; Associate Director of Adult and Adolescent Congenital Heart Disease Clinic, University of Iowa Health Care, Iowa City, Iowa
Marfan Syndrome

Charles M. Myer, III, M.D.
Professor, Department of Otolaryngology, Head and Neck Surgery, University of Cincinnati; Children's Hospital Medical Center, Cincinnati, Ohio
Mastoiditis

E. Kirk Neely, M.D.
Clinical Associate Professor, Division of Pediatric Endocrinology, Stanford University, Stanford, California
Growth Hormone Deficiency

Jeffrey H. Newcorn, M.D.
Associate Professor of Psychiatry and Pediatrics, Director, Division of Child and Adolescent Psychiatry, Mt. Sinai Medical Center, New York, New York
Anxiety Disorders

Jacqueline A. Noonan, M.D.
Professor Emeritus, Pediatric Cardiology, University of Kentucky College of Medicine; Pediatric Cardiologist, University of Kentucky Medical Center, Lexington, Kentucky
Atrial Septal Defect
Congestive Heart Failure

Edward J. O'Connell, M.D.
Professor of Pediatrics, Mayo Medical School; Consultant, Department of Pediatric and Adolescent Medicine, Mayo Clinic and Mayo Foundation, Rochester, Minnesota
Asthma, Management

Chad K. Oh, M.D.
Assistant Professor, Department of Pediatrics, UCLA School of Medicine; Chief, Pediatric Allergy/Immunology, Harbor-UCLA Medical Center, Torrance, California
Anaphylaxis

Bradford W. Olney, M.D.
Clinical Professor of Surgery (Orthopedics), University of Kansas Medical School - Wichita; Pediatric Orthopedics, Wichita Clinic, Wichita, Kansas
Tarsal Coalition

Susan R. Orenstein, M.D.
Professor of Pediatrics, Division of Pediatric Gastroenterology, University of Pittsburgh School of Medicine; Director, Division of Pediatric Gastroenterology, Children's Hospital of Pittsburgh, Pittsburgh, Pennsylvania
Gastroesophageal Reflux

Lauren M. Pachman, M.D.
Professor of Pediatrics, Division of Immunology/Rheumatology, Children's Memorial Hospital, Chicago, Illinois
Dermatomyositis, Juvenile

Frederick B. Palmer, M.D.
Shainberg Professor of Pediatrics, University of Tennessee; Director, Boling Center for Developmental Disabilities, Memphis, Tennessee
Dyslexia (Reading Disorder)

Dana Paquette, M.D.
Dermatology Resident, Boston University School of Medicine, Boston, Massachusetts and Roger Williams Medical Center, Department of Dermatology, Providence, Rhode Island
Ichthyosis

Katherine Parker, M.D.
Fellow, Pediatric Hematology/ Oncology, Indiana School of Medicine, Indianapolis, Indiana
Leukemia, Acute Lymphocytic

Samuel K. Parrish, Jr., M.D.
Director, Student Health and Wellness Center, Johns Hopkins University, Baltimore, Maryland
Inhalants Use

Zbigniew S. Pawlowski, M.D., DTMH
Professor Emeritus in Parasitology and Tropical Medicine, University of Medical Sciences, Poznán, Poland
Trichinellosis (Trichinosis)

David B. Peden, M.D.
Associate Professor of Pediatrics, Division of Pulmonary Medicine and Allergy, and Associate Director, Center for Environmental Medicine and Lung Biology, School of Medicine, University of North Carolina at Chapel Hill, Chapel Hill, North Carolina
Allergic Rhinitis

David H. Perlmutter, M.D.
Donald B. Strominger Professor of Pediatrics, Professor of Cell Biology and Physiology, Washington University School of Medicine; Director, Division of Gastroenterology and Nutrition, St. Louis Children's Hospital, St. Louis, Missouri
Alpha-1-Antitrypsin Deficiency

Jay A. Perman, M.D.
Professor and Chairman, University of Maryland School of Medicine; Pediatrician-in-Chief, University of Maryland Medical Systems, Baltimore, Maryland
Lactose Intolerance

Millicent Winfrey Peterseim, M.D.
Clinical Assistant Professor, Medical University of South Carolina, Charleston, South Carolina
Amblyopia
Refractive Errors (Nearsightedness/ Farsightedness/Astigmatism)

Mary Jane Petruzzi, M.D.
Assistant Professor of Pediatrics, Division of Hematology-Oncology, Children's Hospital of Buffalo, Buffalo State University of New York; Clinical Attending Physician, Roswell Park Cancer Institute, Buffalo, New York
Wilms Tumor

Michael J. Pettei, M.D., Ph.D.
Associate Professor of Pediatrics, Albert Einstein College of Medicine, Bronx, New York; Co-Chief, Division of Pediatric Gastroenterology and Nutrition, Schneider Children's Hospital, Long Island Jewish Medical Center, New Hyde Park, New York
Constipation, Management

Ross E. Petty, M.D., Ph.D.
Professor and Head, Division of Rheumatology, Department of Pediatrics, University of British Columbia; Head, Division of Rheumatology, Department of Pediatrics, British Columbia Children's Hospital, Vancouver, British Columbia, Canada
Reiter Syndrome

William A. Phillips, M.D.
Professor, Orthopaedic Surgery and Pediatrics, Baylor College of Medicine; Chief, Pediatric Orthopaedics and Scoliosis, Texas Children's Hospital, Houston, Texas
Atlanto-Axial Rotary Subluxation (AARS)

Steve Piecuch, M.D., MPH
Clinical Assistant Professor of Pediatrics, State University of New York, Health Science Center at Brooklyn, Department of Pediatrics; Attending Physician, Children's Medical Center of Brooklyn, Brooklyn, New York
Hirschsprung Disease

Harold C. Pillsbury III, M.D.
Professor and Chief, Division of Otolaryngology, Head and Neck Surgery, University of North Carolina School of Medicine, Chapel Hill, North Carolina
Retropharyngeal and Peritonsillar Abscess

Bianca Maria Piraccini, M.D., Ph.D.
Department of Dermatology, University of Bologna, Bologna, Italy
Ingrown Toenail

Peter D. Pizzutillo, M.D.
Professor of Orthopedic Surgery, Professor of Pediatrics, School of Medicine, and Director, Department of Orthopedic Surgery and Pediatrics, St. Christopher's Hospital for Children, Philadelphia, Pennsylvania
Compartment Syndrome, Acute and Chronic

Stanley A. Plotkin, M.D.
Emeritus Professor of Pediatrics, University of Pennsylvania; Medical and Scientific Advisor, Aventis Pasteur, Swiftwater, Pennsylvania
Rubella

Amy Nelson Plumb, M.D.
Assistant Professor of Pediatrics; Director, Pediatric Primary Care Education, Department of Pediatrics, University of Wisconsin, Madison, Wisconsin
Alcohol Use

Cynthia M. Powell, M.D.
Assistant Professor of Pediatrics, Division of Genetics and Metabolism, Medical Director, Cytogenetics Laboratory, University of North Carolina at Chapel Hill, Chapel Hill, North Carolina
Achondroplasia

Dwight A. Powell, M.D.
Professor of Pediatrics, The Ohio State University College of Medicine and Public Health; Chief, Section of Infectious Diseases, Children's Hospital, Columbus, Ohio
Blastomycosis
Mycobacterial Infections, Nontuberous

Keith R. Powell, M.D.
Professor and Chair, Department of Pediatrics, Northeastern Ohio Universities College of Medicine, Rootstown, Ohio; Vice President and Chair of Pediatric Medicine, Children's Hospital and Medical Center of Akron, Akron, Ohio
Fever without a Source (<2 Mos of Age)
Periorbital and Orbital Cellulitis

Arthur L. Prensky, M.D.
Allen P. and Josephine B. Green Professor of Pediatric Neurology, Washington University School of Medicine; Neurologist and Pediatrician, St. Louis Children's Hospital, St. Louis, Missouri
Headache, Migraine, Diagnosis
Headache, Migraine, Treatment

Charles T. Price, M.D.
Surgeon-in-Chief, Nemours Children's Clinic, Orlando, Florida
Fractures, Forearm and Wrist

Howard B. Pride, M.D.
Assistant Clinical Professor, Penn State University College of Medicine, Hershey, Pennsylvania; Associate, Department of Dermatology, Geisinger Medical Center, Danville, Pennsylvania
Seborrheic Dermatitis, Infantile

Neil S. Prose, M.D.
Associate Professor of Dermatology and Pediatrics, Duke University Medical Center, Durham, North Carolina
Alopecia Areata

Simon S. Rabinowitz, Ph.D., M.D.
Clinical Associate Professor, SUNY, Health Sciences Center; Director, Pediatric Gastroenterology, Associate Chairman for Research, Long Island College Hospital, Brooklyn, New York
Esophageal Burns

Wayne R. Rackoff, M.D.
Assistant Medical Director Clinical Affairs, Ortho Biotech Oncology, Raritan, New Jersey
Aplastic Anemia

Michael S. Radetsky, M.D., CM
Clinical Professor of Pediatrics, University of New Mexico School of Medicine; Chair, Department of Pediatrics, Lovelace Clinic, Albuquerque, New Mexico
Shigella Infections

Sharon S. Raimer, M.D.
Professor of Dermatology and Pediatrics, University of Texas Medical Branch, Galveston, Texas
Papular Acrodermatitis of Childhood (Gianotti-Crosti Syndrome)

Gary P. Rakes, M.D.
Assistant Professor of Pediatrics, University of Virginia School of Medicine, Charlottesville, Virginia; Assistant Professor of Pediatrics, University of Virginia Health Sciences Center, Charlottesville, Virginia
Asthma, Status Asthmaticus

Sukhvinder S. Ranu, M.D.
Clinical Assistant Instructor, College of Medicine, SUNY Health Sciences Center at Brooklyn; Fellow in Neonatal-Perinatal Medicine, Children's Medical Center of Brooklyn, Brooklyn, New York
Hirschsprung Disease

Leonard Rappaport, M.D.
Associate Chief, Division of General Pediatrics, Children's Hospital, Boston, Massachusetts
Encopresis

Sarit Ravid, M.D.
Fellow, Pediatric Neurology, North Shore-Long Island Jewish Health System, Schneider Children's Hospital, New Hyde Park, New York
Seizures, Generalized, Myoclonic

Ann M. Reed, M.D.
University of North Carolina, Chapel Hill, North Carolina; Duke University Medical Center, Durham, North Carolina; presently at Mayo Clinic, Rochester, Minnesota
Polymyositis and Dermatomyositis

William F. Reed, M.D.
Assistant Medical Director, Research Blood Centers of the Pacific, Irwin Center, San Francisco; Co-Director, Cord Blood Program, Children's Hospital Oakland Research Institute, Oakland, California
Sickle-Cell Disease Anemia

Thomas S. Renshaw, M.D.
Professor of Orthopaedic Surgery, Yale University, New Haven, Connecticut
Spondylolysis

Frederick J. Rescorla, M.D.
Associate Professor of Surgery, Indiana University School of Medicine, Indianapolis, Indiana; Staff Surgeon, James Whitcomb Riley Hospital for Children, Indianapolis, Indiana
Pectus Excavatum and Pectus Carinatum
Umbilical Abnormalities

Steven D. Resnick, M.D.
Associate Clinical Professor of Dermatology, Columbia University College of Physicians and Surgeons, New York, New York; Chief, Division of Dermatology, Bassett Healthcare, Cooperstown, New York
Scalded Skin Syndrome, Staphylococcal

Marleta Reynolds, M.D.
Associate Professor of Surgery, Northwestern University; Attending Physician, Children's Memorial Hospital, Chicago, Illinois
Thyroglossal Duct Cyst

Karen S. Rheuban, M.D.
Professor of Pediatrics, University of Virginia School of Medicine; Associate Dean, Medical Director, Office of Telemedicine, University of Virginia Health System, Charlottesville, Virginia
Patent Ductus Arteriosus

J. Marc Rhoads, M.D.
Professor of Pediatrics, Department of Pediatrics, University of North Carolina at Chapel Hill, Chapel Hill, North Carolina
Gastroenteritis, Viral

Robert A. Richman, M.D.
Professor of Pediatrics, Division of Pediatric Endocrinology, SUNY Upstate Medical University; Attending Physician, University Hospital, Crouse Hospital, Syracuse, New York
Diabetes Insipidus, Central
Diabetes Insipidus, Familial Nephrogenic, Drug-Induced

Colin Roberts, M.D.
Fellow, Pediatric Epilepsy, Children's Hospital of Philadelphia, Philadelphia, Pennsylvania
Seizures, Complex Partial (Psychomotor, Limbic)

Kenneth B. Roberts, M.D.
Professor of Pediatrics, University of North Carolina School of Medicine, Chapel Hill, North Carolina; Director, Pediatric Teaching Program, Moses Cone Health System, Greensboro, North Carolina
Dehydration

Douglas G. Rogers, M.D.
Head, Section of Pediatric Endocrinology, Cleveland Clinic Foundation, Cleveland, Ohio
Short Stature, Management

Lewis H. Romer, M.D.
Associate Professor of Pediatrics, Cell Biology and Anatomy, and Anesthesiology, University of North Carolina at Chapel Hill, Chapel Hill, North Carolina
Pneumothorax and Pneumomediastinum

Thomas M. Rossi, M.D.
Associate Professor of Pediatrics, State University of New York at Buffalo; Chief, Division of Gastroenterology and Nutrition, Department of Pediatrics, Children's Hospital of Buffalo, Buffalo, New York
Celiac Disease (Gluten-Sensitive Enteropathy)

Marti Jill Rothe, M.D.
Associate Professor of Dermatology, University of Connecticut Health Center and John Dempsey Hospital, Farmington, Connecticut
Ichthyosis

M. Henderson Rourk, Jr., M.D.
Assistant Professor of Pediatrics, Duke University School of Medicine; Director of Recruitment, Pediatric Residency Program, Duke University Medical Center, Durham, North Carolina
Diarrhea Syndrome, Antibiotic-Induced

Dennis R. Roy, M.D.
Professor of Orthopaedic Surgery, University of Cincinnati School of Medicine; Associate Director, Hip Service, Children's Hospital Medical Center, Cincinnati, Ohio
Transient Synovitis

Lorry G. Rubin, M.D.
Professor of Pediatrics, Albert Einstein College of Medicine, Bronx, New York; Chief, Pediatric Infectious Diseases, Schneider Children's Hospital of North Shore-Long Island Jewish Health System, New Hyde Park, New York
Streptococcal Disease, Invasive (Including Fasciitis)

R. Bradley Sack, M.D., ScD
Professor of International Health, Johns Hopkins School of Hygiene and Public Health, Johns Hopkins University, Baltimore, Maryland
Travelers' Diarrhea

Xavier Sáez-Llorens, M.D.
Professor of Pediatrics, Hospital del Nino and University of Panama, Panama City, Panama
Sepsis and Septic Shock

Sameh M. Said, M.D.
Department of Neuropsychiatry, Faculty of Medicine, Alexandria University, Alexandria, Egypt
Neurofibromatosis

Marina Salvadori, M.D., FRCPC
Hospital for Sick Children, Toronto, Ontario, Canada
Cysticercosis

Robert A. Sargent, M.D., FACP, FACS
Associate Clinical Professor, Department of Ophthalmology, University of Colorado Health Sciences Center; Former Chairman, Pediatric Ophthalmology, The Children's Hospital, Denver, Colorado
Foreign Bodies of the Eye

Richard M. Sarles, M.D.
Professor of Psychiatry and Pediatrics, University of Maryland School of Medicine, Baltimore, Maryland
Tics

Frank T. Saulsbury, M.D.
Professor of Pediatrics, Department of Pediatrics, University of Virginia School of Medicine, Charlottesville, Virginia
Kawasaki Disease

Michael S. Schaffer, M.D.
Associate Professor of Pediatrics (Cardiology), University of Colorado Medical School; Director of Arrhythmia Service, The Children's Hospital, Denver, Colorado
Dysrhythmias

Robert Schechter, M.D., FAAP
Infectious Botulism Treatment and Prevention Program, Division of Communicable Disease Control, California Department of Health Services, Berkeley, California; Children's Hospital, Oakland, California
Botulism, Infant

Theresa A. Schlager, M.D.
Associate Professor of Pediatrics and Emergency Medicine, University of Virginia, Charlottesville, Virginia
Urinary Tract Infection, Symptomatic

Barton D. Schmitt, M.D.
Professor of Pediatrics, University of Colorado School of Medicine; Medical Director, General Consultations, The Children's Hospital, Denver, Colorado
School Phobia (School Avoidance or Refusal)

Virginia J. Schreiner, M.D.
Assistant Clinical Professor of Pediatrics, University of North Carolina School of Medicine; Clinical Affiliate, University of North Carolina Hospitals, Chapel Hill, North Carolina
Gingivostomatitis

Gordon E. Schutze, M.D., CAAP
Associate Professor of Pediatrics and Pathology, University of Arkansas for Medical Sciences; Pediatric Residency Program Director, Arkansas Children's Hospital, Little Rock, Arkansas
Tuberculosis, Background/Diagnosis
Tuberculosis, Treatment
Tularemia

Richard H. Schwartz, M.D.
Clinical Professor of Pediatrics, University of Virginia School of Medicine; Inova Fairfax Hospital for Children, Falls Church, Virginia; Clinical Professor of Pediatrics, George Washington University School of Medicine, Washington, DC
Cocaine Use

Sarah Jane Schwarzenberg, M.D.
Associate Professor of Pediatrics, University of Minnesota, Minneapolis, Minnesota
Cholangitis

Mary-Ann B. Shafer, M.D.
Professor of Pediatrics, Associate Director, Division of Adolescent Medicine, University of California, San Francisco, California
Pelvic Inflammatory Disease in the Adolescent

Eugene D. Shapiro, M.D.
Professor of Pediatrics and of Epidemiology and Public Health, Yale University School of Medicine and the Children's Clinical Research Center; Attending Pediatrician, Children's Hospital at Yale–New Haven, New Haven, Connecticut
Lyme Disease
Rocky Mountain Spotted Fever

Vidya Sharma, MBBS, MPH
Associate Professor of Pediatrics; Clinical Associate Professor of Dermatology, University of Missouri at Kansas City; Children's Mercy Hospital, Kansas City, Missouri
Herpes Simplex Virus Infection

Harvey L. Sharp, M.D.
Professor of Pediatrics, Director, Division of Pediatric Gastroenterology and Nutrition, University of Minnesota; Fairview–University Medical Center, Minneapolis, Minnesota
Biliary Atresia
Wilson Disease

David M. Sherman, M.D.
Clinical Assistant Professor, Department of Family Medicine, University of Wisconsin–Madison Medical School, Madison, Wisconsin
Bites, Dog and Cat

Benjamin S. Siegel, M.D.
Professor of Pediatrics and Psychiatry, Boston University School of Medicine; Senior Pediatrician, Boston Medical Center, Boston, Massachusetts
Grief

Richard M. Silver, M.D.
Professor of Medicine and Pediatrics, Director, Division of Rheumatology and Immunology, Medical University of South Carolina, Charleston, South Carolina
Scleroderma

Gerald M. Sloan, M.D.
Ethel F. and James A. Valone Distinguished Professor and Chief, Division of Plastic and Reconstructive Surgery, University of North Carolina School of Medicine, Chapel Hill, North Carolina
Cleft Lip and Cleft Palate

Angela D. Smith, M.D.
Adjunct Professor of Medicine/Sports Medicine, University of Delaware, Newark, Delaware; Attending Faculty, Children's Hospital of Philadelphia, Philadelphia, Pennsylvania
Overuse Injuries of the Lower Leg: Stress Fractures, Shin Splints, and Tendinitis

Bryan W. Smith, M.D., Ph.D.
Clinical Assistant Professor of Pediatrics and Orthopaedics, University of North Carolina School of Medicine; Head Team Physician, James A. Taylor Student Health Services, University of North Carolina at Chapel Hill, Chapel Hill, North Carolina
Sports Injuries/Sprains, Ankle and Foot
Sports Injuries/ Sprains, Wrist

Rebecca R. S. Socolar, M.D., MPH
Clinical Assistant Professor of Pediatrics, University of North Carolina School of Medicine; Medical Director, Child Medical Evaluation, Chapel Hill, North Carolina
Sexual Abuse (Greater Than 72 Hours Postevent)

Shaul Sofer, M.D.
Professor of Pediatrics, Faculty of Health Sciences, Ben-Gurion University of the Negev; Head, Pediatric Intensive Care Unit, Sozoka Medical Center, Beer-Sheva, Israel
Bites, Scorpion

Kit M. Song, M.D.
Assistant Professor, Department of Orthopedics, University of Washington; Assistant Director of Pediatric Orthopaedics, Children's Hospital and Regional Medical Center, Seattle, Washington
Fractures, Ankle and Foot

Alan R. Spitzer, M.D.
Professor of Pediatrics, State University of New York at Stony Brook; Chief, Division of Neonatology, University Hospital at Stony Brook, Stony Brook, New York
Sudden Infant Death Syndrome (SIDS)

Janet E. Squires, M.D.
Associate Professor of Pediatrics, University of Texas Southwestern Medical Center; Director, General Academic Pediatrics, Children's Medical Center of Dallas, Dallas, Texas
Lice
Tetanus

Carl L. Stanitski, M.D.
Professor, Orthopaedic Surgery, Medical University of South Carolina; Children's Hospital, Medical University of South Carolina, Charleston, South Carolina
Sports Injuries, Knee, Acute

Charles A. Stanley, M.D.
Professor of Pediatrics, University of Pennsylvania School of Medicine; Senior Endocrinologist, Children's Hospital of Philadelphia, Philadelphia, Pennsylvania
Hypoglycemia

F. Bruder Stapleton, M.D.
Ford/Morgan Professor and Chair, Department of Pediatrics, University of Washington; Pediatrician-in-Chief, Children's Hospital and Regional Medical Center, Seattle, Washington
Hypercalciuria and Renal Stones

Barbara W. Stechenberg, M.D.
Professor of Pediatrics, Tufts University School of Medicine, Boston, Massachusetts; Vice Chairman, Department of Pediatrics, Director, Pediatric Infectious Diseases, Baystate Medical Center Children's Hospital, Springfield, Massachusetts
Diphtheria

Leonard D. Stein, M.D.
Professor of Pediatrics, University of North Carolina at Chapel Hill; Chief, Pediatric Rheumatology and Immunology, University of North Carolina Hospitals, Chapel Hill, North Carolina
Henoch-Schönlein Purpura (HSP)

Ronald J. Steingard, M.D.
Associate Professor of Psychiatry, Harvard Medical School, Boston, Massachusetts; Acting Chairman, Director, Child and Adolescent Psychiatry, The Cambridge Hospital, Cambridge, Massachusetts
Depression

James A. Stockman III, M.D.
President, American Board of Pediatrics, Chapel Hill, North Carolina
Anemia of Chronic Disease
Hyperlipidemia
Idiopathic Thrombocytopenic Purpura
Neuroblastoma

Alan D. Strickland, M.D., DChem
Researcher, The Dow Chemical Company, Lake Jackson, Texas
Amebiasis

Dennis M. Styne, M.D.
Professor and Section Chief, Pediatric Endocrinology, University of California–Davis Medical Center, Sacramento, California
Hypopituitarism

Ciro V. Sumaya, M.D., MPHTM
Dean and Cox Endowed Chair in Medicine, School of Rural Public Health, Texas A&M University System, Health Science Center, College Station, Texas
Infectious Mononucleosis and Epstein-Barr Virus

Peter J. Sunenshine, M.D.
Resident, New York University Medical Center, New York, New York
Molluscum Contagiosum

Michael D. Sussman, M.D.
Clinical Professor Orthopedic Surgery, Oregon Health Sciences University; Director Postgraduate Education, Shriners Hospital, Portland, Oregon
Scoliosis, Adolescent Idiopathic

Sylvia S. Swilley, M.D.
Assistant Clinical Professor, University of California at Los Angeles; Attending Physician, Kaiser Permanente Hospital, Bellflower, California
Tetralogy of Fallot

Jeffrey E. Taber, M.D.
Associate Professor of Urology, Texas Tech University, El Paso, Texas
Obstructive Uropathy

Bruce Taubman, M.D.
Clinical Professor of Pediatrics, Division of Gastroenterology and Nutrition, University of Pennsylvania School of Medicine; The Children's Hospital of Philadelphia, Philadelphia, Pennsylvania; Cherry Hill Pediatric Group, Cherry Hill, New Jersey
Colic

Lesli A. Taylor, M.D.
Associate Professor of Pediatric Surgery, University of North Carolina at Chapel Hill; University of North Carolina Hospitals, Chapel Hill, North Carolina
Anal Fissure
Hemorrhoids
Intussusception
Perianal and Perirectal Fistula in Ano, Abscess

Jeffrey H. Teckman, M.D.
Assistant Professor of Pediatrics, Washington University School of Medicine; St. Louis Children's Hospital; St. Louis, Missouri
Alpha-1-Antitrypsin Deficiency

Jonathan E. Teitelbaum, M.D.
Fellow, Pediatric Gastroenterology and Nutrition, Combined Program in Pediatric Gastroenterology and Nutrition, Children's Hospital, and Massachusetts General Hospital, Boston, Massachusetts
Diarrhea, Chronic Nonspecific (CNSD) or Toddler's Diarrhea

Michael B. Tennison, M.D.
Professor of Neurology and Pediatrics, University of North Carolina at Chapel Hill, Chapel Hill, North Carolina
Cerebral Edema
Guillain-Barré Syndrome

Stuart W. Teplin, M.D.
Associate Professor of Pediatrics, University of North Carolina School of Medicine; Head, Pediatric Section, Clinical Center for the Study of Development and Learning, University of North Carolina at Chapel Hill, Chapel Hill, North Carolina
Autism

Isabelle Thomas, M.D.
Associate Professor, Dermatology, UMDNJ Medical School, Newark, New Jersey; Chief, Dermatology, EDVAMC, East Orange, New Jersey
Diaper Dermatitis

George H. Thompson, M.D.
Professor, Orthopaedic Surgery and Pediatrics, Case Western Reserve University; Director, Pediatric Orthopaedics, Rainbow Babies & Children's Hospital, Cleveland, Ohio
Metatarsus Adductus (Metatarsus Varus)

Denise M. Tompkins, BSN, MBA
Private Nursing Consultant in Pediatrics, Burns and Accident Prevention, Boston, Massachusetts
Burns, Outpatient

Antonella Tosti, M.D.
Associate Professor, Department of Dermatology, University of Bologna, Bologna, Italy
Ingrown Toenail

R. Franklin Trimm III, M.D.
Professor and Vice Chair of Pediatrics, University of South Alabama College of Medicine, Mobile, Alabama
Divorce and Child Custody

Debra A. Tristram, M.D.
Associate Clinical Professor of Pediatrics, East Carolina School of Medicine, Greenville, North Carolina
Influenza Infections

Sandy S. Tsao, M.D.
Instructor in Dermatology, Harvard Medical School; Beth Israel Deaconess Medical Center, Boston, Massachusetts
Piebaldism, Waardenburg Syndrome, and Tuberous Sclerosis
Vitiligo and Pityriasis Alba

Elaine I. Tuomanen, M.D.
Professor, University of Tennessee; Full Member and Chair, Infectious Diseases, St. Jude's Children's Research Hospital, Memphis, Tennessee
Meningitis, Bacterial

Ronald B. Turner, M.D.
Professor of Pediatrics, Medical University of South Carolina, Charleston, South Carolina
Pneumonia, Viral

Frank J. Twarog, M.D., Ph.D.
Associate Clinical Professor, Harvard Medical School; Senior Associate in Medicine (Immunology), Children's Hospital, Boston, Massachusetts
Serum Sickness

Martin H. Ulshen, M.D.
Professor of Pediatrics, Duke University Medical School, Durham, North Carolina
Abdominal Pain, Chronic: Management
Crohn Disease

David K. Urion, M.D.
Assistant Professor of Neurology, Harvard Medical School; Director, Learning Disabilities/Behavioral Neurology Program, Children's Hospital, Boston, Massachusetts
Hydrocephalus

William F. Vann, Jr, DMD, MS, Ph.D.
Demeritt Distinguished Professor of Pediatric Dentistry, University of North Carolina at Chapel Hill and University of North Carolina Hospitals, Chapel Hill, North Carolina
Bruxism

Karen S. Vargo, M.D.
Director, Adolescent Medicine, Mercy Children's Medical Center, Pittsburgh, Pennsylvania
Tinea Capitis, Corporis, Cruris, and Pedis

Elliott P. Vichinsky, M.D.
Adjunct Professor, University of California, San Francisco, School of Medicine, San Francisco, California; Director, Department of Hematology/Oncology, Children's Hospital Oakland, Oakland, California
Sickle-Cell Disease Anemia

Daniel von Allmen, M.D.
Assistant Professor of Pediatric Surgery, University of Pennsylvania School of Medicine; Attending Surgeon, Children's Hospital of Philadelphia, Philadelphia, Pennsylvania
Appendicitis
Hernia, Inguinal
Lymphagioma

Linda A. Waggoner-Fountain, M.D.
Assistant Professor of Pediatrics, Division of Infectious Diseases and General Pediatrics, University of Virginia School of Medicine and University of Virginia Health System, Charlottesville, Virginia
Epiglottitis
Tracheitis, Bacterial

Kelly M. Waicus, M.D.
Sports Medicine Fellow, University of North Carolina at Chapel Hill, Chapel Hill, North Carolina
Sports Injuries/Sprains, Ankle and Foot

Ellen R. Wald, M.D.
Professor of Pediatrics and Otolaryngology, University of Pittsburgh School of Medicine; Chief, Division of Allergy, Immunology and Infectious Diseases, Interim Chairman, Department of Pediatrics, University of Pittsburgh School of Medicine; Children's Hospital of Pittsburgh, Pittsburgh, Pennsylvania
Sinusitis

Janet L. Walker, M.D.
Associate Professor, Division of Orthopaedic Surgery, University of Kentucky College of Medicine; Attending Surgeon, Shriners Hospitals for Children, Lexington Unit, Lexington, Kentucky
Coxa Vara, Congenital

David K. Wallace, M.D.
Assistant Professor of Ophthalmology and Pediatrics, University of North Carolina at Chapel Hill, Chapel Hill, North Carolina
Glaucoma

Elaine E. L. Wang, M.D., CM, MSc
Associate Professor, Department of Pediatrics, University of Toronto; Clinical Director, Pasteur Mérieux Connaught, Toronto, Ontario, Canada
Pneumonia, Afebrile of Infancy

William C. Warner, Jr., M.D.
Associate Professor and Staff Physician, University of Tennessee, Campbell Clinic, Department of Orthopaedic Surgery, Memphis, Tennessee
Fractures, Hip (Apophysitis/ Hip Pointer), Femoral Neck and Femur

Geoffrey A. Weinberg, M.D.
Associate Professor of Pediatrics, University of Rochester School of Medicine and Dentistry; Director, Pediatric HIV Program, Children's Hospital at Strong Memorial Hospital, Rochester, New York
Histoplasmosis

Louis M. Weiss, M.D., MPH
Professor of Medicine, Division of Infectious Diseases, Professor of Pathology, Division of Tropical Medicine and Parasitology, Albert Einstein College of Medicine; Attending Physician, Weiler Hospital of Montefiore Medical Center and Bronx Municipal Hospital, Bronx, New York
Tapeworm Infestations

Martin E. Weisse, M.D.
Associate Professor and Director, Pediatric Residency Program, Department of Pediatrics, West Virginia University, Morgantown, West Virginia
Thrush, Candidal Diaper Rash, and Other Skin Infections

Brent W. Weston, M.D.
Associate Director of Pediatrics, Division of Pediatric Hematology/Oncology, University of North Carolina; Attending Physician, University of North Carolina Hospitals, Chapel Hill, North Carolina
Wiskott-Aldrich Syndrome (WAS)

William L. Weston, M.D.
Professor and Chairman, Department of Dermatology and Professor of Pediatrics, University of Colorado School of Medicine; Chief of Dermatology, University of Colorado Hospital and the Children's Hospital, Denver, Colorado
Erythema Multiforme
Stevens-Johnson Syndrome

Patience H. White, M.D.
Professor of Pediatrics and Medicine, George Washington University School of Medicine; Chief, Pediatric Rheumatology, Children's National Medical Center, Washington, D.C.
Systemic Lupus Erythematosus

J. Kenneth Whitt, Ph.D.
Professor and Director, Pediatric Psychology/Psychiatry Consultation and Liaison Programs, Departments of Psychiatry and Pediatrics, University of North Carolina School of Medicine, Chapel Hill, North Carolina
Conversion Disorder

Larry W. Williams, M.D.
Associate Professor of Pediatrics, Duke University School of Medicine; Duke University Medical Center, Durham, North Carolina
Food Allergy
Milk Protein Sensitivity

Mary L. Williams, M.D.
Adjunct Professor of Dermatology and Pediatrics, University of California, San Francisco, California
Hypopigmented Lesions
Pigmented Lesions
Vascular Lesions

Roberta G. Williams, M.D.
Department of Pediatrics, University of North Carolina at Chapel Hill, Chapel Hill, North Carolina
Atrial Septal Defect

Douglas F. Willson, M.D.
Associate Professor of Pediatrics and Anesthesia, Chief, Division of Pediatric Critical Care, University of Virginia, Charlottesville, Virginia
Smoke Inhalation and Carbon Monoxide Poisoning

John R. Wingard, M.D.
Professor of Medicine and Pediatrics, University of Florida College of Medicine; Director, Bone Marrow Transplant Program, Shands Hospital, Gainesville, Florida
Bone Marrow Transplantation: Care of the Child Post-Transplantation

Thomas E. Wiswell, M.D.
Professor of Pediatrics, Thomas Jefferson University, Philadelphia, Pennsylvania
Balanoposthitis

Jennifer U. Woelker, M.D.
Senior Resident in Pediatrics, Children's Hospital Medical Center, Cincinnati, Ohio
Marijuana Use

Lawrence C. Wolfe, M.D.
Associate Professor, Pediatrics, Tufts University School of Medicine; Division of Pediatric Hematology/ Oncology, New England Medical Center, Floating Hospital for Children, Boston, Massachusetts
G6PD Anemia
Neutropenia, Autoimmune, Congenital, and Cyclic

Mark L. Wolraich, M.D.
Professor of Pediatrics and Director of Division of Child Development of Vanderbilt University, Nashville, Tennessee
Attention Deficit/Hyperactivity Disorder

Alan D. Woolf, M.D., MPH
Associate Professor of Pediatrics, Harvard Medical School; Director, Program in Clinical Toxicology, Children's Hospital, Boston, Massachusetts
Poisoning: An Overall Approach

Robert J. Wyatt, M.D.
Professor of Pediatrics, University of Tennessee; Professor of Pediatrics, Chief, Division of Nephrology, Le Bonheur Children's Medical Center, Memphis, Tennessee
Hematuria-Proteinuria Evaluation

Robert Wyllie, M.D.
Chairman, Department of Pediatric Gastroenterology and Nutrition, Cleveland Clinic Foundation, Cleveland, Ohio
Helicobacter Pylori Infection
Ulcerative Colitis

Aida Yared, M.D.
Assistant Professor of Pediatrics, Divisions of General Pediatrics and Pediatric Nephrology, Vanderbilt University Medical Center, Nashville, Tennessee
Lactic Acidosis

William F. H. Yee, M.D.
Assistant Professor of Pediatrics, Tufts University School of Medicine; Director, Outpatient Clinics; Director, Pediatric Flexible Fibreoptic Bronchoscopy, Pulmonary and Allergy Division, Cystic Fibrosis Center, Asthma Center, The Floating Hospital for Infants and Children at the New England Medical Center, Boston, Massachusetts
Hydrocarbon Ingestion

Ram Yogev, M.D.
Professor of Pediatrics, Northwestern University Medical School; Director, Section of Pediatric and Maternal HIV Infection, Associate Division Head, Division of Infectious Diseases, Children's Memorial Hospital, Chicago, Illinois
Brain Abscess
Shunt Infections

Christopher W. Zukowski, DO, BS
Assistant Director, Primary Care Sports Medicine Fellowship, Associate Clinical Professor, Uniformed Services University, Bethesda, Maryland; Executive Officer, Sports Medicine, Naval Hospital, Keflavik, Iceland
Bites, Spider

PREFACE

Essence of Office Pediatrics was conceived by the editorial team at W.B. Saunders as a pediatric resource designed to provide—on a single page—a concise description of the essential elements of pediatric disease. We were pleased to be asked to serve as editors for this unique volume, in which the focus is outpatient presentation, evaluation, and management. Once we began working on the project, however, we realized that the interface between outpatient and inpatient management is constantly changing. As a result, the reader will find that some chapters ultimately describe strategies that traditionally have been confined to the inpatient arena.

Each subject is presented in an outline or telegraphic format, with bulleted items for essential content. The reader can then easily scan a page while standing with the open book at a convenient shelf or desk. Material is organized alphabetically by key word or phrase, making it easy to locate each topic quickly. Our intention in preparing this book is to provide clinicians with a quick update or reminder for important topics—not to present exhaustive chapters on all pediatric disorders.

We enlisted a stellar group of contributors for this book, and we are indebted to each of them not only for buying into the concept of this text but also for sharing the essence of his or her knowledge and wisdom within each page. In Chapel Hill, Dylo Mitchell organized the development of the project, and her efforts were essential. Bridget Riordan and Michele Eager also made significant contributions to the preparation of the manuscript. Finally, Judy Fletcher and Dolores Meloni provided leadership from the publisher.

JAMES A. STOCKMAN III, M.D.

JACOB A. LOHR, M.D.

CONTENTS

LIST OF ABBREVIATIONS

Symbols

~	approximately
↑	increase, elevated
↓	decrease, dropping, decline
1°	primary
2°	secondary
μg	microgram
μL	microliter
μmol	micromole
°C	degrees centigrade
°F	degrees Fahrenheit
×	for
2×	twice

A

A-A	alveolar-arterial
ABG	arterial blood gas
ABPA	allergic bronchopulmonary aspergillosis
ABVD	adriamycin, bleomycin, vinblastine, dacarbazine
ac	before eating
ACA	anti-centromere antibody
ACE	angiotensin converting enzyme
AD	attention deficit
AD/HD	attention deficit/hyperactivity disorder
ADD	attention deficit disorder
ADPKD	autosomal dominant polycystic kidney disease
AGA	antigliadin antibodies
AIDS	acquired immune deficiency syndrome
ALT	Alanine aminotransferase
AML	acute myelogenous leukemia
ANA	antinuclear antibody
ANC	absolute neutrophil count
ANCA	antineutrophil antibodies
anti-AChR	anti-acetylcholine receptor
ANUG	acute necrotizing ulcerative gingivostomatitis
AOME	acute otitis media with effusion
AP	anteroposterior
APL	acute promyelocytic leukemia
AR	allergic rhinitis
ARA	antireticulin antibodies
ARBD	alcohol related birth defects
ARDS	adult respiratory distress syndrome
ARF	acute renal failure
ARPKD	autosomal recessive polycystic kidney disease
ARV	antiretroviral
ASCUS	atypical cells of unknown significance
ASO	anti-streptolysin
AST	aspartae aminotransferase
ATR	angle of trunk rotation
AVP	arginine vasopressin

B

BAL	bronchoalveolar lavage
BCAA	branched-chain amino acids
BCKD	branched-chain alpha-ketoacid dehydrogenase
BE	barium enema
bid	twice a day
BIG	botulinum immune globulin
BLL	blood lead level
BMI	body mass index
BMT	bone marrow transplant
BP	blood pressure
BPD	bronchopulmonary dysplasia
bpm	beats per minute
BSA	body surface area
BSAP	brief small amplitude potentials
BUN	blood urea nitrogen

C

C3	complement
CALM	café-au-lait macules
CBC	complete blood count
CBT	cognitive-behavioral therapy
cc	cubic centimeter
CCHB	congenital complete heart block
CDC	Centers for Disease Control
CF	complement fixing
CHD	congenital heart defect
CHF	congestive heart failure
cm	centimeter
CMG	congenital myasthenia gravis
CMN	congenital melanocytic nevi
CMV	cytomegalo virus
CNS	central nervous system
CNSD	chronic nonspecific diarrhea
COPP	cyclophosphamide, onocvin, prednisone
CPK	creatine phosphokinase
CPR	coronary pulmonary resuscitation
CSF	cerebral spinal fluid
CT	computed tomography

D

d	day(s)
DC	direct current
DHE	dihydroergotamine
DHEAS	dehydroepiandrosterone sulfate
DIC	disseminated intravascular coagulation
div	divided

dl	deciliter
DNA	deoxyribonucleic acid
DNPH	2, 4-dinitrophenylhydrazine
DPI	dry-powdered inhaler
DR	drug resistance
DTs	delirium tremens
Dx	diagnosis
DYS-PVS	dysplastic pulmonary valve stenosis

E

EAC	external auditory canal
EACA	epsilon aminocaproic acid
EBV	Epstein-Barr virus
EC	enterocolitis
ECC	emergency contraception
ECHO	echocardiogram
EEG	electroencephalogram
EGW	external genital warts
EHK	epidermolytic hyperkeratosis
EI	erythema infectiosum
EIA	enzyme immunosorbent assay
EKG	electrocardiogram
EM	erythema multiforme
EMA	antiendomysial antibodies
EMG	electromyography
EMLA	eutectic mixture of local anesthetic
EP	erythrocyte protoporphyrin
EPO	erythropoietin
ER	emergency room
ERCP	endoscopic retrograde choangiopancreatography
ES	Ewing sarcoma
esp	especially
ESR	erythrocyte sedimentation rate
ET	epidermolytic toxins

F

FAB	French/American/British
FAS	fetal alcohol syndrome
FB	foreign body
FBN1	Fibrillin-1
FFP	fresh frozen plasma
FSGS	focal segmental glomerular selerosis
FSH	follicle stimulating hormone
ft	feet
FUO	fever of unknown origin
FWLS	fever without localizing signs
FWS	fever without a source

G

g	gram
G6PD	glucose 6 phosphate dehydrogenase
GAS	group A streptococcus
GCT	giant cell tumor
GFR	glomerular filtration rate
GH	growth hormone
GHD	growth hormone deficiency
GI	gastrointestinal

GN	glomerulonephritides
GnRH	gonadotropic-releasing hormone
GVHD	graft-versus-host disease
GYN	gynecology

H

H. flu	*Haemophilus influenzae*
HAE	hereditary angioedema
HAI	hemagglutination inhibition
HAV	hepatitis A virus
Hbc	hepatitis B core antigen
HBIG	hepatitis B immunoglobulin
Hbs	hepatitis B surface antigen
HBV	hepatitis B virus
HCG	human chorionic growth
Hct	hematocrit
HCV	hepatitis C virus
HD	Hirschsprung Disease
HD	hyperactivity disorder
HDCV	human diploid cell vaccine
HDL	high-density lipoids
HEV	hepatitis E virus
Hgb	hemoglobin
HHV	human herpes virus
HIV	human immunodeficiency virus
HMSN	hereditary motor and sensory neuropathy
HPV	human papilloma virus
HR	heart rate
hr(s)	hour(s)
HRIG	human rabies immunoglobulin
hs	at bedtime
HSES	hemorrhagic shock and encephalopathy syndrome
HSIL	high-grade squamous intraepithelia lesions
HSP	Henoch-Schönlein purpura
HSV	herpes symplex virus
Hx	history of

I

I&O	input and output
IBD	inflammatory bowel disorder
ICP	intracranial pressure
ICU	intensive care unit
IDDM	insulin dependent diabetes mellitus
IgA	immunoglobulin A
IgE	immunoglobulin E
IGF	insulinlike growth factor
IgG	immunoglobulin G
IgM	immunoglobulin M
IM	intramuscular
INSS	International Neuroblastoma Staging System
IOP	intraocular pressure
iPTH	intact parathyroid hormone
IT	immunotherapy
ITP	idiopathic thrombocytopenic purpura
IU	international unit

IUD	intrauterine device
IV	ichthyosis vulgaris
IV	intravenous
IVIG	intravenous immunoglobin

J

JN	juvenile nephronophthisis
JRA	juvenile rheumatoid arthritis

K

kcal	kilocalorie
kg	kilogram
KOH	potassium hydroxide
KTWS	Klippel-Trenaunay-Weber syndrome

L

L	liter
lb(s)	pound(s)
LCH	Langerhans-cell histiocytosis
LDH	lactate dehydrogenase
LDL	low-density lipoids
LDL-C	low-density lipoids-cholesterol
LH	luteinizing hormone
LI	lamellar ichthyosis
LOC	level of consciousness
LSIL	low-grade squamous intraepithelia lesions

M

M:F	male to female ratio
MAC	mycobacterium avium complex
MAI	mycobacterium avium-intracellulare
MALT	mucosa associated lymphoid tissue
MASS	myopia, mitral valve, aorta, skin, skeleton
max.	maximum
MBC	minimal bactericidal concentration
MCV	mean corpuscular volume
MDA	metaphysical-diaphyseal angle
MDD	major depressive disorder
MDI	metered-dose inhaler
mEq	milliequivalent
mg	milligram
MG	myasthenia gravis
MI	myocardial infarction
MIBG	meta-iodobenzylguanidine
MIC	minimal inhibitory concentration
min	minute(s)
min.	minimum
mL	milliliter
MLNS	minimal lesion nephrotic syndrome
mm	millimeter
mmHg	millimeters of mercury
MMR	measles, mumps, and rubella
mo(s)	month(s)
MOPP	mechlorethamine, onocvin, prednisone
MPGN	membranopsoliferative glomerulonephritis

MRI	magnetic resonance imaging
MSA	myositis-associated antibodies
MSUD	maple syrup urine disease
MVP	mitral valve prolapse
MWF	Monday, Wednesday, Friday

N

NAPQI	N-acetyl-para-benzoquinoneimine
NARES	nonallergic rhinitis with eosinophils
NBAS	neonatal behavioral assessment scale
NBCIE	nonbullous congenital ichthyosiform erythroderma
NCEP	National Cholesterol Education Program
NCM	neurocutaneous melanosis
NCV	nerve conduction velocities
NG	nasogastric
NIH	National Institutes of Health
NSAID	nonsteroidal anti-inflammatory drug
NTM	notuberculous mycobacterium

O

OB	obstetrics
OCD	ostechondritis dissecans
OE	otitis externa
OR	operating room
ORS	oral rehydration solutions
OSAS	obstructive sleep apnea syndrome
OSD	Osgood-Schlatter disease
OTC	over the counter

P

PAT	paroxysmal atrial tachycardia
pc	after eating
PCA	patient controlled analgesia
PCP	*Pneumocystis carinii* pneumonia
PCR	polymerase chain reaction
PDA	patent ductus arteriosus
PDD	pervasive developmental disorder
PDD-NOS	pervasive developmental disorder not otherwise specified
PEG	polyethylene glycol
PET	positron-emission tomography
PFD	personal flotation devices
PHE	phenylaloanine
PID	pelvic inflammatory disease
PIF	prolactin inhibitory factor
PIGN	post-infectious glomerulonephritis
PKA	phenylketonuria anemia
PKU	phenylketonuria
po	by mouth
PS	penicillin susceptible
PS	primary snoring
PSVT	paroxysmal supraventricular tachycardia
PTA	peritonsillar abscess
PTH	parathyroid hormone
pts	patient/s
PUVA	psoralen with ultraviolet

PVA	polyvinyl alcohol
PVS	pulmonary valve stenosis
PVS-D	domed pulmonary valve stenosis
PWS	port-wine stain

Q

q	every
qam	every morning
qd	every day
qhs	every bedtime
qid	four times a day
qOd	every other day

R

r/o	rule out
RAP	functional abdominal pain (*H. pylori* infection)
RBC	red blood cell
RBF	renal blood flow
RDW	red cell distribution width
RF	rheumatoid factor
RFFIT	rapid fluorescent focus inhibition test
RHF	rheumatic fever
RNA	ribonucleic acid
ROM	range of motion
RPA	retropharyngeal and peritonsillar abscess
RSV	respiratory syncytial virus
RSVIG	respiratory viruses immune globulin
RTA	renal tubular acidosis
Rx	medical prescription

S

S	soluble
SCD	sickle cell disease
SCFE	slipped capital femoral epiphysis
SEA	seronegative enthesopathy-arthropathy
SIADH	syndrome of inappropriate secretion of antidiuretic hormone
SIDS	sudden infant death syndrome
SIL	squamous intraepithelial lesion
SJS	Stevens-Johnson syndrome
SLE	systemic lupus erythematous
SLJD	Sinding-Larsen-Johansson disease
SMX	sulfamethoxazole
SPD	somatoform pain disorder
SPECT	single-photon-emission computed tomography
SSA	anti Ro
SSB	anti La
SSRI	selective serotonin reuptake inhibitors
SSSS	staphyloccal scalded skin syndrome
STD	sexually transmitted disease
STSS	streptococcal toxic shock syndrome

SubQ	subcutaneously
SVT	supraventricular tachycardia
SWS	Sturge-Weber syndrome
Sx	signs and symptoms

T

TAC	transient aplastic crisis
TB	tuberculosis
TBI	total body irradiation
TEN	toxic epidermal necrolysis
THC	tetrahydrocannabinol
TIBC	total iron binding capacity
tid	three times a day
TM	tympanic membrane
TMP	trimethoprim
TNMG	transient neonatal myasthenia gravis
TPN	total parenteral nutrition
TV	tibia vara
Tx	therapy

U

UA	urinalysis
UARS	upper airway resistance syndrome
UGI	upper gastrointestinal
UMCD	uremic medullary cystic kidney disease
UP	urticaria pigmentosa
UPJ	uceteropelvic junction
URI	upper respiratory infection
US	ultrasonography
UTI	urinary tract infection
UVB	ultraviolet

V

VCUG	voiding cystourethrogram
VIP	vasoactive intestinal peptide
VUR	vesicoureteral reflux
VZ	varicella zoster

W

w/	with
w/o	without
WBC	white blood cells
wk(s)	week(s)

X

XLH	x-linked hypophosphatemia
XLI	x-linked ichthyosis

Y

yr(s)	year(s)

EVALUATION

- History:
  - r/o specific etiologies (eg, lactose intolerance)
  - more specific the pain, more likely organic. Exception is functional pain modeled after specific illness (child's resolved acute illness or one experienced by individual close to child, eg, parent's symptoms of cholecystitis)
  - characteristic of functional pain: often child can be distracted
  - time of onset of functional symptoms may correlate w/some life event, ie, loss of someone important
  - time of day of symptoms may correlate w/other events, ie, leaving for school
  - relationship of pain w/eating or bowel movements and response to medications can be helpful in identifying etiology
  - evaluate psychosocial events; consider sexual abuse
- Physical examination:
  - give special attention to diagnoses raised by Hx
  - thorough examination indicates to child and family that symptom receiving serious consideration
  - review weight and height curves
  - include rectal exam to r/o abdominal mass, constipation, and perianal Crohn disease

- Tests:
  - screening—no tests mandatory; when further workup indicated: CBC, sedimentation rate, stool for ova and parasites, urinalysis
  - consider serum liver chemistries, amylase, lipase, albumin, if indicated
  - lactose breath H_2 test for lactose intolerance
  - serum *H. pylori* antibody titer for persistent or recurrent peptic symptoms
- Other studies:
  - radiologic: plain film of abdomen helpful if Hx constipation equivocal. Abdominal ultrasound for hydronephrosis, pancreatitis, gallbladder disease. Upper gastrointestinal or barium enema x rays useful when indicated for symptoms of possible alimentary tract disorder
  - endoscopic: primarily useful for suspected peptic disease or inflammatory bowel disease, biopsy test for *H. pylori*

TREATMENT

- Common specific etiologies:
  - lactose intolerance: lactose-free diet (ie, avoid milk products) +/– lactase replacement (this treatment also test for lactose intolerance)
  - constipation: stool softener (milk of magnesia, mineral oil, lactulose, sorbitol, etc.) +/– additional Tx

  - excessive sorbitol or fructose in diet: sugar-free gum, apple products or fruit juices
  - Crohn disease: anti-inflammatory agents
  - peptic disease: infrequent cause of recurrent abdominal pain in childhood—use acid blocker
  - abdominal migraine: propranolol, amitriptyline, cyproheptadine
- Functional abdominal pain:
  - r/o differential diagnoses developed from Hx and physical exam
  - reassure child and family that serious disorders have been ruled out (often does not require tests)
  - remove secondary gain
  - relaxation technique, psychological counseling, biofeedback may be indicated
  - dysfunctional family: family Tx
  - irritable bowel syndrome: fiber, low-dose antidepressant Tx used in adults w/abdominal pain
  - nonulcer dyspepsia: may respond to acid blockers despite absence of objective evidence of peptic disease

WHEN TO REFER

- Dx uncertain
- Endoscopic procedure indicated
- Parents need reassurance about absence of organic disease or unwilling to accept Dx of functional disease

BACKGROUND

- Acetaminophen most commonly used pediatric antipyretic/analgesic
- Ingestions >150 mg/kg or 7.5 g at risk for liver toxicity
- *Bimodal age distribution:* accidental ingestions in young children/self-destructive, suicidal ingestions in adolescents
- <5% of ingested dose metabolized to N-acetyl-para-benzoquinoneimine (NAPQI). NAPQI reduced by glutathione to a nontoxic metabolite. In overdose glutathione supply exhausted, NAPQI reacts w/cellular macromolecules, causing cell damage
- N-acetylcysteine acts as antidote; replenishes liver glutathione stores
- Young children possibly at lower risk of hepatotoxicity than adolescents and adults
- Single ingestions w/early presentation (<24 hrs postingestion): best prognosis
- Management more complicated/prognosis poorer w/chronic poisoning or late presentations (>24 hrs after ingestion)

CLINICAL MANIFESTATIONS

- *Early Sx* (first 24 hrs): anorexia, nausea, vomiting, malaise—nonspecific and variable; pts may be asymptomatic. Liver damage ongoing during this period; treatment w/N-acetylcysteine prevents morbidity and mortality
- Liver injury signs generally develop in 24–48 hrs
- Liver injury peaks at 72–96 hrs, followed by complete recovery in survivors
- Most often only mild liver tenderness, serum transaminase abnormalities, bilirubin elevations. Occasionally significant serum transaminase elevations, coagulopathy, acidosis, hepatorenal syndrome, hepatic encephalopathy, fulminant hepatic failure observed
- Mortality rate low

LABORATORY FEATURES

- Serum acetaminophen concentration drawn 4–24 hrs after ingestion is plotted on toxicity nomogram. Concentrations on or above the line require treatment; those below the line nontoxic
- Other laboratory tests necessary if serum acetaminophen concentration is in toxic range
- Chronic or late presentations: nomogram not valid in these circumstances
- *Serum transaminases:* first laboratory tests to be elevated in hepatic injury; require further diagnostic testing
- *Serum bilirubin:* elevated in moderate/severe poisoning
- *Coagulation times and serum glucose:* reflect degree of liver damage
- *Electrolytes, BUN, creatinine, pH:* variable abnormalities reflect extent of other organ damaged 2° to hepatotoxicity

DIFFERENTIAL DIAGNOSIS

- *Viral hepatitis:* A, B, C, delta, non-A non-B, herpes, Epstein-Barr, other exotics
- *Idiopathic syndromes:* acute fatty liver of pregnancy, Wilson disease, Reye, Budd-Chiari
- *Metabolic derangements:* hyperthermia, hypoperfusion syndromes (shock liver)
- *Drugs and chemicals:* isoniazid, steroid hormones, valproic acid, carbon tetrachloride, many others
- *Food poisoning:* mushrooms (eg, *Amanita phalloides*) and plants (eg, Pyrrolizidine alkaloid containing such as comfrey)
- *Chronic liver disease:* chronic active hepatitis, cirrhosis (alcoholic, biliary, other), tumors

TREATMENT

- If serum acetaminophen concentration below toxicity nomogram line, only treatment is avoidance of acetaminophen-containing products for 24 hrs
- Oral activated charcoal adsorbs acetaminophen in the GI tract; should be administered within 2 hrs of ingestion at a dose of 1–2 g/kg orally (avoid use of cathartics in children <2 yrs of age
- N-acetylcysteine administered orally as a dilute solution at 140 mg/kg, followed by 70 mg/kg q4h for an *additional* 17 doses
- Potent antiemetics such as ondansetron may be necessary when administering N-acetylcysteine
- IV N-acetylcysteine may be preferable to oral administration in certain cases, and only in consultation w/medical toxicologist or Poison Center
- Specific treatment warranted for severe liver injury
- Poison prevention counseling for parents of younger pts; psychiatric consultation for older pts may be necessary

SPECIAL SITUATIONS

- *Late presentations* (> 24 hrs after acute overdose): measurable serum acetaminophen concentration/evidence of serum transaminase elevation requires N-acetylcysteine treatment, and close monitoring of hepatic function
- *Chronic acetaminophen ingestions:* nomogram not useful in these settings. Evaluation directed at assessing potential for/evidence of liver damage. Treatment involves N-acetylcysteine administration based on multiple evaluations; course of treatment may be prolonged
- Chronic ingestion of alcohol and certain drugs can increase risk of liver injury
- Prolonged fast (> 24 hrs)/poor nutritional state increases risk of liver injury

WHEN TO REFER

- When IV N-acetylcysteine considered
- *Pregnancy:* acetaminophen overdoses in toxic range may harm fetus; IV N-acetylcysteine may be beneficial
- *Hepatic failure:* IV N-acetylcysteine/other therapies may be beneficial
- Liver transplantation has been successful after acetaminophen-induced hepatic failure

ACHONDROPLASIA

CYNTHIA M. POWELL

BACKGROUND

- Most common form of disproportionate short stature
- *Incidence:* 1/26,000–38,000 births
- Usually diagnosed in infancy; prenatal Dx possible by ultrasound at 20+ wks gestation/molecular testing and chorionic villus sampling
- Dx based on physical/radiographic findings
- Autosomal dominant w/75% representing new mutations (neither parent affected)
- Caused by mutation in fibroblast growth factor receptor 3 (FGFR3) gene on short arm of chromosome 4

CLINICAL MANIFESTATIONS

- Rhizomelic (proximal segment) shortening of long bones; redundant skin over proximal segments
- Increased upper to lower segment ratio
- Inability to fully extend at elbow
- Trident hand deformity (inability to approximate, in extension, the tips of fingers, particularly third and fourth)
- Macrocephaly, prominent forehead, depressed nasal bridge, midface hypoplasia w/dental crowding, relative mandibular prognathism
- Infantile hypotonia, persistent joint hypermobility, delayed gross motor milestones
- Normal intelligence
- Average adult height 4 ft

RADIOGRAPHIC FEATURES

- Rhizomelic shortening of long bones
- Radiolucency of proximal femur during infancy
- Decrease in interpedicular distance from upper to lower lumbar spine
- Small and narrow sacrosciatic notch due to hypoplasia of basilar portion of ilia
- Small foramen magnum, megalencephaly, dilated ventricles, occasional hydrocephalus

DIFFERENTIAL DIAGNOSIS

- Other types of short-limbed dwarfism including cartilage-hair hypoplasia, rhizomelic chondrodysplasia punctata, hypochondroplasia, achondrogenesis, hypochondrogenesis, thanatophoric dysplasia
- Important to differentiate due to different natural Hx, genetic causation, risk of recurrence, associated complications
- Most of these conditions easily distinguished w/good radiographic studies

TREATMENT

- No curative treatment
- Monitor and treat complications
- Sleep apnea study in newborn period
- Head support until good head control, which may take several mos
- For infants, avoid soft seats w/o good back support and unsupported sitting until adequate neck and truncal muscle strength
- Monitor hearing and speech development
- Use growth charts appropriate for achondroplasia
- Follow recommendations of American Academy of Pediatrics, Health Supervision for Children with Achondroplasia
- Limb-lengthening procedures experimental
- Referral to support groups such as Little People of America

COMPLICATIONS

- Sudden infant death, apnea (uncommon, but higher than in general population)
- Spinal cord compression at foramen magnum (uncommon)
- Frequent episodes of otitis media (common)
- *Hearing loss:* conductive (common), sensorineural (uncommon)
- Hydrocephalus (uncommon)
- Thoracolumbar gibbus deformity (common in infancy, usually self-correcting, rarely persists)
- Lumbar lordosis (common in older children and adults)
- Spinal stenosis (rare in children, common in adults)
- Obesity (common in older children, adolescents and adults)
- Bowing of legs due to greater longitudinal growth of fibula than tibia (common)
- Hip flexion contractures (common)

WHEN TO REFER

- Refer to geneticist for confirmation of Dx, genetic counseling for parents, long-term management coordination
- Refer to pediatric pulmonary specialist if abnormal sleep study
- Refer to pediatric neurologist or neurosurgeon for evaluation if suspected hydrocephalus or for extreme hypotonia, or other abnormal neurologic signs
- Refer to pediatric orthopedist familiar w/skeletal dysplasias to manage orthopedic complications

REFERENCE

1. Committee on Genetics, American Academy of Pediatrics: Health supervision for children with achondroplasia. Pediatrics 95:443–451, 1995.

ACNE VULGARIS

BERNARD A. COHEN

BACKGROUND

- 25% physician visits for skin disease in US
- Prevalence approaches 100% in teenagers
- First lesions appear at age 11 in boys, 9–10 in girls
- Severe cystic acne peak prevalence in 18–34 yr olds, 0.2% girls, 1% boys
- Activity abates in late teens, but 10% 25–34 yr olds, 2–3% 44 yr olds still w/lesions
- *Risk factors:* 1° relative w/severe disease, XYY genotype, hyperandrogenism (eg, polycystic ovaries, adrenal dysfunction), whites > blacks, Asians

CLINICAL MANIFESTATIONS

- *Comedonal acne:* open comedones (black heads), closed comedones (white heads)
- *Inflammatory acne:* red papules, pustules, cysts, nodules
- *Scarring:* pitting atrophy, postinflammatory hyper/hypopigmentation, cysts, sinus tracts
- *Most common sites:* midface, "V" of chest, upper back, shoulders
- *Acne fulminans:* sudden onset of painful nodulocystic lesions, fever, chills, arthralgias
- *Neonatal and infantile acne:* comedonal/mild inflammatory acne in 20% newborns, infants; self-limiting
- *Acne excoriée:* excoriated, crusted lesions usually in teenage girls (obsessive compulsive disorder)
- *Pomade acne:* comedones at periphery of scalp in pts who use oil-based products in hair

LABORATORY FEATURES

- Usually normal
- *In rare systemic variants:* increased WBC and acute-phase reactants
- In women w/severe disease, androgens (testosterone, DHEAS) may be elevated
- Pelvic ultrasound in women w/severe disease to exclude polycystic ovaries
- *Acne, other signs of hyperandrogenism:* search for congenital adrenal hyperplasia, ovarian tumors, adrenal tumors, Cushing disease

DIFFERENTIAL DIAGNOSIS

- *Acneform rashes:* induced by systemic/topical steroids, anticonvulsants, isoniazid, lithium, vitamin B_{12}; lesions often widespread
- *Radiation-induced acne* at site of administration
- *Folliculitis:* bacterial, candida, pityrosporum, dermatophyte; red papules, pustules, no comedones
- *Acne rosacea:* no comedones; papules, pustules, cysts, erythema, telangiectasias

TREATMENT

- Comedonal acne:
  - tretinoin cream 0.025% or gel 0.01% qhs 10–14 d, increase to qhs as tolerated
  - may add benzoyl peroxide gel 2.5% or 5% am
  - may increase concentration of above products as tolerated
  - may add azeleic acid qd–bid
- Moderate inflammatory acne:
  - as for comedonal acne, but when necessary
  - add topical clindamycin, tetracycline, or erythromycin qd–bid or
  - add tetracycline or erythromycin 500 mg po bid
- Severe inflammatory acne:
  - as for comedonal/moderate acne above
  - consider: oral antibiotics change to tetracycline or erythromycin 500 mg tid, erythromycin 333 tid, minocycline 50–100 mg bid
  - intralesional steroids for cysts
  - 13-cis retinoid acid 1 mg/kg/d × 20 wks (exclude pregnancy) for severe, recalcitrant nodulocystic disease

COMPLICATIONS

- Scarring
- Uncommon reactions to medications used for treatment (dental staining even in teens, blue pigmentation w/oral tetracyclines even in puberty, pseudotumor cerebri w/oral tetracycline and 13-cis retinoic acid)
- Psychosocial

WHEN TO REFER

- Most pts can be managed w/o referral
- Pts w/comedonal or moderate inflammatory acne who do not respond to standard treatment within 3–4 mos
- Pts w/severe nodulocystic acne, scarring, or systemic variants

BACKGROUND

- HIV infection causes progressive immune dysfunction leading to AIDS
- Transmitted in utero, peripartum, breast feeding, sexual contact, contaminated needles
- Untreated, 30% have AIDS by age 18–24 mos; others progress gradually during childhood

CLINICAL MANIFESTATIONS

Acute retroviral syndrome

- Occurs in 30–90% of new adolescent/adult infections; resolves after 2 wks
- *Commonly:* fever, myalgia, sore throat, lymphadenopathy, rash
- *Less commonly:* headache, diarrhea, oral ulcers, neurologic manifestations

Mild and moderate disease progression

- Generalized lymphadenopathy; hepatosplenomegaly
- Parotitis
- Recurrent URI
- Persistent oropharyngeal/cutaneous candidiasis
- Herpes zoster
- Failure to thrive
- Diarrhea, recurrent/chronic
- Lymphoid interstitial pneumonia
- Persistent fever, night sweats

Advanced disease (AIDS)

- Serious bacterial infections, multiple
- Candidiasis, esophageal/pulmonary
- Cryptosporidiosis/isosporiasis w/diarrhea >1 mo
- CMV retinitis, gastroenteritis, hepatitis
- Mycobacterium *tuberculosis*/other species, disseminated
- Pneumocystis carinii pneumonia
- Invasive fungal infections
- *Toxoplasmosis* of the brain: onset >1 mo of age
- Developmental delay
- Malignancy: lymphoma, Kaposi sarcoma
- Organ system disorders (cardiomyopathy, nephropathy, hepatitis, myopathy, neuropathy)

LABORATORY FEATURES

- *HIV antibody:* positive antibody at age >18 mos diagnostic of HIV infection; maternal antibody lost by 18 mos
- *HIV DNA polymerase chain reaction (PCR):* positive in infected infants by age >2 mos; use for early Dx in exposed infants; two negative tests, at age >1 mo and at age >3 mos, presumptively excludes infection; confirm sero-reversion at 18 mos
- *p24 antigen:* use for Dx during acute retroviral syndrome prior to seroconversion
- *Quantitative plasma HIV RNA:* correlated w/risk of disease progression/response to Tx
- *Lymphocyte subsets:* CD4 (helper) T lymphocyte counts ↓; indicates degree of immunodeficiency (see table)
- *Immunoglobulins:* ↑; occasionally hypogammaglobulinemia
- *Chemistries:* liver enzymes often ↑
- *Hematology:* anemia, neutropenia, thrombocytopenia common w/progressive disease

DIFFERENTIAL DIAGNOSIS

- *Acute retroviral syndrome:* Epstein-Barr or cytomegalovirus mononucleosis; 1° toxoplasmosis; 2° syphilis; viral hepatitis; enterovirus, influenza, herpes simplex virus
- *Progressive HIV disease:* hypogammaglobulinemia; severe combined immunodeficiency syndrome; common variable immunodeficiency; other causes of lymphadenopathy/hepatosplenomegaly (eg, EBV, CMV, lymphoma)

TREATMENT

Antiretroviral (ARV) treatment

- Combinations of ARV drugs that fully suppress viral replication
- *Acute retroviral syndrome:* combination ARV treatment may improve prognosis
- *Established infection:* combination ARV recommended for children w/disease progression, all infected infants age <12 mos, most children w/detectable plasma HIV RNA; some experts delay Tx in children w/stable, low-plasma HIV RNA
- *Pregnant women:* offer combination ARV including oral zidovudine (ZDV) after first trimester/IV ZDV during labor
- *Exposed infants:* oral ZDV (2 mg/kg/dose qid) for first 6 wks of life
- *Postexposure prophylaxis:* treatment w/ZDV, lamivudine w/or w/o a protease inhibitor for occupational exposure; consider for nonoccupational exposure in circumstances unlikely to recur (eg, rape)

Prophylaxis for opportunistic infections

- Trimethoprim/sulfamethoxazole (TMP/SMX) to prevent pneumocystis carinii pneumonia (PCP)
- IV immunoglobulin (IVIG, monthly infusions) for recurrent bacterial infections
- Azithromycin, clarithromycin, rifabutin to prevent mycobacterium avium complex (MAC)

Immunizations

- DPT, HIB, hepatitis B per routine schedule
- OPV contraindicated; use all IPV, routine schedule
- MMR at 12 mos if no severe immunosuppression (CD4 category 3 or AIDS); second dose at 1 mo after first dose
- Influenza vaccine every yr after age 6 mos
- Pneumococcus vaccine q3y after age 2 yrs
- Hepatitis A indicated if chronic hepatitis due to HIV/other viruses
- Varicella vaccine not indicated due to insufficient safety/efficacy data

PREVENTION

- Antiretroviral treatment/obstetric intervention prevents 90% of vertical transmission
- Correct use of condoms during sexual contact; avoid sharing sharp personal objects (eg, razors, body-piercing equipment, needles), contact w/blood

WHEN TO REFER

- All children/pregnant women, regardless of disease stage, should be referred to provider w/expertise/managed collaboratively w/primary care provider ,

Immunologic categories based on age-specific CD4 T lymphocyte counts and percentage of total lymphocytes

	Age of child					
	<12 mos		1–5 yrs		6–12 yrs	
Immunologic category	cells/mm³	(%)	cells/mm³	(%)	cells/mm³	(%)
1. No evidence of immune suppression	≥1,500	(≥25)	≥1,000	(≥25)	≥500	(≥25)
2. Moderate immune suppression	750–1,499	(15–24)	500–999	(15–24)	200–499	(15–24)
3. Severe immune suppression	<750	(<15)	<500	(<15)	<200	(<15)

Adapted from Centers for Disease Control. MMWR 1994:43 (No RR-12), p. 4.

ACRODERMATITIS ENTEROPATHICA

PARIS T. MANSMANN

BACKGROUND

- Most frequently found 3 wks–8 mos
- An autosomal recessive mutation, no sexual predominance exists
- Characterized by low plasma zinc levels, dermatitis, hair loss, growth retardation, diarrhea
- Associated w/77% decrease in uptake of zinc into small intestinal biopsies
- *Recovery* >90% w/daily zinc supplement
- *Mortality:* 100% w/o treatment

CLINICAL MANIFESTATIONS

- Progressive bullous-pustular dermatitis (psoriasis-like) of extremities and oral, anal, genital areas
- General alopecia
- Paronychia
- Opthalmologic signs include blepharitis, conjunctivitis, photophobia, corneal opacities
- Chronic malabsorptive diarrhea, steatorrhea, lactose intolerance
- Neuropsychiatric signs include irritability, emotional disorders, tremor, occasional cerebellar ataxia
- Immune dysfunction w/recurrent candida albicans infections, poor wound healing, recurrent boils

LABORATORY FEATURES

- *Blood count:* usually normal; occasionally anemia of chronic disease

- *Plasma zinc levels:* <13.2 µmol/L or 86 µg/dl but more commonly <10.7 and 69.7, respectively
- *Serum zinc levels:* <9.9 µmol/L or 65 µg/dl. Be careful of the 40% diurnal variation in serum zinc levels (best obtained fasting 8–9 am)
- Poor immune function in vivo
- *Skin biopsy:* acrodermatitis enteropathica does not have diagnostic histologic pattern. Early lesions demonstrate loss of granular layer, pallor of keratinocytes, balloonlike keratinocytes w/pyknotic nuclei. Dermis demonstrates lymphocytes and occasionally neutrophils. More developed lesions demonstrate parakeratosis, epidermal hyperplasia, pallorous keratinocytes, slight spongiosis, papillary edema. Subcorneal blisters, necrotic keratinocytes may be present. Developed lesions demonstrate psoriaform hyperplasia. Only three other diseases, essential fatty acid deficiency, necrolytic migratory erythema, pellegra, commonly have pallorous keratinocytes and necrotic keratinocytes together

DIFFERENTIAL DIAGNOSIS

- Zinc-poor total parenteral nutrition (TPN)
- Protein-energy malnutrition
- Hemodialysis-induced acrodermatitis enteropathicalike syndrome
- Cystic fibrosis
- Short bowel syndrome

- Cirrhosis
- Maternal alcoholism
- Advanced HIV infection

TREATMENT

- *Oral supplementation:* infants 0.4 mg/kg/d initially then 0.5 mg/kg/d after 3 mos, monitoring for anemia and irritability. Children 5–8 yrs of age 10 mg/d. Older children 50–150 mg/d. Plasma/serum zinc levels reflect absorption even in severe illnesses
- *Parenteral supplementation:* prematures require 0.35 or 0.4 mg/kg/d IV zinc

COMPLICATIONS

- Neurologic sequelae difficult to reverse
- *Zinc toxicity:* abdominal cramps, nausea, vomiting, headaches, dizziness, chills, flushing, blurred vision, sweating. Premature infants more susceptible to toxicity (irritability, tremor, seizures, tachyarrythmias)

WHEN TO REFER

- Most pts can be managed w/o referral
- Refractory pts may require higher dose therapy
- Uncontrolled immune dysregulation may require aggressive supportive care
- Genetic counseling suggested

BACKGROUND

- Alcohol most widely used drug in US
- 80–90% teens have used alcohol
- 4.6 million teenagers (14–17) problem drinkers
- DUI: leading cause of death among 15–24 yr olds
- 8,000 deaths/45,000 injuries/yr attributed to alcohol-related DUI in adolescents; most deaths in nondependent drinkers
- Widely available/inexpensive
- Central nervous system depressant
- Intoxicating ingredient: ethanol
- Most beers/wine coolers: 5–6% alcohol/ wines: 12–13%/fortified wines: up to 20%/ distilled spirits: 50% alcohol

EFFECTS OF USE

- Used for enjoyment, escape, curiosity/ because of peer pressure
- *Low doses:* behavioral stimulant properties
- *Moderate doses:* sedation, euphoria, decreased inhibitions/impaired coordination
- *Higher doses:* ataxia, confusion, emotional liability/slurred speech
- Toxic levels: unconsciousness, anesthesia, hypoglycemia, hypothermia, respiratory failure, coma/death
- Tolerance/dependence develop over time/ may not occur until early adulthood
- *Withdrawal symptoms:* delirium tremens (DTs)/seizures, uncommon in adolescents

OTHER EFFECTS

- *Physical:* blackouts, accidents, trauma; less frequently gastritis/decreased sexual functioning
- *Social:* trouble w/school/police, dropping out of school, difficulty maintaining interpersonal relationships
- *Drug Interactions:* interferes w/seizure/ diabetes control, potentiates sedative effects of benzodiazepenes, narcotics, other drugs
- *Alcohol-Related Birth Effects:* fetal alcohol syndrome most common/preventable cause of teratogenic mental retardation. Effects include abnormal facies; cardiac, renal, genital, skeletal system abnormalities; mental retardation; small for gestation age infants; irritability/hyperactivity. Maternal alcohol use, even low doses (1–2 drinks/d), may have significant neurobehavioral effects

SCREENING

- Many screening instruments exist
- Assess risk factors: poor school performance, change in friends, family dysfunction
- CAGE questionnaire one of the simplest screening techniques:
  - have you ever felt you ought to *C*ut down on your drinking?
  - have people *A*nnoyed you by criticizing your drinking?
  - have you ever felt bad or *G*uilty about your drinking?
  - have you ever had a drink first thing in the morning to steady your nerves or to get rid of a hangover (*E*ye opener)?

  (Two or more affirmative answers prompt evaluation)
- RAFFT questionnaire: Ask the patient if they use alcohol to *R*elax, when they are *A*lone, what are *F*amily or *F*riends' use and if they have gotten into *T*rouble associated with their use of alcohol
- Quantity/frequency of alcohol consumption used as adjunct questions
- Asking about friend's use may be helpful

TREATMENT: ACUTE INTOXICATION

- Supportive therapy for respiratory system may be required w/toxic levels
- Note: "legal" limit for driving in most states 0.08%–0.10 mg%; 5–6 standard drinks (1 oz distilled spirits = 6 oz wine = 12 oz beer = 12 oz wine cooler) over 1–2 hrs raises blood alcohol level to 0.10 mg% or greater in most teens; 5–6 hrs for blood alcohol level to return to zero

BACKGROUND

- Rare < age 2, increasing incidence thereafter
- Often strong family Hx allergic disease
- Often occurs w/other allergic disorders, including asthma, eczema, allergic conjunctivitis
- Does not respond to antibiotics
- May occur w/distinct seasons or perennially
- May serve to worsen asthma, risk factor for sinusitis
- Little to no mortality, substantial morbidity in terms school absence, lost work productivity, quality of life measures

CLINICAL MANIFESTATIONS

- Sneezing
- Nasal congestion
- Clear rhinnorhea
- May have cough, esp at night
- May have associated snoring, upper respiratory symptoms
- Physical findings may include Dennie's lines (ridge across the bridge of the nose), allergic conjunctivitis, bluish boggy turbinates

LABORATORY/DIAGNOSTIC FEATURES

- Positive epicutaneous skin tests or IgE rast tests to relevant allergens:
  - indoor allergens (esp w/perennial symptoms): dust mites, cockroach, dog, cat, rodents, molds, occupational exposures
  - outdoor allergens: trees in spring, grasses in summer, weeds/molds in fall. Flowering plants requiring insect pollination do not cause symptoms
  - food allergens: almost never occult cause of allergic rhinitis
- Blood tests (rarely needed) consistent w/allergic rhinitis: increased eosinophils, increased total IgE
- Eosinophils on nasal smear (Wright stain) very supportive of allergic rhinitis Dx
- Sinus radiographs useful to r/o sinusitis in cases of refractory disease

DIFFERENTIAL DIAGNOSIS

- Viral URI
- Chronic functional/anatomic nasal congestion (esp infants)
- Sinusitis
- Vasomotor rhinitis
- Nonallergic rhinitis w/eosinophils (NARES)
- Deviation of nasal septum
- Photic sneezing (rare: sneezing response to sudden visual light exposure)
- Rhinitis medicamentosa (due to decongestant overuse)
- Illicit drug abuse

TREATMENT

- Primary treatment:
  - avoidance of relevant allergens, esp indoor pets; shifting activities to the pm hrs (pollen counts higher in am); air conditioning may be useful
  - anti-inflammatory treatment includes topical treatment w/corticosteroids and cromolyn sodium nasal sprays. Cromolyn usually requires tid/qid dosing. Nasal steroids include beclomethasone, flunisoloide, triamcinolone, fluticasone and budesonide. In vitro data suggest latter two steroids more potent w/less systemic absorption
  - allergen immunotherapy ("allergy shots") effective in controlling or eliminating symptoms allergic rhinitis and need for other medications; allergens given in IT preparations should be relevant as determined by *both* assessment of IgE reactivity to the allergen (skin tests or IgE RAST tests) and exposure Hx; relative contraindications for IT include poorly controlled asthma; risks include respiratory reactions (rarely severe); IT should not be given as unsupervised home shots
- Adjunctive treatment:
  - antihistamines: useful for symptom relief, used episodically or chronically. May be adequate for mild disease w/o primary treatment
  - chronic use of nonsedating antihistamines may be needed for more persistent symptoms
  - decongestants: useful for congestive side effects; should not be overused. Topical decongestants associated w/rhinitis medicamentosa, typically w/>3d continuous use
  - topical anticholinergic treatment: ipratropium bromide applied as 2 sprays up to 3×/d
  - treatment of associated allergic conjunctivitis may be useful w/topical decongestants/antihistamines and nonsteroidal anti-inflammatory eye drops

BACKGROUND

- Occurs in children, adolescents; peak incidence at 4–5 yrs
- Family Hx in small percentage pts
- May be associated w/autoimmune thyroid disease and vitiligo
- Self-limited disorder, can recur. May progress to widespread/complete hair loss

CLINICAL MANIFESTATIONS

- One/several completely smooth, bald patches
- *Most common location:* scalp
- *Less common locations:* eyebrow, eyelash, body hair
- Sudden onset—either overnight or over several days
- Rarely progresses to alopecia totalis or alopecia universalis
- Occasional pitting of fingernails

DIFFERENTIAL DIAGNOSIS

- *Tinea capitis:* characterized by scaling in scalp and "black dot" hairs
- *Trichotillomania:* numerous broken hairs in limited area of scalp or eyebrows, Hx pulling hair usually present
- *Traction alopecia:* related to hairstyles w/tight braiding
- *Aplasia cutis congenita:* area of atrophy and hair loss present from birth

TREATMENT

- *Topical and intralesional corticosteroids:* topical corticosteroids preferred in younger children due to pain associated w/intralesional injection
- Dosage:
  - topical: triamcinolone 0.1% or fluocinonide 0.05%, cream or ointment daily
  - intralesional: triamcinolone acetonide suspension (2–4 mg/mL initially) w/maximum 10 mg/mL (no more than 1–2 mL), at 4–6 wk intervals
- Alternative therapies:
  - topical anthralin cream
  - photochemotherapy (Psoralen and Ultraviolet A)

WHEN TO REFER

- Refer children w/large areas of involvement or w/small lesions that do not respond to a brief course of topical corticosteroids

BACKGROUND

- Alpha-1-AT
  - inhibitor of neutrophil elastase
  - acute-phase reactant (plasma concentration increases 3- to 5-fold during host response to inflammation/tissue injury)
  - plasma protein predominantly derived from the liver
- > 75 variants of alpha-1-AT gene. Most variants associated w/alpha-1-AT plasma levels/elastase inhibitory capacity within normal limits ("normal variants")
- Each variant inherited as autosomal codominant
- Variants defined by isoelectric focusing; each variant assigned Pi type (protease inhibitor type)
- Most common normal variant PiM, found 95–98% US population
- Most common deficiency variant PiZ. Homozygous PiZZ alpha-1-AT deficiency affects 1/1,600–1,800 live births. Other deficiency variants rare
- Alpha-1-AT deficiency associated w/85–90% reduction in plasma levels: The most common genetic cause of liver disease in children
- Liver disease affects 10–15% of PiZZ individuals
- The most common genetic cause of emphysema
- Incidence of emphysema among PiZZ individuals unknown but believed to be significantly higher than that of liver disease
- Cigarette smoking increases severity/rate of progression of emphysema > thousandfold
- Controversy whether heterozygotes (PiMZ) develop liver disease/emphysema

CLINICAL MANIFESTATIONS

- Usually presents in infancy w/jaundice, liver enlargement; occasionally cholestasis (particularly pruritus), portal hypertension (edema, ascites, GI bleeding from varices)
- Some small for gestational age; others grow poorly despite born appropriate for gestational age
- Older children: liver enlargement/elevated transaminases on routine exam, portal hypertension w/or w/o severe liver dysfunction

Adolescents: portal hypertension and/or severe liver dysfunction including edema, ascites, spontaneous bacterial peritonitis, GI bleeding, malnutrition, hepatosplenomegaly, hypersplenism

Lung disease/emphysema not manifested until third/fourth decade

LABORATORY FEATURES

- Serum alpha-1-AT level 10–15% of normal
- Pi type ZZ
- Serum transaminases: ~100–300 units/mL
- Serum bilirubin: ~3–5 mg/100 mL (90% conjugated)
- If cholestasis, serum alkaline phosphatase/serum cholestrol ↑
- If liver synthetic dysfunction, serum albumin ↓/prothrombin time ↑
- If chronic GI bleeding, iron-deficiency anemia present
- If hypersplenism, total leukocyte count may ↓ to 3,000–4,000, absolute neutrophil count ↓ to 800–1,600, platelet count ↓ to 20,000–50,000

LIVER HISTOLOGIC FEATURES

- Periodic acid-Schiff-positive, diastase-resistant globules in liver cells
- Cholestasis
- Hepatocellular necrosis/inflammatory cell infiltrate
- Periportal fibrosis/cirrhosis

DIFFERENTIAL DIAGNOSIS

- Infant:
  - biliary atresia
  - choledochal cyst
  - hypothyroidism
  - hypopituitarism
  - sepsis
  - shock
  - congenital infection
  - galactosemia
  - tyrosinemia
  - peroxisomal defects
  - Alagilles syndrome
  - idiopathic "giant cell" neonatal hepatitis

- Older child/adolescent:
  - Wilson disease
  - autoimmune hepatitis
  - drug-induced hepatitis
  - sclerosing cholangitis
  - infectious hepatitis

TREATMENT

- *Avoidance of cigarette smoking:* reduces emphysema risk thousandfold
- *Protein replacement therapy:* not useful in liver disease; used in adults w/established emphysema but little evidence for clinical efficacy
- *Splenorenal shunt:* considered in those w/mild parenchymal liver injury but severe portal hypertension
- *Orthotopic liver transplantation:* excellent results; 90% 1 yr survival/80% 5 yr survival; progression of the liver disease often slow in some affected children who lead relatively normal lives so liver transplantation may not be necessary for years

GENETIC COUNSELING

- Prenatal diagnostic testing using molecular techniques available
- Routine amniocentesis for prenatal diagnosis not always indicated:
  - no evidence that heterozygote is at risk
  - risk of homozygous infant: 1/4
  - risk of liver disease in infant affected ~1/10
  - risk of emphysema decreases dramatically w/avoidance smoking
- Not clear if liver disease/lung disease phenotype breed true in affected families

WHEN TO REFER

- All pts should be seen at least initially by pediatric gastroenterologist. Some will require close/frequent follow-up

BACKGROUND

- Amblyopia ("lazy eye") defined as decreased vision resulting from abnormal visual stimulation during visual development; changes in lateral geniculate nucleus/striate cortex result
- *Incidence:* 2–5% of population
- Risk factors include prematurity, family Hx amblyopia
- Children at risk birth–age 7–8 yrs
- Generally reversible w/patching during this period; becomes permanent after visual development complete
- Dense amblyopia in first 2–3 mos of life left untreated may result in permanent visual loss
- Photoscreeners increasingly accurate in detection of anisometropia, strabismus

ETIOLOGY AND MANIFESTATIONS

- *Anisometropia* (large difference in refractive error of two eyes): eye w/most uncorrected refractive error suppressed, becomes amblyopic; no presenting complaints; found on routine screening exams
- *Strabismus:* eyes not used together; one eye becomes preferred eye and other eye not used becomes amblyopic
- *Visual deprivation:* retina receives blurred/decreased image due to high refractive error, media opacity (such as cataract), occlusion (patching, ptosis, etc). Vision does not return to normal even when obstacle to good vision removed

TREATMENT

- Allow retina to receive clear well-focused image
- If glasses indicated wear at all times
- Media opacity should be treated (cataract removed)
- Young children usually rapidly improve
- In older children (5–8 yrs), longer patching regimens (many months) required
- Continued until the vision equal in both eyes
- Child w/Hx amblyopia at risk for recurrence until visual maturity
- In some situations, penalization of good eye accomplished by atropine drops or spectacle blur
- Surgery generally deferred until amblyopia treated

PREVENTION AND WHEN TO REFER

- Any child whose care providers notice eye wandering/abnormal appearance of one/both eyes should have ophthalmologic evaluation as soon as possible
- Child w/family Hx strabismus/amblyopia/who was premature should be referred for ophthalmologic evaluation by at least 3. The younger the child, the better treatment success
- All children should have reliable visual screening w/each eye covered by age 4–5 (as early as possible); any decreased vision/difference between eyes: refer for ophthalmologic evaluation
- Any child who has suffered eye injury, undergone any patching for eye injury: screen for visual acuity after treatment or refer for ophthalmologic evaluation as appropriate

ALAN D. STRICKLAND

BACKGROUND

• 10% worldwide infected; <5% US, >75% parts of Southeast Asia
• *Peak incidence:* 2–3 yrs of age/> 40 yrs of age
• Infection passed through fecal-oral route; only mammals infected
• Cysts/trophozoites found in colon; invasive intestinal amebiasis when trophozoites invade colonic wall
• Extraintestinal invasive disease when trophozoites penetrate colonic wall, enter bloodstream, migrate to liver; amebic liver abscess usually first extraintestinal site of amebic involvement
• From liver, ameba may infect pericardium, cerebrum, pleura, lung, abdominal cavity, bladder via hematogenous spread/direct invasion

CLINICAL MANIFESTATIONS

• *Noninvasive intestinal amebic infestation:* asymptomatic; found during stool parasitic examinations for other organisms
• *Intestinal amebiasis:* symptomatic when invades bowel wall; invasive trophozoites cause painful diarrhea w/blood/mucus; <50% w/invasive amebiasis associated w/fever. Proctoscopy: 1–10 mm friable ulcerations filled w/mucus/active trophozoites; mucosa between ulcers normal
• *Extraintestinal amebiasis in children:* hepatic abscess w/high fever, abdominal distention, irritability, tachypnea but little pain (unlike adults). Amebic hepatic abscess usually solitary mass. Organisms found only in wall of abscess; fluid sterile on culture. Abscesses increase in size quickly; pts deteriorate within days
• Hepatic amebic abscess may lead to pulmonary, pleural, pericardial amebiasis. Any combination of these may present w/no additional symptoms beyond those of hepatic disease or may cause increased tachypnea. Pts w/cerebral amebiasis usually so ill from hepatic infection that no neurologic symptoms can be attributed solely to cerebral abscesses

LABORATORY FEATURES

• Amebic cysts/trophozoites found in 60% if three stools examined after fixation in polyvinyl alcohol (PVA); proctoscopy (see above)
• Multiple serologic tests available; most diagnose >90% extraintestinal amebiasis, but <50% if disease limited to intestine

DIFFERENTIAL DIAGNOSIS

• *Invasive intestinal amebiasis:* inflammatory bowel diseases such as ulcerative colitis, Crohn disease, bacillary dysentery, tuberculous colitis, eosinophilic gastroenteritis
• *Invasive hepatic amebiasis:* hepatic bacterial abscesses, hepatic tumors, hepatic failure from viral/metabolic causes

TREATMENT

• *Intraluminal intestinal amebiasis:* either diloxanide furoate 20 mg/kg/d in 3 doses × 10 d (call CDC at 404-639-3670/after hours 404-639-2888) or paromomycin 25–30 mg/kg/d in 3 doses × 7 d (not available in US). More dangerous drug is iodoquinol 30–40 mg/kg/d in 3 doses × 20 d. Antibiotics (tetracycline/oral aminoglycosides) may help but usually not needed
• *Invasive amebiasis* (intestine, liver, other organs): metronidazole 35–50 mg/kg/d in 3 doses × 10 d followed by diloxanide furoate 20 mg/kg/d in 3 doses × 10 days for intestinal therapy. Alternative to metronidazole: dehydroemetine 1–1.5 mg/kg/d (max. dose 90 mg/d) in 2 IM doses/d × 5 d (obtain from CDC at above telephone number). Dehydroemetine should be followed by 2–3 wks treatment w/oral chloroquine phosphate 10 mg base/kg/d (max. dose 300 mg base) or diloxanide furoate. Extraintestinal invasive amebiasis may also be treated by tinidazole 50 mg/kg/d (max. dose 2,000 mg) in one daily dose × 5 d followed by an intraluminal agent (drug not available in US)

COMPLICATIONS

• Bowel perforation (in 30% of deaths), hepatic abscess rupture (in 40% of deaths) w/resultant peritonitis or pleural fluid
• Bacterial superinfection (in 10% of deaths), esp after needle aspiration hepatic abscesses
• Fistula formation
• Arterial erosion w/massive hemorrhage (usually into intestine)

PREVENTION

• Good sanitation procedures. Chlorination of drinking water/waste water

WHEN TO REFER

• Every pt w/amebic infection outside the bowel/liver should be referred to center where infectious disease specialist and surgeon available. Any pt w/invasive diseases who does not become afebrile within 1–2 d on metronidazole should be referred to tertiary center

BACKGROUND

- Primary amenorrhea usually defined as absence of menses by age 16
- Incidence ~1%
- Onset of menses should be correlated w/pubic hair/breast development (commences by age 14 in most girls)
- Girls w/serious chronic illness or involved in competitive sports (such as gymnastics/track) may have delayed menses

PERTINENT HISTORY

- Age at start of pubertal development
- Growth progression from annual growth charts
- Previous/current medications, irradiation, surgery, chemotherapy
- Family Hx including age of menarche/fertility of mother, sisters, other female relatives; heights of immediate family members; Hx endocrine disorders; Hx autoimmune disorders; Hx ovarian malignancy
- Review of systems focusing on past/current weight changes, eating/exercise habits, substance abuse, emotional stressors, travel, competitive sports participation, hirsutism, abdominal pain, bowel habits, headaches, other neurologic symptoms including sense of smell
- Sexual activity, sexual abuse
- Perinatal Hx including birth weight, neonatal course, lymphedema, other congenital anomalies, maternal ingestion of hormones

PHYSICAL EXAMINATION

- Height/weight on growth chart
- Blood pressure
- Fundoscopic examination
- Assessment of olfaction
- Palpation of thyroid
- Tanner staging of breast development, assessment for galactorrhea
- Cardiac examination
- Abdominal examination
- Tanner staging of genitalia, thorough examination for anomalies, clitoromegaly, estrogenization, hymenal configuration
- Recto abdominal examination in virginal girls to palpate uterus/cervix
- Pelvic examination in sexually active girls
- Assessment for hirsutism, facial anomalies, body habitus
- *Thorough* neurologic examination including visual fields

LABORATORY STUDIES

- For all patients to assess for evidence of chronic illness:
  - CBC
  - erythrocyte sedimentation rate
  - electrolytes, BUN, creatinine
  - liver function tests
  - urinalysis
- Normal breast development and uterus present:
  - pregnancy test
  - prolactin level: high in pituitary adenoma, hypothyroidism
  - TSH/free T4: abnormal w/hyper/hypothyroidism
  - luteinizing hormone/follicle stimulating hormone (LH/FSH): elevated w/premature ovarian failure, low in hypothalamic/pituitary abnormalities
  - MRI if vaginal outflow tract abnormal
- No breast development but presence of uterus:
  - LH/FSH: low/normal in hypoganadotropic hypogonadism; high in hypergonadotropic hypogonadism
  - karyotype (if LH/FSH high): XO—gonadal dysgenesis (Turner syndrome); XY—Swyer syndrome; XX—need to refer for ACTH stimulation test (normal in premature ovarian failure/resistant ovary syndrome, abnormal in adrenal enzyme deficiency, hermaphroditism)
- Breast development but no uterus:
  - total testosterone: female levels indicate Muellerian dygenesis; male levels w/XY karyotype indicate testicular feminization

DIFFERENTIAL DIAGNOSIS

- Chronic disease (Crohn disease, cystic fibrosis, diabetes, sickle-cell anemia, systemic lupus erythematosus, renal failure)
- Hypothalamic disease or tumor
- Pituitary tumor
- Hypopituitarism
- Kallman syndrome
- Laurence-Moon-Biedl syndrome
- Thyroid disease
- Cushing syndrome
- Hermaphroditism
- Hypergonadotropic hypogonadism (Turner syndrome, Turner syndrome mosaic, structural anomaly one X chromosome, gonadal dysgenesis, resistant ovary syndrome, 17-alpha hydroxylase deficiency, autoimmune ovarian failure, premature menopause, ovarian failure 2° to chemotherapy/radiation, Swyer syndrome)
- Hypogonadotropic hypogonadism (athletic amenorrhea, eating disorders, medications (phenothiazines, amitriptyline, benzodiazepines, haloperidol, cimetidine, reserpine, prostaglandins, methyldopa, metoclopramide), stress
- Genital anomalies (imperforate hymen, vaginal septum, Mayer-Rokitansky-Kuster-Hauser syndrome)

TREATMENT

- Treatment based on etiology
- Optimal treatment may induce puberty/subsequent menstruation
- Estrogen replacement therapy warranted in girls w/ovarian dysgenesis, ovarian failure, Kallman syndrome, athletic amenorrhea, anorexia nervosa; will induce development of secondary sexual characteristics, produce cyclic vaginal bleeding, prevent osteoporosis. After initial estrogen replacement, cyclic estrogen/progestin therapy should be instituted

WHEN TO REFER

- Pts need referral to pediatric specialist based on etiology of primary amenorrhea for treatment of underlying disorder
- Pts who require neuroendocrine testing, have growth delay, have Turner syndrome or a variant warrant referral to pediatric endocrinologist for initial assessment/treatment

AMENORRHEA, SECONDARY

ELIZABETH M. ALDERMAN

BACKGROUND

- Defined by absence of menses for 3 mos after menarche has occurred w/regular menstrual cycles
- Many conditions that cause secondary amenorrhea also cause primary amenorrhea, irregular menses/oligomenorrhea
- Amenorrhea/oligomenorrhea may be normal in a girl within 2 yrs of menarche
- R/O pregnancy, most common cause of secondary amenorrhea

PERTINENT HISTORY

- Age of menarche
- Last menstrual period
- Characteristics of previous menstrual cycles (frequency, duration, dysmenorrhea)
- Sexual activity, contraception methods, recent pregnancy
- Recent Hx travel, stress, weight loss/gain, medications
- Participation in strenuous athletics
- Hx chronic illness
- Review of systems including headache, galactorrhea, hirsutism, acne, visual disturbances, change in voice/libido

PHYSICAL EXAMINATION

- Access weight/height
- Vital signs: pulse and blood pressure
- Dermatologic examination for acne, hirsutism
- Head/neck examination, visual fields, thyroid palpation, acanthosis nigrans
- Breast exam for galactorrhea
- Abdominal exam
- Gynecologic exam, assessment for pregnancy, clitoromegaly, ovarian cysts, virilization
- Pelvic examination to assess for pregnancy

LABORATORY STUDIES

- Initial study:
  - serum pregnancy test
- If amenorrhea >3 mos, pt not pregnant, or as indicated by physical examination:
  - Provera challenge: 10 mg/d × 10 d to induce withdrawal bleeding
- If pt has withdrawal bleed:
  - *Luteinizing hormone (LH)/follicle stimulating hormone (FSH):* If ratio LH:FSH >3:1, polycystic ovarian syndrome likely. ↓ LH/FSH indicate hypothalamic disorder, stress, weight-related problem. ↑ LH/FSH suggest ovarian dysfunction. *Prolactin:* If ↑, pituitary adenoma. *Thyroid function tests:* May indicate hyper/hypothyroidism
- With hirsutism or virilization:
  - free/total testosterone: elevated in polycystic ovarian syndrome/androgenizing tumor
  - DHEAS: ↑ in polycystic ovarian syndrome, adrenal tumor, abnormality in adrenal steroidogenesis
  - 24 h urine 17 ketosteroids: ↑ in disorders of adrenal steroidogenesis
  - androstenedione: ↑ in polycystic ovarian syndrome, other virilization states
  - pelvic ultrasound: to assess for ovarian cysts/masses
  - ACTH stimulation test: to assess adrenal steroid production
  - dexamethasone suppression test: to assess hypothalamic-pituitary axis
- If pt does not have withdrawal bleed w/Provera:
  - LH, FSH, thyroid function tests, prolactin but must consider neurologic imaging/refer for neuroendocrine testing

DIFFERENTIAL DIAGNOSIS

- Pregnancy: intrauterine/ectopic
- Stress
- Weight loss secondary to eating disorder
- Excessive weight gain
- Chronic illness (diabetes mellitus, inflammatory bowel disease, sickle-cell anemia)
- Thyroid disease
- Pituitary adenoma
- CNS tumor
- Pituitary infarction
- Empty sella syndrome
- Adrenal tumor
- Cushing disease
- Partial 21-OH deficiency
- Polycystic ovarian syndrome
- Gonadal dysgenesis
- Autoimmune oophoritis
- Ovarian tumor
- Asherman syndrome
- Previous chemotherapy/radiation
- Medroxy-progesterone/oral contraceptive usage

TREATMENT

- Treatment based on underlying cause
- Treat polycystic ovarian syndrome w/oral contraceptives (Provera as second choice)
- Treat secondary amenorrhea due to obesity w/Provera q3mos to induce withdrawal bleed, oral contraceptive pills, esp if pt sexually active, to prevent endometrial hyperplasia

WHEN TO REFER

- Depends on underlying cause
- To endocrinologist if thyroid disease, pituitary adenoma, or need for ACTH stimulation tests/dexamethasone suppression test
- To eating disorder specialist if anorexia nervosa/bulimia
- To appropriate specialist if chronic illness
- To OB/GYN if pregnant

BACKGROUND

• Tear of anal mucocutaneous junction usually due to hard stool, although stool may be normal or even soft; rare in breast-fed infants
• Peak incidence age 6–24 mos

CLINICAL MANIFESTATIONS

• Tear of anal mucocutaneous junction, posterior in midline or anterior in midline
• Sentinal tag if chronic
• Pain on defecation
• Withholding of stool due to pain
• Constipation
• Streak of blood
• 2° trauma to fissure from hard stool

LABORATORY FEATURES

• No studies indicated

DIFFERENTIAL DIAGNOSIS

• Anorectal abuse w/ fissures, wide dilatation of anus, venous engorgement, perianal hematoma, edema
• Skin tag may mimic warts, condyloma acuminatum
• Pruritis ani, other inflammatory conditions may cause superficial cracks that do not extend into anal canal
• Crohn disease, ulcerative colitis, intestinal tuberculosis

TREATMENT

• Avoid digital exams, enemas, suppositories
• Medical:
    – establish regular defecation w/ stool softener, laxatives, high-fiber diet
    – soap and water bath after each stool for max hygiene
    – warm sitz baths for comfort
    – local anesthetic cream difficult to use and not recommended
    – fissure from Crohn disease or leukemia best treated w/ metronidazole
• Surgical:
    – exam and digital anal dilatation under general anesthesia as outpt
    – dilatation relieves spasm of internal sphincter, which allows painless defecation and normal bowel habits
    – skin tag need not be excised
    – biopsy if fissure looks atypical
    – fecal disimpaction if indicated
    – lateral sphincterotomy as last resort; rarely needed in children

COMPLICATIONS

• If inadequately treated, chronic constipation and attendant psychosocial problems may develop
• 5–10% inadequately treated or recur

WHEN TO REFER

• If stool softener, high-fiber diet, laxative ineffective

BACKGROUND

- *Anaphylaxis:* acute, generalized allergic reaction w/simultaneous involvement of several organ systems, usually cardiovascular, respiratory, cutaneous, gastrointestinal
- Immunologic event, whereas anaphylactoid reaction a nonimmunologic response. Although of different causes, clinical manifestations of two types of reactions similar and require same treatment
- Occurs at rate of 0.4 cases/million/yr in general population; in hospitals prevalence 0.6/1,000 pts
- *Recovery:* most pts recover w/o complications
- *Mortality:* fatal anaphylaxis to penicillin or bee sting ~0.002%. Early administration of epinephrine significantly reduces mortality rate
- Representative causes of anaphylaxis and anaphylactoid reactions:
  - food: nuts and seeds, legumes, fish, shellfish, egg, grains, milk
  - food additives: aspartame, monosodium glutamate
  - biologicals: insulin, corticotropin, chymotrypsin, allergen extracts, blood, gamma globulin
  - drugs: antibiotics, chemotherapeutics, muscle relaxants
  - diagnostics: iodinated radiographic contrast media
  - physical stimuli: exercise, cold
  - other: latex, bisulfites, preservatives, insect stings, animal antiserum (eg, horse serum)

CLINICAL MANIFESTATIONS

- *Reaction:* begins within seconds or minutes after exposure to allergen
- *Cardiovascular system:* hypotension, shock, cardiac arrhythmias
- *Respiratory tract:* nasal congestion, nasal mucosa/hyperemia, profuse watery rhinorrhea, itching of nose, palate
- *Skin:* generalized pruritus, erythema, urticaria, angioedema
- *GI system:* crampy abdominal pain, nausea, diarrhea
- *Others:* disseminated intravascular coagulation, thrombocytopenia, convulsions

LABORATORY FEATURES

- Laboratory tests seldom necessary or helpful initially
- Blood cell counts may be elevated because of hemoconcentration
- Eosinophilia may be present
- *Chest x ray:* hyperinflation w/ or w/o areas atelectasis
- *Electrocardiogram:* conduction abnormalities; atrial or ventricular dysrhythmias, ST-T wave changes of myocardial ischemia or injury, acute cor pulmonale

DIFFERENTIAL DIAGNOSIS

- Anaphylactic shock must be differentiated from other causes of circulatory failure, including primary cardiac failure, endotoxin shock, reflex mechanisms
- Vasovagal collapse
- Jarish-Herxheimer reaction
- Aspirin, NSAIDs, sulfite additives in certain foods may affect some asthmatics w/a similar anaphylactic-like reaction

TREATMENT

- Treatment must be started promptly, so high index of suspicion necessary and Dx must be made rapidly
- Once anaphylaxis suspected, aqueous epinephrine, 1:1000 solution, injected IM or SubQ in dose of 0.2–0.5 mL for adults or 0.01 mL/kg of body weight for children. Dose repeated in 15–30 min if necessary. If reaction caused by insect sting or injected drug, 0.1–0.2 mL epinephrine, 1:1000 solution, infiltrated locally to retard absorption of residual allergen
- When anaphylaxis occurs in pt receiving beta-adrenergic blocking drug, reaction may be esp resistant to epinephrine, so higher doses may be required
- Tourniquet should be applied proximally if injection or sting on extremity

COMPLICATIONS

- Death from laryngeal edema, respiratory failure, shock, or cardiac arrhythmia usually occurs within minutes after onset of the reaction, but in occasional cases irreversible shock persists for hrs
- Permanent brain damage may result from hypoxia of respiratory or cardiovascular failure
- Urticaria or angioedema may recur for mos after penicillin anaphylaxis
- Myocardial infarction, abortion, renal failure other potential complications

WHEN TO REFER

- Identification and/or confirmation of causative allergen needed
- Desensitization of causative allergen indicated
- Serious complication occurs

ANCYLOSTOMIASIS

BACKGROUND

- Human hookworm disease caused by *Nectar americanus/Ancylostoma duodenale,* both of worldwide distribution
- Common in tropics/subtropics; in US restricted to southern states
- *A. duodenale* only human hookworm in central/northern Asia, Mediterranean coast, Europe
- Adult worm finally attaches to intestinal mucosa
- 0.03 mL of blood lost/worm/d by *N. americanus*/0.2 mL by *A. duodenale* for life span of 5 y
- Eggs passed in feces, hatch in soil; rhabditiformlarvae undergo number of molts, emerge as infective filariform larvae/penetrate skin (usually bare feet), enters venous circulation, carried to lung, penetrate alveoli, move up respiratory tree to pharynx, swallowed, settle in duodenum/jejunum

CLINICAL MANIFESTATIONS

- Severe itching at site of penetration (ground itch)
- Erythematous papular/papulovesicular rash on feet most common site of infection
- Generalized urticaria, 2° infection may occur
- Respiratory symptoms, cough/wheezing due to migration of parasite

- GI symptoms include abdominal pain, nausea/vomiting, diarrhea, flatulence
- Iron deficiency anemia most characteristic finding; degree of anemia depends on parasite load/duration of infection

DIAGNOSIS

- Ova of parasite found in stools

TREATMENT

- Mebandazole, 100 mg as single dose effective; in heavier infections, 100 mg bid × 3 d repeated in 2 wks advisable
- Albendazole, 400 mg/d × 3 d also effective/w/o toxicity

STRONGYLOIDIASIS

BACKGROUND

- Larva migrans/Strongyloidal ground itch caused by *S. stercorales,* widely spread in warm/damp climates
- Life cycle similar to hookworm, but eggs hatch in intestine/larvae not eggs seen in stools
- Larvae develop into infectious stage find another human host, develop into adults in soil, propagate w/o human host
- Alternatively, infectious larvae may penetrate intestinal mucosa/perineal skin, migrate back to lung, resume migratory cycle, maintain, multiply infection in host (hyperinfection)

- Larvae may also migrate in SubQ tissue, usually of abdomen/buttocks; many larvae may migrate in skin at same time, leading to crisscross appearance
- Infection may subside in few weeks/can be persistent for up to 45 y

CLINICAL MANIFESTATIONS

- Intense papular/papulovesicular eruption at site of penetration
- Urticaria/nonspecific eruptions may occur
- Abdominal pain, diarrhea if severe weight loss/stunting of growth in children
- Tracks seen on abdomen/buttocks but do not extend beyond knees/nipples
- W/ hyperinfections constitutional symptoms more severe, leading to electrolyte loss mental changes, severe pulmonary symptoms, shock

DIAGNOSIS

- Demonstration of larvae in stools requires concentration techniques
- Examination of jejunal contents/jejunal biopsy higher yield
- In some centers antibody tests for strongyloides available
- Eosinophilia common

TREATMENT

- Thiabendazole, 25 mg/kg bid × 3 d po (if necessary by gastric tube)
- Albendazole, 400 mg/d × 3 d also effective

BACKGROUND/CHARACTERISTICS

- Develops slowly (usually over 1 mo)
- Anemia in association w/:
  - ↓ plasma iron
  - ↓ total plasma iron-binding capacity
  - ↓ plasma transferrin saturation
  - ↑ normal reticuloendothelial iron
  - ↑ normal plasma ferritin

ETIOLOGY

- Always 2° to some underlying disease/disorder
- Common associations:
  - cancer
  - lymphoma
  - collagen vascular disease
  - severe tissue injury
  - renal failure
  - infectious diseases (many types: particularly common w/HIV)
  - other inflammatory states

DIFFERENTIAL DIAGNOSIS

- Characteristic laboratory findings specific for anemia of chronic disease; sometimes difficult to determine cause
- Iron deficiency anemia (generally lower MCV; ↓ plasma iron/↑ iron-binding capacity; ↓ plasma ferritin; absent marrow iron stores)
- Thalassemia trait disorders (generally lower MCV; iron studies normal; Hgb electrophoresis may be abnormal depending on type)

CLINICAL FEATURES

- Anemia mild; Sx may not be present
- If anemia moderate: easy fatigability, difficulty concentrating, ↓ appetite
- In certain disorders, ↓ Hgb, even if mild, may aggravate underlying chronic fatigue/↓ appetite (eg, chronic renal failure, HIV infection)

LABORATORY FEATURES

- ↓ Hgb mild to moderate; if severe, examine for other causes (blood loss/hemolysis); Hct rarely <30% in adults, <20% in children w/chronic disease
- ↓ reticulocyte count
- MCV normal/slightly ↓; if significantly ↓, consider iron deficiency/thalassemia trait
- Peripheral blood smear generally unremarkable
- WBC count usually normal; may be abnormal depending on underlying disease
- Platelet count usually normal; may be ↑ in inflammatory states, ↓ in malignancy
- Bone marrow examination rarely needed for Dx; generally normal appearance; ↑ sideroblasts w/iron stain
- Perform appropriate studies for Dx of underlying disorder

TREATMENT

- If anemia mild/pt asymptomatic, no treatment needed; correction of underlying disease resolves anemia
- Iron Tx not needed unless deficiency confirmed; even if iron deficiency present, may not respond to iron Tx
- Recombinant erythropoietin (EPO) usually reserved for anemia associated w/chronic renal failure/specific infections such as HIV in association w/easy fatigability, poor appetite
- *EPO dose:* 150–300 U/kg, 3×/wk SubQ/IV initially until Hct ↑ to 35%; then 15–125 U/kg 3×/wk to maintain Hct
- Transfusions rarely needed unless unresponsive to EPO

WHEN TO REFER

- Anemia associated w/chronic diseases/disorders rarely requires referral
- Refer to pediatric hematologist if Dx in doubt/need advice on management

BACKGROUND

- Urticaria and angioedema related conditions; often occur together (50% pts have both, 40% only urticaria, 10% only angioedema)
- Both disorders characterized by vasodilation, increased vascular permeability, extravasation of fluid, protein caused by mast cell–derived mediators or complement-derived activators. Urticaria involves superficial dermis; angioedema takes place in submucosa, deep dermis, subcutaneous tissue
- Urticaria and angioedema have many causes that may be classified as follows:
  - IgE mediated: foods (eg, shellfish, peanuts, eggs, wheat, milk), drugs (eg, penicillin, sulfonamides), infection (eg, viral, streptococcal), insect stings (eg, *Hymenoptera*), parasites, animal dander
  - circulating immune complexes: serum sickness, hepatitis B infection, systemic lupus erythematosus, Epstein-Barr virus infection
  - drug induced: direct stimulant effect on mast cells (eg, codeine, radiocontrast media, hyperosmolar solutions, etc), abnormalities of arachidonic acid metabolism (symptoms worsen in 20–40% pts w/urticaria, angioedema who takes NSAIDs), angiotensin-converting enzyme inhibitors (may cause severe life-threatening symptoms in pts w/preexisting angioedema)
  - physical stimuli: eg, cold, sunlight, pressure, vibration
  - hereditary angioedema (HAE): uncommon autosomal dominant disorder that results in decreased levels of C1 inhibitor (Type I, 85% cases) or dysfunctional C1 inhibitor (Type II, 15% cases). Rarely, C1 inhibitor deficiency acquired in association w/lymphoproliferative disorders (eg, chronic lymphocytic leukemia)
  - idiopathic
  - association w/rare syndromes: eg, mastocytosis, facial angioedema, eosinophilia
- Urticaria and angioedema classified as acute if process lasts <6 wks (most common form in children) or chronic if present for >6 wks (more likely to occur in middle-aged pts)

CLINICAL MANIFESTATIONS

- Diffuse, often well-demarcated, nonpitting swelling w/predilection for periorbital and perioral areas where there is loose subcutaneous tissue, or hands, feet
- Skin overlying area of angioedema is normal
- Pruritus often absent but burning sensation may be appreciated
- In urticaria, individual lesions are transient, lasting 24 hrs or less; angioedema may resolve more slowly
- Systemic symptoms generally absent but direct involvement of viscera may cause hoarseness, respiratory distress, vomiting, diarrhea, abdominal pain, arthralgias, headache, syncope, hypotension, shock
- Recurrent episodes of angioedema *w/o* urticaria, particularly if accompanied by systemic involvement or family Hx similar problems, should raise concern about existence of HAE

DIFFERENTIAL DIAGNOSIS

- Atopic dermatitis
- Cellulitis
- Lymphedema
- Idiopathic edema, idiopathic scrotal edema
- Melkersson-Rosenthal syndrome

LABORATORY FEATURES

- *Acute angioedema, urticaria, no systemic symptoms:* in children, most cases are produced by acute infection (eg, viral streptococcal), foods, medications. Laboratory studies to determine etiology should be directed by Hx, physical examination
- *Chronic angioedema, urticaria, no systemic symptoms:* unusual presentation in children and adolescents; no etiology found in most cases (75–90%). Laboratory studies directed by Hx, physical examination. Some authorities recommend performance of minimal laboratory evaluation, including CBC, sedimentation rate, chemistry panel, urinalysis
- *Angioedema w/o urticaria:* Should suggest HAE, particularly in presence of systemic symptoms or family Hx of similar problems. Studies to perform:
  - C4: in pt w/HAE, C4 almost always abnormally low between and during attacks
  - C1 inhibitor level: perform if C4 low

TREATMENT

- Remove or avoid identified precipitant
- Antihistamines first line of therapy:
  - begin w/first-generation H_1 antagonist (eg, hydroxyzine, 2–5 mg/kg/d, div qid [10–25 mg qid for adolescents]); increase dose as tolerated to control symptoms. Alternately, a second-generation, nonsedating H_1 antagonist such as cetirizine (5–10 mg daily for children 6–11 yrs of age, 10 mg for those ≥12 yrs) or loratidine (10 mg once daily for pts ≥6 yrs of age); others may be selected, although comparatively much more expensive
  - if pt experiences intolerable drowsiness w/first-generation H_1 antagonist, change to second-generation, nonsedating antihistamine. Bedtime dose of first-generation antihistamine may be used to provide additional control of symptoms while limiting daytime sedation
  - if response not optimal, consider one or more of following: change to another class of first-generation H_1 antagonist, add doxepin, which possesses H_1 antagonist effects [10–25 mg hs in pts 12 yrs of age or older], use an H_2 antagonist (eg, cimetidine or ranitidine) in conjunction w/H_1 antagonist: some pts benefit from this combined therapy (H_2 antagonists not used alone in management of urticaria and angioedema)
- *Corticosteroids:* corticosteroids generally not required to manage acute urticaria and angioedema. However, short courses of agents (eg, prednisone 1 mg/kg/d) may be of assistance in management of occasional pts whose symptoms not controlled by antihistamines. Corticosteroids not used to manage pts w/chronic urticaria
- *Special situations:* in general, evaluation and management of following situations require consultation w/or referral to allergist/immunologist or dermatologist:
  - angioedema, urticaria w/episodes of respiratory difficulty: provide pt w/injectable epinephrine (eg, EpiPen or EpiPen, Jr), and refer
  - angioedema w/generalized urticaria or respiratory difficulty following insect sting: provide pt w/injectable epinephrine, refer for possible desensitization
  - chronic urticaria: consultation w/or referral to specialist indicated
  - HAE:
    ○ Management of acute episodes (1) Supportive care, airway management (including intubation when appropriate). Epinephrine, antihistamines, corticosteroids may be of limited benefit but often employed. (2) Administration of epsilon aminocaproic acid (EACA), or attenuated androgens (eg, danazol or stanozolol) after onset of angioedema of questionable benefit. (3) Fresh frozen plasma (FFP) may be of benefit; however, complement components present in preparation may further angioedema process. (4) C1 inhibitor concentrate: available in Europe and on a research basis in US. Infusions can attenuate attacks within 30 min w/complete resolution of 24 hrs. Clinical effect lasts 3–5 d
    ○ Prophylaxis (1) Surgical procedures (particularly involving oral cavity where precipitation of laryngeal edema likely): EACA, attenuated androgens, FFP, C1 inhibitor concentrate beneficial. (2) Long-term prevention of attacks: Few pts require long-term prophylaxis; indications for Tx include episode of laryngeal obstruction, repeated episodes of face, neck edema or frequent debilitating attacks (eg, abdominal pain). In children, EACA probably drug of choice for prophylaxis. Attenuated androgens effective but interference w/growth and virilization preclude use in pediatric patients. C1 inhibitor infusions used prophylactically with excellent results

WHEN TO REFER

- See treatment section

ANKYLOSING SPONDYLITIS, JUVENILE AND OTHER SERO-NEGATIVE ARTHRITIDES

RONALD M. LAXER

BACKGROUND

- Second most common group of chronic rheumatic disorders in children (next to JRA)
- Various incidence/prevalence figures suggest ~50% that of JRA to almost as common as JRA
- Usually seen in "older" children (>8 yrs of age)
- Much more common in males
- Made up of several distinct entities, overlapped by peripheral and axial joint inflammation, enthesitis, skin and mucous membrane involvement, positive family Hx, presence of HLA B27
- Entities include juvenile ankylosing spondylitis, seronegative enthesopathy-arthropathy (SEA) syndrome, some types of psoriatic arthritis, some types of arthritis associated w/ inflammatory bowel disease, Reiter disease, reactive arthritis
- Some follow bacterial (GI or genitourinary) infection

CLINICAL MANIFESTATIONS

- *Peripheral arthritis:* pauciarthritis or monoarthritis, usually of lower limb (knee, ankle, hip)/monoarthritis
- Dactylitis (swollen tendon sheath) w/ sausage digit appearance common
- Enthesitis (inflammation of tendon, ligament, joint capsule insertion to bone); most commonly affected sites: achilles tendon, plantar fascia, quadriceps tendon, patellar tendon insertions
- Inflammatory spine pain (early morning stiffness, improvement w/ movement) not common but occasionally present; flattening of thoracolumbar spine on forward flexion important sign

- Signs of psoriasis (skin, scalp, nails) and inflammatory bowel disease must be searched for
- Extraarticular symptoms include uveitis (acute, symptomatic vs. pauciarticular JRA, which is chronic and asymptomatic), aortic valve insufficiency (uncommonly symptomatic)
- Reiter syndrome includes urethritis and conjunctivitis
- Joints in reactive arthritis may be red and very painful (more so than in JRA), and child may be febrile

LABORATORY FEATURES

- None diagnostic
- HLA B27 in 50–90% (depending on seronegative entity)
- ↑ ESR
- ↑ serum immunoglobulins, esp IgA
- Negative ANA, rheumatoid factor
- Joint fluid inflammatory (in Reiter/reactive, may be >50,000 cells/mm^3

DIFFERENTIAL DIAGNOSIS

- Depends on presentation
- Septic arthritis
- Malignancy
- Rheumatic fever
- Juvenile rheumatoid arthritis
- Fibromyalgia
- Mechanical syndromes
- Orthopedic (eg, slipped capital femoral epiphysis, osteochondritis dissecans)

TREATMENT

- *Principles:* reduce inflammation, preserve function

- NSAIDs drugs of first choice; indole acetic class of agents seem to work best (tolectin 30 mg/kg/d in 3 doses, indomethacin 2–3 mg/kg/d in 3 doses—watch primarily for GI side effects; rarely allergy or hepatic, renal dysfunction)
- Local treatments w/ intraarticular corticosteroid very effective (up to max 3×/1 y), triamcinolone hexacetonide, 10–40 mg per joint
- Role of second-line agents (if above ineffective) not clear, eg, sulfasalazine, 50 mg/kg/d in 2 div doses, methotrexate, 10 mg/m^2/1×/wk
- Rarely need for systemic steroid
- Aggressive physical Tx, esp to maintain ROM of spine and hips
- Orthotics for enthesitis
- Surgical management if disease uncontrolled (eg, hip replacement)

COMPLICATIONS

- Weakness of muscles around inflamed joint; ligamentous instability and muscle wasting
- Joint contractures
- Cartilage destruction
- Potential for fibrous and ultimately bony ankylosis
- Ultimate spinal stiffening

WHEN TO REFER

- All should be referred to physical Tx program, esp to maintain spinal motion
- If Dx unclear
- If pt fails to respond to NSAIDs

BACKGROUND

- *Prevalence:* 1/100 adolescent girls, higher in ballet dancers, gymnasts (wrestlers, swimmers in young men)
- 90–95% cases young women from *all* socioeconomic groups. Bimodal age distribution peaks at 14 and 18 yrs; 25% cases <13 yrs of age
- Originally restricted to Western cultures; however, more common throughout world as Western concept of excessive thinness becomes ideal of feminine beauty
- Equal prevalence among Caucasian and Hispanic females; more frequent in Native Americans; less frequent among African and Asian American females
- *Risk factors:* poor self-esteem, early maturation, enmeshed overprotective families, excessive focus on body ideal by family or peers
- Onset sometimes associated w/developmental challenge (puberty, college) or negative life event (divorce, death)
- *Pathogenesis:* biopsychosocial maladaptation
- Outcomes improved w/early intervention:
  – course of treatment 3–4 yrs before weight, menses restoration
  – good outcome 50–75% cases
  – adolescent boys have poorer outcomes
  – severely ill women requiring acute hospitalization have very poor 10 yr outcomes (only 25% fully recovered) and long-term mortality of 10% (starvation, suicide, electrolyte imbalances, cardiac arrhythmias)
  – progression to bulimia anorexia in 10–50% cases

CLINICAL MANIFESTATIONS

- Intense fear of fat or gaining weight
- Distorted body image (weight, size, shape)
- Amenorrhea, usually secondary to weight loss
- Abnormal body weight for age, secondary to actual weight loss or failure to grow (common pattern w/onset prepubertally). Less than 85% of ideal body weight for age or less than 5th percentile body mass index for age
- Presence/absence of binge eating or purging determines subtype: anorexia nervosa, restricting or anorexia nervosa, binge eating/purging
- *Associated findings:* bradycardia, hypothermia, postural hypotension, peripheral edema, lanugo, obsessive exercise, binging, induced vomiting, purging w/laxatives or enemas, unusual handling/hoarding of food, sleep disturbance/deprivation, constipation, high academic achievement
- *Comorbidities:* affective and anxiety disorders, more frequently w/disease onset >14 yrs of age

LABORATORY FEATURES

- Usually normal
- Anemia, leukopenia common
- Dehydration w/elevated BUN, LFTs, cholesterol
- Low zinc, magnesium, phosphorus
- Low thyroid, estrogen levels
- Metabolic alkalosis 2° to induced vomiting
- Metabolic acidosis 2° to chronic laxative use
- Hypercarotenemia, transaminitis *not* useful screens

DIFFERENTIAL DIAGNOSIS

- Occult malignancies
- HIV/AIDS
- Serious depression
- Superior mesenteric artery syndrome
- Bulimia (near-normal body weight)
- Undiagnosed chronic illness

TREATMENT

- Goals must include all of following:
  – correction of anorexic's underlying misconceptions of body size, shape
  – support of adolescent's sense of autonomy
  – restoration of family function
  – achievement of appropriate weight gain
- Intervention requires active collaboration between primary care practitioner and experienced mental health professional (social worker, psychologist, psychiatrist). Treatment must target all above goals and include identified adolescent pt and family
  – nutritional restitution
  – appropriate nutritional counseling: weight gain is objective measure (not quantity or quality of food consumed). Goal (after initial correction of hydration) should be consistent 0.5–1.0 lbs/wk; is pt's contracted responsibility. IV or enteral feeding in hospital w/experienced staff only when required for medical complications
  – individual psychotherapy: ego-oriented individual Tx focusing on fact finding. Cognitive-behavioral techniques to reinforce food intake, self-monitoring, reframing, adolescent autonomy, assertiveness training
  – family Tx
  – behavioral family systems Tx

  – hospitalization: preferably on adolescent unit w/staff experienced in management of eating disorders should be considered for body weight <75% of ideal body weight for age, failure of outpatient treatment and/or for acute management of dehydration, electrolyte balance, medical complications listed below
  – psychopharmacology to treat symptoms of associated depression, anxiety, or obsessive-compulsive disorder may provide adjunct but *not* primary intervention. Appetite stimulants *not* helpful

COMPLICATIONS

- Complications reflect effects of chronic starvation and/or refeeding process (intracellular shifts of Mg and PO$_4$)
  – skeletal: bone loss, fractures, short stature
  – cardiac: prolonged QT interval, other EKG manifestations, reduced left ventricular mass, mitral valve prolapse, sudden death
  – GI: esophagitis, necrotizing colitis, gastric perforation
  – CNS: seizures, myopathy, delirium secondary to hypophosphatemia, attention and learning problems
  – renal: nephrogenic diabetes insipidus
  – skin: hypercarotenemia, alopecia
  – dental: dental enamel erosion, increased cavities
  – sensory: olfactory dysfunction

PREVENTION

- Challenge cultural norms of beauty
- Support healthy nutrition and exercise practices
- Anticipatory guidance for all early adolescents and their families about normal body changes at puberty
- Identify prepubertal pts and families at risk for targeted intervention

WHEN TO REFER

- At presentation, immediate referral and collaboration w/experienced mental health care professional experienced w/treatment of eating disorders for joint management
- Refer to adolescent medicine specialist if pattern of consistent weight gain *not* established after 1 mo office care, for management of serious complications or when Dx in doubt
- Hospitalization on adolescent unit w/interdisciplinary treatment approach for failure of outpatient care, correction of acute dehydration or electrolyte imbalance, medical complications of starvation

SUSAN LURIE AND JEFFREY H. NEWCORN

BACKGROUND

- Among most common psychological disorders
- 8–15% of children and adolescents at least one anxiety disorder
- May not appear in isolation, may occur w/other anxiety disorders, major depressive disorder, ADHD, disruptive behavior disorders
- Must be differentiated from normal fears and worries
- Isolated subclinical anxiety symptoms common (eg, fear of dark, harm to attachment figures, overconcern about competence, excessive need for reassurance, somatic complaints)

RISK FACTORS

- Temperamental trait of behavioral inhibition to the unfamiliar—unusually shy, show fear and withdrawal in novel situations
- Insecure mother-child attachment
- Family Hx anxiety and depressive disorders
- Variety of family and environmental stressors

CLINICAL MANIFESTATIONS

- *Separation anxiety disorder (SAD):* esp marked anxiety about separation from significant others or home; 75% of children w/SAD manifest school refusal
- *Generalized anxiety disorder (overanxious disorder in DSM-III-R):* marked unrealistic worry about variety of situations (eg, future events, past behavior, competence, physical symptoms); worry difficult to control
- *Specific phobia:* excessive, unreasonable, persistent fear of stimulus w/avoidant behavior; interferes w/normal functioning
- *Obsessive-compulsive disorder:* recurrent obsessions, compulsions: unwanted, and cause marked distress; washing, checking, ordering rituals common
- *Post-traumatic stress disorder:* exposure to traumatic event(s), child experiences significant

fear, helplessness, horror; persistent reexperiencing of event; avoidance of stimuli associated w/trauma; flashbacks uncommon in childhood; may engage in play using themes of past trauma; sleep problems and other symptoms of increased arousal (eg, irritability, difficulty concentrating, hypervigilance, exaggerated startle response)
- *Panic disorder:* discrete episode of intense fear, w/physical and psychological symptoms, including feelings of unreality, fear of losing control, or dying; uncommon before puberty, can occur in young children; may/may not be accompanied by agoraphobia; peak age of onset 15–19 yrs
- *Social phobia:* excessive anxiety about social or performance situations when individual exposed to unfamiliar people or possible scrutiny; onset most common early to mid adolescence; selective mutism may be form of social phobia
- *Adjustment disorder w/anxiety:* significant anxiety developing within 3 mos of exposure to clear-cut psychosocial stressor; acute if symptoms last <6 mos; chronic if symptoms last >6 mos in response to chronic stress

Note: Dx is made only if symptoms excessive, interfere w/child's functioning, and persistent. Symptomatology below diagnostic level common, and may still be focus of clinical attention.

PHYSICAL SYMPTOMS

- Tachycardia, tachypnea, sweating, tremulousness, chest pain, nausea, abdominal distress, dizziness, lightheadedness
- May present to ER fearing "heart attack"

DIFFERENTIAL DIAGNOSIS

- *Other psychological conditions:* mood disorders, ADHD, borderline or other personality disorders, eating disorders, pervasive developmental disorders
- *Physical conditions mimicking anxiety disorders:* hypoglycemia, hyperthyroidism, cardiac

arrhythmias, caffeinism, pheochromocytoma, seizure disorders, migraine, CNS pathology such as delirium, brain tumor
- *Medication reactions:* antihistamines, antiasthmatics, sympathomimetics, steroids, antidepressants, benzodiazepines (paradoxical reaction), neuroleptics, diet pills, cold medications
- *Substance abuse:* including alcohol, nicotine, marijuana, cocaine, stimulants, inhalants, hallucinogens, including substance abuse

Note: Virtually all on the DDX list can also occur comorbidly with the anxiety disorders.

ASSESSMENT

- Hx from child, parent, other pertinent informants
  – environmental family stressors (eg, disorganized home, abuse, neglect, mental or physical illness, exposure to danger/violence)
  – comorbid psychopathologic symptoms
  – impact of symptoms on daily life (ie, impairment)
  – social/family reinforcers of symptoms
  – developmental Hx, w/attention to temperament, quality of attachment, stranger and separation responses, childhood fears
  – medical Hx medical disorders, medications
  – school Hx
  – peer relationships
  – family Hx (including child's role, stresses, coping style, psychological Hx)
- Interview child; in mental status exam note following:
  – child's report of symptoms, including self-assessment of impairment
  – objective physical signs of anxiety (eg, motor tension, autonomic hyperactivity, vigilance and scanning, variations in speech patterns and production, separation difficulty)
  – communication of anxiety through play drawings in very young

THERAPY

Individual psychotherapy using cognitive behavioral techniques, behavior Tx, or psychodynamic Tx; family counseling or Tx; pharmacotherapy; or combinations of the above; SSRIs preferred over tricyclics due to potential for cardiovascular and other side effects w/TCAs. Tricyclics require EKG monitoring at baseline and above 3 mg/kg

Medication	Indications	Dose
Antihistamines	short-term Rx for insomnia	diphenhydramine 25–100 mg qhs; hydroxyzine 25–100 mg qhs
Benzodiazepines	short-term Rx for moderate to severe anxiety symptoms	clonazepam 0.25–0.5 mg bid or tid; lorazepam, 0.5–1 mg bid to tid
	short-term Rx for insomnia	qhs dosing only
Selective serotonergic reuptake inhibitors	longer term Rx of moderate to severe anxiety disorders, including OCD	fluoxetine, 5–20 mg qam; sertraline, 25–50 mg bid; paroxetine, 5–20 mg qhs
Tricyclic antidepressants	longer term Rx of moderate to severe anxiety disorders	nortriptyline, 10–100 mg qhs; imipramine, 25–200 mg qhs; clomipramine, 25–200 mg qhs. Divided doses are preferable in young children
Alpha adrenergic agents	short- to long-term Rx of moderate to severe anxiety disorders; may be particularly useful for the arousal symptoms of PTSD	clonidine, 0.025–0.1 mg bid or tid
	moderate to severe insomnia	qhs dosing only

OFFICE TREATMENT

- Establish Dx, monitor course
- Reassurance, supportive counseling, and brief family interventions, esp if anxieties are in normal developmental range or pathology less severe

- Short-term anxiolytic medication, if situation warrants

WHEN TO REFER

- Symptoms persistent
- Multiple domains affected, requiring additional intervention

- Severe pathology requiring large time commitment
- Child in significant distress
- More comprehensive assessment needed

BACKGROUND

- Aplasia results from absent or defective production of terminally differentiated blood cells
- May occur any age
- May be acquired/inherited
- Inherited syndromes associated w/aplastic anemia:
  - Fanconi anemia: physical anomalies, chromosomal breakage
  - Shwachman-Diamond syndrome: exocrine pancreatic insufficiency
  - dyskeratosis congenita: dermatologic manifestations
  - amegakaryocytic thrombocytopenia: thrombocytopenia in infancy
  - reticular dysgenesis: absent cellular and humoral immunity
  - familial aplastic anemia
- Acquired aplastic anemia associated w/exposure to chemicals (eg, benzene derivatives), viruses (eg, hepatitis B), drugs (eg, chloramphenicol). However, no causative factor found in as many as 50% of pts

CLINICAL MANIFESTATIONS

- Insidious onset, as opposed to acute leukemia, idiopathic thrombocytopenic purpura
- Bleeding due to thrombocytopenia often first manifestation
- Infections
- *Complications of anemia:* pallor, fatigue

LABORATORY FEATURES

- Severe acquired aplastic anemia defined by presence of moderate to severe hypocellularity on examination of bone marrow biopsy plus two of following:
  - neutrophil count <500mm^3
  - platelet count <20,000/mm^3
  - reticulocyte count <1% (corrected for Hct) or absolute reticulocyte count <50,000/mm^3
- Mean corpuscular volume (MCV), fetal Hgb level may be elevated, esp in inherited syndromes associated w/aplastic anemia
- Definitive Dx made by examination of bone marrow aspirate, biopsy

DIFFERENTIAL DIAGNOSIS OF PANCYTOPENIA

- Preleukemia/Monosomy 7 syndrome
- Leukemia/lymphoma
- Infiltration of bone marrow space by solid tumor
- HIV-related disease

TREATMENT

- Supportive care that may be provided by the generalist pediatrician:
  - transfusion RBCs, platelets should be minimized to reduce risk of alloimmunization, esp in pts who are bone marrow transplant candidates
  - all blood products should be negative for cytomegalovirus, irradiated to 1,500 cGy, given through leukocyte depletion filter
  - fever, neutrophil count of <1,000/mm^3 should prompt thorough evaluation to identify source of infection. Empiric treatment w/broad-spectrum antibiotics should begin while awaiting results of blood cultures, other diagnostic tests
- Specific Tx provided under the direction of a pediatric hematologist:
  - bone marrow transplantation: if HLA-matched sibling available, current treatment of choice for severe acquired aplastic anemia, some of inherited aplastic anemias
  - immunosuppressive therapy for severe *acquired* aplastic anemia: if an HLA-matched family member not identified, anti-thymocyte globulin, cyclosporine, methylprednisolone given
  - hematopoietic growth factors: GM-CSF, GCSF stimulate increased neutrophil production in most pts
  - androgen therapy:
    - not effective for pts w/severe acquired aplastic anemia
    - treatment of choice for some inherited bone marrow failure syndromes

PROGNOSIS

- In some centers cure rate for severe acquired aplastic anemia >80% for pts who receive bone marrow from HLA-matched sibling. Results of bone marrow transplantation using HLA-matched unrelated donors and partially matched family members are less encouraging (survival rates 30–60%)
- Immunosuppression effective in 50–60% pts w/severe acquired aplastic anemia
- Prognosis for inherited syndromes associated w/bone marrow failure variable

WHEN TO REFER

- Referral to pediatric hematologist for accurate Dx, specific treatment essential
- For pts w/severe acquired aplastic anemia, pediatric hematologist will contact recognized pediatric bone marrow transplantation center to assist in HLA typing of family members, to make arrangements for transplantation if donor identified

APPENDICITIS

DANIEL VON ALLMEN

BACKGROUND

- *Incidence:* all ages—11 cases/10,000 population/yr. Age 10–19 yrs—23 cases/ 10,000 population/yr
- *Pathophysiology:* luminal obstruction by fecalith, lymphoid hyperplasia, parasites, tumor, foreign body. Luminal distention results in vascular compromise, appendiceal gangrene, ultimately perforation

CLINICAL PRESENTATION

- *Abdominal pain:* classically migrates to right lower quadrant from periumbilical area
- *Anorexia:* 50–75%
- *Nausea:* 65–95%
- *Vomiting:* 40–70%
- *Diarrhea:* 9–16%

PHYSICAL EXAM

- Low-grade fever
- Tenderness to palpation in right lower quadrant (93–100%)
- *Peritoneal irritation signs:* guarding, Rovsing sign, percussion tenderness (80–91%)
- Obturator/psoas sign may indicate retroperitoneal inflamed appendix
- Tenderness on rectal exam suggests pelvic appendix
- Dx frequently made on basis of Hx and physical exam alone w/o laboratory or radiologic exams

LABORATORY

- Mild to moderate increase in WBC count w/left shift
- Urine analysis may show WBC or leukocyte esterase but not organisms

- Plain abdominal x ray: fecalith, mass effect, or local ileus. May be normal
- Ultrasound useful to r/o other pathology in equivocal cases. Most helpful in postmenarchal females

DIFFERENTIAL DIAGNOSIS

- Gastroenteritis
- Mesenteric adenitis
- Salpingitis
- Ectopic pregnancy
- Ruptured ovarian follicle (Mittelschmerz)
- Pyelonephritis/urinary tract infection
- Inflammatory bowel disease
- Constipation
- Pneumonia (right lower lobe)
- Tumor

	Duration Sx	Temp	WBC	Exam
Acute appendicitis	24–48 hrs	mildly elevated	8–12,000, left shift	tender in right lower quadrant
Perforated appendicitis	3–5 d	spiking fevers	12–20,000 w/left shift	diffuse pain, peritoneal signs

TREATMENT

- *Acute appendicitis:* appendectomy w/perioperative antibiotics. Hospital discharge when tolerating oral intake (24–48 hrs)
- *Perforated appendicitis:* appendectomy w/4–7 d broad-spectrum IV antibiotics
- Appendiceal abscess:
  - early operation w/appendectomy and drainage followed by broad-spectrum antibiotics
  - broad-spectrum antibiotics w/percutaneous drainage of abscess. Interval appendectomy 6 wks after initial Tx

COMPLICATIONS

- *Misdiagnosis:* 10% overall w/higher rates in teenage females 15–40%, lower rates in males (5–10%)
- *Perforated appendicitis:* 25–30% of all pts. Higher rates in young children <5 yrs of age (50–75%)
- *Wound infection:* 0–2.4% w/primary wound closure
- *Intra-abdominal abscess:* 1.7–5% w/broad-spectrum antibiotics

WHEN TO REFER

- Pts w/clear signs of appendicitis should be referred immediately for surgical evaluation. Pts w/equivocal findings should be referred within 12–24 hrs if symptoms have not resolved

ASCARIASIS

BACKGROUND

- Acquired by ingesting eggs of *A. lumbricoides* found in soil, hence vegetables
- Larvae 0.2–0.3 mm hatch from eggs in upper small intestine, migrate in intestinal wall, reach blood vessels carried to right heart/lungs where they molt into third stage (1–2 mm) then migrate through bronchioles to pharynx, swallowed/molt again in intestine, reach adulthood
- Females 20–35 cm/males 15–31 cm × 6 mm width
- Eggs (200,000)/d passed in feces/repeat cycle

CLINICAL MANIFESTATIONS

- Worldwide distribution except in very cold climates
- Infection asymptomatic; in heavy migration in lung Loffler's syndrome/pneumonitis may occur
- Nutritional deprivation, loss of weight, appetite, abdominal pain
- May penetrate intestine/cause peritonitis, bile duct obstruction, intestinal obstruction, pancreatitis
- Urticaria/erythema annulare centrifugum common cutaneous symptoms

DIAGNOSIS

- Ova may be demonstrated in stools
- Adult worms appear in stools rarely
- Eosinophilia

TREATMENT

- Pyrvinium pamoate as single dose in children
- Mebendazole, 100 mg am/pm × 3d, pyrentel pamoate, 11 mg/kg (max 1 g), both for pts >2 yrs of age
- Piperazine citrate (Antipar), 75 mg/kg not to exceed 3–4 g for any 2 consecutive d
- Prognosis good; recurrence possible; personal hygiene important

ENTEROBIASIS (PINWORMS)

BACKGROUND

- Most common human intestinal infection worldwide
- Prevalent in cold/temperate climates
- Common in children (30%)/adults (16%)
- Prevalent in whites
- Worms develop in cecum/appendix, also colonize colon/rectum
- Male worms rarely seen, female 8–13 mm deposit eggs in anal/perineal areas; eggs hatch in 6 hrs/infective, hence autoinoculation
- Reinfection by direct/indirect contamination of hands, fomites, clothing, dust

CLINICAL MANIFESTATIONS

- Pruritus, intense at times leading to scarification, lichenification. Repeated attacks of abdominal pain, nervousness, loss of sleep, anorexia, weight loss
- Vaginitis produced by irritation from migrating worms in girls

DIAGNOSIS

- Dx suspected because of itching
- Worms/eggs may be seen in anal/perineal areas
- Cellophane tape smears should be prepared in am before pt washes ×3 consecutive d/until ova found

TREATMENT

- Mebandazole, 100 mg as single dose cures 90% infections; however 100 mg bid ×3/d more efficient. Repeat treatment in 2–3 wks advisable
- All family members should be treated
- Pyrvinium pamoate as single dose in children
- Topical antipruritic treatment
- Personal hygiene essential to prevent reinfection

BACKGROUND

- Aspergillosis refers to disease caused by environmentally ubiquitous fungi of genus *Aspergillus* (most commonly *A. fumigatus* or *A. flavus*)
- Portal of entry usually through respiratory tract, resulting in either allergic reaction to aspergillus conidia, or tissue invasion by hyphae
- Allergic bronchopulmonary aspergillosis (ABPA) occurs in pts w/chronic lung disease. Up to 10% of pts w/cystic fibrosis may develop ABPA
- Invasive pulmonary aspergillosis occurs in pts w/neutrophil defects, chronic neutropenia, immunosuppression due to chemotherapy or organ (esp bone marrow) transplantation

MANIFESTATIONS

- Allergic bronchopulmonary aspergillosis:
  - wheezing, cough common. Fever unusual, and suggests infectious etiology
  - worsening pulmonary function from baseline clinical disease
- Invasive pulmonary aspergillosis
  - fever may be only symptom
  - variable presence of cough, pleuritic chest pain, hemoptysis
  - other symptoms develop if secondary sites involved due to dissemination: neurologic changes; necrotic nasal septum; raised, erythematous cutaneous lesion w/central eschar

LABORATORY FEATURES

- Allergic bronchopulmonary aspergillosis:
  - peripheral blood eosinophilia, otherwise normal CBC, differential

  - positive skin test to aspergillus antigens
  - positive serum precipitating antibodies to *A. fumigatus*
  - elevated total serum IgE
  - elevated serum IgG and IgE antibodies specific to *A. fumigatus*
  - fleeting pulmonary infiltrates on chest x ray
- Invasive aspergillosis:
  - neutropenia or normal CBC, differential, depending on underlying immune deficiency
  - chest x ray may show single pulmonary nodule or diffuse interstitial infiltrates
  - respiratory tract cultures not helpful in establishing Dx
  - blood cultures almost always negative

DIFFERENTIAL DIAGNOSIS

- Allergic bronchopulmonary aspergillosis:
  - asthma
  - exacerbation of chronic lung disease
- Invasive pulmonary aspergillosis:
  - pneumonias due to other organisms common to immunocompromised hosts: bacterial pneumonia; *Pneumocystis carinii* pneumonia; other fungi: *Candida sp.*, *Pseudallesceria boydii*, *Penicillium sp.*

TREATMENT

- Allergic bronchopulmonary aspergillosis:
  - systemic corticosteroids: prednisone, 2 mg/kg/d in 2 or 3 div doses × 4 wks, followed by slow taper to qOd dosing
  - alternative: beclomethasone dipropionate, 2 puffs by inhalation 2 or 3 times/d. Note: limited experience in children for this indication

  - adjunctive: itraconazole, 100–400 mg po qd (4–8 mg/kg/d) may reduce burden of fungal hyphae for pts heavily colonized w/*Aspergillus sp.* Limited data on pharmacokinetics of itraconazole in children
- Invasive pulmonary aspergillosis
  - amphotericin B, 1.5 mg/kg/d. Toxic, requires inpatient treatment initially w/careful monitoring of renal status and serum potassium
  - alternatives: liposomal amphotericin B—less nephrotoxic, but less experience. Itraconazole—better tolerated, given po. May be as effective as amphotericin B

COMPLICATIONS

- Allergic bronchopulmonary aspergillosis:
  - relapses frequent. Side effects from systemic corticosteroids
- Invasive pulmonary aspergillosis:
  - often progressive and fatal unless immune defect corrected

WHEN TO REFER

- Pts w/ABPA should be referred to pediatric pulmonologist for management of chronic lung disease
- Pts w/invasive aspergillosis should be referred to center w/expertise in management of infections in immunocompromised host

BACKGROUND

- Incidence of aspirin poisoning in children declined sharply after use curtailed following observation of association w/Reye syndrome
- Aspirin converted in body to salicylate, which produces observed therapeutic, toxic effects
- Some preparations of salicylate, such as methyl salicylate (ie, oil of wintergreen), extremely concentrated; parents often unaware of salicylate content
- Salicylate acidic (pKa = 3.5), and can only cross cell membranes in nonionized form, causing concentration in basic environment (ion trapping)
- Hepatic enzyme systems responsible for majority of salicylate metabolism saturated in overdose, slowing rate of salicylate elimination, and raising proportion eliminated unchanged in urine
- Salicylate poisons Kreb's cycle, substantially reducing usable energy produced from glucose metabolism, increasing glucose metabolism, resulting in hypoglycemia and generation of significant heat. Final result increased fat metabolism, increased ketone body formation, ultimately development of ketoacidosis
- Important to distinguish acute single salicylate ingestion from chronic salicylate poisoning. Chronic salicylate poisoning results from long-term ingestion of excessive doses or decrease in drug elimination (due to drug-drug interaction, decreased hepatic or renal clearance, etc). Acute poisoning generally well tolerated, but chronic poisoning difficult to treat; associated w/high morbidity and mortality

CLINICAL MANIFESTATIONS

- *Metabolic:* hypermetabolic state, tachycardia, tachypnea, hyperthermia, fluid losses
- GI: vomiting, hypoglycemia, erosive gastritis, increased serum transaminases
- CNS: tinnitus, agitation, confusion, lethargy, seizure, coma, death
- Pulmonary: noncardiogenic pulmonary edema
- *Hematological:* increased coagulation times, platelet dysfunction
- *Renal:* protinuria, renal failure

LABORATORY FEATURES

- Obtain measurements of electrolytes, BUN, creatinine, blood glucose, arterial blood gases in all but trivial ingestions; young children can have significant derangements while still appearing clinically well
- Concomitant centrally induced respiratory alkalosis (direct brain stem effect) and metabolic acidosis result in complex mixed acidemia
- Presence of respiratory acidosis due either to pulmonary edema or extremely decreased sensorium; indicates severe poisoning w/poor prognosis
- Increased coagulation times (PT, PTT) and platelet dysfunction due to direct toxic effects also possible
- Although salicylate acidic, serum content itself contributes little to acid-base balance. Serum salicylate concentration measurement early after acute ingestion reflects total body burden; later, or following a chronic ingestion, salicylate redistributes into body tissues, rendering serum measurements less useful. Pt's clinical status, laboratory abnormalities, serial serum salicylate concentration determinations used to guide treatment decisions

DIFFERENTIAL DIAGNOSIS

- Differential Dx acute salicylate poisoning includes all causes of increased anion gap metabolic acidosis:
  - poisoning: methanol, ethylene glycol, paraldehyde, phenphormin/metphormin, iron
  - uremia
  - diabetic, other metabolic causes of ketoacidosis
  - lactic acidosis
- Chronic salicylate poisoning generally presents as altered sensorium; difficult to distinguish from sepsis, meningitis, metabolic disease, other drug overdoses

TREATMENT

- Gastric lavage effective at removing aspirin from stomach within first 2 hrs after ingestion
- Oral activated charcoal at dose of 1–2 g/kg (may follow gastric lavage) acts by adsorbing aspirin remaining in stomach. Due to possibility of concretion formation in stomach, pts may need to have activated charcoal repeated (0.5–1 g/kg q2–4 hrs) until passage of charcoal stool
- Sorbitol (or another cathartic) safely used w/first dose of activated charcoal in children 2 yrs of age and older; generally not given in subsequent doses of activated charcoal
- In overdose, increased proportion of salicylate eliminated in urine; possible to enhance renal elimination by alkalinization of urine. Goal of urinary alkalinization: raise urine pH above (make more basic than) serum pH that "traps" acidic salicylate ion in urine. Method only works when pt has normal hydration status, normal renal function
- Restoration of fluid and electrolyte balance similar to treatment of diabetic ketoacidosis, except glucose-containing solution used to compensate for significant hypermetabolic state. Urinary alkalinization then initiated w/IV bolus of 1–2 mEq/kg of sodium bicarbonate, followed by 150 mEq of sodium bicarbonate (3 ampoules of 8.4% [1 mEq/mL]) in 1 L D_5W at 2 × maintenance requirements. Goal of treatment: raise urine pH to 8.0 or higher w/o raising serum pH significantly out of normal range
- Essential to keep serum potassium in normal range, but >4.0 mEq/L, as ability of kidney to excrete bicarbonate depends on adequate potassium stores

COMPLICATIONS

- Sequelae of salicylate poisoning due to cellular damage in organs most sensitive to disruption of glucose metabolism. Central nervous system, liver, kidney most often affected
- Most damage reversible; some permanent

WHEN TO REFER

- Complex cases of salicylate poisoning require hemodialysis, excellent (although invasive) therapy for salicylate poisoning, which efficiently removes salicylate from serum while restoring fluid, electrolyte, acid-base homeostasis. Indications for hemodialysis: shock, noncardiogenic pulmonary edema, renal failure, reliable Hx acute ingestion of >450 mg/kg of salicylate, increasing serum salicylate concentrations despite appropriate treatment, clinical deterioration (ie, decreased sensorium, worsening acid-base imbalance, etc) despite appropriate treatment, serum salicylate concentration of 100 mg/dl at any time, chronic salicylate ingestion w/significant clinical manifestations even in setting of low serum salicylate concentration
- Clinical improvement w/falling serum salicylate concentration indicates recovery; clinical deterioration w/falling serum salicylate concentration indicates high salicylate concentration in brain, end organs; signals need for hemodialysis

BACKGROUND

- Asthma considered most common chronic condition of toddlers, children, adolescents, affecting 5–10% of population
- Common cause of absenteeism from school and work, ER visits, hospitalizations
- *Common manifestations:* cough (may be sole manifestation), wheeze, dyspnea
- *Most frequent triggering factors:* include viral upper respiratory tract infections, exercise, allergens (cats, house dust mites, pollen, mold), exposure to smoke
- *Asthma classified as follows: mild intermittent,* brief symptoms <2×/wk; *mild persistent,* symptoms >2×/wk but < once daily; *moderate persistent,* daily symptoms, occasional nocturnal asthma; *severe persistent,* continual symptoms, interference w/sleep, activity

CLINICAL MANIFESTATIONS

- *Cough:* repeated frequent coughing episodes occurring day and night. Most episodes triggered by upper respiratory tract infection. Cough or wheezing usually worsens w/exercise
- Wheezing and dyspnea may occur, often interfere w/sleep
- Physical examination:
  - often, examination reveals only cough w/few other findings, but some pts have frank wheezing, dyspnea
  - frequently, nasal edema, rhinorrhea present as result of upper respiratory tract infection, allergic reaction
  - some pts have eczema

LABORATORY FEATURES

- *Spirometry:* results often normal when pt asymptomatic. FEV_1 can be reduced, flow volume curve scooped out; if reduced and improvement of 10–15% or more after use of bronchodilator such as albuterol, asthma very likely
- *Peak expiratory flow rate:* normal to reduced
- Chest radiograph usually negative but may show hyperinflation
- CBC count: peripheral eosinophilia may be found

DIFFERENTIAL DIAGNOSIS

- Cystic fibrosis
- Foreign body aspiration
- Pertussis syndrome

- Gastroesophageal reflux
- Habit cough
- Pneumonitis
- Congestive heart failure
- Monitoring:
  - peak flow monitoring instituted as early as possible after diagnosis. Three zones established to help monitor and treat pts: *green zone:* normal breathing and personal best minus 20%; *yellow zone (caution):* from minus 20% of the personal best to minus 50%; and *red zone (danger):* 50% or more below personal best. Treatment plan designed for pt on basis of zones

TREATMENT

- Treatment proportional to severity of asthma
- Environmental control first step, including elimination of exposure to cigarette smoke. For pts w/specific allergic factors, reduce exposure to pets, institute precautions for house dust mites (ie, encase mattress, pillows; wash bedding in hot water). If pollen or mold allergy factor, air conditioning can be used
- Pts should have written "Asthma Action Plan" available at home for reference, used at time of flares
- All pts w/asthma should have access to bronchodilator such as albuterol
- All pts should have plan for management of acute asthma, including use of prednisone, if necessary (1–2 mg/kg/d × 5 d)

Mild intermittent asthma

- Young child (2–6 yrs of age) can start treatment w/albuterol orally w/syrup (dose, 0.1–0.2 mg/kg per dose 3×/d; maximum of 12 mg/d) or have nebulizer treatments (dose, 0.15–0.3 mg/kg q1–4 hrs). The older child or adolescent can use an albuterol metered-dose inhaler (MDI) w/spacer device

Mild persistent asthma

- Pts w/this type of asthma should already have bronchodilator (relief medication) such as albuterol, given on as-needed basis orally or by MDI or nebulizer. Anti-inflammatory agent (controlling or preventing medication) is added to treatment; should be given on regular daily basis for months
- NSAIDs:
  - cromolyn (Intal) MDI, 2 puffs 4×/d or 3 puffs 3×/d; nebulizer, one vial 4× or 3×/d; or nedocromil (Tilade), 2 puffs 4×/d; after pt well controlled, dosage can be decreased to 2 puffs 2×/d

- Corticosteroid anti-inflammatory agents (typical starting doses):
  - beclomethasone (42 μg/puff), 2–8 puffs/d; triamcinolone (100 μg/puff), 2–6 puffs/d; flunisolide (250 μg/puff), 2, 3 puffs/d; fluticasone (44 μg/puff), 2–4 puffs/d

Moderate persistent asthma

- Use of bronchodilators established; there is plan to manage flares. Dose of anti-inflammatory agents increased as follows: beclomethasone (42 μg/puff), 8–16 puffs/d; triamcinolone (100 μg/puff), 8–12 puffs/d; flunisolide (250 μg/puff), 4, 5 puffs/d; fluticasone (110 μg/puff), 2–4 puffs/d

Severe persistent asthma

- Treatment same as for moderate asthma w/higher doses of inhaled anti-inflammatory medications. Pts need more frequent, longer courses of oral corticosteroids for control. Inhaled corticosteroids: beclomethasone (84 μg/puff), 4–8 puffs/d; triamcinolone (100 μg/puff), >12 puffs/d; flunisolide (250 μg/puff), >5 puffs/d; fluticasone (110 μg/puff), >4 puffs/d
- Leukotriene modifiers: may be used for mild persistent asthma or added to inhaled steroids for moderate and severe persistent asthma

| Montelukast (Singulair) | 6–13 yrs: 5 mg at bedtime
≥ 14 yrs: 10 mg at bedtime |
| Zafirlukast (Accolate) | ≥ 12 yrs: 20 mg bid,
1 hr before meals or 2 hrs after meals |

COMPLICATIONS

- Absenteeism from school, work common
- Complications due to frequent use of oral corticosteroids, including growth failure, cushingoid features, related problems
- Pneumothorax
- Atelectasis
- Death

WHEN TO REFER

- Many pts w/mild asthma managed w/o need for referral
- If moderate to severe asthma requiring frequent use of corticosteroids, ER visits, unscheduled office visits, or hospitalizations, referral may be necessary
- For pts in whom environmental or pollen allergen suspected, referral appropriate

Daily dosages for inhaled corticosteroids

Drug	Low dose	Medium dose	High dose
Beclomethasone dipropionate, μg/puff	84–336 μg	336–672 μg	>672 μg
42	2–8 puffs	8–16 puffs	>16 puffs
84	1–4 puffs	4–8 puffs	>8 puffs
Budesonide Turbuhaler, 200 μg/dose	100–200 μg	200–400 μg 1–2 inhalations, 200 μg	>400 μg >2 inhalations, 200 μg
Flunisolide, 250 μg/puff	500–750 μg	1,000–1,250 μg	>1,250 μg
	2–3 puffs	4–5 puffs	>5 puffs
Fluticasone	88–176 μg	176–440 μg	>440 μg
MDI: 44, 110, 220 μg/puff	2–4 puffs, 44 μg	4–10 puffs, 44 μg OR 2–4 puffs, 110 μg	>4 puffs, 110 μg OR >2 puffs, 220 μg
DPI: 50, 100, 250 μg/dose	2–4 inhalations, 50 μg	2–4 inhalations, 100 μg	> 4 inhalations, 100 μg OR >2 inhalations, 250 μg
Triamcinolone acetonide, 100 μg/puff	400–800 μg	800–1,200 μg	>1,200 μg
	4–8 puffs	8–12 puffs	>12 puffs

Abbreviations: DPI, dry-powder inhaler; MDI, metered-dose inhaler.

Source: From Guidelines for the Diagnosis and Management of Asthma. National Institutes of Health, National Heart, Lung, and Blood Institute, No. 97–4051, 1997.

BACKGROUND

- *Definition:* severe asthma exacerbation unresponsive to usual treatment, including bronchodilators, corticosteroids
- Can occur w/o warning, but often presaged by progression of asthma symptoms and medication requirements
- Precipitants include viral infections, allergen exposure, environmental triggers, noncompliance w/or lack of access to medical care
- Asthma prevalence (>7% of children), mortality (342 pediatric asthma deaths in 1993) ↑ in US

CLINICAL MANIFESTATIONS

- Respiratory distress w/anxiety, wheezing, shortness of breath (unable to speak clearly), chest discomfort/pain
- ↑ work of breathing on exam, w/nasal flaring, suprasternal/intercostal retractions, use of accessory muscles (neck, stomach)
- *Auscultation:* wheezing (may be absent w/severe air-flow limitation), diminished breath sounds, prolongation of expiration. Wheezes primarily expiratory
- Tachycardia, diaphoresis, "pounding chest." May have pulsus paradoxicus (>15 mm Hg drop in systolic BP w/inspiration)

LABORATORY FEATURES

- Required:
  - peak flow measurements: <50% of pt's predicted or personal best
  - pulse oximetry: usually <90% saturated on room air
- Optional (indications: poor response to initial Tx or if indicated by exam/Hx):
  - chest x ray: marked hyperinflation, often w/areas of atelectasis. Possible findings include pneumomediastinum, pneumothorax, pneumonia
  - arterial blood gas: frequently reveals ↓ PaO_2 (<60 mm), $PaCO_2$ slightly low or normal, normal pH. Progression, danger of respiratory failure indicated by evidence of metabolic acidosis, respiratory acidosis
  - CBC, differential: WBC often mildly ↑, esp after corticosteroid use. Many children w/asthma have eosinophilia (>500 cells/mm³). On corticosteroids, eosinophil count should be ≤100 cells/mm³—if otherwise, consider noncompliance, poor responsiveness to steroid Tx
  - serum theophylline level, if drug part of child's medication regimen

DIFFERENTIAL DIAGNOSIS

- Foreign body aspiration
- Bronchiolitis (respiratory syncytial virus, adenovirus)
- Viral or bacterial lower respiratory tract infection
- Viral laryngotracheobronchitis (croup)
- Pneumothorax
- Hyperventilation syndrome
- Laryngo/tracheomalacia (infants)
- Cystic fibrosis exacerbation
- Aspiration syndromes
- Pulmonary embolism
- Cardiac/CHF
- Epiglottitis

TREATMENT

Primary (Emergency Department/Hospital)

- O_2: Administer by nasal cannula or mask to keep O_2 saturations ≥90%
- Bronchodilation:
  - albuterol solution (5 mg/ml diluted to 3 ml with saline, or 2.5 mg/3 ml unit dose) by nebulizer at dose of 0.15 mg/kg/dose (min. 2.5 mg, max. 5 mg) every 20 min for 3 doses, then 0.15-0.3 mg/kg/dose (max. 10 mg) every 1–4 hrs as needed. May give instead as 0.5 mg/kg/hr continuous nebulization (max. 10–15 mg/hr)
  - consider ipratropium bromide (0.5 mg/2.5 ml) by nebulizer at dose of 0.25–0.5 mg in combination with albuterol every 20 min for 3 doses and then every 2–4 hrs
  - if on theophylline, consider continuing po or aminophylline infusion (check level)
- Corticosteroids:
  - prednisone (tab or syrup), prednisolone (syrup), or methyprednisolone (tab or IV) 1 mg/kg every 6 hrs for 48 hrs then 1–2 mg/kg/d in 2 div doses (max. 60 mg/day) for 3–10 d (goal: peak flow 70% of personal best)
- Peak flow monitoring before and after bronchodilator treatments or at frequent intervals
- *Hydration:* Mild dehydration common: po or IV fluid resuscitation, then maintenance
- *Antibiotics:* only in case of sinusitis or probable bacterial pneumonia

Secondary

- Bronchodilation (alternatives to nebulized medications):
  - albuterol MDI (90 mcg/puff) 4–8 puffs by spacer/holding chamber every 20 min for 3 doses then every 1–4 hrs as needed May be equivalent or superior to nebulized albuterol *if used with good technique*
  - epinephrine (1:1000; 1 mg/ml) 0.01 mg/kg (up to 0.3–0.5 mg) subcutaneously every 20 min for 3 doses
  - terbutaline (1 mg/ml) 0.01 mg/kg (up to 0.25 mg) subcutaneously every 20 min for 3 doses then every 2–6 hrs as needed

- Intensive care recommended for continued/worsening work of breathing and distress, hypoxia, peak flow <50% baseline and/or pCO_2 ≥42 mm
- Intubation and mechanical ventilation for respiratory fatigue (often marked by progressive hypoxia and/or hypercarbia, metabolic acidosis, and pulsus paradoxicus >30 mm)

COMPLICATIONS

- Respiratory failure/mechanical ventilation; death
- *Atelectasis:* segmental or lobar, affecting right middle lobe most commonly
- Pneumothorax, pneumomediastinum, interstitial emphysema (esp w/mechanical ventilation)
- *Bacterial infections:* pneumonia, sinusitis
- Side effects of commonly used drugs:
  - albuterol: possible side effects include tremors, nervousness, tachycardia, arrhythmias, ↓ serum potassium, magnesium, phosphate
  - corticosteroids: immediate side effects can include hypokalemia, hyperglycemia, hypertension, mood swings/psychoses
  - methylxanthines (theophylline, aminophylline): nervousness, nausea/vomiting, diarrhea, headache, tachycardia. At high levels: arrhythmias, convulsions

PREVENTION

- Comprehensive pt/family education about asthma followed by regular healthcare visits, measurement of lung function
- Identification, avoidance of allergens and "triggers"
- Effective, simple medication regimens emphasizing correct use of inhalers, other asthma medications
- Peak flow monitoring, effective recognition of "warning signs"
- Institution of asthma care plan for school, home

WHEN TO REFER

- Acutely, if child w/status asthmaticus does not readily respond to initial Tx, then consultation w/asthma care specialist and/or intensivist recommended
- Specialist referral as part of initial or long-term outpt care encouraged if 1° care provider unable to provide key elements of asthma care (see Prevention)

WILLIAM A. PHILLIPS

BACKGROUND

- Most frequently 2–12 yrs of age. Occurs more commonly in girls than boys
- Most commonly associated w/either minor trauma, such as fall rarely severe enough to result in fracture, or with upper respiratory infection. AARS also reported following tonsillectomy and other head and neck surgical procedures. No known cause determined for some cases
- Pathogenesis unknown but thought related to increased ligamentous laxity commonly seen in children along w/more horizontal orientation of cervical facet joints of children
- Prognosis varies w/duration of symptoms prior to treatment. Usually operative intervention required only in children seen >1 mo after onset of symptoms

CLINICAL MANIFESTATIONS

- Children frequently present w/minimum discomfort but may complain of neck pain. Neurologic examination usually normal
- Torticollis (chin tilted toward one shoulder and ear tilted toward the opposite shoulder) present. Sternocleidomastoid muscle spasm noted on chin side. Differs from congenital torticollis where sternocleidomastoid muscle on ear side tight

LABORATORY FEATURES

- *Routine radiography:* flexion-extension lateral radiographs of cervical spine obtained to r/o instability. Should be active motion only and may be limited by muscle spasm. Open mouth view of odontoid attempted. Asymmetry of lateral masses both in contour and in distance from dens can be diagnostic. Unfortunately, frequently impossible to get satisfactory open-mouth view in these children. Lateral x rays of cervical spine may be suboptimal due to difficulty positioning w/head tilt. In this condition, lateral radiographs of skull may give better view of upper cervical spine
- *Dynamic CT:* also used and often preferred study. Thin slices taken from base of skull through bottom of second cervical vertebra w/head laterally rotated to each side as much as possible. As w/flexion-extension views, care taken to make this active study and not attempt to range neck more than child comfortable moving. In AARS relationship between C1 and C2 fixed and does not alter regardless of head rotation. Other studies such as MRI would be indicated only in presence of neurologic deficit

DIFFERENTIAL DIAGNOSIS

- Congenital torticollis present from birth and most often due to fibrosis in sternocleidomastoid muscle. Uncommon causes of torticollis in infants include upper cervical spine malformations seen in Klippel-Feil syndrome
- Infants can also develop condition known as benign paroxysmal torticollis w/intermittent rather than fixed torticollis. Intermittent nature of condition distinguishes it from AARS, which is fixed
- Tumors, particularly in posterior fossa or upper cervical spinal cord, as well as other disorders of CNS such as syringomyelia and Arnold-Chiari malformation, may present w/torticollis. Careful Hx and neurologic examination usually detects some abnormality. Findings in syringomyelia may be as subtle as intrinsic wasting of hands as only sign
- Fractures, osteomyelitis or neoplasms of upper cervical spine should also be considered. Careful review of radiographs should rule these out
- Fourth cranial nerve palsy can cause child to assume torticollislike position to minimize diplopia

TREATMENT

- Treatment usually determined by duration of symptoms

Duration of symptoms	Recommended treatment	Comments
<1 wk	Symptomatic treatment w/soft cervical collar	Follow-up essential
<1 mo	Chin-halter traction, either at home or in hospital supplemented w/muscle relaxant such as diazepam, 2–5 mg tid. Discontinue traction when lateral rotation to each side equal	Once torticollis resolves, soft cervical collar should be worn until full motion returns and lateral flexion-extension radiographs normal
> 1 mo	Chin-halter traction attempted but may not be successful. Halo traction w/3–5 lbs attempted. Refractory or recurrent cases may require operative stabilization by posterior arthrodesis from C1 to C2	Formal manipulative reduction can result in catastrophic injury and should not be attempted

COMPLICATIONS

- Failure to recognize AARS and manage properly increases likelihood of need for cervical arthrodesis. Recurrence rare in cases recognized and treated promptly. Arthrodesis usually successful in resolving head tilt, but also permanently limits cervical motion

PREVENTION

- AARS cannot be prevented, but delay in recognition can increase complexity of treatment and reduce chance of full recovery

WHEN TO REFER

- Majority of cases recognized early resolve w/simple treatment described above
- Long-standing cases of acquired torticollis (>1 mo) or cases where initial treatment failed usually referred

CYNTHIA GUZZO

BACKGROUND

- Common, chronic inflammatory skin disorder prevalent in childhood
- Cumulative incidence of 10%, up to 14 yrs of age
- 95% of cases apparent by 5 yrs of age
- Typically associated w/personal Hx (1/3 pts) or family history (2/3 pts) of atopy (allergic rhinitis or asthma)
- Etiology unknown but underlying abnormalities include increase in CD4+ TH2 helper T-cell subset resulting in elevated serum IgE levels; fluctuating abnormalities in beta-adrenergic responsiveness; mediator excesses associated w/histamine and prostaglandins
- *Potential exacerbating factors:* cold weather, excessive humidity and sweating, wool and lanolin exposure, house dust mites, food allergies, *Staphylococcus aureus* infection, stress
- *Outcome:* generally improves w/age resulting in resolution or more localized disease
- *Risk factors associated w/persistent adult disease:* late onset of disease, family Hx of atopy, presence of severe dermatitis

MANIFESTATIONS

- *Lesion morphology variable:* generally presents as erythematous papulovesicular eruption that progresses to scaly lichenified dermatosis 2° to persistent excoriation
- *Distribution:* facial, extensor involvement in infants; flexural (popliteal, antecubital regions), neck, facial involvement in childhood; localized disease, particularly w/affected hands, and sensitive, unstable skin in adulthood
- *Diagnostic criteria:* pruritus; chronically relapsing course; typical morphology of skin lesions; personal or family Hx atopy; duration >6 wks
- *Associated cutaneous features:* xerosis, pityriasis alba (hypopigmented macules appearing in darkly pigmented individuals after eczema resolves), palmar hyperlinearity, keratosis pilaris, recurrent conjunctivitis, Dennie-Morgan infraorbital fold

LABORATORY FEATURES

- Serum IgE level frequently elevated but not necessary to obtain for Dx if clinical presentation and Hx consistent
- Tzanck smear and culture of vesicular lesions or punched-out erosions to r/o herpes simplex
- Bacterial culture and sensitivity of the skin if *S. aureus* infection suspected and unreponsive to routine antibiotic Tx
- *Skin biopsy:* hyperkeratosis, parakeratosis, acanthosis and spongiosis of epidermis; mixed perivascular dermal infiltrate

DIFFERENTIAL DIAGNOSIS

- Irritant or allergic eczematous contact dermatitis
- Nummular dermatitis
- Psoriasis (esp palmoplantar)
- Scabies
- *Immunodeficiency syndromes in infants:* Wiskott-Aldrich syndrome, ataxia-telangiectasia, Swiss-type agammaglobulinemia
- Hyperimmunoglobulin-E syndrome
- Histiocytosis X
- Phenylketonuria

TREATMENT

- *Nonspecific measures:* limited bathing in tepid water; restricted use of mild soap; frequent application of lubricating ointment or cream, particularly after washing; use of lightweight, nonocclusive clothing; avoidance of extremes of temperature and humidity
- *Corticosteroids:* topical agents mainstay of Tx; midstrength corticosteroids (0.1% triamcinolone ointment) on body, low-potency preparations (1.0% hydrocortisone cream or ointment) on face or intertriginous regions; w/improvement reduce steroid strength and frequency to prevent side effects, esp in infants; avoid systemic steroids if possible to prevent adverse affects of chronic usage
- Antihistamines for pruritus particularly at nighttime
- *Systemic antibiotic:* control *S. aureus* colonization or infection; erythromycin, 30–50 mg/kg div q6h (max. 1 g); if ineffective, dicloxacillin, 12.5 mg/kg div q6h (max. 1 g) or culture and sensitivity followed by appropriate antibiotic
- Antiviral agents for herpes simplex infections, po limited skin lesions, IV disseminated disease (eczema herpeticum)
- *Diet:* specific food allergies can trigger flare of skin disease; frequent offending foods—eggs, milk, peanuts, soy, and wheat; avoidance of specific foods if allergy documented by careful testing
- *Phototherapy:* both ultraviolet B (UVB) and psoralen w/ultraviolet A (PUVA) effective in those unresponsive to routine regimen; UVB preferred in pediatric population; requires treatment 3×/wk over several months
- Hospitalization for severe cases

COMPLICATIONS

- Cutaneous infection rate increased: *S. aureus;* herpes simplex; dermatophytes; warts; molluscum contagiosum; chicken pox
- *S. aureus* infection: bacterial density increased in involved and uninvolved skin; produces erythema, weeping, and crusting; deeper infections uncommon
- Kaposi varicelliform eruption (eczema herpeticum): disseminated herpes simplex infection w/widespread vesicles, hemorrhage, crusting; associated w/systemic toxicity
- *Erythroderma:* diffuse erythema and scaling covering majority of body surface area; often associated w/lymphadenopathy, fever, chills, tachycardia, excessive heat loss, protein loss, bacterial sepsis; often results from irritation or infection; frequently requires hospitalization
- *Cataracts:* uncommon complication; usually in those w/severe disease

WHEN TO REFER

- Pts w/widespread disease on presentation should be referred
- Referral also recommended when Dx in doubt, if constant use of topical steroids required to control disease, when widespread disease appears or complications listed above develop

ATRIAL SEPTAL DEFECT

JACQUELINE A. NOONAN

BACKGROUND

- Relatively common cardiac malformation comprising 9% of all cardiac defects
- Female predominance; F:M ratio 2:1
- Secundum defect most common type, defect in fossa ovale
- Usually recognized after infancy
- Dx may be delayed until adulthood

CLINICAL MANIFESTATIONS

- Often asymptomatic
- Large defects may cause fatigue, rarely CHF
- Pulmonary ejection systolic murmur most common presenting sign
- To distinguish from innocent flow murmur, left chest prominence, hyperdynamic precordial activity helpful
- Widely split S_2 important clinical finding
- Mid diastolic murmur at lower left sternal border frequent additional finding

LABORATORY FEATURES

- *EKG:* right axis deviation, rsR' (incomplete right bundle branch block)
- *Chest x ray:* may appear normal or show right-sided enlargement, prominent pulmonary arteries, ↑ pulmonary vascularity
- *Cardiac echocardiogram w/color flow Doppler:* dilated right ventricle, left-to-right shunt across atrial opening definitive laboratory study
- *Cardiac catheterization:* rarely indicated unless associated cardiac problems suspected

DIFFERENTIAL DIAGNOSIS

- Innocent "flow" murmur
- Physiologic "flow" murmur (eg, anemia, fever, thyrotoxicosis)
- Mild pulmonary valve stenosis

TREATMENT

- Closure of ASD indicated if shunt >1.5 to 1
- Surgical closure carries mortality <1%, low morbidity, good long-term results
- Nonsurgical closure by catheter intervention feasible for selected pts
- Catheter treatment limited to institutions involved in clinical studies assessing results, risk of variety of devices currently available to close atrial defects

COMPLICATIONS

- Pulmonary hypertension w/Eisenmenger physiology occasional complication in unoperated adult
- Paradoxical embolus possible complication w/any atrial opening
- Atrial arrhythmias frequent in untreated adults
- Atrial arrhythmias in occasional pt in spite of successful closure of defect

WHEN TO REFER

- If atrial defect suspected, referral to pediatric cardiologist appropriate

PITFALLS

- Doppler studies so sensitive that patent foramen ovale may be misdiagnosed as atrial septal defect
- Nearly 25% newborns studied in first week of life have small (3–8 mm) atrial opening
- >90% these defects spontaneously close by 1 yr of age
- Delay closure of ASD past infancy unless significant cardiac symptoms present

ATTENTION DEFICIT/HYPERACTIVITY DISORDER

MARK L. WOLRAICH

BACKGROUND

- Some symptoms present <7 yrs of age and present for >6 mos. (Symptoms such as hyperactivity may be noted in utero)
- Symptoms continue throughout life span but most frequently diagnosed in elementary school–aged children (5–11 yrs of age)
- Prevalence 3–5%; M:F ratio: 2–4:1
- Occurs more frequently in family members but no clear genetic pattern identified
- Symptoms can be related to CNS insults, eg, closed head trauma, lead intoxication, in utero exposure to alcohol
- Prognosis worsened by inadequate treatment, dysfunctional family environment, presence of comorbid condition, eg, conduct disorder

CLINICAL MANIFESTATIONS

- *Predominantly inattentive subtype of AD/HD* categorized by "often" occurrence of at least 6/9 of following behaviors:
  - careless mistakes
  - difficulty sustaining attention
  - seems not to listen
  - fails to finish tasks
  - difficulty organizing
  - avoids tasks requiring sustained attention
  - loses things
  - easily distracted
  - forgetful

- *Predominantly hyperactive/impulsive subtype of AD/HD* categorized by "often" occurrence of at least 6/9 of following behaviors:
  - hyperactivity: fidgeting, unable to stay seated, moving excessively (restless), difficulty engaging in leisure activities quietly, "on the go," talking excessively
  - impulsivity: blurting answers before questions completed, difficulty awaiting turn, interrupting/intruding on others, (meeting criteria on both dimensions)
- *Combined subtype of AD/HD* categorized by "often" occurrence of at least 6/9 of behaviors in each of dimensions

LABORATORY FEATURES

- No laboratory tests or neuroimaging of clinical benefit in making Dx
- Hearing, vision need to be screened
- Continuous performance tests not diagnostic by themselves, not required for Dx
- Most children require psychological testing to help define comorbidity
- Parent and teacher behavior rating scales aid in Dx management

DIFFERENTIAL DIAGNOSIS

- Anxiety or mood disorders
- Learning disabilities
- Absence seizures
- Pervasive developmental disorder

COMORBID CONDITIONS

- Learning disabilities
- Oppositional defiant or conduct disorder
- Anxiety or mood disorders
- Language and communication disorders
- Developmental coordination disorder
- Tourette syndrome or chronic tic disorder
- Generalized unresponsiveness to thyroid hormone

TREATMENT

- Appropriate treatment requires multimodality approach
- Physicians need to work in coordination w/pt's school program
- Psychopharmacologic treatment predominantly w/stimulant medications
  - methylphenidate—start 5 mg, ↑ max. of 0.6–0.8 mg/kg/dose 2–3×/d
  - dextroamphetamine—start 2.5 mg, ↑ max. 0.3–0.4 mg/kg/dose 2–3×/d
  - mixed salts of amphetamines, start 5 mg ↑ max. 0.3–0.4 mg/kg/dose, 1–2×/d ↑ max. 112.5 mg usually 1×/d
- Behavior modifications programs at school, home
- Social skills training

WHEN TO REFER

- Presence of significant cormobidity
- Significant family dysfunction
- Inadequate response to treatment

BACKGROUND

- Biologically based, heterogeneous, CNS disorder, often idiopathic, sometimes associated w/specific genetic (eg, Fragile X syndrome, tuberous sclerosis, phenylketonuria) and nongenetic (eg, congenital rubella, perinatal complications) conditions
- Genetic influences strongly implicated; risk of recurrence in siblings estimated 3–5%
- Onset usually occurs <3 yrs of age, typically by 18–24 mos. Children w/higher functioning autism (eg, Asperger syndrome) may not be detected until school age
- *Prevalence:* estimated 4–20/10,000 depending on inclusion criteria
- *M:F ratio:* 3–4:1

CLINICAL MANIFESTATIONS

- *Triad of dysfunctions:* qualitative impairments in (1) reciprocal social interaction and (2) verbal and nonverbal communication; (3) restricted range of activities/interests (see table for examples)
- Some experts prefer term "autism spectrum disorder," highlighting broad range of function
- Mental retardation ~75%
- Seizures ~15–35%
- *Other variable features:* unusual sensory responses, short attention span, emotional lability, occasional "savant" skills (eg, hyperlexia, high-speed math calculations)
- Showing or accepting affection w/familiar people does *not* r/o autism

Examples of clinical features of autism

Impaired social interaction	Verbal and nonverbal communication dysfunction	Restricted, repetitive interests and behaviors
• poor eye contact • little or no interest in establishing friendships • difficulty w/reciprocal social interaction • limited pretend play	• diminished or absent verbal expression or gestures; poor comprehension of others' speech and body language • when child verbal, language often stereotyped, echolalic, or rote • ineffective "pragmatics" of initiating/sustaining conversation	• perseveration or preoccupation w/certain topics; • restricted interests (eg, weather, schedules) • preference for routines; need for sameness • fascination w/parts of toys, rather than usual function of toy • stereotypic behaviors (e.g. hand flapping)

LABORATORY FEATURES

- Most cases have no identifiable etiology. Selective tests should be considered, but none universally indicated
- Hearing testing always part of initial workup
- Karyotype, DNA study for Fragile X, metabolic testing, EEG may be appropriate when indicated by specific clinical, historical features
- Brain imaging generally *not* helpful, unless additional symptoms coexist

DIFFERENTIAL DIAGNOSIS

- Autism considered (*DSM-IV,* 1994) a subcategory of Pervasive Developmental Disorder ("PDD"). Other PDD conditions include:
  - Asperger syndrome: form of high-functioning autism
  - Rett syndrome: neurodegenerative disorder of females
  - childhood disintegrative disorder: later onset of autistic symptoms
  - PDD-NOS (PDD—Not Otherwise Specified): subthreshold or atypical PDD
- Non-PDD conditions to consider:
  - hearing impairment
  - mental retardation
  - specific language disorders
  - extreme shyness
  - social deprivation
  - obsessive-compulsive disorder
  - Tourette syndrome
  - disorders of attention
  - other learning disorders

MANAGEMENT

- Help family build on child's strengths and provide structured, predictable environments
- Refer child and family for appropriate evaluative, educational, treatment, support services/resources (see "When to Refer"). Educational services should emphasize communication, socialization. Interventions tailored to identified needs, not simply to diagnosis of "autism"
- Behavioral management counseling to decrease symptoms, improve social interaction
- Psychopharmacological treatments sometimes helpful for targeted symptoms (eg, self-injurious behaviors, compulsive behaviors, hyperactivity/short attention span, aggression), but rarely affect core features of autism. Careful monitoring of side effects necessary
- Parent involvement w/national and local family support/advocacy groups (eg, Autism Society of America, Bethesda, MD; 800-328-8476)
- Resources for parents (eg, Siegel, B: *The World of the Autistic Child.* Oxford University Press, 1996)

PROGNOSIS

- Lifelong disorder w/changing nature and severity of symptoms over time
- Documented advantages to early Dx and referral for services
- IQ and educational intervention influence adult functioning, degree of independent living
- Higher functioning autistic adolescents at risk for secondary depression

WHEN TO REFER

- As soon as autism suspected, referral to interdisciplinary team of professionals w/expertise in autism indicated for full diagnostic assessment, intervention recommendations. Periodic reassessments helpful as developmental needs change
- Mental health professionals can help teach parents behavioral management techniques, provide social skills training, counsel stressed parents or siblings when needed, help treat secondary depression in higher functioning autistic adolescents
- Referral to child psychiatrist or developmental pediatrician helpful when complex psychopharmacological treatments considered

BACKGROUND

- *Two forms:* transient (most frequent) and chronic
- Age of onset in first 4 yrs of life in majority of transient, <50% chronic
- Conflicting reports on M:F ratio. Males more frequent and less likely chronic
- Follows viral illness, mycoplasma infection, immunizations, or drugs (rare in children)
- *Underlying diseases:* (F>M) SLE, JRA, or lymphomas; (M = F) HIV infection
- *Recovery:* transient—most recover in 3–6 mos; chronic—persists for yrs
- *Mortality:* 9–19% acutely from severe anemia or hemorrhage w/thrombocytopenia; higher in chronic cases and due to underlying disorder

CLINICAL MANIFESTATIONS

- Acute tiredness, pallor, jaundice, dark urine, abdominal pain, sometimes fever. Severe cases: tachycardia, tachypnea, or shock. Slower onset suggests chronic course
- Mild hepatosplenomegaly common in both forms
- Skin may have livedo reticularis after cold exposure

LABORATORY FEATURES

- *Anemia:* Hct <20% in most
- *Reticulocytes:* elevated in half, may be decreased initially
- *Platelets:* associated thrombocytopenia (Evan syndrome) rare
- *WBC count:* usually normal or elevated
- *Peripheral smear:* spherocytes, polychromasia, nucleated RBC, rarely phagocytosis of RBC by macrophages, rouleaux formation
- *Bone marrow:* not usually indicated; erythroid hyperplasia common
- *Serologic tests:* Direct Coombs' Test for IgG, complement (C3), and IgM. "Warm agglutinin" = IgG ± complement; "cold agglutinin" = IgM + complement. Note: these tests may be negative initially; should be repeated. May need to order a more sensitive (radiolabeled) method or test for IgA-mediated hemolysis
- *Other:* Cold agglutinin titer (be sure to store blood at 37° C to prevent false negative result), antinuclear antibody (Lupus "panel"), complement, antiviral titers
- Sedimentation rate not indicated: it could be abnormally elevated by anemia

DIFFERENTIAL DIAGNOSIS

- Drug-induced hemolysis or secondary immune reactions
- Hemolytic uremic syndrome
- Collagen vascular disease
- Hepatitis
- Blood group incompatibility
- Aplastic anemia
- Malignancy
- Paroxysmal nocturnal hemoglobinuria

TREATMENT

- Principal options include no treatment, corticosteroids, IV gamma globulin, or in emergency, transfusion of washed, packed red cells
- *No treatment:* when anemia is mild such that pulse and respiratory rate not above normal for age and when treatment of underlying disease can control manifestation
- *Warmth:* if IgM-mediated, avoid cold environments, food
- *Corticosteroids:* best with IgG-mediated hemolysis: 2–10 mg/kg/d. Usually works within 5 wks of starting. When pt responds, begin *gradual* taper over several wks or months. Use qOd dose as soon as possible. May require high doses (30 mg/kg/d) for IgM-mediated, or IgG type unreponsive to lower doses. Consider other Tx if pt requires >10–25 mg/d
- *Intravenous gamma globulin:* when IgG-mediated form steroid unresponsive. Use 0.5–1 gm/kg/d × 5 d. May need to repeat in 3–4 wks
- *Red cell transfusions:* for emergency stabilization. Difficult because of common antibodies. Tell blood bank to get "most compatible" units and wash (to remove complement). Consider steroids and benadryl. Keep well hydrated. Monitor closely for renal complications. *If IgM-mediated, use blood warmer on infusion line*
- *Splenectomy:* indicated for persistent hemolysis unresponsive to steroids and immunoglobulin or other Tx, esp when toxicity of steroids is a major concern. Response rate: 5-–70%, may only be transient because liver is also site of hemolysis. Need *pneumococcal, hemophilus, and meningococcal* immunizations before splenectomy and penicillin prophylaxis postsplenectomy
- *Alternative therapies:* plasmapheresis, immunosuppressive therapy including cytostatic agents (6-mercaptopurine, cyclophosphamide, chlorambucil, vincristine, vinblastine), cyclosporine, danazol

COMPLICATIONS

- Steroid-associated toxicity
- Transfusion-associated toxicity
- Postsplenectomy sepsis
- Associated thrombocytopenia w/hemorrhage

WHEN TO REFER

- Pt hemodynamically unstable: elevated pulse and respirations from anemia
- Mild case initially controlled by steroids stops responding
- When Dx in doubt
- Referral generally indicated

	Transient	**Chronic**
Onset	Sudden—hours or days	Slowly—days or wks
Age	Most 2–4 yrs of age	More <2 yrs or >12 yrs
Prodome infection	Common	Rare
Hemoglobinuria	Common	Rare
Diagnosis	Anemia, reticulocytosis, + Direct Coombs' Test	Same
Type of + serology	Most IgM +	>85% IgG, no complement
Other labs	↑ Indirect bilirubin, ↑ BUN	Same
Steroid response	Good if IgG mediated; poor if IgM mediated	Inconsistent—may work initially or require high doses

BACKGROUND

- *Balanitis:* inflammation of glans; posthitis: inflammation of prepuce (foreskin); balanoposthitis: inflammation of both glans and prepuce
- Most common "penile problem" seen in male children; rarely seen in females (who have a fold of skin akin to prepuce over glans of clitoris)
- 5- to 10-fold more common in uncircumcised compared to circumcised males
- Occurs throughout childhood and adulthood; although likely underreported, at least 6–16% uncircumcised boys have balanoposthitis during childhood
- Likely due to several factors: poor genital hygiene, presence of smegma and epithelial debris, warm, moist environment, maceration, opportunistic organisms
- Infectious agents associated w/balanoposthitis include *Candida albicans, Staphylococcus aureus,* groups A, D nonhemolytic streptococci, groups A, B beta-hemolytic streptococci, several gram-negative enteric organisms. In sexually active adolescents and adults, sexually transmissible organisms that cause balanoposthitis include *Trichomonas vaginalis, Chlamydia trachomatis,* human papilloma virus, syphilis, mycoplasmas, and *Gardnerella vaginalis*
- Balanoposthitis may be presenting symptom of diabetes mellitus
- *Recovery:* in >95% essentially self-limited cellulitis that responds to topical antibiotic ointments, oral antibiotics, good hygiene

CLINICAL MANIFESTATIONS

- Pain, erythema, edema, dysuria, urinary frequency, occasionally fever, pruritis
- Malodorous, purulent discharge may be present; occasionally, discharge may be serosanguinous
- Erosions, ulcerations occur
- Balanoposthitis secondary to group A, beta-hemolytic streptococci has been associated w/concurrent perianal streptococcal dermatitis

LABORATORY FEATURES

- *Streptococcal antibody titers:* elevated if group A, beta-hemolytic streptococcus causative organism

- *Culture:* discharge may yield single etiologic agent or multiple organisms
- WBC count and differential: generally normal
- *Urinalysis:* WBCs and RBCs often present; if underlying diabetes mellitus, may be glucosuria
- *Other:* other studies considered when trying to identify etiologic agent:
  - KOH smear to examine for budding yeast, hyphae
  - Gram stain
  - wet mount prep to examine for trichomonas
  - if adolescent affected or if suspicion of sexual abuse, consider diagnostic studies for sexually transmissible organisms

DIFFERENTIAL DIAGNOSIS

- Allergic dermatitis
- Seborrheic dermatitis
- Edema, inflammation 2° hair or thread wrapped around sulcus of corona of glans
- Irritant dermatitis from detergent or soap retained under prepuce
- Mechanical trauma from normal genital manipulation common in young children
- Recently (<1 wk) circumcised penis commonly demonstrates edema and erythema of wound site, as well as yellow (nonpurulent) exudate over surface of glans
- In females, consider vaginitis 2° to foreign body, infection
- Urinary tract infection
- *Balanitis xerotica obliterans:* chronic, sclerosing, atrophic disorder of glans penis and preputial skin. Begins as erythematous lesions, which eventually form thickened white plaques. Histologically resembles lichen sclerosus et atrophicus, may be precursor of squamous cell carcinoma of penis
- Fixed drug reactions have predilection for glans penis, esp those due to tetracycline, sulfonamides

TREATMENT

- Mild to moderate balanoposthitis (localized erythema, edema, minimal discharge): topical antibacterial ointments (or topical antifungal agent if KOH smear or culture indicative of candidal infection), oral antibiotics for 7–10 d (amoxicillin or erythromycin appropriate initial agents pend-

ing culture, sensitivity results), warm soaks, attention to local hygiene
- Severe balanoposthitis (cellulitis spreading proximally up shaft of penis or beyond, profuse discharge, Sx systemic disease): broad-spectrum parenteral antibiotic Tx
- Dorsal slit of foreskin may relieve severe edema
- In adolescents, if causative organism trichomonas, candida, or other probable sexually transmitted agent, sexual partners should be investigated, treated
- Circumcision prevents recurrent balanoposthitis

COMPLICATIONS

- Recurrent balanoposthitis may cause scarring, fibrosis which leads to pathologic phimosis
- <5% may progress to more diffuse cellulitis, which can spread to perineum or abdominal wall and may cause life-threatening bacteremia (a toxic shock–like illness, staphylococcus scalded skin syndrome, etc)
- Potential for poststreptococcal sequelae such as acute glomerulonephritis
- Severe edema associated w/untreated balanoposthitis may cause acute urine outflow obstruction or ischemia of glans
- Gangrenous balanoposthitis is result of anaerobic fusospirochetal infection of glans. A profuse, malodorous discharge present. Gangrenous changes may occur in both glans and shaft of penis

WHEN TO REFER

- Most pts managed w/o referral
- Refer if either balanitis xerotica obliterans or gangrenous balanoposthitis suspected
- Refer if urine outflow obstruction suspected (2° edema or scarring) or if disorder fails to respond readily to initial management
- Refer if circumcision recommended or requested

BACKGROUND

- *Definition:* no lumen exists in some portion of extrahepatic biliary tree; excludes loss of intrahepatic bile ducts w/intact extrahepatic biliary tree
- Usually presents as asymptomatic cholestasis during infancy
- Incidence in range of 1:8,000–20,000 live births
- Etiology and pathogenesis not well defined
- Fatal in 1–2 yrs, median 12 mos, prior to development of hepatic portoenterostomy (Kasai procedure)
- Rare occurrence in subsequent siblings; may be discordance in twins

CLINICAL MANIFESTATIONS

- Jaundice during infancy; stools become acholic (may have yellow coating)
- Hepatomegaly early; splenomegaly later
- Usually full term w/normal birth weight
  - initially normal growth and development w/only 10% having insignificant failure to thrive
- When laterality sequence present—*assume* Dx:
  - associated common anomalies include abdominal situs inversus; intestinal malrotation; anomalies of portal vein, hepatic vein, inferior vena cava; cardiovascular defects; polysplenia, asplenia
- Other common anomalies include urinary system, small bowel atresia

DIAGNOSIS

- Helpful tests or procedures:
  - fractionated bilirubin w/elevation of conjugated or direct form
  - hepatobiliary scintography 4 d after phenobarbitol 10 mg/kg/d: excretion into bowel r/o complete biliary obstruction; nonexcretion does not rule in extrahepatic atresia
  - percutaneous or open liver biopsy demonstrating bile duct and ductular proliferation w/minimal giant cell transformation and extramedullary hematopoiesis; indeterminant when significant giant cell transformation and/or extramedullary hematopoiesis present. Accuracy up to 95%
  - demonstration of bile contents by duodenal aspiration or string test
  - lack of biliary tree by inspection or no excretion in bowel by cholangiogram
- Misleading tests or procedures:
  - routine liver tests
  - liver ultrasound
  - endoscopic retrograde cholangiography

DIFFERENTIAL DIAGNOSIS

- Infections:
  - viral—TORCH; rarely A, B, C, D, E hepatitis viruses
  - bacterial—urinary tract infection; sepsis
- Genetic:
  - alpha-1-antitrypsin deficiency
  - progressive familial intrahepatic cholestasis (Types I, II, III)
  - arteriohepatic dysplasia (Alagille syndrome)
  - cystic fibrosis
- Less common:
  - galactosemia; fructosemia; tyrosinemia
  - sphingomyelin—cholesterol lipidosis, bile acid, peroxisomal disorders
  - cholestasis w/lymphedema (Aägenaes syndrome)
  - trisomy 21, 17–18
- Choledochal cyst, bile duct perforation, stenosis (focal)
- Inspissated bile syndrome from hemolytic anemia
- Neonatal hepatitis (unknown etiology in association with hypopituitarism)

TREATMENT

- Hepatoportoenterostomy preferably <8 wks of age; forget >4 mos of age. Cure—*rare* because of progressive intrahepatic disease exacerbated by cholangitis. When successful, serum bilirubin will normalize. Ten-year survival up to 90%—*if* bilirubin returns to normal
- Potentially helpful:
  - choleretics or anti-inflammatories: steroids, Actigall, phenobarbitol
  - prophylactic sulfamethoxazole-trimethoprim (minimal data)

CURE

- Liver transplantation—85% 2 yr survival

WHEN TO REFER

- As early as possible when initial screening tests for infantile cholestasis not diagnostic—ie, *within 1 wk of detectable cholestatic jaundice*
- For liver transplantation evaluation:
  - failure of portoenterostomy or too late for Kasai procedure to be done
  - persistent cholestasis or pruritus
  - recurrence of elevated bilirubin after normalization
  - failure to thrive
  - cholangitis
  - complications of portal hypertension

HELPFUL MEDICAL THERAPIES

- Vitamins K, D, E, A
- Medium-chain triglycerides; medical gastroesophageal reflux regimen
- Actigall, rifampin for pruritus
- Diuretics for ascites
- Prophylactic penicillin to prevent sepsis

HELPFUL INTERVENTIONAL THERAPY

- Banding of esophageal varices for bleeding

BITES, DOG AND CAT

STEPHEN C. ARONOFF AND DAVID M. SHERMAN

BACKROUND

- 1–2 million bites/yr, $30 million/y, 1% all ER visits
- Dog bites account for 80–90% bites w/25 fatalities/y
  - most common complication functional damage
- Cat bites account for 5–10% bites
  - most common complication infection

CLINICAL MANIFESTATIONS

- Dog bites:
  - usually occur on extremities (50–80%), w/head and neck involved 15–30%
  - in victims < 4 yrs of age, 60% bites involve head and neck; associated w/higher mortality rate
  - seemingly minor neck injuries may be associated w/significant underlying vascular damage
  - apparently superficial puncture wounds, esp to hands and feet, may have underlying tendon, nerve, bone, joint injury
- Cat bites:
  - predominantly puncture wounds

LABORATORY FEATURES

- Cultures, Gram stains of uninfected wounds not predictive of development of infections
- Clinically infected bite wounds should have aerobic and anaerobic cultures obtained from within wounds. Notify lab it is bite wound culture, and ask that sample be kept for at least 7–10 d because some bite wound pathogens slow growing
- Radiographs indicated in dog bites to head and face to r/o facial fractures and penetration of skull, and when foreign matter or involvement of other bones suspected

TREATMENT

- Cleanse w/1% povidone-iodine solution; use local or regional anesthesia if necessary
- Irrigate forcefully w/at least 200 mL sterile saline using 18–19 gauge needle/catheter and 30–60 cc syringe, or water pick
- Explore all wounds for underlying tendon, bone, joint, nerve involvement
- Debride devitalized tissue
- Primary closure acceptable for dog bites resulting in nonpuncture wounds <24 hrs old that do not involve hands, feet, joints, and have occurred in immune-competent host. Cosmetically important cat bites to face can be closed if no sign of infection
- Delayed closure recommended for all other cat bites; puncture wounds; all hand, foot, joint injuries; wounds >24 hrs; clinically infected wounds
- Elevate all wounds, esp those involving hands, joints
- Rabies and tetanus prophylaxis as indicated
- Prophylactic antibiotics indicated for all cat bites; delayed closures; hand, foot, joint wounds; bites seen >8 hrs after injury; severe crush injuries; bone or tendon involvement; immunocompromised individuals, including diabetics
  - *drugs of choice:* Augmentin (amoxicillin/clavulanate) 40 mg/kg/d div bid; cefuroxime 30 mg/kg/d div bid
  - *if penicillin allergic:* trimethoprim/sulfamethoxazole 5 cc susp./10 kg, each dose bid
- Follow up all wounds, esp those w/sutures, in 48 hrs

COMPLICATIONS

- Infectious:
  - local wound infections: 5% dog bites, 30–50% cat bites
  - other infections include osteomyelitis, tenosynovitis, septic arthritis, abscess formation
  - asplenic, immunocompromised individuals suffering dog bites can develop overwhelming sepsis from *C. canimorsus* and *P. multocida*
  - rabies, tetanus rare
- Noninfectious:
  - cosmetic and functional damage
  - hemorrhagic shock
  - intracranial hemorrhage
  - undetected vascular injury, esp w/dog bites to neck

PREVENTION

- Children, particularly young children, should be supervised when interacting w/animals
- Avoid dog breeds responsible for majority of fatal attacks, ie, German shepherds, Chows, Rottweilers, pit bulls, and animals w/Hx aggression
- Spay/neuter all dogs
- Teach children to never approach unknown dog, not to run away or scream, and not to disturb dog sleeping, feeding, caring for puppies
- Report stray animals to authorities

WHEN TO REFER

- Significant injuries to hand, foot, face, head, neck
- Suspected bone, joint, tendon, nerve involvement
- Injuries requiring complicated repairs, grafting
- Extensive infection

CHARLES M. GINSBURG

BACKGROUND

- Precise incidence unknown
- Equal incidence in children <2 yrs of age; male predominance during preschool and elementary school years; <12 yrs of age, two-thirds human bites occur in females
- Majority occur in late afternoon, early evening
- In contrast to adults who often seek delayed medical attention for bite injuries, >75% of childhood victims brought for medical care within 12 hrs of injury
- Similar to adults, upper extremities most common bite site; however, proportion of face, neck bites larger in children than adults
- Incidence of infection, other complications after human bites larger than from dog, cat bites

CLINICAL MANIFESTATIONS

- Three types of wound injuries:
  - abrasions: most common, two-thirds of injuries in children
  - punctures: most serious; generally clenched-fist injuries
  - lacerations: least common
- Two major mechanisms of injury:
  - occlusional:
    ○ most common
    ○ child or sexual abuse considered when multiple occlusional injuries present, particularly in young children
  - clenched fist:
    ○ most serious human bite injury; large incidence of infection
    ○ occur when closed fist of individual meets teeth of another (fights, contact sports)
    ○ most commonly injure third metacarpophalangeal joint of dominant hand
    ○ generally small (3–8 mm)
    ○ almost always ignored until Sx of infection present

DIFFERENTIAL DIAGNOSIS

- Differentiating between child abuse and accidental injury
- Differentiating between infected and noninfected wounds

LABORATORY FEATURES

- Routine hematologic and radiologic studies generally unncessary
- *Wound cultures:* because of large incidence of infection following human bites, samples for aerobic, anaerobic bacterial cultures obtained from clinically infected wound, puncture wounds, wounds >8–12 hrs old
- Bacteriology of human bite wounds reflect mouth flora of humans; larger incidence of anaerobic bacteria recovered from human bite wounds than from animal bite wounds
- *Eickenella corrodens* isolated from 25% of human bite wounds

TREATMENT

- *Cleansing:* all wounds meticulously cleansed w/1% providone-iodine solution
- *Irrigation:* mainstay of therapy; wounds thoroughly irrigated w/copious amounts normal saline. Pressure irrigation avoided in deep puncture wounds
- Two controversial areas:
  - antibiotic prophylaxis: although commonly used, no clear evidence of efficacy, particularly for noninfected abrasional injuries, simple lacerations that come to medical attention within 6–8 hrs after injury. Although not proven effective for preventing infection, antibiotics considered for pts w/deep puncture wounds, clenched-fist injuries, lacerations involving deep subcutaneous tissue
  - primary wound closure: increasing evidence primary closure of noninfected wounds, regardless of anatomic site, does not increase likelihood of secondary bacterial infection provided wound meticulously irrigated, debrided prior to closure
- Radiographs obtained when suspicious of tooth fragment in the wound, on clenched-fist injuries, on occlusional bite of hand severe enough to have invaded bone or joint space, when soft tissue infection present in close proximity to bone, joint
- Moderate or severe injuries of extremities elevated for first 24 hrs
- Immobilization of hand in position of function considered for moderate to severe hand wounds

COMPLICATIONS

- Potential for soft tissue, bone, joint infection w/flora from human mouth
- Cosmetic deformity

ANTIMICROBIAL THERAPY

- *Oral:* amoxicillin/clavulanate potassium (Augmentin) 20–40 mg/kg/d div q8h × 5–7 d
- *Parenteral:* ampicillin/sulbactam (Unasyn) 100–200 mg/kg d div q6h

WHEN TO REFER

- All puncture and infected bite wounds of hand evaluated by hand surgeon
- Surgical consultation obtained for infected wound
- Moderate to severe wounds of face evaluated by plastic surgeon

BITES, INSECT, AND STINGS

PAUL A. CARBONARO AND CAMILA K. JANNIGER

BACKGROUND

- Insects that commonly bite or sting: lice, flies, mosquitoes, bedbugs, fleas, bees, wasps, ants
- Children at increased risk due to greater outdoor exposure and more frequent close contacts (eg, schools, nurseries) w/insects that cause infestations
- *Papular urticaria,* a pruritic, papular, hypersensitivity reaction to arthropods (including insects), arthropod products, most commonly seen in infants and children
- Insect bites medically important because of possible disease transmission, anaphylaxis, superinfection of excoriations

CLINICAL MANIFESTATIONS

- Often multiple, grouped or linear, pruritic, erythematous papules, occasionally w/a central punctum; however, insect bites may present as vesicles, bullae, any combination
- Bites more often found on areas of skin not covered by clothing
- Commonly occur after outdoor exposure in summer mos, or discovered upon arising in morning
- Often multiple household members affected
- Presence of household pet increases suspicion of insect bites
- Papular urticaria presents as diffuse, intensely pruritic, papular eruption, most often on arms, trunk, legs; frequently, excoriations become secondarily impetiginized
- Pruritus of scalp and pubic area in case of head lice and pubic lice, respectively, w/presence of "nits" or eggs in both cases; local lymphadenopathy may be present
- Stings from bees, wasps, ants typically produce intense local pain, w/"wheal-and-flare" reaction (raised, erythematous papule w/surrounding halo of erythema)
- Pts stung by bees, wasps, ants may present w/large, local, indurated areas that persist for days
- Pts may present w/frank anaphylaxis

LABORATORY FEATURES

- Blood work usually unnecessary
- Skin scrapings may be very useful in detection of scabies mite (member of the class Arachnida)

DIFFERENTIAL DIAGNOSIS

- Variety of differential diagnoses exist, given enormous variety of insects and other arthropods and various responses to bites and stings; some include:
  - contact dermatitis
  - varicella (in case of papular urticaria)
  - impetigo
  - urticaria
  - linear IgA bullous dermatosis
  - noninsect bites/infestations (mites, spiders, ticks)
  - delusions of parasitosis
  - neurotic excoriations
  - lichen simplex
  - folliculitis
  - drug eruption
  - tinea capitis/corporis
  - seborrheic dermatitis (in case of head lice)

TREATMENT

- Wounds should be cleansed thoroughly w/soap and water; most important in fly bites, as flies vectors for multitude of infectious agents
- Pruritus controlled w/topical agents containing phenol, camphor, menthol; topical corticosteroids used to quickly control pruritus; systemic antihistamine also of benefit; sedating properties of first-generation antihistamines helps control nocturnal pruritus
- Bacterial superinfections treated empirically w/antistaphlococcal/antistreptococcal, such as mupirocin 2% ointment, applied 2–4×/d, several d
- Lice treated w/insecticides such as malathion 0.5% lotion, permethrin 0.5% lotion, 1% gamma-benzene hexachloride lotion for pubic lice; treatment repeated after 1 wk to kill surviving lice; scabies mite also eliminated w/5% permethrin cream; most importantly, all household contacts treated in case of infestations; clothing and bedding washed w/hot water; pets may need to be treated by veterinarian for fleas, mites, other infestations
- Stings of bees, wasps, ants treated w/simple analgesics, antihistamines. Large, local reactions may additionally require short course of oral corticosteroid. Anaphylaxis due to insect stings treated like anaphylaxis due to any cause: children require 0.01 ml epinephrine per kg body weight, not exceeding 0.3 ml per dose, SubQ, q20 min as needed

COMPLICATIONS

- Anaphylaxis due to injected venom
- Disease transmission, eg, viral encephalitides
- Bacterial superinfection at site of excoriation

WHEN TO REFER

- Most insect bites treated empirically and successfully; treatment failure may indicate that one not dealing w/insect bites
- Important component of treatment includes eradicating source of pests; pts may need help of veterinarian for proper pet treatment
- Bronchospasm, angioedema, nausea, vomiting should prompt referral to local ER

SHAUL SOFER

BACKGROUND

- Scorpion sting common medical hazard in various parts of world; common in southwestern US
- Sting may cause severe envenomation that may lead to organ failure, death
- Venom of different species varies in toxicity
- Venom complex substance containing several neurotoxins, which following the sting may rapidly enter serum and body tissues provoking severe adrenergic and cholinergic response and cell destruction
- Severity of intoxication related to amount and composition of venom as well as age and size of victims; thus infants and children more prone to severe intoxication
- Most victims presenting to well-equipped medical facility, shortly after being stung, survive, recover completely

CLINICAL MANIFESTATION

- Following sting, most victims only experience local pain at site of sting, which may vary in intensity. Others may develop general intoxication, which also varies in severity
- Sx may start within minutes after sting and may include:
  – CNS-related symptoms: irritability, tremor, muscle rigidity, nystagmus, hypothermia or hyperthermia, coma, convulsions
  – symptoms related to stimulation of sympathetic nervous system: tachycardia, hypertension, midriasis, excessive sweating, urinary retention
  – symptoms related to stimulation of parasympathetic nervous system: excessive secretions, bradycardia, hypotension, miosis, priapism in males

– GI symptoms, including abdominal pain, nausea, vomiting common and may be attributed to (transient) pancreatitis
  – Sx usually resolve within 24 hrs
- Respiratory failure occurs in ~15–20% of symptomatic children stung by most toxic species. May be of several origins: (1) acute (hypertensive) encephalopathy w/apneic episodes and bradypnea; (2) allergic subglottic swelling w/inspiratory stridor and expiratory wheeze; (3) myocardial hypokinesia w/heart failure, pulmonary edema, and cardiogenic shock; (4) acute lung injury and ARDS (rare)

LABORATORY AND IMAGING

- Leukocytosis, hyperglycemia most common laboratory findings
- Elevated CPK and SGOT, as well as mild metabolic and respiratory acidosis
- EKG may show elevated T waves and occasionally elevated P waves, S-T changes and rhythm disturbances
- In cases of heart failure and shock, echocardiography characterized by myocardial hypokinesia w/decreased fractional shortening, mitral regurgitation

DIFFERENTIAL DIAGNOSIS

- When Hx (scorpion) sting lacking, other intoxications (organophosphate compounds) and encephalopathies from other etiology considered

TREATMENT

- Pts w/local pain only may require general analgesics, cryotherapy, and occasionally local infiltration w/lidocaine. If symptoms of general intoxication do not develope within 6 hrs of arrival, pts may be discharged

- Children w/systemic intoxication given IV maintenance fluid
- Children severely agitated given sedatives (eg, midazolam) and analgesics
- Pts w/hypertension given sublingual nifedipine (0.5 mg/kg) or IV hydralazine (0.2 mg/kg)
- Respiratory insufficiency, heart failure, shock treated conventionally
- Atropine sulphate not given routinely, but considered in pts w/severe bradycardia, excessive secretions
- Specific serum immunoglobulins available in many endemic areas. Their titer, dosage, route of administration, effectiveness vary. In US, antisera not approved by FDA but used in Arizona by special action of Arizona State Board of Pharmacy

COMPLICATIONS

- Respiratory and heart failure ~15–20% of children w/general intoxication
- Brain ischemia and hemorrhage occasionally reported

PREVENTION

- Scorpions nocturnal animals. Do not attack humans. In endemic areas, wear high shoes and refrain from inserting hands between rocks and stones

WHEN TO REFER

- Infants and children should be rushed to hospital
- If >6 hrs have passed from sting and no signs of general intoxication, no need for referral or specific therapy (other than analgesics)

BACKGROUND

- Poisonous snakebites occur in ~2,500 children in North America each year
- Most poisonous snakebites in US from pit vipers
- Poisonous snakes indigenous to US are among two families: Crotalidae (or pit vipers) and Elapidae
- Snakes in Crotalidae family include rattlesnake, water moccasin, copperhead. Responsible for 99% of poisonous snakebites in US
- Coral snakes only members of the Elapidae family found in US
- Children often experience more severe symptoms than adults due to larger dose per kg injected venom
- Snake variables that affect toxicity include size of snake, amount/potency of venom
- Mortality <0.2%

CLINICAL MANIFESTATIONS

- Local symptoms may appear within minutes of envenomation:
  - intense pain
  - swelling at site of bite
  - enlargement of regional lymph nodes
  - necrosis of skin w/bullae formation, discoloration
- Systemic symptoms vary depending on species. Bites by Crotalidae family result in mostly hemorrhagic symptoms; bites by Elapidae family result in mostly neurotoxic symptoms (see table)

- Helpful tools on examination include:
  - measure distance between fang marks to judge size of snake: <8mm indicates small snake, >12mm indicates large snake
  - serial circumferential measurement of affected limb in 2–3 places q20–30 min helps judge progression of symptoms (>0.5 cm/hr considered rapid progression and requires antivenin administration)

LABORATORY FEATURES

- *CBC:* potential for thrombocytopenia, anemia
- *Coagulation studies:* potential for activation of coagulation cascade or fibrinolysis
- *Electrolyes, BUN, creatinine:* potential for nephrotoxicity

DIFFERENTIAL DIAGNOSIS

- Only 200/3,500 species of snakes worldwide poisonous. Not all poisonous snakes inject venom
- Other bites and stings

TREATMENT

- Remove clothing, jewelry on involved limb and immobilize limb
- Avoid exercise to ↓ lymphatic spread of venom
- Constriction bands (instead of tourniquets) should be applied 5–10 cm proximal to bite. Should be loose enough to maintain distal pulses (and admit a finger) but constrict venous return
- Irrigation of wound (Note: Incision, suction not generally recommended)
- Analgesia as needed
- IV access and fluids
- Tetanus as needed
- Broad-spectrum antibiotics for prophylaxis of superinfection
- Antivenin indications based on presence of systemic symptoms, laboratory abnormalities, and/or rapid progression of local signs
- Antivenin has maximal binding effects if given within 4 hrs of bite and has questionable benefit if given after 12 hrs
- Amount of antivenin given based on severity of symptoms, *not* on pt weight
- Skin testing mandatory prior to administration of antivenin (9–25% have acute hypersensitivity, including anaphylaxis). Almost universal delayed reactions such as serum sickness

COMPLICATIONS

- Compartment syndrome of affected limb (not common)
- Shock
- Life-threatening bleeding diathesis
- Respiratory insufficiency
- Renal failure

WHEN TO REFER

- If compartment syndrome suspected, surgical consultation should be sought
- Positive skin tests to antivenin warrants consultation w/a medical herpetologist

General	Hemorrhagic	Neurotoxic
Metallic taste	Oozing from bite and venipuncture sites	Drowsiness
Nausea/vomiting	Epistaxis	Slurred speech
Muscle fasciculations	Hematuria	Diplopia
Sweating	Hypotension/shock	Motor weakness/paralysis
Chills	Disorientation/coma	Seizures
Oliguria	Acute respiratory insufficiency	Coma
	Seizures	Death usually 2° to respiratory paralysis
	Death usually 2° to intracranial hemorrhage	

BROWN RECLUSE SPIDER— LOXOSCELES RECLUSA

BACKGROUND

- *Where:* central and southern US, except Pacific Northwest. In Pacific Northwest common aggressive house spider is hobo spider (Tegenaria Agrestis)
- *Environment:* nocturnal, likes hot, dry, dark, quiet areas; wood piles, rock piles, etc
- *Appearance:* shades of brown, 1–5 cm long, 25% of which is body, violin-shaped mark on cephalothorax, 3 pairs of eyes, instead of 4

CLINICAL MANIFESTATIONS

- Bite frequently unnoticed
- Toxic effects begin in 2–6 hrs
- *Effects:* local pain only to full thickness necrosis
- Progression:
  – local induration, mild pain, pruritis, occasional ring of pallor
  – erythema gives way to violaceous color over 24 hrs, then develops blisters
  – after 24–48 hrs area can expand to full thickness necrosis up to 30 cm diameter
  – eschar forms, then ulceration
- *Systemic reaction:* uncommon, delayed 24–72 hrs after bite
  – malaise, nausea, vomiting, fever, chills, arthralgias; rarely, DIC, convulsions, massive hemolysis, hemoglobinuria, renal failure, death

LABORATORY STUDIES

- Serial CBCs, w/smears to look for hemolysis
- UA—hemoglobinuria
- PT, PTT, platelets—DIC

- Focal vasculitis, thromboembolic phenomena, factitious injection

TREATMENT

- Tetanus, good wound care
- Symptomatic therapy, ice pack
- Curettage of wound, late surgical debridement
- Systemic steroids usually helpful
  – prednisone 1–2 mg/kg/d × 3 div doses

- Dapsone—seems to be effective but w/side effects, esp hemolytic reactions in neonates, G6PD deficiency; dose: 50–100 mg in adults, correspondingly smaller doses in children

WHEN TO REFER

- Children w/systemic Sx, evidence of necrosis should be considered for hospitalization/surgical evaluation

BLACK WIDOW SPIDER— LATRODECTUS MACTANS

BACKGROUND

- *Where:* continental US except Alaska
- *Environment:* warm, dry areas; under stones, logs, debris, outhouses
- *Appearance:* black w/hourglass marking in red/yellow on ventral abdomen, body up to 0.5 in diameter w/overall leg span of 2 in. Only bites of female clinically significant

CLINICAL MANIFESTATIONS

- Neurotoxin, causes release of massive amount of acetylcholine, epinephrine, norepinephrine, blocks reuptake of neurotransmitters
- *Pain:* minimal to sharp
- Bite may go unnoticed, may have two small fang marks
- *No tissue reaction!*
- 15 min–4 hrs: muscle fasciculations/ spasm, initially around bite, then spreads to regional muscle; may become generalized
- Pain peaks in 2–3 hrs, lasts 12–48 hrs
- *Symptoms:* pain, muscle spasms, parasthesias/cutaneous hyperesthesia, autonomic stimulation (sweating, increased salivation, fever, chills, urinary retention, priapism), nausea, vomiting, ptosis, headache, hypertension, dizziness. Symptoms may mimic acute abdomen. Muscle spasms may be severe enough to cause respiratory compromise
- *Delayed hypersensitivity:* 2–3 d after envenomation, intense pruritis w/or w/o ecchymosis
- Prolonged neurologic dysfunction—parasthesia, "neurasthenic syndrome"—weakness, headache, body pains, sleeplessness, fatigue; may last for several wks

TREATMENT

- Tetanus, good wound care, ice pack
- Symptomatic Tx:
  – acetaminophen
  – 10% calcium gluconate, 0.1 mg/kg q2–4h for muscle spasm/pain
  – consider narcotics/muscle relaxants
- *Specific Tx:* antivenin indicated for moderate to severe envenomations; prevents prolonged neurologic dysfunction
  – skin test first: inject 0.02 mL into, not under, skin, evaluate in 10 min; positive result: urticarial wheal surrounded by zone of erythema
  – if skin test negative, inject one entire vial IM/alternatively dilute to 10–50 mL, IV over 15 min
  – expect rapid relief within 1 hr
  – acute anaphylaxis rare, delayed serum sickness occurs but usually mild

PREVENTION

- Caution in typical environment areas for spiders. Sprays/other interventions to decrease spider population/their food sources also recommended

WHEN TO REFER

- Children requiring more than acetaminophen for pain control should be considered for hospitalization

---

BLASTOMYCOSIS

DWIGHT A. POWELL

BACKGROUND

- Uncommon infection occurring as sporadic cases or in outbreaks
- Sporadic cases occur mainly in adult males; outbreaks more often involve children, have equal distribution of males/females
- Most cases occur in north and south central, southeastern US; individuals w/outdoor exposure to wooded areas around waterways appear at highest risk of infection
- Infection follows inhalation of conidial spores of dimorphic fungus *Blastomyces dermatitidis* w/resulting pneumonitis; yeast cells may then disseminate to any other organ in body

CLINICAL MANIFESTATIONS

- Infection may remain asymptomatic, result in mild illness, or cause acute or chronic pulmonary disease w/or w/o disseminated extrapulmonary disease
- Most mild illness has been defined in context of outbreaks where individuals may experience self-limited flulike symptoms w/myalgias, arthralgias, chills, fever
- Acute pneumonia most common illness in children, presenting as fever, chills, cough, chest pain. Hemoptysis rare
- Chronic pulmonary disease most common in adults and characterized by several months of weight loss, cough, fever, night sweats
- Disseminated disease may occur w/or w/o pulmonary illness; most common sites of dissemination in children skin and bones. Infection of prostate or epididymus common in adult males

- Skin lesions usually verrucous or ulcerative. Osteolytic lesions most commonly involve long bones, ribs, vertebrae
- Infection in immunocompromised hosts, including those w/AIDS, rare, but accompanied by high incidence of meningitis or brain abscess formation

LABORATORY FEATURES

- Most common radiographic appearance of acute pneumonia lobar or segmental alveolar infiltrates. Multiple lobes may be involved. Pleural effusions present <25% of time; hilar lymphadenitis uncommon
- W/chronic lung disease cavitation or mass lesions that mimic bronchogenic carcinoma occur almost as frequently as alveolar infiltrates. Calcification following resolution of blastomycosis very unusual
- Dx confirmed by isolation of fungus from any clinical specimen; fungal growth slow, requiring up to 4 wks
- Dx probable if characteristic broad-based budding yeast cells identified in KOH or calcofluor stained smears of infected material such as sputum or pleural fluid
- No skin test available and serologic methods (complement fixation, immunodiffusion) not sensitive or specific

DIFFERENTIAL DIAGNOSIS

- *Pulmonary disease:* bacterial, mycoplasmal, chlamydial, fungal pneumonia; tuberculosis, malignancy
- *Skin disease:* pyoderma gangrenosum, *Mycobacterium marinum* infection, giant keratoacanthoma, squamous cell carcinoma
- *Bone disease:* bacterial osteomyelitis, tuberculosis, malignancy

TREATMENT

- For non-life-threatening, nonmeningeal forms of blastomycosis, itraconazole effective Tx. Adult doses: 200 mg/d × 6 mos; doses may be increased up to 400 mg/d in refractory cases. No approved pediatric dosage recommendations; some authors use 3–5 mg/kg/d
- For meningitis or other severe forms of infection, amphotericin B treatment of choice. Dose: 1 mg/kg/d IV × at least 4 wks

COMPLICATIONS

- Mortality rare w/proper Dx, Tx
- Extrapulmonary dissemination may occur in up to 80% pts, particularly if not diagnosed during acute pulmonary phase of illness

PREVENTION

- No simple preventative measures, since sporadic disease infrequent and outbreaks have not followed predictable seasonal or geographic pattern

WHEN TO REFER

- Infectious disease consultation appropriate for most cases to help establish Dx and determine proper Tx

PAULETTE MEHTA AND
JOHN R. WINGARD

BONE MARROW TRANSPLANTATION: CARE OF THE CHILD POST-TRANSPLANTATION

BACKGROUND

- *More children undergo BMT:* greater number of diseases responsive to BMT, greater numbers of stem cell sources
- *More children survive:* better HLA matching of donors, better control of graft-versus-host disease (GVHD), improved prophylaxis/treatment cytomegalovirus (CMV) infections, improving care of fungal infections

POSSIBLE CONSEQUENCES OF BMT

- Immunodeficiency for first 12 mos
- Infections (esp related to central venous catheters), CMV, candidiasis, aspergillosis, varicella-zoster virus. Sinus infections frequent
- Myelosuppression first 2–3 mos
- Growth/development delay common, less with non–total body irradiation (TBI) regimes, "catch-up" may occur
- *gonadal failure:* 50% prepubertal, 90% postpubertal girls
- Pulmonary/cardiac complications, usually subclinical
- Cataracts ↑ risk w/TBI/high-dose steroids
- *Neurologic complications:* leukoencephalopathy, learning disabilities
- ↑ *risk of secondary malignancies:* skin, lung, mouth cancers, leukemia, lymphoma, myelodysplastic syndrome, esp if treated at younger ages
- Hearing loss 2° to platinum/aminoglycoside drugs

- Bone abnormalities including avascular necrosis
- *Acute GVHD first 100 d:* skin rash, ↑ liver enzymes, diarrhea
- *After 100 d, chronic GVHD:* ↑ autoimmunity, collagen-vascular disease, wasting, rashes, joint contractures, alopecia, Sjögren sicca syndrome, lichen planus lesions in mouth, pneumonitis, bronchiolitis obliterans
- Sun exposure can activate GVHD
- Blood transfusion–derived infections
- *Graft rejection:* occasionally seen in pts w/aplastic anemia
- *Psychological complications:* anxiety, depression, drug abuse

LABORATORY FEATURES

- Immune function (eg, lymphocyte subsets) tests abnormal in first year
- Infection manifested by positive bacterial, fungal, viral cultures
- *Abnormal chest x rays:* interstitial pneumonia
- ↓ serum magnesium 2° to cyclosporine, platinum use
- laboratory features of GVHD include anemia, thrombocytopenia, auto-antibodies, typical skin, liver, GI biopsy findings
- Abnormal FSH, LH, estradiol, testosterone levels, provocative tests for GH

TREATMENT

- Mask isolation for 6 mos post-transplant
- Prompt treatment for infections

- *IV acyclovir for varicella zoster (VZ) virus infections:* first year post-transplant
- VZIG IV to seronegative pts exposed to VZ in first year post-transplant
- In-hospital treatment for interstitial pneumonias
- *PCP prophylaxis:* septra or dapsone, 6 mos post-transplant, longer if chronic GVHD
- No work/school until 3–6 mos post-transplant
- Sunblocking creams (SPF ≥15)
- Avoid barnyard animals, swimming in public pools/lakes 3–6 mos; household pets, plants OK
- Vaccinations at 1 yr (tetanus, diphtheria toxoids, inactivated polio), MMR after 2 yrs, siblings need inactivated polio vaccine
- Transfusions as needed (irradiated)
- Treat growth hormone/other hormone deficiencies
- Observation for secondary malignancies
- Endocarditis prophylaxis for dental procedures, first year post-transplant
- *Pregnancy possible post-BMT:* birth control information as needed, post-BMT ↑ risk for obstetric complications

WHEN TO REFER

- Serious infections
- GVHD/suspicious skin lesions
- Hormone deficiency/secondary malignancy

BACKGROUND

- Multiple entities
- Hx, plain x ray essential to narrow differential Dx
- X rays must be read by orthopedist familiar w/bone tumors or skeletal radiologist to avoid needless biopsy, overtreatment, improper Dx
- Benign bone tumors much more common than malignant tumors
- Children of all ages affected, but lesions have age predilections

MANIFESTATIONS

- Painful mass fixed to bone malignancy until proven otherwise. Refer urgently
- Painless mass fixed to bone usually benign
- Incidental x ray finding usually benign
- Most common presentations:
  - dull aching, gradually worsening pain
  - insidious onset
  - painless limp
- Common in benign and malignant tumors:
  - pain at rest
  - nocturnal pain
  - pathologic fracture (often no pain prodrome in benign tumors)
- Painful scoliosis often associated w/benign tumor

DIFFERENTIAL DIAGNOSIS

- *Epiphyseal lesions:* giant cell tumor (GCT), chondroblastoma:
  - lytic lesions w/poorly defined borders
- GCT:
  - Larger tumor (epiphysis and metaphysis)
  - skeletally mature pt
  - pathologic fracture into joint
- Chondroblastoma:
  - seldom >3 cm
  - speckled calcifications on x ray
- *Bone-forming tumors:* osteoid osteoma, osteoblastoma:
  - painful lesion in adolescent

- sclerotic on x ray, hot on bone scan
  - osteoid osteoma:
    - <2 cm
    - often long bones
  - osteoblastoma:
    - >2 cm
    - common in posterior spinal elements
- Eosinophilic granuloma:
  - any bone w/hematopoietic marrow
  - present as pain, pathologic fracture, deformed bone
  - punched-out holes w/o borders on x ray
  - flattened vertebral body (vertebra plana) frequent presentation
  - lateral skull x ray showing additional lesion confirm Dx; biopsy not necessary
  - may be manifestation of systemic histiocytosis
- Enchondroma:
  - common childhood hand tumor
  - pathologic fracture, deformity phalanx, metacarpal
  - expansile lesion w/speckled calcifications
- Simple (unicameral) bone cyst:
  - proximal femur, humerus, tibia most common
  - usually metaphyseal abutting growth plate
  - pathologic fracture w/o pain common; may present w/dull pain
  - slight expansion of bone, thinned cortex, fine large trabecular pattern
- Aneurysmal bone cyst:
  - arise de novo or in combination w/other tumors
  - any bone involved
  - pain and swelling w/mass common—may mimic malignancy
  - lytic, expansile; soft tissue expansion w/thin rim of bone
- Fibrous cortical defect (nonossifying fibroma):
  - incidental finding in metaphysis
  - may develop stress fracture or complete fracture
  - eccentric position in bone
- Fibrous dysplasia:

- single or multiple lesions
  - yellow or brown skin patches occur w/multiple lesions
  - multiple lesions plus skin changes, precocious puberty in girls; Albright syndrome
  - long bones, ribs, jaw, skull affected
  - pain, deformity (femoral neck), defective growth common presentations
  - defined areas of deficient cortex, sometimes w/sclerotic rim
- Osteochondroma (osteocartilaginous exostosis):
  - common
  - mass near joint, painless unless causing bursitis
  - pedunculated lesion w/cortical bone often pointing away from joint

TREATMENT

- Treatment initiated only after consultation w/an orthopedist familiar w/lesion. May not need to refer pt
- Lesions often treated by observation if no symptoms: osteochondroma, eosinophilic granuloma, simple cyst, enchondroma, nonossifying fibroma, and fibrous dysplasia. Serial x rays and exams at 3 mo intervals for 1–2 y if no change
- Lesions treated surgically: giant cell tumor, chondroblastoma, osteoblastoma, aneurysmal bone cyst
- Treatment depends on symptoms: osteoid osteoma, simple bone cyst

COMPLICATIONS

- Pathologic fracture
- Recurrence after surgery

WHEN TO REFER

- Growth of lesion, worsening of symptoms, recurrence after surgery

ROBERT SCHECHTER AND STEPHEN S. ARNON

BACKGROUND

- Intestinal colonization by *Clostridium botulinum,* almost unique to infants, leads to sustained toxemia by phenomenally potent botulinum neurotoxin. Neurotoxin causes enzymatic damage of presynaptic cholinergic motor neurons, resulting in progressive, descending flaccid paralysis most evident in cranial nerves
- Risk factors include exposure to honey (only 5% of cases), slow intestinal transit (<1 bowel movement per day)
- Breast-fed infants more likely to be hospitalized, less likely to die at home from infant botulism than formula-fed infants
- Occurs in all races during first year of life, primarily 1–7 mos of age
- *M:F case ratio:* 1:1
- Type A botulinum toxin causes most cases in western US; type B botulinum toxin predominates in eastern US. Approximately half of recognized cases occur in California;
- Mean hospital stay: 5 wks (range 0–43 wks); mean cost ~$100,000
- *Mortality:* death in hospitalized pts rare. Number of infants dying undiagnosed prior to hospitalization unknown
- *Prognosis:* full recovery in absence of hypoxic CNS injury or other severe complications
- Botulism also can occur at any age from consumption of neurotoxin in tainted food (food-borne botulism) or from toxemia caused by wound contaminated w/*C. botulinum* (wound botulism)

CLINICAL MANIFESTATIONS

- Decreased frequency of stools, which may be acutely malodorous; increased flatus
- Progressive inability to feed from weakness of latch, suck, swallow. Drooling while adequately hydrated; gurgling on pooled secretions in pharynx
- Feeble cry, persistent moaning
- Poor head control
- Flattened facial expression
- Progressive ptosis, dysconjugate gaze, ophthalmoplegia
- Generalized weakness, hypotonia
- Apnea from upper airway obstruction, eg, flexion for lumbar puncture, inadequate suctioning
- In severe cases, progressive respiratory distress, failure
- Pupillary mydriasis, sluggishness and hypo- or areflexia often lag behind other findings
- Significant variability in severity, rapidity of onset. Typical course characterized by increasing weakness during first days to weeks, followed by lengthy nadir of maximal paralysis, followed by lengthy recovery period. Within this pattern, daily mild waxing and waning of strength, tone; fatigability w/repetitive activity clinical hallmark in all types of botulism

LABORATORY FEATURES

- Routine laboratory tests unremarkable in absence of aspiration or secondary infections
- *WBC and differential:* normal unless secondary infection present
- *Hemoglobin:* appropriate for age of illness, which spans physiologic nadir
- *Serum electrolytes:* bicarbonate level reflects hydration status
- *CPK:* normal
- *Cerebrospinal fluid:* normal levels RBCs, WBCs, glucose. Protein level occasionally mildly elevated for age due to dehydration
- Identification of botulinum toxin and isolation of *C. botulinum:* contact state health department promptly to arrange testing and for (legally required) reporting of case:
  – stool sample provides highest yield, but collection limited by constipation. If pt does not defecate spontaneously or after glycerine suppository, administer enema of 30 cc sterile water (as used for feeding). Collect, refrigerate all effluent. Save, refrigerate subsequent stools for possible confirmatory testing
  – serum sample (5 cc blood) also may be requested
- Following frequently superfluous unless clinical presentation ambiguous:
  – electromyogram: yield highest in symptomatic muscles. Affected motor units may demonstrate brief small amplitude potentials (BSAPs). High-frequency repetitive nerve stimulation at 20–50 HZ may demonstrate facilitated response of >40%. Sensory nerves and conduction display normal function
  – others: imaging of brain, spinal cord; Tensilon test; muscle, nerve biopsies; chromosomal testing for spinal muscular atrophy; organic, amino acid panels

DIFFERENTIAL DIAGNOSIS

- *"Rule out sepsis":* most frequent Dx at admission
- *CNS infections:* myelitis including polio, meningo-encephalitis
- Guillain-Barré syndrome
- Immune or familial myasthenia gravis
- Spinal muscular atrophy (including Wernig-Hoffmann disease)
- Rare to nonexistent for infants: tick paralysis, Eaton-Lambert syndrome

TREATMENT

- Mainstay of treatment nutritional and respiratory support. Assistance needed depends on severity of illness (mild oral motor weakness to total flaccid paralysis)
- *Fluids and nutrition:* feeding by nasoenteral tube provides adequate fluid and nutrition while minimizing aspiration risk. Expressed breast milk preferred to maximize peristalsis, to promote bowel flora hostile to *C. botulinum,* and to provide immune factors to limit secondary infection

- *Respiratory support:* proper positioning minimizes labor of respiration, risk of aspirating oropharyngeal secretions. Place infant on back, head of bed elevated to 30 degrees, on flat surface w/thin neck roll. Half of hospitalized pts require mechanical ventilation. Meticulous care in intubation and toilet obviates tracheostomy placement
- *Constipation:* constipation often first symptom to appear, last to recede. Infrequent, hard stools often remain problem after infant returns home. Softening agent (eg, lactulose) along w/glycerin suppositories helpful to achieve soft daily bowel movements
- *Immunotherapy of botulinum toxemia:* botulinum equine antitoxin efficacious in reducing severity of botulism in adults; not given to infants because of potential allergic reactions. For information on therapy w/human Botulinum Immune Globulin (BIG), call California Department of Health Services at (510) 540-2646 (24 hr)
- Complications during hospitalization may present as increased weakness after period of stability or improvement
- *Antibiotics:* if no evidence of secondary infection, avoid use of antibiotics. Pts frequently develop secondary respiratory or urinary tract infections. Two antibiotic categories have relative contraindications: (1) aminoglycosides may increase neuromuscular blockade. (2) clostridiocidal antibiotics (beta-lactams, clindamycin) may lead to additional toxin release upon bacterial cell death. If secondary infection suspected and coverage appropriate, select trimethoprim-sulfamethoxazole, as *C. botulinum* resistant to this antibiotic
- *Hyponatremia:* one-quarter of intubated pts develop hyponatremia akin to SIADH manifesting as increased paralysis or seizures. Monitoring of I&O serum sodium helpful for early intervention. Responds rapidly to fluid restriction or additional sodium

COMPLICATIONS

- Complications during hospitalization discussed above
- *Strabismus:* dysconjugate gaze may persist after recovery; requires usual evaluation and treatment to preserve vision

WHEN TO ADMIT

- All pts at risk of progressive, life-threatening paralysis in hours to days following presentation. Observation in hospital setting appropriate until pt clearly recovered from maximal paralysis. Proximity or admission to critical care services preferable

---

All material in this chapter is in the public domain, with the exception of any borrowed figures or tables.

BACKGROUND

- Congenital lesions most frequently found in neck of children 2–10 yrs of age
- Result of epithelial remnants of the brachial clefts
- Anomalies of 1st, 2nd, 3rd, 4th brachial clefts occur, w/>95% 2nd brachial cleft derivatives
- Subsets of brachial cleft anomalies include *cyst* (isolated mass within neck w/no drainage tracts), *sinus* (saclike structure w/single drainage site, most typically to skin), or *fistula* (tract extending from intraoral cavity through to neck)
- Lesions generally change in size; often first detected after upper respiratory tract infection, which causes enlargement of mass
- Concern for complications associated w/lesions, most commonly infection, main reason for removal

CLINICAL MANIFESTATIONS

- First brachial cleft anomalies (two subtypes):
  - type I:
    - various degrees of atresia of external auditory canal
    - often begins in external auditory canal; can extend through to posterior tonsillar pillar
      - associated w/microtia or anotia
      - one-third bilateral
      - most common presentation: cystic swelling below lobule of ear
      - often detected as pit or dimple within external auditory canal
  - type II:
    - open onto anterior aspect of neck; typically above hyoid bone, anterior to sternocleidomastoid. Intraoral component ends at posterior tonsillar pillar
    - surgical treatment, particularly for type II, very difficult because of close association w/parotid gland and potential of injury to facial nerve
- Second brachial cleft anomalies:
  - opening on skin found at junction of lower and middle third of anterior border of sternocleidomastoid muscle
  - internal opening in region of tonsillar fossa
  - tract passes lateral to hypoglossal and glossopharyngeal nerves; enters superior to both
  - tract extends between internal and external carotid artery
- Third brachial cleft anomalies:
  - often indistinguishable from second cleft anomalies
  - cutaneous opening at junction of middle and inferior third of sternocleidomastoid
  - tract extends posterior to both internal and external carotid arteries between glossopharyngeal nerve and hypoglossal nerve
  - tract enters at level of piriform sinus
- Fourth brachial cleft anomalies:
  - debate regarding existence: if exist, extremely rare
  - cutaneous opening would be at same position as second, third brachial cleft anomalies. Tract would course over hypoglossal nerve, then descend to go under subclavian artery on right or under aortic arch on left. Opening would then be in either upper esophagus or pyriform sinus

LABORATORY FEATURES

- When infected, increased WBC count typical
- CT, MRI most useful in narrowing differential Dx
- Radiologic evaluation most helpful w/cystic brachial cleft anomalies
- W/fistula or sinus tract, imaging studies may not delineate lesion as collapsed tract very small in diameter

DIFFERENTIAL DIAGNOSIS

- Cervical lymphadenopathy
- Neck abscess
- Preauricular cyst
- External laryngocele
- Thyroglossal duct anomaly (more typically midline)
- Epidermal cyst
- Dermoid
- Malignancy (lymphoma most likely in children)

TREATMENT

- When acutely infected:
  - treatment similar to cervical lymphadenopathy; often difficult to distinguish between the two
  - oral antibiotics used if no fluctuance noted and pt nontoxic
  - IV antibiotics used if child has had poor response to oral antibiotics, appears toxic, or lesion rapidly enlarging
  - if fluctuance noted or imaging studies demonstrate abscess formation, surgical drainage necessary followed by appropriate antibiotic treatment based on cultures obtained intraoperatively
- When noninfected:
  - no treatment
    - generally reserved for pts ≤10 mos of age, after which anesthetic risks lower
    - occasionally type II first branchial cleft anomalies followed rather than removed if lesion seems stable and surgical risk of injury to facial nerve high
  - surgical intervention
    - generally accepted as treatment of choice for brachial cleft anomalies
    - essential to remove opening of lesion as well as entire tract to avoid recurrence

COMPLICATIONS

- Recurrent infection
- Abscess formation
- Deep neck space infection
- Airway compromise secondary to expansion
- Surgical
  - nerve injury
  - vascular injury
  - recurrence

WHEN TO REFER

- Most pts initially managed w/o referral when acutely infected and no evidence of abscess formation
- Abscess formation requires referral for surgical drainage
- Eventually almost all lesions require referral for surgical excision

BACKGROUND

• *Most common mechanism in infants:* traction of head and neck during delivery
• *Incidence:* 2/1,000 births. Risk factors: excessive lateral traction on neck, breech presentation, increased birth weight, shoulder dystocia, complicated labor, low forceps deliveries, neuromuscular hypotonia
• Prognosis: 70–95% experience full recovery

MANIFESTATIONS

• Four types of nerve injury. *Avulsion:* nerve torn at cord; no recovery. *Rupture:* nerve torn, not at cord. *Neuroma:* scar tissue around injury. *Praxis:* nerve damaged but not torn; complete spontaneous recovery. Improvement should be seen within 3 mos
• *Upper brachial plexus injury (Erb's type):* 5th, 6th cervical nerve roots. Most common type. Infant's arm extended, humerus tightly adducted and internally rotated, forearm pronated, wrist flexed. Over pull of extensors places arm in "waiter's tip" position. Fingers uninvolved, hand grasp present. Absent biceps and radioperiosteal reflexes. Unilateral Moro reflex
• *Lower brachial plexus injury (Klumpke's type):* 8th cervical, 1st thoracic nerve roots. Very rare. Infant's arm flexed, shoulder relatively normal, forearm supinated, wrist and fingers flaccid. Clawlike deformity of hand w/hyperextension of wrist and fingers may be present. Weakness of forearm extensors, flexors of wrist and fingers, and intrinsic muscles present. Triceps reflex may be diminished. Other deep tendon reflexes spared. Grasp reflex usually absent. Horner syndrome (ptosis, miosis, anhydrosis) often present due to involvement of first thoracic nerve sympathetic fibers. There may be delayed pigmentation of iris on affected side
• *Combined upper and lower brachial plexus injury:* all three trunks of brachial plexus involved. Flaccidity and no movement or reflexes on affected side. Sensory deficits accompanying injury to any segments may be variable and may be difficult to determine. Sensory loss does not correspond to extent of motor involvement; its recovery may lag return of motor function

• *Associated birth injuries:* clavicle, humerus or skull fractures, sternocleidomastoid hematoma, ipsilateral facial palsy, diaphragmatic paralysis, scalp and facial bruising, cephalhematoma, Horner syndrome, scapula winging

LABORATORY FEATURES

• Radiographs of upper limb and clavicle if fractures suspected

DIFFERENTIAL DIAGNOSIS

• Pseudoparalysis from fractures or osteomyelitis/septic arthritis
• Hemiplegia
• See associated birth injuries
• Damage to spinal cord may produce symmetrical signs of upper motor neuron lesion
• Klumpke paralysis-thoracic outlet tumors, cystic hygromas, postop cardiac surgery
• Moro reflex present w/shoulder girdle fractures differentiating pseudoparalysis from brachial plexus injury

TREATMENT

• Impossible at birth to predict who will have persistent deficits. Faster the recovery, more complete the eventual function. For maximum functional status, spontaneous recovery should be evident 2nd–6th mo of age. No spontaneous recovery by 3 mos predictive of significant residual deficits
• *First 7–10 days:* Document precise injury, follow serial physical exams; pay attention to associated injuries. Protect arm from further injury by pinning forearm in sleeve to clothing over anterior trunk. Use of orthotic devices/splinting not recommended. Arm and hand should be kept in functional position for first 7–10 days. Passive movements should be avoided due to pain from traumatic neuritis
• *10 d–2 mos:* Gentle range of motion exercises should be done at home 2–3 ×/d to maximize recovery; will decrease joint immobility, atrophy and contracture. Surgical intervention during this phase not demonstrated to achieve better results than conservative management. Infant that shows

improvement before 2 wks will achieve full recovery by 1 mo, no later than 5 mos. Infants who show partial recovery, improvement begins after 2 wks
• *2–4 mos:* Time to resolution or plateau of objective findings averages 4.5 mos. Minimal improvement of symptoms noted after 4–6 mos. 92% pts recover completely by 3 mos of age; poor prognosis likely in pt who does not demonstrate significant improvement by this time. Recovery rates 70–95%; 90–95% recover w/o surgery; ~10% need treatment-exercise therapy or surgery. Surgery may help in children who do not recover by 4 mos of age and most effective ages 4–12 mos; 50–90% show improvement. After 1 yr surgery may not be successful. Neurosurgical techniques include neuroplasty, external neurolysis, internal neurolysis, nerve grafting, neuroma dissection and removal, and direct end-to-end nerve anastomosis. Children w/persistent palsy may benefit from surgical procedures that improve activities of daily living by allowing better control of hands; indicated after 1–2 yr, when no further recovery expected. Long-term pts may require release of joint contracture, tendon transfer, other orthopedic/plastic surgery to improve function

COMPLICATIONS

• Persistent long-term brachial plexus dysfunction rare but results in muscle atrophy, decreased bone growth, joint contractures, scapular winging, weakness of shoulder girdle, persistent loss of sensation, and lack of awareness of arm by infant. Child may be left w/"Erb engram" in which flexion of elbow accompanied by abduction of shoulder

PREVENTION

• Avoid obstetrical risks

WHEN TO REFER

• To neurologist if recovery does not occur in 2 wks. Surgical nerve repair should be considered if no signs of recovery observed by 4–5 mos

BRAIN ABSCESS

BACKGROUND

- Relatively rare disease (very rare in children <2 yrs except as complication of bacterial meningitis)
- *Peak incidence:* 4–7 yrs
- M:F ratio: 2:1
- Predisposing factors:
  - contiguous infection (eg, bacterial meningitis, sinusitis, chronic otitis media, mastoiditis, orbital cellulitis)
  - cyanotic congenital heart disease
  - hematogenous spread (eg, endocarditis, bacterial pneumonia, bronchiectasis [esp in cystic fibrosis], dental abscess)
  - other (ie, hereditary hemorrhagic telangiectasia)
- Infectious agent depends on predisposing factor. Most common pathogens: streptococci (aerobic, anaerobic, and microaerophilic, ie, *S. milleri, S. intermedius*), staphylococci, Enterobacteriaceae (eg, *E. coli, Klebsiella, Enterobacter*). Mixed infections common
- In pts w/immunodeficiency, fungal organisms (eg, *Candida, Aspergillus*) *L. monocytogenes* more commonly found

CLINICAL MANIFESTATIONS

- Frequently insidious/nonspecific
- Triad of fever, headache, focal neurologic deficit: strong indicator, but infrequently present (<30%)
- Fever, vomiting, headache are most common symptoms (>50% each), followed by mental status changes (30–40%), seizures (25–35%), focal neurologic deficit (25–35%). Coma in only 15–20%
- *Common physical examination findings:* papilledema (30–40%), meningeal signs (25–35%), hemiparesis (20–30%), ataxia (5–15%)
- Location of abscess suggested by Sx (eg, aphasia and hemianopsia—temporal lobe; dysphasia, dyspraxia—parietal lobe; forced grasping, sucking and/or behavioral changes—frontal lobe)

LABORATORY FEATURES

- *Most important diagnostic tests:* CT scan or MRI
- Routine blood tests including CBC and differential, sedimentation rate and culture frequently unhelpful
- Lumbar puncture contraindicated until increased intracranial pressure has been excluded by imaging study; CSF analysis (ie, WBC and differential, glucose, protein) rarely helpful for Dx

DIFFERENTIAL DIAGNOSIS

- *Other infections:* meningitis, encephalitis, subdural or epidural abscesses, cysticercosis, tuberculoma
- *Vascular:* hemorrhage (intracerebral, subdural, subarachnoid), infarct, venous sinus thrombosis, migraine
- *Tumor:* primary/metastatic (eg, lymphoma, neuroblastoma)

TREATMENT

- Antibiotic Tx alone appropriate for pts:
  - w/short period of symptoms (<2 wks) who are clinically stable and have relatively small abscess (<3 cm)
  - w/multiple abscesses
  - w/abscess in critical area difficult to approach surgically (eg, brain stem, thalamus, basal ganglia)
  - who are poor surgical candidates
- Stereotactic aspiration should be used to identify pathogen or if inadequate response to antibiotics alone within 1–2 wks
- Excision of abscess reserved for:
  - multiloculated abscess
  - posterior fossa abscess
  - fungal or helminthic abscess
- Antibiotic choice based on predisposing factors:
  - brain abscess associated w/otitis media, sinusitis, cyanotic heart disease. Drugs of choice: ceftriaxone (100 mg/kg/d) or cefotaxime (200 mg/kg/d) *w*/metronidazole (30 mg/kg/d). Alternatively, penicillin (400,000 units/kg/d) w/chloramphenicol (100 mg/kg/d) or ampicillin-sulbactam (200 mg/kg/d)
  - brain abscess associated w/head trauma, postneurosurgery, endocarditis, immunocompromised host. Drugs of choice: vancomycin (60 mg/kg/d) w/ceftriaxone (or cefotaxime) and, possibly, metronidazole
- *Recommended duration of therapy:* 4–6 wks
- Corticosteroids only if reduction of edema or intracranial pressure considered potentially lifesaving

COMPLICATIONS

- *Mortality:* 5–15%
- *Seizures (yrs later, in some cases):* 10–25%
- *Hemiparesis:* 7–15%
- *Cranial nerve palsy:* 5–10%
- *Hydrocephalus:* 5–10%
- *Behavior disorders:* 3–10%
- *Ataxia, visual deficits, spasticity:* rarely

PREVENTION

- High index of suspicion/prompt Dx
- Early/appropriate treatment of predisposing factors (eg, antibiotics for contiguous infectious sites)

WHEN TO REFER

- Referral indicated if:
  - disease suspected or part of differential Dx
  - antibiotic treatment alone fails to improve condition (eg, clinical Sx do not improve, reduction in abscess size not seen within 1 wk)

BRAIN ABSCESS

BACKGROUND

- Most common malignant brain tumor of childhood. Represents ~20% of all brain tumors seen in pediatric age group. Peak incidence: 5 yrs of age. Bimodel distribution seen initially at 3–4 yrs of age and again at 8–9 yrs of age
- Reported M:F ratio varies from 1.3:1–4.8:1. Associated w/number of inherited syndromes including Turcot syndrome

MANIFESTATIONS

- Classical presentation includes vomiting, headache, ataxic gait. Obstruction of fourth ventricular outlet results in signs of increased intracranial pressure, specifically headache, vomiting, lethargy, papilledema. Vomiting typically seen when child awakens in morning
- Cerebellar involvement produces progressive clumsiness and awkwardness, ultimately w/inability to stand or walk w/o support

RADIOGRAPHIC FEATURES

- MRI particularly sensitive for disease evaluation in posterior fossa. Medulloblastoma usually appears as midline enhancing lesion on gadolinium MRI

TREATMENT: SURGICAL

- Surgical intervention initial treatment w/attempt at gross resection. Total gross resection enhances survival

STAGING

- All pts should undergo tumor staging to define extent of tumor spread. Appropriate studies include postoperative MRI of head, MRI of spine, bone scan, CSF for cytopathology, bone marrow aspiration

RADIOTHERAPY

- Craniospinal radiotherapy conventionally used for all children >3 yrs of age. Children w/standard risk disease (no residual disease evident on MRI, no metastases) treated w/2,400 cGy to whole brain and spine w/boost to 54–5,600 cGy to the posterior fossa in conjunction w/chemotherapy. Children w/high-risk medulloblastoma require <3,600 cGy to whole brain and spine w/similar posterior fossa boost, plus chemotherapy

CHEMOTHERAPY

- Chemotherapy now considered standard intervention for pts w/standard risk or high-risk medulloblastoma
- Active agents include cisplatin, cyclophosphamide, vincristine, VP-16, possibly CCNU
- High-dose chemotherapy w/concomitant bone marrow or peripheral stem cell rescue may be curative in pts w/localized recurrent medulloblastoma

PRICE OF INTERVENTION

- Children treated for medulloblastoma require attention to neuropsychologic, endocrinologic, neoplastic consequences of treatment
- All children w/medulloblastoma, indeed all w/brain tumors, should be treated by comprehensive team seeing at least 25 children w/brain tumors/year

BACKGROUND

- Inflammatory conditions of the breast uncommon in children or adolescents
- Mastitis, breast abscess may occur in the adolescent breast, typically in association w/lactation, but may result from spread of cutaneous infections (folliculitis of periareolar hairs, eczema, foreign bodies), chronic illness, epidermal cysts, trauma
- Although rare, neonates, infants 2 wks– 6 mos of age also can develop infection of the mammary region w/subsequent abscess or life-threatening necrotizing fasciitis if not promptly treated. This usually follows local trauma (eg, milking of "witch's milk" from hypertrophied neonatal breast) or a surgical wound. It also can occur in early childhood
- Breast infections may be deep, more extensive than outward appearance would suggest
- Fluctuant breast abscess is late finding
- *Staphylococcus* most frequent causative organism, w/lactational abscesses almost exclusively due to *Staphylococcus aureus*. *Streptococcus, E. coli, Pseudomonas,* other anaerobes also contribute, esp in nonlactational abscesses

CLINICAL MANIFESTATIONS

- Breast pain and erythema, warmth, edema of the overlying skin
- Usually unilateral
- Single or multiple areas of focal induration w/or w/o palpable mass suggests *Staphylococcus*
- Diffuse spreading infection suggests *Streptococcus*
- Axillary adenopathy often present
- Infants also have fever, may appear septic

LABORATORY FEATURES

- Gram stain, aerobic, anaerobic cultures, sensitivities of aspirates of frank abscesses or "tissue fluid" from areas of cellulitis should be sent
- Ultrasound-guided needle aspiration, if ultrasound demonstrates pus, may aid in obtaining specimen for culture, also be therapeutic

DIFFERENTIAL DIAGNOSIS

- Localized infarcts of breast tissue (may follow trauma or be common during third trimester of pregnancy)
- Fibrocystic breasts often become tender premenstrually w/pronouncement of their cordlike nodularity
- Other breast cysts may present as tender mass
- Cyclic mastodynia, as name suggests, recurs w/menstrual cycle, but no erythema or warmth
- Neonatal breast hypertrophy, common finding in newborns resulting from transmitted maternal hormone stimulation; erythema, tenderness, fever not present in simple hypertrophy

TREATMENT

- Analgesics, warm compresses used for pain, although ice may be more helpful first 24 hrs if trauma is precipitant
- Penicillinase-resistant penicillin should be given po × 2–4 wks; consider broader-spectrum coverage if pt not lactating
- Ultrasound-guided needle aspiration to drain, reduce pressure may be additional effective measure if accumulation of pus seen on ultrasound. Repeat aspiration may be necessary in some after antibiotic Tx
- Incision, drainage of fluctuant abscesses should be done promptly in OR under anes-thesia, not in office because may be extensive, difficult to drain adequately
- Inflammatory masses w/o evidence of pus treated w/antibiotics alone
- For infants, broad-spectrum IV antibiotics, warm compresses, incision and drainage of palpable fluctuance. Unlike adults, pediatric pts do not require excision of involved glandular tissue, and must not have excision if breast deformity, atrophy to be avoided. Approach should be through circumareolar, not radial, incision to prevent deformity from scar contraction

COMPLICATIONS

- *Recurrent abscesses:* 40–50% of subareolar location, less often w/peripheral position
- *Scarring:* more common when trauma the precipitant or w/recurrent abscesses
- Sinus tract formation or mammary duct fistulas
- Necrotizing fasciitis may develop in infants not treated promptly

PREVENTION

- Good nipple hygiene should be taught to avoid cracking of nipples during breast-feeding and thereby reduce portal of entry for bacteria
- Nipple ring piercing or breast tattoos should be discouraged
- New mothers should be educated about normality of neonatal breast hypertrophy and dangers of attempting to express milk from neonate's breast

WHEN TO REFER

- Surgical referral should be made for neonates, for any fluctuant abscess, or if ultrasound reveals collection of pus

BACKGROUND

- Benign type of passing out, lasting <1 min
- Occurs 1/2 ×/d–1/2 ×/mo
- *Peak age of onset:* 6 mos–2 yrs of age
- *Spontaneous resolution:* by 5–6 yrs of age
- *Incidence:* 4–5% of children
- *Cause:* abnormal reflex that causes prolonged involuntary holding of breath. ↓ venous return to heart following forceful breath holding leads to reduced cerebral blood flow, ↓ O_2
- Temper tantrums nonessential, contributing factor

CLINICAL MANIFESTATIONS

- Precipitated by upsetting event, such as anger about limit setting, fear, or injury (eg, falling down, bumping head)
- Starts w/child giving out 1 to 2 long cries
- Then holds breath in expiration until cyanosis occurs (blue spell)
- Then passes out and often becomes stiff or rigid (opisthotonos common)
- One-third of children progress to having few twitches or myoclonic jerks during some attacks
- Then resumes normal breathing and becomes fully alert in <1 min
- 10% are pallid spells. Due to hyperresponsive vagal reflex that causes transient bradycardia

LABORATORY FEATURES

- Iron deficiency lowers threshold for breath-holding spells. Obtain CBC in high-risk cases. Caution: may occur w/o anemia
- EKG if precipitated by exercise or excitement. R/o prolonged QT interval or other arrhythmia
- EEGs normal, not indicated

DIFFERENTIAL DIAGNOSIS

- Seizure disorder
- Cardiac arrhythmia
- Infantile apnea
- With above, no precipitating event or crying. Also no breath holding, except w/apneic episodes

TREATMENT

- Reassure parent that attacks harmless, always stop by themselves
- If child starts to have attack while standing near hard surface, advise parent to go to child quickly, help lower to floor
- During attack, have child lie flat. Position ↑ blood flow to brain, may prevent some of clonic jerks that concern parents
- Apply cold, wet washcloth to child's forehead until he or she starts breathing again. May help parent more than child
- Time length of a few attacks, using watch w/second hand because it is difficult to estimate length of attack accurately. Attacks always seem to last longer than they actually do
- Many parents overreact. Advise them not to start resuscitation or call 911; not to put anything in child's mouth; not to shake baby (risk of subdural hematomas)
- After attacks advise parents to give child brief hug and go about their business. If child has temper tantrum that progressed to breath-holding spell because child wanted own way, do not give in after attack because may cause deliberate breath-holding spells

COMPLICATIONS

- None from attack itself. No ↑ incidence of seizures or learning disabilities
- Head injury or other injury may occur from fall during a spell

PREVENTION

- Iron Tx may reduce or eliminate spells in 50% of children
- Try to remove unnecessary frustration and tantrums, which can trigger breath-holding spells
- Avoid exhaustion, hunger w/properly timed naps, snacks
- Avoid games or toys beyond child's ability
- Avoid activities or events (eg, concert) beyond child's attention span
- Avoid excessive rules, restrictions. Reasonable limits, however, essential
- Do not give in to tantrums or crying. Will lead to more testing, tantrums, breath-holding spells in future

WHEN TO REFER

- Age <3 mos
- Pallid breath-holding spells. Refer to cardiologist to r/o occult arrhythmia
- Atypical spell, such as unconsciousness lasting >1 min. R/o seizure disorder
- Frequent attacks that do not respond to oral iron or behavioral treatment

BRONCHIOLITIS

GERALD M. LOUGHLIN

BACKGROUND

- Viral infection of small airways
- Respiratory syncytial virus (RSV) most common etiologic agent
- Adenovirus, parainfluenza, influenza, also potential pathogens
- Commonly affects infants <1 yr of age
- Recurrence w/RSV possible
- Increased morbidity, mortality in pts w/underlying cardiopulmonary disease

CLINICAL FEATURES

- *Apnea:* early apnea—specific for RSV; late apnea—marker of respiratory failure
- Tachypnea, tachycardia
- Increased work of breathing (retractions, nasal flaring, rib cage paradox)
- Rales (late inspiratory)
- Wheezing—may be variable finding
- Cyanosis

LABORATORY FEATURES

- Gas exchange
  - ↓ $PaCO_2$ and O_2 sats
  - ↑ $PaCO_2$—respiratory failure
- CBC
  - nonspecific ↑ WBC
- Chest x ray
  - hyperinflation
  - diffuse infiltrates
  - atelectasis
- Viral cultures
  - results available in several days
- Rapid viral diagnostics
  - antigen detection by Elisa or immunofluorescence—results available in hrs

DIFFERENTIAL DIAGNOSIS

- Status asthmaticus
- Cystic fibrosis—acute infection
- Aspiration
- Heart failure
- In general, since bronchiolitis occurs during respiratory viral season in characteristic epidemic fashion w/classic clinical presentation, establishing Dx fairly straightforward

TREATMENT

- Accepted:
  - rest
  - adequate hydration—may need to restrict oral feedings
  - supplemental O_2
  - routine antibiotics *not* indicated
- Controversial:
  - sympathomimetics:
    ○ racemic epinephrine—evidence accumulating the inhaled epinephrine may be beneficial. More data needed on frequency, duration, side effects of Tx. Nonetheless, trial of inhaled racemic epinephrine indicated as initial Tx for pts w/severe disease (dose 0.05 ml/kg/dose of 2.25% solution q2–4 hrs; add saline to bring volume to 3 cc) as tolerated
  - beta agonist:
    ○ variable responses to conventional doses. Trial of inhaled beta agonist indicated. If no response after 24 hrs consider stopping (dose 0.1 mg/kg/dose for infants)
  - Steroids:
    ○ no clear-cut benefit shown for systemic or inhaled steroids. In child w/wheezing and positive family Hx of asthma, trial of steroids (2 mg/kg/d, prednisone) warranted

  - role of theophylline and ipratropium bromide unclear, generally not indicated
  - ribavirin:
    ○ "use highly controversial." Antiviral therapy not recommended for mild disease. AAP recommendation (1995) "should be considered in infants w/bronchopulmonary dysplasia, cystic fibrosis, immunodeficiencies, congenital heart disease (esp those w/pulmonary hypertension); infants w/severe disease; infants at risk for complications from RSV
    ○ no established benefit in ventilated pts

PREVENTIVE MEASURES

- Good handwashing
- RSV Ig-monoclonal antibody (15 mg/kg IM) q monthly during RSV season or pooled gammaglobulin (RSV-IG-IV) in small, premature infants with significant chronic lung disease (750 mg/kg, IV q monthly during RSV season). See AAP guidelines, Nov. 1998

COMPLICATIONS

- Acute:
  - respiratory failure
  - apparent life-threatening event
- Chronic:
  - increased airway hyper-reactivity
  - bronchiolitis obliterans
  - possible precursor of chronic lung disease in adults

DEFINITION

- Chronic lung disease in neonates requiring positive pressure ventilation or supplemental O_2 beyond 1 mo of age

BACKGROUND

- Most common chronic lung disease in childhood (except asthma)
- *Incidence:* ~20% of premature infants w/hyaline membrane disease or ~2–3/1,000 live births
- *M:F ratio:* 1.5:1
- Lung injury attributed to O_2 toxicity and barotrauma in immature lung
- Typically follows hyaline membrane disease; may follow meconium aspiration, neonatal pneumonia, asphyxia, apnea or congenital heart disease
- Most infants surviving neonatal period improve by 6–12 mos of age
- Airway obstruction and airway reactivity may persist for yrs

CLINICAL MANIFESTATIONS

- Tachypnea and increased work of breathing
- Wheezing—usually bronchodilator responsive
- Hypoxemia—worse during sleep, feeding, crying
- Intermittent pulmonary edema
- Pulmonary hypertension
- Poor growth

LABORATORY AND RADIOGRAPHIC FEATURES

- Arterial blood gas (ABG) values reflect hypoventilation, respiratory acidosis, hypoxemia
- *Acceptable baseline ABG values:* pCO_2 50–70 mmHg (if compensated w/pH > 7.30); pO_2 55–60 mmHg; O_2 saturation 92–95%
- *Chest radiographic findings:* hyperinflation w/multiple fine, lacy densities; typically improve progressively over first years of life

DIFFERENTIAL DIAGNOSIS

- Viral pneumonitis
- Recurrent aspiration
- Pulmonary interstitial emphysema
- Congenital heart disease w/pulmonary edema
- Pulmonary hemorrhage
- Wilson-Mikity syndrome
- Cystic fibrosis
- Pulmonary lymphangiectasia

OUTPATIENT MANAGEMENT

- *Modify according to disease severity:* many infants go home on supplemental O_2, diuretics, bronchodilators
- *Optimize nutrition:* may require 150 kcal/kg/d for adequate weight gain
- *Optimize oxygenation:* maintain pO_2 >55 mg Hg and O_2 saturation at 92–95% using supplemental O_2 administered by nasal cannula
- *Minimize bronchospasm:* nebulized albuterol or ipratropium (avoid theophylline, if possible, because of side effects)
- *Minimize pulmonary edema:* chronic use of hydrochlorothiazide (0.5–1.5 mg/kg/dose, po, bid) and spironolactone (0.5–1.5 mg/kg/dose), po, bid; intermittent use of furosemide (1.0–2.0 mg/kg/dose) (avoid chronic daily use of furosemide because of side effects)
- *Minimize airway inflammation:* nebulized cromolyn, inhaled corticosteroids and/or burst of systemic corticosteroids (avoid prolonged use of systemic corticosteroids)
- *Optimize airway clearance:* chest physiotherapy; avoid cough suppressants
- *Minimize additional pulmonary insults:* immunize (routine and influenza virus vaccines); consider immunoprophylaxis for respiratory syncytial virus (RSV) using palivizimab (15 mg/kg IM, administered monthly during RSV season; control gastroesophageal reflux; avoid day-care setting, other sites of exposure to respiratory viruses; control exposure to cigarette smoke, other irritants
- *Monitor for associated disorders:* neurodevelopmental delays, apnea, retinopathy of prematurity, hearing deficits, gastroesophageal reflux, tracheo- and broncho-malacia, subglottic stenosis

COMPLICATIONS

- Right-sided heart failure
- Respiratory failure, esp w/RSV pneumonitis
- Subglottic stenosis from chronic intubation

WHEN TO REFER

- Persistent wheezing and labored breathing
- Episodes of cyanosis or hypoxemia
- Deterioration during viral respiratory infection
- Stridor (for evaluation of subglottic stenosis)
- Inadequate growth (may reflect hypoxemia)

BACKGROUND

- Transmitted from animals to humans through direct contact w/infected animal
- Also acquired (most common in children) by ingesting unpasteurized milk, milk products (cheese) from infected cattle, goats
- Caused by *Brucella* species, a small, gram-negative, nonmotile, non-spore-forming coccobacillus
- Four species involved in human infection: *B. abortus* (cattle), *B. suis* (swine), *B. melitensis* (goats), *B. canis* (dogs)
- Brucella organisms obligate intracellular parasites; multiply in lymphocytes, monocytes. Localize and tend to form granulomas in bone marrow, lymph nodes, spleen, liver
- Brucellosis primarily occupational disease
- Uncommon in children in US

CLINICAL MANIFESTATIONS

- Incubation period: few days/few wks
- Fever most common finding. When disease becomes chronic, afebrile periods alternate w/febrile ones (undulant fever)
- Arthralgia, arthritis, general body aches common
- Splenomegaly and/or hepatomegaly most common physical findings
- Lymphadenopathy occurs
- Chronic brucellosis can continue for months, years

LABORATORY FEATURES

- WBC count usually normal or low
- Erythrocyte sedimentation rate normal or mildly elevated
- Liver enzymes generally elevated
- Blood culture may be positive early in disease; organism may take as long as 2 wks to grow
- Bone marrow, urine, CSF may also yield positive cultures
- Brucella serum agglutinin titer (SAT) often positive at presentation of disease, but may have to be repeated in few weeks if negative initially. 1:160 considered positive titer

DIFFERENTIAL DIAGNOSIS

- Fever of unknown origin
- Juvenile rheumatoid arthritis
- Infectious mononucleosis
- Tuberculosis
- Systemic lupus erythematosus
- Salmonellosis
- Hepatitis

TREATMENT

- Prolonged antimicrobial therapy keystone to therapy
- *Tetracyclene:* 30–40 mg/kg/d (max. 2 g/d) in 4 div doses po 4–6 wks preferred treatment for children >9 yrs of age
- *Doxycycline:* 5 mg/kg/d (max. 200 mg/d) in 2 div doses po 4–6 wks more convenient; also only for children >9 yrs of age
- Oral trimethoprim-sulfamethoxazole drug of choice for children <9 yrs of age. Dose: trimethoprim 10 mg/kg/d (max. 480 mg/d); sulfamethoxazole 50 mg/kg/d (max. 2.4 g) in 2 div doses 4–6 wks
- Second drug added for the first 7–14 d for treatment of serious infection and complications; either gentamicin 5 mg/kg/d or streptomycin 20 mg/kg/d IM. Rifampin 20 mg/kg/d used as second or third drug in very severe cases, particularly for treatment of meningitis

COMPLICATIONS

- Relapse common if initial therapy <4 wks
- Infective endocarditis rare but serious complication
- Meningitis another rare, serious complication
- Osteomyelitis, suppurative arthritis occur
- Untreated, brucellosis may become chronic, last for months or years

PREVENTION

- Avoidance of raw milk, products made from raw milk, cheese in particular, esp in parts of world where animal brucellosis common

WHEN TO REFER

- If meningitis or endocarditis present, infectious disease consultation indicated

WILLIAM F. VANN, JR.

BACKGROUND

- Bruxism defined as habitual grinding, gnashing, clenching of teeth at times other than for mastication of food. In children bruxism occurs mostly during sleep; thus often called night grinding
- Bruxism sometimes categorized as behavior disorder, sleep disorder, self-mutilation, but term *oral habit* best description for most tooth grinding seen in children
- Prevalence of bruxism 15% in children. Clinical examination and positive parental report indicate bruxism in 5 and 6 yr old children; 15.4% exhibited clinical signs in absence of positive parental report, suggesting parents unaware of habit
- Different entity than adults or adolescents w/full complement of permanent teeth. Exhibited in comatose children and those w/musculoskeletal disorders or mental handicaps; etiology for these pts distinctly different from otherwise normal, healthy children
- In children, etiology somewhat obscure; factors can be categorized as follows:
  - intraoral factors: cuspal interferences, malocclusion, mobile teeth, premature contacts
  - systemic factors: allergies, endocrine disorders, intestinal parasites, subclinical nutritional deficiencies. Threefold incidence in bruxism in allergic children vs. nonallergic controls matched by age, sex, race reported
  - psychological factors: response to stress, nervous habit, inability to express emotions (ie, anxiety, rage, hate, aggression, sadism, libidinous desires)
- Bruxism in normal preschool children thought to have no significant psychological significance
- Relatively common; often exists w/o parental knowledge and no apparent etiology

CLINICAL MANIFESTATIONS

- Most children unaware they grind teeth. Forceful bruxism sometimes generates characteristic tooth grinding noise worrisome to parents; noise may keep parents, siblings awake at night
- Usually biting (occlusal) surfaces of teeth reveal flattened appearance most pronounced on molar, canine teeth. Occasionally tooth wear significant and encroaches tooth's pulp (nerve, circulation)
- Some children complain of tenderness in muscles of mastication—rare manifestation

LABORATORY FEATURES, DIFFERENTIAL DIAGNOSIS (N/A)

TREATMENT

- Treatment should begin simply. Local occlusal interferences eliminated, occlusion equilibrated and stabilized, systemic contributions ruled out
- If wear advanced to extent that child experiences tooth sensitivity or compromises tooth vitality, tooth restoration and/or appliance, Tx may be needed
- Although habit appears self-limiting, appliance therapy most popular treatment modality. Mouth guard or soft plastic splint used at night to protect teeth, disrupt grinding habit. Topical fluorides used inside appliance to desensitize symptomatic teeth
- Appliance Tx also successful in eliminating tooth grinding noises noxious to parents and siblings
- In adolescents or older children, significant wear on permanent teeth should signal concern; often related to malocclusion; occasionally related to psychological factors. Treatment focused on transitional splint Tx and comprehensive diagnostic assessment for malocclusion

COMPLICATIONS

- Complications uncommon except in rare instances where primary teeth must be restored or extracted due to excessive wear

WHEN TO REFER

- Most children should be managed by team approach; pediatric dentist assesses for intraoral etiological factors while pediatrician assesses for systemic factors

BACKGROUND

- *Prevalence:* 1–3% of adolescent girls; increasing in college-aged populations; 10–50% adolescent girls report occasional binge eating and/or self-induced vomiting
- *Age distribution:* onset late adolescence or early adulthood; 90–95% young women from all socioeconomic groups
- *Risk factors:* Hx premorbid obesity (higher association in boys) or anorexia nervosa, low self-concept, self-rejection, self-neglect, increased life stress, positive family Hx for eating disorders, alcoholism, depression
- *Pathogenesis:* maladaptive biopsychosocial response to perceived need for weight loss and/or traumatic life event. Cycle of binge eating, subsequent purging symbolizes loss and regain of control over one's body
- Mood disturbances, distorted body images persist chronically in nearly 50%. Clinical course stabilizes by 4 yrs. Poorer outcomes associated w/substance abuse and borderline personality disorder
- Mortality associated w/daily cycles and multiple methods of purging w/resultant electrolyte imbalances, ipecac use, suicide

CLINICAL MANIFESTATIONS

- Binge eating associated w/shame, secrecy
- Inappropriate compensatory behaviors to prevent weight gain: most commonly self-induced vomiting, also excessive laxative or diuretic use, fasting, excessive exercise, enemas
- Recurrent pattern of above cycle (binge, purge), often several times weekly
- Normal or increased weight
- Self-evaluation unduly related to body size, shape
- Subtypes distinguished by presence or absence of purging
- *Comorbidities:* ~30–50% associated borderline personality disorder (associated with poor prognosis), ~30% associated w/ substance abuse (tobacco, alcohol, stimulants), associated depression (more frequent in purging type), seasonal affective disorder, anxiety, obsessive-compulsive disorders

- *Associated findings:* subconjunctival hemorrhages, esophagitis, abdominal cramps, dental enamel erosion (esp lingual aspect of anterior incisors), chipped teeth, dental cavities, calluses on knuckles (Russell sign), parotid gland hypertrophy, amenorrhea, diarrhea, constipation

LABORATORY FEATURES

- Hyponatremia, hypokalemia, hypochloremia
- Metabolic alkalosis 2° to vomiting
- Metabolic acidosis 2° to laxative abuse

DIFFERENTIAL DIAGNOSIS

- Anorexia nervosa, binge-eating/purge type
- Kleine-Levin syndrome
- Major depression

TREATMENT

- Goals must include:
  - control over binge-purge cycles
  - restoration of family function
  - support of adolescent's sense of autonomy, self-worth
  - treatment of comorbid conditions
  - appropriate nutritional intake, exercise
- Intervention requires active, ongoing collaboration between primary care practitioner and experienced mental health professional (social worker, psychologist, psychiatrist)
- Treatment must target above goals and include pt, family
- Individual psychotherapy
  - ego-oriented individual psychotherapy to focus on facts of health, nutrition, adolescents tasks
  - cognitive behavioral techniques to decrease frequency, intensity of binge-purge cycles, reframing, stimulus control, food diaries, coping strategies, assertiveness training
- Family therapy
  - behavioral family systems therapy
- Nutritional counseling
- Psychopharmacology

- SSRIs to decrease binge frequency, sertraline hydrochloride (Zoloft) starting at 50 mg/d w/increases weekly to maximum of 200 mg/d. Effect may take several wks. Consult psychiatry if failure of effect by 6 wks
  - avoid benzodiazepines (Xanax, Valium, Ativan, Tranxene) due to risk of abuse and addiction
- Hospitalization
  - preferably on adolescent unit w/staff experienced in management of eating disorders for treatment of acute dehydration, electrolyte imbalances, medical complications listed, and/or failure of outpatient treatment

COMPLICATIONS

- *Cardiac:* arrhythmias (2° to electrolyte imbalance), myopathy (2° to ipecac abuse), orthostatic hypotension
- *GI:* esophageal tears, gastric perforation, acute pancreatitis, hematemesis, hematochezia

PREVENTION

- Support healthy nutrition, exercise practices
- Anticipatory guidance about weight loss, substance abuse, sexuality, adolescent autonomy
- Careful management of pts w/anorexia nervosa to prevent conversion to bulimia nervosa

WHEN TO REFER

- At presentation, immediate referral, ongoing collaboration w/experienced mental health professional
- Refer to adolescent medicine specialist if no improvement in pattern of binge-purging after 1 mo office care, for management of medical complications, when Dx in doubt
- Hospitalization on adolescent unit w/interdisciplinary approach for failure of outpatient care, management of acute medical complications, detoxification or suicidal ideation

BACKGROUND

- Pts w/burns of <10% body surface area (BSA) of 1° and 2° safely treated as outpatients unless unsuitable home situation noted. Burn injuries treated in outpatients 10 times as frequent as hospital admission for burns
- Use the "rule of palm" to determine %BSA for small burns; palm of child, not including fingers, equals 1% BSA
- Scald burns have highest incidence of burns in children <3 yrs of age
- Scald and contact burns may be result of child abuse and/or neglect
- Contact burns from touching hot radiators or woodstoves and stepping on hot charcoal, seasonal accidents
- Aesthetic outcome of most small 2° burns good if wounds heal within 2 wks
- Highest complications from biting on electrical extension cord, which causes arc and burn to upper and lower lip and usually adjacent oral commissure. (This is not high-tension electrical burn)
- Most burn deaths caused by residential fires; associated w/severe inhalation injury

LABORATORY FEATURES

- Burns >10% BSA, obtain CBC, electrolytes, serum glucose, BUN, creatinine
- Carboxy hemoglobin if Hx includes possible smoke inhalation
- Skeletal survey if suspect trauma
- EKG if Hx high-tension electrical injury

DIFFERENTIAL DIAGNOSIS

- Accurate and complete Hx accident for burn Dx
- Ensure Hx matches clinical picture to r/o child abuse/neglect, esp in scald, contact burns. Definitive line of demarcation of burn wound is red flag

TREATMENT

- *Emergency care:* stop burning process, remove any clothing, particularly diapers and plastic coverings that may retain heat and cause deeper injury. Rinse affected area w/cool water for at least 15 min. If chemical involved, check w/poison control center for best neutralizing agent and repeat washing process until all chemical removed
- Clean wound w/water. Leave blisters intact. Only debride devitalized tissue after blister bursts. For tar burn, remove tar w/mineral oil
- Burns on trunk and extremity: apply 1% silver sulfadiazine cream, mafenide acetate or povidone-iodine cream for partial thickness burns, secure w/clean gauze bandage and stockinette. Change dressings twice daily; remove any remaining cream before reapplying. If creams unavailable wrap w/clean gauze and bandage. Elevate injured area
- For facial burns use neomycin or bacitracin. Protect from sun exposure
- For electric cord injury to oral commissure, use neomycin ointment tid. Gently rinse area w/water after eating. Instruct family to pinch affected area if rapid bleeding occurs and go to nearest ER
- See pt daily or qod until healing under way
- Burn wound care may be done at home using clean technique, but topical cream must be removed w/each cleansing before reapplying and redressing
- Provide pain relief w/analgesics; usually acetaminophen sufficient
- Use emollient cream once burn wound healed to lubricate and protect skin. Protect from sun exposure with clothing and sunblock
- Tetanus prophylaxis indicated only when immunizations not up to date

COMPLICATIONS

- Persistent deep burn wound infection causes further epithelial destruction and conversion of 2° burn to full thickness burn, which requires skin grafting
- Electrical burn to mouth may cause severe bleeding from lip artery when eschar separates and detaches from surface usually 14–21 d postinjury

PREVENTION

- Counsel parents on injury prevention at routine pediatric visits:
  - use smoke detector—change batteries when you change clocks
  - plan fire escape route with meeting place outside; practice
  - do not drink hot liquids when holding or feeding infant
  - use care when using front burners of stove, have kitchen fire extinguisher
  - keep pot handles on stove turned in
  - do not store any items of interest to children above stove
  - keep temperature of hot water boiler set below 120° F
  - cover radiators to prevent contact burn
  - insulate stove door
  - dispose of hot charcoal properly after use
  - promote educational programs in schools and professional groups on burn prevention

WHEN TO REFER

- Burn >10% BSA
- Respiratory burn potential or actual
- Electrical burn, high-tension wire accident
- Full thickness burn >2 in diameter
- Burn to areas of body where dressings difficult to apply at home, eg, face, perineum
- Inadequate home situation
- Injuries caused from child abuse and/or neglect

CLINICAL MANIFESTATIONS

	Cause	Surface appearance	Pain and temperature	Histologic depth	Healing time
First Degree	Scald, flash, flame, contact, chemical, ultraviolet light	Dry, no blisters Minimal or no edema Erythematous	Very painful Rapid heat loss	Epidermal layers only	2–5 d w/*no* scarring. May have some discoloration
Second Degree Partial thickness	Scald, flash, flame, contact, chemical, ultraviolet light	Moist blebs, blisters Underlying tissue mottled pink and white Good capillary refill	Very painful Rapid heat loss	Epidermis, papillary, reticular layers of dermis. May include domes of subcutaneous layer	Superficial: 5-ʼ grafting. D 21–35 d infeʼ tʼ
Third Degree Full thickness	Scald, flash, flame, contact, chemical, electrical	Dry, leathery, eschar. Mixed white, waxy, pearly, khaki, mahogany, soot stained	Insensate Less rapid heat loss	Down to and may incluʼ fat, subcutaneous tiʼ May include fascʼ bone	

60

BACKGROUND

- *Synonyms:* Sever disease, painful heel syndrome in children
- Most frequently found 7–15 yrs of age, peak incidence 9–13 yrs
- Most frequent in boys, children active in sports, overweight children
- Sports requiring cleated, hard-soled shoes risk factor. Soccer most common
- Recovery universal. Duration difficult to predict, typically 2–6 mos. Recurrent symptoms may occur, but uncommon

ETIOLOGY

- Basically pediatric overuse syndrome similar to Osgood Schlatter disease
- Secondary ossification center; appears 4–7 yrs of age in girls and 6–9 yrs in boys. Initial ossification starts in several irregular fragments that unite within few mos to form single, somewhat semicircular disc of bone at posterior aspect of calcaneus. Insertion of Achilles tendon at superior aspect and plantar fascia at inferior end imparts significant stress to calcaneal apophysis, manifested on plain radiographs as increased sclerosis (result of mechanical stress). Role of weight-bearing stress further elucidated by nonambulators who demonstrate both delayed development of this apophysis and marked reduction of its sclerosis (density)
- Repetitive stress causes micro-fracturing of calcaneal apophysis. At completion of growth, weak link eliminated as relatively elastic physis absorbed. Muscle forces acting on calcaneus then distributed through larger portion of heel and marked sclerosis of posterior calcaneus disappears
- Transverse fragmentation lying at midportion of calcaneal apophysis may be observed in normal children, but CT scans document increased association of this finding in symptomatic children, further supporting role of repetitive trauma as cause of calcaneal apophysitis

CLINICAL MANIFESTATIONS

- Indolent onset of posterior heel pain
- No specific injury but symptoms increase w/activity, decrease w/rest
- Tenderness posterior aspect calcaneus increased w/medial and lateral compression
- No skin changes, swelling, or palpable abnormalities
- Mild restriction of dorsiflexion, 5–10°, common, but otherwise range of motion and alignment of foot, ankle normal
- Bilateral involvement common, as much as 50% in some studies

LABORATORY FEATURES

- No definitive radiographic features. Sclerosis of calcaneal apophysis normal and routine radiographs have not demonstrated significant difference in normal and involved children
- Radiographs not necessary in typical case w/bilateral involvement. Obtain lateral radiograph of heel in child w/unilateral involvement to exclude possibility of unicameral bone cyst, etc

DIFFERENTIAL DIAGNOSIS

- Tumors (unilateral)
- Osteomyelitis of calcaneus (unilateral)
- Enthesitis such as Achilles tendinitis or plantar fascitis (associated w/Reiter syndrome or other seronegative spondyloarthropathy)

TREATMENT

- Short-term modification or restriction of activity most important, allowing healing of microscopic stress fractures
- Stretching exercises for Achilles tendon if dorsiflexion restricted
- Shoe modifications to style w/shock absorbent or cushion heel features
- Other shoe modification such as heel lift or heel cup also helpful
- Parents must understand variable nature of disorder and effect this has on when child will be able to resume competitive sports activities. Most important w/parents overinvolved in child's athletic activities ("special" parents)

COMPLICATIONS

- No long-term sequelae

WHEN TO REFER

- Not needed, except w/"special" parents
- Suspicion of tumor

CARDIOMYOPATHY

CHARLES E. CANTER

BACKGROUND

- Dilated cardiomyopathies:
  - ↑ left ventricular volume, insufficient compensatory ↑ in wall thickness, impaired systolic function
  - frequently (20%) associated w/familial cardiomyopathy
  - cause most commonly idiopathic; can be associated w/myocarditis, muscular dystrophies, toxins (adriamycin ipecac), hyperthyroidism, disorders of fatty acid and carbohydrate metabolism

- Hypertrophic cardiomyopathies:
  - massive myocardial hypertrophy often with asymmetrical involvement of the interventricular septum, normal systolic function w/or w/o subaortic stenosis
  - familial hypertrophic cardiomyopathy associated w/autosomal dominant inheritance pattern w/variable expression and penetrance
  - may spontaneously regress in infants of diabetic mothers

- has been associated w/Friedrich ataxia, Noonan syndrome, and metabolic diseases as dilated subtype
- annual mortality rate 3–6% in children
- syncope and positive family Hx risk factors for sudden death
- Restrictive cardiomyopathies (rare):
  - normal ventricular size and systolic function w/marked atrial enlargement, diastolic dysfunction

CLINICAL MANIFESTATIONS

	Dilated	Hypertrophic	Restrictive
exercise intolerance	+	+	+
chest pain		+	
murmur	+	+	
palpitations	+	+	
syncope	+	+	
heart failure	+	+	+
pulmonary edema	+		+
sudden death	+	+	
Laboratory Features			
cardiomegaly on x ray	+	±	
EKG			
ventricular hypertrophy	+	+	
atrial enlargement	+	+	+
ventricular arrhythmias	+	+	
atrial arrhythmias	+	+	+

DIFFERENTIAL DIAGNOSIS

- Congenital coronary artery anomalies (dilated)
- Incessant atrial tachycardia (dilated)
- Ventricular hypertrophy from athletic training (hypertrophic)
- Constrictive pericarditis (restrictive)

TREATMENT

- Prohibit strenuous activities, competitive sports
- Dilated cardiomyopathy:
  - vasodilators
    - captopril: 0.1–2 mg/kg/dose po q8–12h
    - enalapril: 0.04–0.1 mg/kg/dose po q12–24h
    - should be started at low dose, titrated as tolerated
    - risk of renal failure when used in infants
    - hydralazine: 0.5–2 mg/kg po q6–8h

  - Digoxin: 0.4 mg/kg total digitalizing dose div 1/2–1/4–1/4 q8h; maintenance dose 0.004 mg/kg q12–24h
  - diuretics:
    - furosemide: 0.5–2 mg/kg po, IV q8–24h
    - Aldactazide: (hydrochlorothiazide/spironolactone) 0.5–2 mg/kg each drug po q8–12h
  - intravenous gamma globulin (myocarditis): 2 g/kg IV over 24 hrs
  - beta blockers (experimental)
  - cardiac transplantation
- Hypertrophic cardiomyopathy:
  - no therapy shown ↓ risk of sudden death
    - beta blockers: propranolol: 0.5–2 mg/kg po q6–8h
    - calcium channel blockers: verapamil: 1–3 mg/kg po q8h
    - surgical myectomy
- Restrictive cardiomyopathy:
  - diuretics/vasodilators used cautiously

COMPLICATIONS

- Ventricular arrhythmias (dilated, hypertrophic)
  - antiarrhythmics used only for symptomatic arrhythmias
- Atrial flutter/fibrillation (dilated, hypertrophic, restrictive)
  - controlled to maximize ventricular stroke volume
- Thromboembolism (dilated) anticoagulate

WHEN TO REFER

- To pediatric cardiologist at time of Dx
- To pediatric cardiologist:
  - pts w/Hx familial cardiomyopathy
  - pts w/symptoms observed w/cardiomyopathies

BACKGROUND

- Congenital:
  - accounts for 20% students in schools for blind
  - 1/3 inherited, 1/3 disease syndromes, 1/3 unknown
  - maternal infection embryopathy (ie, TORCH exposure)
  - associated ocular disease/anomalies
- Juvenile:
  - trauma induced: blunt/penetrating trauma
  - uveitis: JRA
  - drug exposure: corticosteroids, phenothiazines, metallic foreign body, busulfan, benzenes, triparanol, naphthalene, triparanol
  - radiation

CLINICAL EVALUATION

- Visual function assessed by Hx, fixation, following reflexes both binocularly and monocularly, electrophysiologic tests
- Red reflex geminii test compares red reflexes simultaneously

- Complete cataracts may present w/leukocoria (white pupil)
- Infants w/bilateral congenital cataracts often demonstrate decreased visual interest/delayed development
- Nystagmus can result from early vision deprivation, an ominous sign of poor visual potential
- Any central opacity >3 mm visually significant
- Age of formation of cataract determines location/severity
  - nuclear/central occurs in early gestation
  - zonular/lamellar occur later; may not need surgery
- Monocular cataracts generally not metabolic

LABORATORY

- TORCH titers/serology
- Aminoaciduria: galactosemia, homocystinuria, Lowe syndrome
- Urine examination for Alport syndrome (hematuria), Fabry disease (sediment), Wilson disease (copper)

- *Special:* RBC G6PD, galactokinase, WBC mannosidosis, phytanic acid (Refsum syndrome), fibroblast cystathionine synthetase

TREATMENT AND PROGNOSIS

- Surgery in first 8 wks for monocular congenital cataracts, and by 4 mos for binocular congenital cases
- Bilateral involvement has less amblyogenic potential
- Children >2 yrs of age often receive intraocular lenses for ideal visual rehabilitation
- Prognosis best w/early Dx/prompt intervention

J. JEFFREY MALATACK

BACKGROUND

- Most frequently found in children 2–18 yrs of age (87%); reported in infants and octogenarians
- *M:F ratio:* 1:1
- 3–5 d after exposure to cat (most often an immature cat <1 yr of age) papule develops at site of integument injury or directly on mucous membrane (inoculation site)
- Infectious agent causing majority of cases of clinical cat scratch disease *Bartonella henselae.* Small number of cases may be due to *Afipia felis*

Unusual manifestations based on 1,587 pts (1957–1988)

Diagnosis	Frequency
Parinaud oculoglandular syndrome	6.1%
Encephalopathy (radiculopathy)	2.1%
Systemic disease, severe, chronic	1.8%
Erythema nodosa	0.75%
Neuroretinitis	0.5%
Thrombocytopenic purpura	0.34%
Primary atypical premia	0.20%
Breast tumor	0.10%
Angiomatoid papular	0.10%
Osteomyelitis	0.06%
	12.00%

Source: Adapted from Margileth AM, Hatfield TL. Contemp Pediatr. Table 2, page 30, Dec. 1990

- *Recovery:* complete in virtually all pts not suffering from some comorbid process, particularly immunodeficiencies. Lymph node enlargement may, in severe cases, take mos to resolve
- *Mortality:* no reported mortality in immunocompetent pts

CLINICAL MANIFESTATIONS

- Papule (inoculation site) appears on skin 3–5 d after exposure to infection-carrying cat. Cat vector not ill
- Papule evolves to vesicle, then crusts in 2–3 d
- Mild flulike illness occurs in 75% pts at time of appearance of adenopathy

- 1–2 wks after appearance of inoculation papule lymphadenopathy (cold lymphadenitis) develops at site of lymphatic drainage of inoculation papule; on occasion, nodes tender, red, very large; ⅓ cases may suppurate. Usually single node involved (85%). Less frequently 2, 3, 4 regional nodes affected
- Axillary node single most frequently involved node. Coupled w/epitrochlear nodes, upper extremity nodes involved in 45–50%. High frequency consistent w/fact most cat contact w/hands. Neck and then inguinal adenopathy second and third in frequency
- Atypical presentations seen in 10–15% (table) usually occur in conjunction w/classic features. Visceral disease w/granulomatous hepatitis and systemic symptoms seen in absence of adenopathy. Paurinaud oculaglandular syndrome, most frequent unusual presentation, due to inoculation of conjunctiva. Mucous membranes inoculation does not require integument break. Conjunctival inoculations associated w/ipsilateral preauricular adenopathy (lymph node that drains periorbital area)
- Other unusual manifestations include transverse myelitis, cerebral arteritis, osteomyelitis, encephalitis

LABORATORY FEATURES

- *Antibodies to Bartonella Henselae:* only reliable diagnostic test. When seen in significant titer 1:64 in conjunction w/Sx cat scratch disease, test nearly 100% specific and sensitive. Positive control pts probably represent asymptomatic or mildly symptomatic past infection
- *Other:* organism detected by PCR of CSF if CNS involved; number of standard laboratory tests used to support Dx. Erythrocyte sedimentation rate often elevated during first few wks of disease. Leukocyte count often mildly to moderately elevated w/eosinophilia occurring in some pts. Epstein-Barr virus, cytomegalovirus, toxoplasmosis, and in appropriate geographic regions, histoplasmosis titers useful in differential Dx
- *Imaging studies:* both CT scan and MRI occasionally useful, particularly when hepatic, splenic involvement exist

DIFFERENTIAL DIAGNOSIS

- Pyogenic lymph node infection
- Atypical mycobacterial infection
- Tularemia
- Early Hodgkin disease
- Early tuberculosis
- Malignancy

TREATMENT

- No treatment indicated in classic mild disease
- *Local treatment:* it pt suffering local discomfort due to swollen node, local application of moist saline compresses for 3–5 d may provide relief. Needle aspiration w/18–19 gauge needle relieves painful adenopathy, provides material for culture
- *Antibiotic treatment:* antibiotic treatment indicated in immunoincompetent host or w/certain unusual manifestations including systemic illness w/visceral disease, encephalopathy, atypical pneumonia. Oral trimethoprem/sulfamethoxozole, rifampin, ciprofloxacin have demonstrated in vitro activity and in vivo efficacy. In severely ill child, parenteral gentamicin 6–7.5 mg/kg/d div q8h very effective

COMPLICATION

- Recovery complete in most pts within several months. Fatal complications and irreversible sequelae not documented in immunocompetent pt. Life-threatening disease and persistent sequelae noted in immunocompromised pts, particularly those w/HIV

PREVENTION

- Avoidance of handling and close contact w/cats reduces risk of developing cat scratch disease

WHEN TO REFER

- Most pts managed w/o referral
- Referral indicated for serious disease or when Dx in doubt

CAVOVARUS FOOT

JAMES C. DRENNAN

BACKGROUND

- *Pes cavus:* fixed equinus deformity of forefoot relative to hindfoot that results in abnormally high arch. Other terms describe changes in hindfoot position, eg, equinocavovarus
- Intrinsic (lumbricales, interossei) muscles stabilize metatarsophalangeal joints, permitting long toe flexors and extensors to coordinate movement of each digital joint. Loss of metatarsophalangeal stability results in hyperextension of metatarsophalangeal joints and flexion of interphalangeal joints (claw toes). Inelastic fascia that spans plantar surface of foot attaches to proximal phalanges. Contracture of plantar fascia forces forefoot into fixed equinus; rigid cavus deformity results

LABORATORY FEATURES

- Lateral weight-bearing radiographs may demonstrate marked plantar flexion of first metatarsus relative to long axis of talus. Measurement of tibiocalcaneal angle determines hindfoot position
- A-P and lateral radiographs of entire spine needed to r/o spinal dysraphism
- Electromyography distinguishes myopathic, neuropathic conditions
- Motor nerve conduction studies necessary

DIFFERENTIAL DIAGNOSIS

- Spinal cord anomaly:
  - diastematomyelia
  - lipomeningocele
  - myelomeningocele
  - spinal cord tumor
- Anterior horn cell:
  - arthrogryposis
  - poliomyelitis
- Spinal cerebellar tract:
  - Friedreich ataxia
- Peripheral nerves:
  - hereditary motor and sensory neuropathy (HMSN)
  - metabolic neuropathies
- Post-traumatic cavus feet may develop following tibial fractures w/associated compartment syndrome
- *Most common etiology of pes cavus:* HMSN Type I (70%) and HMSN Type II (15%)

	HMSN I	HMSN II
Genetic patterns	Autosomal dominant	Autosomal dominant
Chromosome locus	17p	1p
Pathology	Hypertrophic	Neuronal
Onset symptoms	2d decade	3rd–4th decade
Foot deformity	Cavovarus	Calcaneo-cavus
EMG	Neuropathic	Neuropathic
Nerve conduction	Low velocity	Normal velocity

TREATMENT (HMSN I)

- *Teenage yrs:* Intrinsic and plantar fascial release plus nighttime ankle-foot-orthotics (AFOs)
- *Older teen/adult:* above release plus corrective osteotomies
- Tendon transfers, tibialis posterior, considered for weakness of lateral dorsiflexors
- Triple arthrodeses contraindicated; 90% unsatisfactory outcome after 20 yrs from degenerative joint disease, ankle instability and subluxation
- Ankle-foot-orthotics, custom shoes important
- Physical therapy emphasizes strengthening dorsiflexors and everters. Power-building program for pelvic girdle may be needed to correct functional weakness caused by abnormal gait

COMPLICATIONS

- Progressive foot deformity develops
- Forefoot becomes supinated, adducted
- Weight bearing becomes limited to lateral forefoot, which increases precariousness of upright activity in pts w/decreased proprioception
- Initial hindfoot functional inversion becomes fixed when plantar fascia contracts
- Loss of adult ambulation can occur from progressive pedal deformity, pain under lateral border of forefoot
- Fat pads under metatarsal heads can be lost
- Ankle instability can lead to degenerative joint disease

WHEN TO REFER

- To establish Dx
- Presence of increasing deformity or excessive shoe wear
- Complaint of pain
- Earlier referral, less likely major foot surgery required

BACKGROUND

- Disease produced in susceptible individuals by gluten, storage protein found in endosperm of wheat, barley, oats, rye
- Most pts tolerate oats (contains avenin instead of gliadin, alcohol-soluble portion of gluten). Toxicity of avenin not definitively established
- Gluten probably injures mucosa of small intestine by attaching and exposing epitopes on surface epithelium allowing immune system to recognize normal tissue antigens as foreign
- Symptoms correlate w/age at presentation; age at presentation parallels age at introduction of gluten
- Early onset disease presents w/GI (malabsorption symptoms) and develops at 9–18 mos of age; most commonly few mos after gluten introduced into diet
- Late onset disease presents >5 yrs of age w/growth failure w/or w/o GI complaints
- Incidence of overt disease high in Europe and Mediterranean area (1/400–1/4,000). Incidence in US of overt disease much less (1.29/10,000 live births). Frequency of asymptomatic disease may be similar in these areas
- 10% family members asymptomatic and possess villus atrophy
- Associated conditions: dermatitis herpetiformis, diabetes mellitus (4%), Down syndrome

MANIFESTATIONS

- Progressive development of Sx malabsorption (frequent, malodorous stools, abdominal distention, eventual malnutrition)
- *Constipation:* 10%

Clinical features of celiac disease

Early presentation (<2 yrs of age)

Diarrhea	Malnutrition
Weight loss	Growth failure
Vomiting	Pallor
Anorexia	Delayed development
Abdominal distention	Bruising
Irritability	Rickets
Apathy	
Constipation	

Late presentation (>5 yrs of age)

Lactose intolerance	Clubbing
Abdominal pain	Short stature
Anorexia	Anemia
Growth failure	Osteopenia
Pubertal delay	Bruising
Diarrhea	Enamel hypoplasia
Arthritis/arthralgia	

LABORATORY FEATURES

- Diagnostic criteria require characteristic small bowel biopsy in addition to either serum antigliadin (AGA), antireticulin (ARA), or antiendomysial (EMA) antibodies
- Small intestine biopsy features severe villus atrophy, intense inflammation w/plasma cells and lymphocytes and deep crypts
- *AGA:* wide range of sensitivity, specificity for celiac disease, have been found in normal controls, other diseases
- *ARA:* more specific for celiac disease than AGA, but not all celiacs express ARA
- *EMA:* considered most specific, sensitive serologic marker for celiac disease. Specificity, sensitivity approach 100%, titres fall to zero w/3–6 mos strict gluten-free diet, rise on challenge w/gluten. For diagnostic purposes, pts must be receiving gluten in diet. Also useful in following compliance to diet
- *Iron deficiency anemia:* serum iron low and mean corpuscular volume low
- *Megaloblastic anemia:* RBC folate level low
- *Hypoproteinemia:* serum albumin levels <3 g/dL in severe cases
- *Vitamin deficiency:* prolonged prothrombin time reflects vitamin K deficiency secondary to malabsorption. Prothrombin time corrects within 12–24h following SubQ administration of vitamin K. Vitamin A and carotene levels may be low
- Fecal fat excretion >5–7% of ingested dietary fat
- D-xyose absorption low 0.35 g/kg—usually 5 g and not >25 g of D-xylose administered po. One hr serum level <20 mg/dL in celiac disease reflecting villus atrophy
- Elevated AST and ALT

DIFFERENTIAL DIAGNOSIS

- Cystic fibrosis, other forms of pancreatic insufficiency
- Sucrase isomaltase deficiency
- Abetalipoproteinemia
- Intestinal lymphangiectasia
- Chronic active hepatitis

TREATMENT

- Gluten-free diet for life generally recommended
- Improvement in clinical symptoms within days to wks following gluten-free diet
- Continuation or recurrence of symptoms in 7–30%. May reflect lactase deficiency; associated either deliberate or inadvertent gluten ingestion may be operative. Serum AGA, ARA, or EMA should be monitored to help evaluate dietary compliance
- Severe cases may require elemental diets ie, vivonex, or even TPN. Pharmacological therapy w/immunosuppressive agents such as corticosteroids, azathioprine, or cyclosporine may be necessary

PREVENTION

- Breast feeding and delay in introduction of gluten in diets of infants has been associated w/delay in onset of disease

COMPLICATIONS

- Intestinal lymphoma occurs at greater rate than in general population. One study indicates as many as 14% celiacs develop lymphoma; may be overstated. Association established but incidence not
- Dental enamel hypoplasia
- Arthritis/arthraglia
- Behavioral problems, irritability in infants, young children resolve w/institution of gluten-free diet
- Recurrent apthous ulcers
- Rickets
- Growth failure

WHEN TO REFER

- Refer for diagnostic small bowel biopsy and suspicion of enteropathy, ie, infants and children w/Sx malabsorption or positive AGA, ARA, or EMA

BACKGROUND

- Bacterial skin infections (impetigo, ecthyma, folliculitis, furuncles, boils, and cellulitis) common in pediatric practice
- Cellulitis invasive bacterial infection of dermis and surrounding subcutaneous tissues. Erysipelas, preseptal cellulitis, buccal cellulitis, perianal cellulitis represent specific clinical presentations of cellulitis usually associated w/particular organisms. For example, erysipelas rapidly progressive form of cellulitis often caused by *Streptococcus pyogenes* characterized by intensely red, well-demarcated area of tender, brawny edema and induration
- Lymphangitis consists of red streaks (inflamed small lymphatic vessels) which extend proximally from primary area of cellulitis. Small lymphatic vessels allow bacterial organisms and/or extracellular products, toxins to spread
- Pathogenesis depends on introduction of bacteria into subcutaneous tissues by either hematogenous spread, or by direct extension from superficial infection, or skin trauma (cuts, abrasions, bites, burns, puncture wounds, etc). Once present, bacteria multiply and challenge host defenses by producing potent toxins and enzymes which damage tissue and cause inflammation and spread to contiguous sites
- Bacterial organisms which cause cellulitis (table)

Frequent causes	Unusual/special circumstance, causes
Streptococcus pyogenes	*Pseudomonas aeruginosa*
Staphylococcus aureus	*Pasteurella multocida*
Haemophilus influenza type B	Atypical mycobacteria
Streptococcus pneumoniae	Anaerobes and other bacteria*

*A variety of bacterial organisms can cause cellulitis in special circumstances

CLINICAL MANIFESTATIONS

- Localized erythema, swelling, induration, tenderness
- Lymphangitis
- Fever in severe or complicated cases
- Signs of preceding skin trauma or superficial infection

LABORATORY FEATURES

- *WBC count and differential:* WBC often elevated, differential has predominance of polymorphonuclear leukocytes, band forms
- *Blood culture:* often positive in severe or complicated cases
- *Culture of primary site:* open lesions (denuded skin, vesicles/bullae, pustules, burn areas, etc) usually positive for causative organism. Aspirates of primary sites (leading edge or center of site) may or may not be positive, depending on technique of aspiration and concentration of organisms per unit volume of tissue

DIFFERENTIAL DIAGNOSIS

- Venomous bite or sting
- Viral or fungal cutaneous infection
- Contact dermatitis
- Septic arthritis, osteomyelitis
  - if area of suspected cellulitis in close proximity to joints or metaphyses of long bones
- Trauma

TREATMENT

- Uncomplicated (minimal toxicity; all signs localized; no concern about bacteremia or exotoxin production)
  - oral antibiotic w/effectiveness for *Streptococcus pyogenes* and *Staphylococcus aureus* (cephalexin, nafcillin, dicloxicillin, amoxicillin/clavulanate)
- Complicated (impressive toxicity; generalized signs of bacteremia or exotoxin production; evidence of invasive disease)
  - hospitalized for intensive care to manage fluids, shock, sepsis. Treat w/parenteral antibiotics to cover *Streptococcus pyogenes* and *Staphylococcus aureus* (IV oxacillin or nafcillin). Add other antimicrobial agent if pathogens, in addition to *S. pyogenes, S. aureus* considered)

COMPLICATIONS

- Usually seen w/virulent and/or exotoxin producing strains of *Streptococcus pyogenes* or *Staphylococcus aureus*
- Bacteremia/sepsis
- Toxic shock syndrome (TSS)
- Staphylococcal scalded skin syndrome (SSSS)
- Severe invasive disease due to virulent *Streptococcus pyogenes*. Generalized toxicity, sepsis, myositis, fascitis, gangrene may result

- Abscess formation due to *Staphylococcal aureus* may require surgical drainage

PREVENTION

- HIB vaccine has greatly reduced all types of invasive HIB disease, including cellulitis
- Varicella vaccine (by reducing the incidence of varicella) prevents many cases of varicella-associated cellulitis
- Prompt cleansing and evaluation of burns, puncture wounds, animal bites, etc, may reduce incidence of secondary cellulitis. In severe skin trauma, prophylactic antibiotics may be considered

WHEN TO REFER

- Signs of toxicity, TSS, SSSS, severe invasive disease or sepsis
- Difficulty in distinguishing cellulitis and either septic arthritis or osteomyelitis
- Abscess formation, which may need surgical drainage

CEREBRAL EDEMA

MICHAEL B. TENNISON AND JOHN DOUGLAS MANN

BACKGROUND

- Three major types of cerebral edema:

Type	Mechanism	Examples
Cytotoxic	Swelling of neurons, glia	Hypoxia, encephalitis, trauma
Vasogenic	Breakdown of blood-brain barrier	Tumor, abscess, trauma
Interstitial	Blocked CSF pathways	Obstructive or communicating hydrocephalus, pseudotumor cerebri

- Pts may have more than one type of brain edema
- Brain swelling within confines of rigid container (skull) leads to elevation of intracranial pressure (ICP), which impairs cerebral vascular perfusion
- Cerebral perfusion pressure = mean arterial pressure − ICP; must be maintained to prevent cerebral infarction
- Shifts in intracranial contents (herniation syndromes) lead to permanent cerebral damage 2° to venous hemorrhage or arteriolar/venous thrombosis
- Rapid progression of edema most common w/head trauma and infection

CLINICAL MANIFESTATIONS

- Headache may/may not be present
- *Vital signs:* ↑ BP (widened pulse pressure) and ↓ HR (<50 in older child)
- Periodic breathing patterns—frequent sighing and yawning progressing to Cheyne-Stokes respirations
- Bulging fontanel in infants
- Papilledema may be absent early
- Observe for signs of head trauma: bruising, skull deformity, blood behind tempanic membranes
- *Encephalopathy:* altered content (confused, combative) and level (lethargy, coma) of consciousness

- Asymmetrical pupils w/larger pupil sluggish or fixed suggests third nerve palsy of uncal herniation syndrome
- *VI nerve paresis:* nonlocalizing sign of increased ICP
- *Focal neurologic findings:* hemiparesis, extensor plantar response

LABORATORY FEATURES

- CT/MRI head imaging
- *EEG:* nonspecific diffuse or focal slowing. Always normal in pseudotumor
- Hyponatremia from SIADH may be present
- *LP: should not be done* if brain edema suspected

Type of edema	Findings
Cytotoxic	diffuse brain swelling, small ventricles, loss of gray/white junction
Vasogenic	enhancing lesion(s)—tumor, abscess, infarction, encephalitis nonenhancing lesion(s)—subdural/epidural hematoma
Interstitial	hydrocephalus small ventricles w/pseudotumor

DIFFERENTIAL DIAGNOSIS

- *Metabolic encephalopathy:* hyperglycemia, ingestion, electrolyte disturbance
- *Seizure disorder:* postictal state or nonconvulsive status epilepticus
- *Complex migraine*
- *Psychogenic:* fugue state, catatonic reaction, conversion, somatoform disorder

TREATMENT

- *Goals:* maintenance of cerebral perfusion pressure, arrest and reversal of herniation syndromes, treatment of underlying causes. Most pts benefit from ICU-based monitoring. Acute treatment w/mannitol, steroids may buy time for diagnostic studies, transfer to ICU, surgery
- *Hyperosmolar agents* (vasogenic edema/cytotoxic): mannitol 0.5–1.0 g/kg given as slow IV push. Repeat 0.25–0.5 g/kg q4h as needed
- *Steroids* (vasogenic): dexamethasone IV 1–2 mg/kg (max. 10 mg) loading dose followed by 1 mg/kg/d (max. 16 mg) div q4–6h
- *Reduction in CSF formation* (interstitial—pseudotumor): acetazolamide 15–30 mg/kg/24h po in 3 div doses
- *Body positioning* (all types): head up 30°, maintain in midline to promote venous drainage
- *Hyperventilation* (all types): intubate, maintain pCO$_2$ 25–30 mmHg to decrease intracranial vascular volume

WHEN TO REFER

- W/exception of pseudotumor cerebri, all pts w/suspected brain edema should be transferred to tertiary care center promptly
- Refer all pts w/pseudotumor cerebri to ophthalmologist to monitor optic nerve function
- Refer pseudotumor nonresponders to neurologist

CEREBRAL PALSY

JAMES A. BLACKMAN

BACKGROUND

- Static, nonprogressive disorder of movement and posture
- Caused by injury to brain pre-, peri-, or postnatally (through first several years of life)
- Diverse etiologies include developmental abnormalities of brain, infection, trauma, hypoxia, stroke, intracranial hemorrhage
- Incidence ~2/1,000 live births

CLINICAL MANIFESTATIONS

- Delayed or deviant motor skills
- Hyper- or hypotonia
- Motor quotient (gross motor age ÷ chronological age × 100) <50
- Persistent primitive reflexes (eg, Moro, asymmetric tonic neck reflex)
- *No loss of skills*—static brain injury
- Types:
  – spasticity: 60%. Associated w/lesions of pyramidal tract, motor cortex, related areas of brain. Flexors in upper, extensors and adductors in lower extremities most affected. Associated signs include hyperactive deep tendon reflexes, clonus, positive Babinski. With rapid stretch of spastic muscles, "catch" and release characteristic (clasped-knife phenomenon)
  – dyskinesia (extrapyramidal): 20%. Associated w/lesions of basal ganglia. Reduced inhibition results in choreoathetoid or dystonic movements. Dysarthria commonly present
  – ataxia: 1%. Associated w/lesions of cerebellum. Imbalance may not be apparent until child ambulatory
  – Remaining cases may be of rigid, hypotonic, or *mixed* type w/one type predominating
- Distribution:
  – diplegia: involvement of legs more than arms
  – hemiplegia: involvement of one side of body only
  – quadriplegia: involvement of arms, legs, head, trunk
- Degree:
  – mild: minimal impairment
  – moderate: some impairment, improved w/therapy and/or assistive devices
  – severe: significant impairment, less improved w/therapy and/or assistive devices

LABORATORY FEATURES

- Head ultrasound, CT, or MRI may show various abnormalities, ie, neuronal migration defects, cerebral hemiatrophy, periventricular leukomalacia, porencephalic cysts, ventricular dilatation—or may be unremarkable
- No laboratory findings diagnostic. Cerebral palsy a clinical Dx

DIFFERENTIAL DIAGNOSIS

- Degenerative diseases of white matter (eg, leukodystrophies)
- Mass lesions impinging on descending motor fibers
- Infections, metabolic disorders, toxins, traumatic injuries, vascular diseases may cause movement disorders mimicking cerebral palsy. *Key difference: new and/or progressive*

TREATMENT

- Goal of treatment: reduce disability, facilitate function
- Multisystem disorder requires interdisciplinary management
- Primary care physician provides medical home
- Tertiary center interdisciplinary team provides comprehensive assessment, care suggestions
- Parents, child integral to decision making
- Main treatment involves physical therapy, orthopedics, orthotics, assistive technology
- Additional treatments may involve occupational and speech therapy, special education, nutrition
- Options for medical treatment of hypertonia include muscle relaxant drugs (diazepam, dantrolene, baclofen), botulinum toxin injections into selected muscles, intrathecal baclofen pumps, selective dorsal rhizotomy
- Medical subspecialists consulted as needed: ophthalmology, ENT, dentistry, gastroenterology, neurology (depending on complications)

COMPLICATIONS

- *CNS:* seizures, mental retardation, cortical blindness
- *Eyes:* strabismus, refraction errors
- *Ears:* recurrent otitis media, middle ear effusions, conductive hearing loss
- *Mouth:* drooling, dental caries, gingivitis, chewing and swallowing difficulties
- *Lungs:* recurrent aspiration pneumonia w/dysphagia or reflux
- *GI tract:* esophagitis from reflux, constipation
- *Musculoskeletal:* joint contractures, hip dislocation
- *Psychosocial:* isolation, education and career misopportunity, dependence, sexual frustration

PREVENTION

- Primary prevention:
  – optimize pre-, peri-, postnatal care
  – prevent known causes of infantile brain injury: meningitis w/vaccines, child abuse w/counseling, automobile-related injury w/restraints
- Secondary prevention:
  – minimize effect cerebral palsy has on failure to achieve full potential
  – reduce likelihood or severity of complications

WHEN TO REFER

- When suspected by Hx or exam, refer to developmental specialist or neurologist to confirm Dx, r/o other Dx
- Obtain comprehensive interdisciplinary evaluation
- Refer for indicated therapies, sometimes available through community early intervention or school programs
- Consult medical specialists as complications arise or suspected

CHARCOT-MARIE-TOOTH DISEASE

JAMES C. DRENNAN

BACKGROUND

- Charcot-Marie Tooth disease historical name for two most common forms of inherited progressive peripheral neuropathy. Hereditary motor sensory neuropathies (HMSN) most common cause of progressive cavus. Current classification subdivides Charcot-Marie-Tooth disease into HMSN I (hypertrophic) and HMSN II (neuronal) (see table)
- Major clinical problem progressive cavus deformity. Term *cavus* describes weight-bearing plantar flexed forefoot compared to hindfoot, which can be plantar flexed, (equinocavus), dorsiflexed (calcaneocavus), or in neutral position (cavus)
- May be later onset loss of peripheral proprioception, loss of fine motor function in upper extremities
- All types HMSN have autosomal dominant inheritance w/exception of type III, which is autosomal recessive. Most types commonly present in second decade w/symmetrical involvement. Involved persons demonstrate slow centripetal progression of weakness. May be varying degrees of clinical severity within given family. Life expectancy normal

TYPE I (75% HMSN)

CLINICAL MANIFESTATIONS

- Mild cavus deformity or clawing of toes may be first clinical manifestation in second decade of life
- Abnormal foot position initially flexible. Increasing peroneal and intrinsic involvement leads to equinocavovarus deformity w/high medial arch. Pt gradually develops weakness in all muscles distal to knee leading to drop-foot gait
- Pt may develop pain under lateral metatarsal heads during weight bearing and experience difficulty in running

- Atrophy of intrinsic hand muscles and later radially innervated muscles of forearm result in progressive loss of fine motor activities
- Type I pts have generalized tendon areflexia; more distal sensory deficits; more frequent hip and spinal deformities than other types

LABORATORY FEATURES

- Normal weight-bearing lateral x ray should demonstrate that line drawn through long axis of talus passes through long axis of first metatarsus confirming normal medial longitudinal arch. Angle of Meary created when forefoot plantar flexed relative to hindfoot
- EMG neuropathic w/increased amplitude and duration of response
- Motor nerve conduction velocities frequently one-half expected rate
- Histologic evaluation of sural nerve biopsy demonstrates formation of an "onion-bulb" cross-sectional appearance secondary to repetitive demyelinization and remyelinization of peripheral nerve
- Genetic analysis of HMSN type I demonstrates DNA duplication of portion of short arm of chromosomes 17 in region of p11.2–p12. Human peripheral myelin protein-22 gene contained within duplication. Felt to be either point mutation in peripheral myelin protein-22 or duplication of region containing peripheral myelin protein-22 gene

TYPE II

CLINICAL MANIFESTATIONS

- Clinical onset generally delayed until 2nd or 3rd decade of life w/more profound distal lower extremity weakness than type I
- Characteristic stork leg appearance caused by atrophy of distal third of quadriceps and hamstrings

- Flail foot progresses to calcaneocavus deformity, which shortens foot w/majority of weight bearing on heel
- Upper extremity involvement less pronounced

LABORATORY FEATURES

- Weight-bearing lateral x rays show progressive calcaneal pitch to hindfoot associated w/forefoot plantar flexion
- EMG neuropathic
- Motor nerve conduction velocities either slightly reduced or normal

DIFFERENTIAL DIAGNOSIS

- Friedrich ataxia
- Other forms of peripheral neuropathies
- Spinal cord lesions
- Idiopathic cavus (rare)

TREATMENT

- Surgery limited to forefoot correction when clinical heel varus demonstrated to be flexible. Accomplished by block test (1 in block placed beneath 4th and 5th rays while permitting first metatarsus to assume weight-bearing position and assessing whether clinical heel varus remains fixed or corrects to neutral or valgus position)
- When heel demonstrates flexibility, correction limited to intrinsic release and introduction of ankle-foot-orthotics. Tendon transfers may be necessary to manage drop-foot gait or may be used w/interphalangeal fusions for rigid claw toe deformities
- Lateral displacement calcaneal osteotomy added when heel has fixed varus position. Anthrodeses contraindicated

WHEN TO REFER

- Evidence of progression of cavus deformity

Hereditary motor sensory neuropathies

Type	Term	Inheritance
I	Charcot-Marie-Tooth (hypertrophic form)	Autosomal dominant
II	Charcot-Marie-Tooth (neuronal form)	Autosomal dominant
III	Dejerine-Sotta disease	Autosomal recessive
IV	Refsum disease	Autosomal dominant
V	Inherited spastic paraplegia	Autosomal dominant
VI	Peroneal muscular atrophy w/optic atrophy	Autosomal dominant
VII	Retinitis Pigmentosa w/distal muscle atrophy	Autosomal dominant

BACKGROUND

- ~3 million cases reported, 1 million cases substantiated annually
- Includes physical abuse, sexual abuse, emotional abuse, neglect. Neglect more common than abuse
- Etiology multifactorial. Associated w/ social isolation; parental Hx abuse; parental drug, alcohol abuse; domestic violence
- Children of all ages affected; mortality greatest in infants, young children

Clues to possible physical abuse

- Significant injuries unaccompanied by Hx trauma
- Hx does not explain injuries identified
- Unexpected and unexplained delay in seeking care
- Hx injury changes w/ time
- Injuries to multiple organs that are pathognomonic of abuse

CLINICAL MANIFESTATIONS

Physical abuse

- *Bruises:* patterned, isolated to unusual areas, multiple, in nonambulatory infants
- *Burns:* tap water scald burns, immersion burns, patterned contact burns
- *Fractures:* single or multiple, various stages of healing, nonambulatory infants
- *Abdominal trauma:* liver injuries, pancreatitis, duodenal hematoma, intestinal perforations. Bruising to abdominal wall often absent
- *Shaking impact syndrome:* subdural hemorrhage, brain injury, retinal hemorrhage, w/ or w/o extracranial injuries (rib, metaphyseal fractures, bruises). Presenting symptoms include seizures, lethargy, irritability, vomiting, coma. High mortality rate

Sexual abuse

- Symptoms nonspecific, including withdrawal, acting out, hypersexual behaviors, depression
- Hx from child most important diagnostic tool
- Genital examination often normal
- STDs possible, not frequent

Neglect

- Environmental malnutrition (FTT), unexplained lack of medical or dental care, supervision, clothing, education

LABORATORY FEATURES

- *Skeletal survey:* for children <2 yrs of age w/ any suspicious injury. Occult, healing fractures in setting of other injury suggestive of abuse
- *LFTs, amylase, lipase, UA, CPK:* screen for intraabdominal trauma
- *CT scan:* imaging method of choice for acute head or abdominal injury
- MRI more sensitive than head CT in detecting subtle or old brain injuries
- Genital cultures needed for symptomatic sexually abused children
- Forensic evidence collection indicated within 48 hrs of sexual assault

DIFFERENTIAL DIAGNOSIS

- *Bruises:* accidental bruises, coagulopathy, Mongolian spots, folk remedies
- *Burns:* accidental burns, rashes, diaper dermatitis, phytophotodermatitis, impetigo, toxin-mediated diseases
- *Fractures:* accidental fractures, metabolic bone diseases
- *Shaking impact syndrome:* accidental trauma, coagulopathy, arteriovenous malformation
- *Sexual abuse:* vulvovaginitis, urethral prolapse, lichen sclerosis et atrophicus, anatomic variations

TREATMENT

- All physicians *mandated* to report suspected child abuse to child welfare agency for investigation
- Police involvement necessary for serious physical abuse, sexual abuse
- Remain nonaccusatory when discussing possibility of abuse w/ family. Focus discussion on well-being of child
- Treatment options include supportive services for family and pt (most common), kinship or foster care (less common)

COMPLICATIONS

- Reabuse of children previously known or not known to child welfare. Majority of fatally injured children have evidence of previous abuse at time of death

PREVENTION

- Many preventive strategies have not been rigorously studied. Successful 1° prevention includes universal home visitation for new parents. Preventive efforts focus on offering support and monitoring of families

WHEN TO REFER

- Refer all cases of suspected abuse and neglect to state's child welfare agency. Police notification needed for serious physical and all sexual abuse
- Refer acute sexual assault if forensic evidence collection needed
- Referral to specialist for second opinion does not relieve you of your mandate to report children w/ suspected abuse

CHOLANGITIS

SARAH JANE SCHWARZENBERG

BACKGROUND

- Inflammation of biliary tree: infectious or noninfectious
- Most common in pts w/preexisting biliary surgery (extrahepatic biliary atresia, post Kasai) or autoimmune disease
- Infectious agent most commonly involved: enteric bacteria, both aerobes and anaerobes

CLINICAL MANIFESTATIONS

- Fever, usually w/o localizing source
- Jaundice or worsening of preexisting jaundice
- Right upper quadrant abdominal pain
- Deterioration of hepatic function, as measured by coagulation studies
- Sepsislike picture w/or w/o DIC
- May be asymptomatic, w/laboratory changes as only diagnostic clue
- Primary sclerosing cholangitis may precede onset of inflammatory bowel disease

LABORATORY FEATURES

- Elevated biliary (alkaline phosphatase, gamma-glutamyl-transpeptidase 5'-nucleotidase) and hepatocellular (SGOT, SGPT) enzymes. May be elevation above baseline in pt w/preexisting liver disease
- Conjugated hyperbilirubinemia
- *Coagulation studies:* prolongation of prothrombin and partial thromboplastin time and/or prolongation of thrombin time (if DIC develops)
- Positive blood cultures in 75% if cultures performed 15 min after liver biopsy
- *Hepatic ultrasound:* may demonstrate ductal dilatation, gallstone, or enlarged gallbladder
- Liver biopsy
- *WBC and differential:* usually elevated w/predominance of neutrophils
- *Other:* specific autoimmune marker and nonspecific markers of inflammation may be elevated

DIFFERENTIAL DIAGNOSIS

- Infections:
  - postoperative, after surgery for extrahepatic biliary atresia (EHBA), choledochal cyst, other biliary anomaly
    - cholecystisis, w/or w/o cholelithiasis
    - HIV
- Noninfections:
  - autoimmune
  - primary sclerosing cholangitis
  - drug induced: intrahepatic arterial infusion w/5-fluorodeoxyuridine (FUDR)
  - post–liver transplantation w/hepatic artery thrombosis (may include infectious component)

TREATMENT

- *Infectious:* IV antibiotic therapy 10–14 d followed by weekly liver enzymes and bilirubin for 1 mo
- *Obstructive:* endoscopic retrograde cholepancreatography w/sphincterotomy to relieve biliary obstruction and to biopsy biliary tree for opportunistic organisms *and* IV antibiotics as above. Operative management required in some cases
- *Autoimmune:* appropriate immunosuppression, usually w/combination of corticosteroids and 6-mercaptopurine

COMPLICATIONS

- Progressive inflammatory destruction of hepatic parenchyma w/development of cirrhosis
- Biliary structure
- Metabolic consequences of cholestasis (deficiencies of fat-soluble vitamins, bone disease, and dietary fat malabsorption)

WHEN TO REFER

- Consultation w/pediatric gastroenterologist/hepatologist essential in all cases, both for Dx and management

CHOLECYSTITIS

EUGENE D. McGAHREN III

BACKGROUND

- Refers to inflammation of gallbladder secondary to obstruction of cystic duct
- May occur any age
- Most common cause: occlusion of cystic duct by gallstones or biliary sludge
- In ambulatory population, gallstones usually idiopathic cholesterol stones, or pigmented stones resulting from hemolytic diseases
- Infants and children receiving total parenteral nutrition (TPN) may also be prone to cholestasis and subsequent development of gallstones
- Other less common causes of gallstones and/or cholecystitis include inflammatory bowel disease, cystic fibrosis, pregnancy, oral contraceptives, obesity, female gender, trauma, and genetic influences

CLINICAL MANIFESTATIONS

- Infants and younger children tend to present w/relatively chronic symptoms. Recurrent abdominal pain common although these pts cannot normally localize their pain
- Older children and adolescents may present with either acute or chronic symptomatology and are more able to localize their pain to right upper quadrant area of abdomen
- Other presenting signs may include fever, vomiting, dehydration
- If common bile duct has been occluded by gallstone, jaundice, darkened urine, light color stool may result

LABORATORY FEATURES

- *WBC count:* likely elevated in acute cholecystitis; may be normal in chronic cholecystitis
- *Bilirubin:* normal or slightly elevated. Level more significantly elevated if common bile duct obstruction present
- *Alkaline phosphatase, amylase:* likely elevated if common bile duct obstructed
- *Ultrasonography:* best study to demonstrate presence of gallstones or sludge in gallbladder, inflammation of gallbladder, degree of dilatation, if any, of extra hepatic biliary system
- *Biliary scintigraphy:* may be useful in confirming cystic duct obstruction by showing absence of dye in gallbladder, or common duct obstruction by showing absence of drainage into duodenum

DIFFERENTIAL DIAGNOSIS

- Any of variety of causes of abdominal pain in infants and children constitute differential Dx for cholecystitis
- Some of more common causes of abdominal pain include gastroenteritis, appendicitis, Meckel diverticulitis, urinary tract infection, lower lobe pneumonia, pancreatitis, incarcerated hernia, ovarian torsion, hepatitis, abdominal tumors, mesenteric cysts, bowel duplications, pyelonephritis, choledochal cyst

TREATMENT

- Generally, cholecystitis treated by removal of gallbladder
- Removal can be accomplished by either open laparotomy or laparoscopy
- Need for intraoperative cholangiography or common bile duct exploration depends upon presenting symptoms, laboratory values, and degree of suspicion for common bile duct involvement
- Usually, mild episodes of cholecystitis in infants and young children receiving TPN may be managed expectantly, since associated sludge or gallstones often resolve when TPN discontinued

COMPLICATIONS

- Sepsis
- Injury to common bile duct during surgery
- Pancreatitis

WHEN TO REFER

- Severe or persistent right upper quadrant pain in older children and adolescents
- Chronic abdominal pain w/o obvious source
- Jaundice
- Significant fever, vomiting, dehydration

BACKGROUND

- Abnormal dilatations of extrahepatic and/or intrahepatic biliary system
- Cysts have thick walls of dense connective tissue w/little smooth muscle; may be significant surrounding inflammation
- Most frequently found in females, people of Asian descent
- Etiology unclear but may be related to reflux of pancreatic secretions into biliary tree due to abnormal entrance of main pancreatic duct into common bile duct above sphincter of Oddi
- 5 types
  - type I: cystic dilatation of common bile duct
  - type II: diverticular malformation of common bile duct
  - type III: choledochocele at level of sphincter of Oddi
  - type IV: cystic dilatation of intrahepatic and extrahepatic ducts
  - type V: single or multiple intrahepatic ductal dilatation (also known as Caroli disease)

CLINICAL MANIFESTATIONS

- Infants usually present w/jaundice. Palpable mass may be felt
- In older children, pain and jaundice most common presenting symptoms. Classic triad of pain, jaundice, palpable mass described; however, <30% have all three symptoms
- Children may also present w/pancreatitis

LABORATORY FEATURES

- *Bilirubin and alkaline phosphatase:* usually elevated, indicating bile duct obstruction
- *Amylase:* frequently elevated
- *Ultrasound:* best initial imaging study to determine presence of choledochal cyst
- *CT:* helps delineate relationship of cyst to surrounding structures
- *Biliary scintigraphy:* helps determine degree of intrahepatic pathology and degree of bile outflow obstruction
- *Endoscopic retrograde cholangiopancreatography (ERCP):* definitive study for outlining cyst anatomy. May not be needed if other studies give adequate information

DIFFERENTIAL DIAGNOSIS

- Hepatitis
- Unconjugated bilirubinemia
- Biliary atresia
- Cholestasis from drugs or TPN
- Alpha-1-antitrypsin deficiency
- Pancreatitis or pancreatic mass
- Cholecystitis or gallbladder hydrops
- Any other cause of jaundice

TREATMENT

- Surgical excision of cystic area (essentially encompasses extrahepatic biliary tree) w/choledochojejunostomy at most proximal portion of common bile duct optimal when possible. Gallbladder also removed. If outer wall of cyst too inflamed, inner lining may be removed. Strategy works best for types I, II, IV
- Type III cysts (choledochocele) unroofed by transduodenal approach
- Type V cysts usually managed similarly to types I, II, IV. However, abnormal tissue left behind within liver. If disease limited to one lobe, lobectomy considered. If disease widespread and affecting liver function, transplant considered
- Any cyst epithelium left behind is at risk of developing into adenosquamous carcinoma. Thus type V cysts most worrisome
- Outcome generally good for types I–IV

COMPLICATIONS

- Stricture or leakage of biliary-enteric anastomosis
- Damage to pancreatic duct during dissection of cyst
- Pancreatitis
- Cholangitis
- Adenosquamous carcinoma in cyst epithelial remnants

WHEN TO REFER

- Jaundice
- Persistent abdominal pain
- Pancreatitis
- Abdominal mass

CHRONIC FATIGUE SYNDROME

DAVID S. BELL

BACKGROUND

- Incidence in adolescents depends on criteria used, one estimate of 40/100,000; estimates in children <12 yrs of age unknown but felt to be less common
- Diagnostic criteria for adolescents same as for adults; criteria for children <12 not yet established
- Most frequently follows nonspecific acute viral illness; gradual or insidious onset may be more common in children than in adults
- Noted to follow specific infectious agents (EBV infection, Lyme disease, Q fever), also trauma, stress
- Long-term outcome unknown; estimated half of adolescents recover within 2 yrs

CLINICAL MANIFESTATIONS

- Dx requires unexplained chronic fatigue of new onset for at least 6 mos significantly limiting activity and not alleviated by rest *and*
- 4 of following 8 symptoms, which did not predate fatigue: (1) cognitive dysfunction, (2) recurrent sore throat, (3) tender cervical or axillary lymph nodes, (4) muscle pain, (5) multijoint pain w/o swelling or redness, (6) headaches of new pattern, (7) unrefreshing sleep, (8) postexertional malaise lasting >24 h
- Dx cannot be made in presence of major depression, anorexia, bulimia, school phobia
- Mild depression, fibromyalgia may coexist and do not preclude Dx
- Tender lymph nodes w/o adenopathy, mild abdominal tenderness, mild pharyngitis, low-grade fever often seen on physical examination

LABORATORY FEATURES

- Laboratory evaluation used to exclude other disorders causing fatigue, not to make a diagnosis of CFS
- Exclusionary testing includes CBC, ESR, urinalysis, chemistries including blood sugar, liver function tests, tests of thyroid function
- Mantoux skin test, chest x ray, Lyme serology, ANA, RF, and other testing as clinically indicated
- Detailed immunological workup, MRI of brain; SPECT scanning may be of value in research protocols but not clinically indicated

DIFFERENTIAL DIAGNOSIS

- Medical causes of fatigue including anemia, hypothyroidism, diabetes mellitus, hepatitis, chronic infection
- Rheumatoid arthritis, lupus erythematosis, autoimmune disease
- Primary depression, somatization disorder and anxiety disorders; careful evaluation of psychosocial status important

Differences between chronic fatigue syndrome and major depression		
	CFS	Depression
Fatigue	flulike malaise	anhedonia
Motivation	high	low
Exercise	worsens symptoms	improves symptoms
Hopelessness, despair	0	+++
Depression	+–+++	+++
Headaches, sleep disturbance	+++	++
Cognitive disturbance	++	++
Abdominal pain	+++	+
Muscle, joint pain	+++	0
Lymphodynia, sore throat	+++	0
Fever, night sweats	+++	0

TREATMENT

- Ongoing medical and emotional support w/emphasis on realistic scheduling, improved coping skills, development of autonomy
- Symptomatic treatment of somatic symptoms ie, headache, muscle/joint pain, abdominal pain, lymphodynia
- Treatment of sleep disorder w/sleep hygiene techniques and nonpharmacologic Tx if possible
- Treatment of coexisting depression if present
- Educational support, w/modification of school schedule as needed (eliminate physical education, reduced classroom time, home tutoring if necessary)
- Encourage increased activity w/graded activity/exercise plan as tolerated
- Ongoing evaluation of potential medical causes of fatigue
- Ongoing evaluation of psychosocial status

COMPLICATIONS

- Depression
- Educational disruption
- Social isolation
- Disruption of autonomy development

WHEN TO REFER

- Majority of children w/CFS managed by primary care personnel
- Referral useful when depression or family dysfunction clouds Dx
- Referral useful if abnormal behavior patterns (enmeshment, disruption of autonomy, poor coping patterns) complicate Dx or recovery

CLEFT LIP AND CLEFT PALATE

GERALD M. SLOAN

BACKGROUND

- Clefting among most common of major congenital malformations
- Frequency of clefting in US ~1/600 term newborns, w/variation by racial or ethnic group
- Clefting can occur in lip alone, palate alone, or both
- Cleft lip plus cleft palate most frequent manifestation (~40% of cleft cases), followed by isolated cleft palate (35%) and isolated cleft lip (25%)
- Cleft lip more common in males (M:F ratio: 3:2); cleft palate more common in females (M:F ratio: 2:3)
- Cleft lip can occur unilaterally on either side (left more common than right by 2:1) or bilaterally (only one-tenth as common as unilaterally)
- Substantial portion (15–60%) of clefts occur as part of recognizable syndrome, which may have prognostic and genetic implications

CLINICAL MANIFESTATIONS

- Dx of cleft lip obvious at birth, and may even be suspected prenatally on ultrasound
- Cleft lip can be "complete" (extending through one or both sides of lip and into nose) or "incomplete" (w/an intact tissue bridge under nostril)
- All newborns should be examined for cleft palate by directly visualizing entire length of anterior ("hard") and posterior ("soft") palates
- Small, incomplete cleft palate, involving only posterior soft palate, can be missed if entire length of palate, including uvula, not well visualized
- Cleft palate must be suspected whenever nasal regurgitation of feedings, inability to adequately breast or bottle feed, and/or failure to thrive occur
- Subset of cleft palate pts, those w/Pierre Robin sequence (micrognathia, wide U-shaped cleft palate, glossoptosis), can have early and severe airway as well as feeding problems, which may require urgent or emergent endotracheal intubation and/or surgical management

LABORATORY FEATURES

- Not generally applicable

DIFFERENTIAL DIAGNOSIS

- Early effort should be made to distinguish syndromic from nonsyndromic clefting, based on presence or absence of other congenital anomalies
- >200 disorders that include cleft lip or cleft palate have been identified, including Mendelian (autosomal dominant, autosomal recessive, and X-linked), chromosomal, sporadic, environmental causes

TREATMENT

- Surgical lip repair usually performed at 2–3 mos of age and 10 lbs body weight
- For bilateral cleft lip, both sides repaired at same operation to achieve better symmetry
- Bilateral cleft lips almost always require separate operation to lengthen columella (central strut between nostrils) of nose; some surgeons do this 2–4 wks before lip repair; others prefer to do it 2–4 yrs after lip repair
- Surgical palate repair performed at 9–18 mos of age and 20 lbs body weight, usually closing hard and soft palate at same operation
- Secondary lip and/or nasal correction, when indicated, performed anywhere from preschool years to late teens or early 20s
- Secondary palate surgery, when indicated, should be performed as early as need established, typically 3–6 yrs of age; most common procedures: pharyngeal flap, pharyngoplasty, palatal lengthening
- Alveolar bone grafting, to stabilize upper dental arch and allow proper permanent tooth eruption at cleft site, performed at 6–9 yrs of age, when indicated, in conjunction w/experienced cleft orthodontist
- Orthodontic treatment may be needed early in childhood and/or later during preteen and teenage years
- Orthognathic surgery, to correct upper and lower jaw discrepancies, when necessary, performed in teens in females, late teens to early 20s in males

COMPLICATIONS

- Airway problems, particularly w/Pierre Robin sequence, may require immediate attention in newborn
- Feeding problems occur in virtually all newborn cleft palate pts but can almost always be successfully managed using proper cross-cut nipple w/or w/o squeeze bottle
- Direct breast feeding rarely successful w/cleft palate, but maternal breast milk may be expressed and fed via soft cross-cut nipple
- Cleft palate repair can be complicated by upper airway obstruction in early postop period, particularly w/Pierre Robin infants
- Secondary palate surgery, such as pharyngeal flap, can be complicated by acute or chronic (obstructive sleep apnea) airway problems, which usually improve over time but occasionally require surgical division of flap

PREVENTION

- In family w/Hx clefting, genetic consultation important for evaluation of recurrence risk, prenatal testing, discussion of diet and other preventive measures

WHEN TO REFER

- Birth of child w/cleft can be psychologically devastating to family
- Airway problems require immediate attention and consultation
- Feeding next priority, family should quickly be referred to experienced cleft team
- Advantages of multispecialty, experienced cleft team, including pediatric plastic surgery, genetics, pediatric otolaryngology, orthodontics, pediatric dentistry, feeding expertise, speech pathology, and audiology, as well as other specialists such as prosthodontics, psychology, and oral surgery well established and documented

BACKGROUND

- *Synonyms:* congenital talipes equinovarus, equinovarus congenita, congenital idiopathic clubfoot
- Although recognized for thousands of years, etiology remains unknown
- Occurs in 1–1.5/1,000 live births in Caucasians; less common in Asians, more common in Polynesians
- Males affected twice as often as females
- Bilateral ~50% affected people
- Uncorrected clubfoot results in weight bearing on dorsum (top) of foot; is unsightly, painful, and results in ulceration

CLINICAL MANIFESTATIONS

- The 4 components of clubfoot: (1) equinus of ankle (foot plantar flexed), (2) varus of hindfoot (heel turned inward), (3) cavus of midfoot (excessively high arch), (4) adductus of forefoot (front of foot turned inward)
- Foot stiff. Although varying amounts of passive motion present, foot *can not* be positioned in normal weight-bearing position
- Foot smaller and calf thinner than normal side

HERITABILITY

- 33% identical twins concordant
- 3–4% fraternal twins concordant
- If one child has clubfoot, 3–4% chance of sibling having clubfoot
- The more affected people in family, the higher recurrence risk
- Single major gene effect best explanation for inheritance pattern of clubfoot. However, many families have only one affected member. Idiopathic clubfoot probably etiologically heterogeneous

DIFFERENTIAL DIAGNOSIS

- *Postural equinovarus:* Rarely occurs; feet have components of clubfoot but are passively correctable into normal weight-bearing position. Follow-up mandatory as these feet may become stiff and behave like true clubfeet. Most resolve spontaneously
- *Metatarsus adductus:* These feet may have severe, rigid inward position of forefoot, but they lack other components of clubfoot
- *Neuromuscular clubfoot:* Clubfoot deformity may occur in association w/myelomeningocele, arthrogryposis multiplex congenita, other systemic neuromuscular disorders
- *Syndromic clubfoot:* Clubfoot deformity may occur in association w/many syndromes both w/and w/o cytogenetic abnormalities
- Careful general and neurologic examination necessary to exclude nonidiopathic clubfoot

TREATMENT

- Manipulation and casting should begin as early as possible—first week of life
- Ponseti method of manipulation and casting corrects 80–90% of idiopathic clubfeet. Other techniques have much lower success rates. Correction obtained in 8–16 wks weekly cast changes. Tenotomy of Achilles tendon may be required for complete correction
- Clubfeet uncorrectable by manipulation require surgical correction; usually performed 4–12 mos of age
- Most children can be expected to wear normal shoes and run/play nearly normally

COMPLICATIONS

- Clubfoot foot and leg always small
- Clubfoot always less supple than normal foot
- Recurrence of foot corrected by manipulation and casting may occur until age 5–7
- Surgical releases may result in flat foot deformities, incomplete correction and/or weakness of calf muscles, causing difficulties w/running, easy fatigability

WHEN TO REFER

- Referral should be made in first week of life to orthopedist experienced in treatment of clubfoot

BACKGROUND

- Occurs ~2/10,000 births; M:F ratio ~1.5:1
- *Definition:* obstruction of systemic blood flow by usually discrete and juxtaductal site of aortic narrowing
- Develops due to diminished prenatal blood flow through left heart and aortic isthmus and postnatal constriction of periaortic ductal smooth muscle
- Dx may be difficult to exclude in newborn, even by echocardiography, due to incomplete closure of ductus
- Occurs as isolated abnormality (simple, 60%) or w/associated defects (complex, 40%)
- *Common associated defects:* bicuspid aortic valve, PDA, VSD, aortic or subaortic stenosis, mitral stenosis, Turner syndrome
- *Recurrence risk:* 3–4% for 1° relatives

Bimodal clinical presentation

	Newborn–2 wk old	Older infants and children
Clinical picture	Heart failure or shock/acidosis	Incidental heart murmur, poor pulses or hypertension
Symptoms	Dyspnea/tachypnea w/feeds	None, exercise intolerance; rarely, claudication, headaches
Signs	Pallor, weak pulses, rales; hepatomegaly; 4 extremity BPs may be similar	Absent leg pulses or radiofemoral delay; posterior thoracic bruit, upper extremity hypertension
CXR	Pulmonary edema +/– cardiomegaly	normal or "3 sign" +/– rib notching
EKG	usually *right* ventricular hypertrophy	normal or *left* ventricular hypertrophy
Differential diagnosis	hypoplastic left heart, critical aortic stenosis, interrupted aortic arch; myocarditis/cardiomyopathy	essential hypertension

DEFINITIVE DIAGNOSIS

- *Echocardiography:* often sufficient (persistent ductus complicates interpretation)
- *MRI:* adjunctive or sufficient in older children
- *Cardiac catheterization and angiography:* reserved for assessment of associated defects, interventional procedures, or when above imaging modalities inconclusive

TREATMENT

- Stabilization of critically ill newborn:
  – prostaglandin E$_1$ (Prostin VR): 0.05–0.1 mcg/kg/min
  – sodium bicarbonate, 4.2% neonatal solution: 1 mEq/kg or 2 mL/kg
  – inotropic support, eg, dobutamine: 5–10 mcg/kg/min
- *Surgical repair:* usually, resection with end-to-end anastomosis; less commonly, subclavian flap or patch aortoplasty; 15–40% incidence of late recurrent coarctation when primary repair performed in infancy
- *Balloon angioplasty:* standard and 75–80% efficacious for postop recurrent coarctation; controversial for native, unoperated coarctation
- *Chronic antihypertensive therapy:* usually, beta blockers or ACE inhibitors, necessary in some pts, usually after late diagnosis and repair beyond age 5 yrs or w/residual coarctation not amenable to further intervention

COMPLICATIONS AND PREVENTION

- Acute perioperative morbidity and mortality low (~1% simple, ~5% complex)
- office-based primary care providers most often encounter pts years after surgery or angioplasty w/following issues in some pts:
  – exercise prescription: exercise testing identifies subset of pts w/normal resting hemodynamics but marked hypertension w/exercise. Limit participation in collision sports and intense isometric training
  – hypertension management
  – endocarditis prophylaxis
  – left ventricular dysfunction (particularly w/associated defects)
  – rare, late occurrence of aortic aneurysms, dissection or intracranial hemorrhage
- Long-term postop surveillance

WHEN TO REFER

- Heart failure in infancy
- Heart murmur not clearly innocent (any age)
- Upper extremity hypertension (older children)
- Difficulty palpating lower extremity pulses (any age)

BACKGROUND

- Potent alkaloid stimulant euphoriant drug; prepared from leaves of coca plant; purified to cocaine hydrochloride (often adulterated w/lidocaine or ephedrine); ingested by snorting into nose and by IV injection
- Cocaine freebase (also known as crack or base) smoked in special pipe
- Cocaine effect self-reinforcing, rapidly leading to loss of control over use and binge use; highly addicting

PHARMACOLOGY

- Onset of intense euphoria 8 sec, inhaled cocaine freebase; 30 sec, IV cocaine hydrochloride injection; several minutes for intranasal cocaine hydrochloride
- Duration of euphoria 15–20 min crack, 60–90 min cocaine hydrochloride
- Difficult to modulate effects of drug, titrate desirable effects, resist intense craving to repeat immediately cocaine-induced euphoria
- Use of cocaine highly predictive of polydrug use, often to modulate sympathomimetic effects of cocaine
- Metabolized by plasma cholinesterase (pseudocholinesterase)

MECHANISM OF ACTION

- Inhibition of reuptake of major neurotransmitters (eg, dopamine, serotonin, norepinephrine)
- Stimulates reward centers causing irresistible intense euphoria
- Binging or chronic use exhausts dopamine reserves, leading to intense dysphoria/irresistible craving to regain euphoric effect and mask highly unpleasant rebound exhaustion, mental depression

EUPHORIC PROPERTIES

- Subjective effects
  – fools brain: powerful stimulation of reward center, reinforcement. Euphoric, enraptured, elated, energized (wired), optimistic, overconfident, contented, gregarious, affable, garrulous, alert, hypervigilant
- Adverse effects:
  – pharmacologic: tolerance, binging, craving, high dependence potential
  – hypothalamic dysfunction: continued use leads often to disorders of appetite, sexual function, sleep
  – psychiatric: hypomania, jitteriness, depression, anxiety, mental exhaustion, suspiciousness, unpredictable mood swings, explosive temper disorder
  – neurologic: syncope, seizures, headache, fine tremor, stroke
  – cardiovascular: chest pain, arrhythmias, ischemia, hypertension
  – metabolic: hyperthermia, rhabdomyolysis

  – behavioral: major erosion of ethical, social, academic, vocational goals. Motor vehicle accidents, homicide, STDs (including syphilis), AIDS. Status offenses include running away, promiscuity, truancy, academic failure, antisocial behaviors (including stealing, dealing drugs, prostitution)

CLINICAL MANIFESTATIONS

- Abuse, dependency syndromes
- Increasing part of life devoted to planning, purchase, storing, use, selling, avoiding detection, partying, treating adverse effects of drug and social consequences from its use
- Use occurs despite adverse social, vocational, scholastic, criminal consequences
- Vows of abstinence repeatedly broken; gives up important social, vocational, recreational activities to use cocaine
- Distorted hierarchy of importance (drug first, self second, money third, loved ones fourth, society last)

COCAINE EFFECTS IN CERTAIN GROUPS

- *Newborns:* small for dates, low birth weight (<2,500 g), reduced head circumference, irritability and feeding problems, risk for SIDS, inattentive maternal care, abandonment, inconsistent or absent prenatal care, failure to thrive, syphilis of newborn
- *Children:* neurologic symptoms (eg, syncope or seizures), ataxia, behavioral problems
- *Adolescents:* oppositional, defiant, conduct disorder (eg, stealing, lying), antisocial personality disorder, explosive temper disorder, attention deficit disorder, STDs (esp syphilis), accidents, injuries, suicide, homicide, pregnancy, AIDS, incarceration, malnutrition, depression, psychosis, offenses against property and persons, binging, expense of drug treatment program, high risk of failure to complete treatment or relapse, initiation of siblings, friends to drug use
- *Pregnant females:* vascular accidents (abruptio placenta), hypertension, STDs, irresponsibility w/prenatal care, fetal wastage, syphilis and gonorrhea during pregnancy, AIDS

DIAGNOSIS

- High index of suspicion when behavioral and/or medical adverse effects suggest possibility of cocaine use. Unkempt, unhygienic appearance, "druggie" attire, including tattoos and key chains dangling from back pocket. Close association w/known drug users
- Urine toxicology screens important in ER setting, hospital admission, and newborn nursery
- Discussion of possibility of drug abuse w/adolescent, parents, teachers, drug counselor or psychiatrist

DIFFERENTIAL DIAGNOSIS

- Major mood disorders, oppositional-defiant adolescent, hyperanxiety disorder, amphetamine, PCP, alcohol, marijuana abuse, major causes of syncope, seizures, conduct disorders, aggression, explosive temper outbursts

TREATMENT

- No specific antidotes. Medical treatment based on treating specific adverse behavioral, psychiatric, metabolic, cardiac, neurologic complications
- Seizures and psychomotor agitation treated w/benzodiazapine, psychosis w/haloperidol or antidepressants such as desipramine (norpramine), malignant hypertension w/sodium nitroprusside, chest pain w/coronary vasodilators

DRUG TREATMENT

- Treatment programs of escalating intensity and duration matched to severity of abuse or dependence, stability of significant others such as parents, comprehensiveness of health insurance plan, local community resources for drug treatment, financial resources of parent
- Treatment programs include 12-step programs, highly structured long-term day care, residential programs, therapeutic communities, w/monitored abstinence for all illicit drugs, tranquilizers, alcohol
- Aftercare component usually essential. Serial urine tests for drugs of abuse mandatory. High rate of dropout and relapse for cocaine dependence
- Concomitant antidepressant, antianxiety medication may be useful

WHEN TO REFER

- Major medical or psychiatric adverse effect, signs of cocaine abuse or dependency of polydrug abuse, out of control conduct disorder, extreme oppositional/defiant attitude
- Cocaine abuse during adolescence often copathologic w/major depression, poor self-image, attention deficit disorder, learning disabilities, post-traumatic stress disorder, parent-child conflict; significant comorbidity may require referral

BACKGROUND

- Occurs 10–15% infants
- Usually begins first 2–3 wks of life
- Originally thought result of abdominal pain and/or gas; however, no well-designed studies support this hypothesis
- Resolves in most cases by 3 mos of age
- Effective treatments based on hypothesis that cause results from combination of three factors:
  - parental misconception of infant behavior, leading to
  - misinterpretation of infant cries, in an
  - infant whose temperament such that when needs not met infant cries to point of extreme agitation and inconsolability

CLINICAL MANIFESTATIONS

- Excessive crying that parents unable to console
- Infants cry in manner that leads parents to think infant crying because of pain
- Parents often think abdomen source of pain
  - Infants have no symptoms other than crying and passing of flatus
  - No vomiting, diarrhea, blood in stool, poor feeding, inadequate weight gain

LABORATORY FEATURES

- All laboratory tests normal

DIFFERENTIAL DIAGNOSIS

- All conditions that cause pain in infancy should be considered:
  - milk protein allergy suspected if vomiting, diarrhea, poor feedings, poor weight gain, blood present in stool
  - constipation
  - incarcerated hernia
  - hair cutting into digit
  - foreign body in eye

TREATMENT

- Dispel common myths about colic, eg, infant in pain, result of milk protein allergy, caused by gas
- Determine if parents have misconceptions about infant behavior that would lead to misinterpretation of infant cries:
  - need to limit frequency of feedings
  - need for strict sleeping schedule
  - pacifiers should not be used
  - only way to get infant to sleep is to walk and rock child
  - holding infant too much spoils child
- Educate parents concerning infant behavior and needs

- Counsel parents to treat infant's fussing and crying as infant's way of communicating needs
- Inform parents of five basic reasons for infant crying: hunger, tiredness, need to be held, need to suck, need for stimulation
- Instruct parents to respond quickly to infant cries before baby becomes agitated and inconsolable
- Often difficult to determine how parents misinterpreting infant cries and to counsel them effectively w/o use of behavioral diaries (refer to *Why Is My Baby Crying* by Bruce Taubman, Simon & Schuster)

COMPLICATIONS

- Interferes w/development of healthy maternal-infant attachment

PREVENTION

- Counsel parents to treat crying and fussing in healthy baby as communication not sign of pain or gas
- Educate parents about infant's needs: ie, to feed on demand, to be held, to suck, for stimulation, sleep

WHEN TO REFER

- Referral to subspecialist not necessary

COMMON COLD

J. OWEN HENDLEY

BACKGROUND

- Defined as acute, self-limited respiratory illness caused by virus
- Colds occur because of acquisition of virus from another human, not reactivation of indigenous viral flora
- Cold virus transmission normally occurs in "family contact" settings, suggesting direct contact or large droplet aerosol usual route for spread
- Colds common because two attributes of causative viruses:
  - some viruses (ie, respiratory syncytial virus, parainfluenza viruses, coronaviruses) can reinfect child or adult multiple times
  - other viruses (ie, rhinoviruses, adenoviruses, Coxsackie A and B, echoviruses) infect individual only once in life, but multiple serotypes of each virus exist. As result, some 200 different viral serotypes available to infect, each serotype only one time
- In 1950s preschool-age children averaged ~8 viral respiratory infections/yr, w/first infection at ~4 mos of age. W/daycare attendance, average number of colds per year in normal children now presumed to be ≥10–12/yr

CLINICAL MANIFESTATIONS

- Most cold symptoms in adults (nasal obstruction, scratchy/sore throat, sinus fullness, malaise) subjective, w/o associated physical findings
- Subjective symptoms in young children often missed by parents; objective findings such as fever, rhinorrhea (clear, white, yellow or green), anterior cervical adenopathy, cough *may* be noted
- Fever common in preschool age children in first 3–4 d of viral respiratory infections. In contrast, fever rarely occurs in adults infected w/same viruses
- Colds in children regularly last 10–14 d, whereas in adults symptoms abate by 5–7 d
- Eustachian tube dysfunction, evidenced by retracted or immobile eardrums w/serous fluid, common part of viral colds in preschoolers

LABORATORY MANIFESTATIONS

- *WBC count and differential:* normal
- PMNs and sloughed ciliated cells expected to be present in nasal secretions but rarely sought
- Paranasal sinuses by coronal CT imaging usually abnormal (≥80%) in adults w/viral colds; sinuses would also be expected to be abnormal in children
- Tympanometric evaluation usually abnormal during viral colds as reflection of eustachian tube dysfunction

COMPLICATIONS

- Secondary bacterial infection of middle ear (5% of colds in children) or paranasal sinuses (0.5% of colds in adults) difficult to differentiate from common involvement of ear and/or sinuses in viral infection
- Bacterial otitis media may be heralded by secondary fever and/or bulging tympanic membrane w/pus behind it
- Secondary bacterial sinusitis suggested by prolonged (>10–14 d) rhinorrhea and/or cough
- Exacerbations of asthma frequently precipitated by viral colds

TREATMENT

- Variety of medications may be useful in alleviating symptoms of cold:
  - acetaminophen/ibuprofen: helpful in running doses early in illness for fever and/or malaise
  - antihistamine/decongestant (many preparations): alone or in combination
  - dextromethorphan: to suppress nonproductive cough awakening child or parents at night
  - guaifenesin: expectorant to loosen secretions
  - vaporizer in bedroom at night
- *Antibiotics: deleterious* in viral respiratory infections, since virus not killed and antibiotics always select resistant normal bacterial flora (ie, penicillin-resistant pneumococcus)

WHEN TO REFER

- "Recurrent infections": 10–12/y viral respiratory infections each lasting 2 wks norm in preschoolers, so referral *not* necessary except for possible allergic component or for ≥2 bacterial pneumonias

COMPARTMENT SYNDROME, ACUTE AND CHRONIC

PETER D. PIZZUTILLO AND

MARTIN J. HERMAN

BACKGROUND

- A compartment is closed fascial space, eg, deep posterior compartment of calf
- Compartment syndrome is clinical manifestation of increased tissue pressure in this fixed space and its effects on function of muscles, nerves, blood vessels contained within that anatomic space
- Common etiologies:
  - trauma (fracture, contusion, wringer injury)
    - vascular injury/occlusion
    - tight cast
    - bleeding disorders (hemophilia)
    - burns
    - snakebites
    - intensive muscle use
- Most commonly seen in forearm after supracondylar elbow fractures or radius and ulna fractures, and in calf after tibia fractures. Can occur in any compartment of upper and lower extremity, including compartments of hand and foot
- Recovery excellent if recognized and appropriately treated. Late or missed Dx can result in significant limb dysfunction

CLINICAL MANIFESTATIONS

- Persistent, progressive pain out of proportion to clinical situation
- Tenseness to palpation of limb within boundaries of compartment
- Weakness of muscles contained within compartment
- Numbness or reduced sensation in anatomic distribution of compressed nerves contained within compartment
- *Hallmark of Dx:* pain on passive stretch of muscles contained within compartment
- *Warning:* unless vascular injury is etiology, distal pulses and capillary refill may remain intact despite severe compartment syndrome

LABORATORY

- No specific laboratory tests indicated
- Useful as adjunct in establishing specific etiology and guiding treatment, eg, factor levels in hemophilia or radiographs in trauma
- Measurement of intracompartmental pressures (by consultant)

DIFFERENTIAL DIAGNOSIS

- Soft tissue injury w/o elevated intracompartmental pressure
- Arterial laceration or occlusion
- Neuropraxia

TREATMENT

- If Dx suspected:
  - careful, well-documented examination of limb to include compartment palpation, motor, sensory, vascular assessment, passive muscle stretch testing
  - release or complete removal of all circumferential dressings, casts, etc
  - elevation of limb *at level of heart*
  - Sx not improved promptly, transport pt immediately to ER for evaluation
  - measurement of intracompartmental pressure by surgical consultant to confirm Dx (if necessary)
- If Dx compartment syndrome:
  - immediate surgical release of all involved compartments

COMPLICATIONS

- Ischemic injury to muscle and nerve occurs within 4–6 hrs onset of compartment syndrome
- Late/missed Dx (chronic compartment syndrome) can result in permanent muscle necrosis and contracture and nerve insensibility. If muscle necrosis complete when diagnosed, surgical decompression not useful. Appropriate rehabilitation, late reconstruction indicated

WHEN TO REFER

- Refer suspected compartment syndrome promptly. *Maintain high index of suspicion, low threshold for referral*

CONCUSSION

DAVID M. McKALIP AND STEVEN K. GUDEMAN

BACKGROUND

- Short-lasting, reversible neurologic disturbance w/o evidence of pathology following mild head injury
- Use of helmets during sporting and recreational activities (bicycling, skating, motorcycling, use of all-terrain vehicles) can minimize effects of minor head injuries

CLINICAL MANIFESTATIONS

- Spectrum of disturbances after mild head injury ranging from confusion w/or w/o varying depths and duration of *amnesia* and/or *loss of conscisouness*
- *Infants:* seldom w/loss of consciousness (LOC). More common is brief, wide-eyed immobility followed by crying and possible irritability, lethargy, poor oral intake, and/or vomiting
- *Children:* more classic symptoms, longer recovery phase
- Transient focal neurologic deficits may appear, including weakness, altered sensation, dysphasias
- May display brief respiratory, circulatory, autonomic disturbances
- At least half of children vomit once. Persistent vomiting may occur

DIFFERENTIAL DIAGNOSIS

- Hx accidental minor head injury uncertain, or trauma may have been *precipitated* by change in consciousness, consider following:
    - postictal confusion following seizure
    - drug intoxication
    - metabolic disturbance/hypoxia
    - meningitis/encephalitis
    - CNS structural lesion (tumor, hemorrhage)
    - hydrocephalus
    - syncope
    - child abuse

RADIOLOGIC FINDINGS

- Head CT indicated for loss of consciousness, focal neurologic deficits, persistent vomiting, skull fracture, seizure following head injury. High index of suspicion warranted in children w/coagulation disorders, CSF shunts, or congenital cerebral malformations, even if head injury minor
- Negative scan consistent w/Dx of concussion

TREATMENT

- Pt should be admitted for 24–48 hr period of observation and frequent neurologic checks in presence of following:
    - significant post-traumatic amnesia
    - deteriorating LOC
    - moderate to severe headache
    - drug or alcohol intoxication
    - skull fracture
    - CSF leak
    - significant associated injuries
    - abnormal head CT
    - no reliable companion at home
    - frequent vomiting necessitating IV fluids
    - seizures
- Otherwise, pt may be discharged home in care of reliable companion w/"Head" sheet describing warning signs of neurologic deterioration (pupilary changes or decreased LOC). Pt should be aroused q2h for next 12–24 hrs
- Follow-up clinic appointment in 1 wk

COMPLICATIONS

- Early, self-limited "impact" seizures may occur. Usually not multiple and occur immediately or within first few hrs of injury
- Pediatric concussion syndrome: acute pallor, diaphoresis, varying levels of diminished responsiveness. Usually clears spontaneously and rapidly
- Postconcussive syndrome may persist for months, usually in children and adolescents. Consists of one or more of following: headaches, fatigue, memory impairment, dizziness, visual aberrations, changes in mood

WHEN TO REFER

- Pts w/post-traumatic seizures, fractures, abnormal head CT, diminishing mental status, focal neurologic deficits, CSF leaks should be evaluated by neurosurgeon

BACKGROUND

• Conduct disorders characterized by serious, persistent, deliberate violations of rules/behavioral norms. Causes clinically significant impairment in functioning and often would result in arrest of an adult demonstrating parallel behaviors. Many of these children at high risk for future difficulties

– prevalence believed 6–10% males and 2–9% females

– childhood onset type occurs <10 yrs of age, more often in males, usually includes aggressive behaviors, associated w/worse prognosis

– adolescent onset type occurs >10 yrs of age and rarely has its onset after 16; associated w/better prognosis

– pathogenesis unknown but believed to be multifactorial

– predisposing factors include (1) genetic: increased incidence in twins and in families with Hx antisocial behavior, substance abuse, affective disorders, (2) organic: CNS or cognitive compromise including lower IQ, learning disabilities, ADHD, communication disorders, substance abuse, affective disorders, difficult temperaments, (3) environmental: harsh discipline, abuse, neglect, early institutional living, association w/delinquent groups

• *Significance:* impaired development and achievement w/greater likelihood of adult antisocial disorder, substance abuse, affective and somatoform disorder. Family disruption common; marked costs to society

CLINICAL MANIFESTATIONS

• Three or more symptoms in any of following areas:

– bullies or intimidates
– initiates fights
– used weapon
– physically cruel to people
– cruel to animals
– confrontational stealing
– forced sex
– fire setting
– destruction of property
– breaking and entering
– lies
– nonconfrontational stealing
– staying out all night
– running away
– truancy

• *Associated finding:* anger, hostility, lack of empathy for others, little guilt or remorse, externalization of blame ("it's not my fault"), and low self-esteem common. Often associated w/early onset of substance abuse and sexual activity. Suicidal ideation, attempts, completions greater than expected

LABORATORY FEATURES

• Generally noncontributory except for Dx associated disorders or disabilities though appropriate assessment

DIFFERENTIAL DIAGNOSIS

• Principal differential diagnosis lies between conduct disorder (CD) and other disruptive behavior disorders (ADHD and oppositional defiant disorder, ODD). Key elements: if misbehavior appears volitional, likely ODD or CD. If behavior would result in adult arrest, conduct disorder. If disregard for social rules, probably ODD. Both disorders can occur comorbidly w/ADHD, which if alone, does not typically appear as deliberate misbehavior

• Other possible Dx include adjustment disorders w/disturbance of conduct (must be precipitant and time limitations of 6 mos) and manic episodes in which underlying disturbance in affect and thinking generally quite obvious

• Comorbid disorders include: ADHD, learning disorders, substance abuse, depression. Should all be screened for by Hx or appropriate testing

TREATMENT

• Multimodal using an integrated bio-psycho-social model

• Identify and treat any underlying, associated, comorbid feature: ADHD, learning disorder, substance abuse, depression, abuse, neglect, etc

• Children w/CD action oriented and cost/benefit sensitive. Almost universally have poor problem-solving skills. Action-oriented interventions employing clear rewards and punishments coupled to enhanced, cognitively based problem-solving strategies are individual treatments of choice

• Family/parent interventions to develop improved management and problem solving

• Milieu management in school or residential school as indicated

• Hospitalization may be needed to stabilize most severe cases

• Medications generally target associated disorders. Primary trials of stimulants, antidepressants, anticonvulsants, lithium, may help but literature equivocal on utility

• *Complications/prognosis:* majority of children w/CD do not become adult antisocial characters but >25% do. Early onset (<10 yrs of age), violent offenses, increased numbers of offenses, comorbid disorders all associated w/worse prognosis

• Increased incidence of substance abuse, depression, suicide, somatoform disorders all associated

PREVENTION

• Early identification of at-risk children w/individual risk factors (ADHD, LD, depression) or environmental risk factors (abuse, neglect, harsh discipline, gang involvement) followed by appropriate intervention

WHEN TO REFER

• Differential diagnostic evaluation of children w/suspected CD can be undertaken in the office. If underlying disorders, ODD or ADHD, found, office treatment may be appropriate. Majority of children/adolescents w/CD require multimodal, intense interventions that do not fit context of most pediatric practices. Collaborative, coordinated work w/mental health professionals intervention of choice

BACKGROUND

- *Cardiac failure:* heart unable to deliver oxygen to tissues at rate sufficient to meet body's needs
- Underlying causes:
  - intrinsic heart muscle dysfunction, eg, myocarditis or cardiomyopathy
  - structural heart disease, eg, congenital heart malformation
  - sustained tachycardia
  - reduced afterload, eg, anemia, thyrotoxicosis, malnutrition
  - systemic hypertension
  - pulmonary hypertension (cor pulmonale)
  - acute heart failure in infancy medical emergency
  - role of primary care pediatrician: recognize heart failure
  - needs referral for specific Dx and treatment

CLINICAL MANIFESTATIONS

- Depends on underlying cause, but common findings include:
  - tachypnea
  - tachycardia
  - hepatomegaly
  - peripheral edema

SPECIFIC MANIFESTATIONS

- Neonate w/ductal dependent lesion, eg, hypoplastic left heart, coarctation, critical aortic stenosis
  - ductal constriction causes abrupt low cardiac output w/:
    ○ poor color
    ○ decreased pulses
    ○ decreased perfusion
    ○ metabolic acidosis

- Infants w/large left-to-right shunts often present w/:
  - failure to thrive
  - prominent sweating
  - wheezing

LABORATORY FEATURES

- No specific laboratory test
- Hemoglobin usually normal unless severe anemia underlying cause
- *WBC count and differential:* normal
- *Urinalysis:* ↑ specific gravity, albuminuria, ↓ volume
- *Electrolytes:* ↓ serum sodium
- Hypoglycemia and hypercalcemia in young infants
- *Chest roentgenogram:* usually cardiac enlargement and may show pulmonary edema
- *EKG:* helpful in Dx underlying cause of heart failure
- *Echo:* helpful in Dx structural heart disease and evaluation of cardiac function

DIFFERENTIAL DIAGNOSIS

- Sepsis (esp neonates)
- Pneumonia
- Renal disease
- Liver disease

TREATMENT

- Hospitalization for treatment of acute heart failure in all infants and most children
  - general measures:
    ○ reduce metabolic needs: bed rest, supplemental O_2, sedation if needed
    ○ identify underling cause of heart failure
    ○ inotropes to improve cardiac contractility
    ○ diuretics to relieve fluid retention
    ○ ACE inhibitors for afterload reduction
  - specific measures:
    ○ prostaglandin E, to dilate ductus in neonate w/ductal-dependent lesion
    ○ adenosine or cardioversion for sustained supraventricular tachycardias
    ○ correction of structural heart disease if feasible
- appropriate treatment of underlying cause whenever possible

AMBULATORY MANAGEMENT

- *Digoxin maintenance:* 10 mg/kg qd or div q12h
- *Diuretics:* furosemide 1–2 mg/kg qd. K⁺ sparing spironolactone may be added. 1.5–3 mg/kg/d in 2–3 div doses
- *Captopril or other afterload reduction drugs:* 1–5 mg/kg/d (div 2–3 doses)
- *Nutrition:* no-added-salt diet for children. Infants: milk not to exceed 24 cal/oz. May need tube feedings to obtain adequate caloric intake

COMPLICATIONS

- *Electrolyte imbalance:* monitor to avoid hypokalemia
- *Drug toxicity:* digoxin levels not needed routinely, but drug interactions must be noted and any arrhythmia should prompt digoxin level
- Mortality significant if underlying cause of cardiac failure not successfully treated

WHEN TO REFER

- Cardiac failure requires referral for specific Dx and treatment. Follow-up management requires collaboration between pediatrician and consultant

CONJUNCTIVITIS (ACUTE BENIGN INFECTIOUS CONJUNCTIVITIS)

JACOB A. LOHR

BACKGROUND

- No precise incidence rates available
- Vision rarely threatened except in unusual cases of *Herpes simplex* conjunctivitis
- Can be highly contagious in home, daycare, school settings
- Etiologic agents:
  - common misconception: "most cases are viral"
  - bacterial: nontypeable *Haemophilus influenzae, Streptococcus pneumoniae, Moraxella catarrhalis, Staphylococcus aureus* (rare cause except in surgical pts)
  - viral: adenovirus (can present as pharyngoconjunctival fever)
- Concombinant/subsequent otitis media may occur (most frequently associated w/ *H. influenzae* infection)

CLINICAL MANIFESTATIONS

- Initial sign usually hyperemia of conjunctival vessels
- Itching, burning, photophobia
- Complaint of foreign body sensation
- Discharge (water, mucopurulent, purulent); matting of eyelashes w/discharge, most noticeable when child awakens from sleep
- Fever usually not present unless associated w/ other site(s) of infection
- *Common misconception:* "One can tell difference between viral/bacterial cases based on presentation"

LABORATORY FEATURES

- Gram/giemsa stain of specimen from conjunctival sac or from scraping of conjunctiva usually not helpful in identifying etiologic agent
- Obtaining conjunctival cultures probably not cost effective

DIFFERENTIAL DIAGNOSIS

- Allergic conjunctivitis most easily confused Dx
- R/o foreign body
- Vesicles/ulcerations suggest *Herpes simplex* conjunctivitis
- Toxicity suggests systemic illness (eg, measles, Kawasaki disease, toxic shock syndrome)

TREATMENT

- Topical antibiotic treatment of bacterial conjunctivitis results in:
  - earlier clinical improvement than would naturally occur within 5–10 d
  - earlier eradication of specific etiologic bacterial agent from conjunctivae, probably interrupting contagion
- Many topical antibacterial agents available:
  - polymyxin B sulfate-bacitracin/polymyxin B sulfate-trimethoprim sulfate considered topical agents of choice; polymyxin B sulfate-bacitracin ophthalmic ointment applied to conjunctival sac q4h (5 doses/d) × 7–10 d; polymyxin B sulfate-trimethoprim sulfate ophthalmic solution instilled (1 drop) q3h (6 doses/d) × 7–10 d; medications difficult to apply if child uncooperative; may cause irritation; serious side effects rare; avoid neomycin-containing agents because of known hypersensitivity reactions
- Oral antibiotic Tx probably effective but not fully studied
- No specific treatment of adenovirus conjunctivitis available

COMPLICATIONS

- Serious complications rare

PREVENTION

- Hand washing by caretakers after contact w/ infected child
- Avoidance of sharing of toys, washcloth, towel used by infected child
- No proven benefit of prophylactic use of topical/oral antimicrobial

WHEN TO REFER

- Initial visit:
  - foreign bodies not readily removable
  - Hx penetrating ocular injury
  - recent ophthalmologic surgery
  - loss of acuity
  - significant pain
  - contact lenses
- During course of Tx:
  - symptoms that progress rapidly in first few days
  - development of excessive pain
  - development of decreased acuity
  - no improvement in first week Tx

BACKGROUND

- 3% general pediatric clinic visits; 10–25% pediatric gastroenterology visits
- Most cases chronic functional constipation; "encopresis" denotes chronic constipation w/overflow soiling
- Age of onset frequently <1 yr old/highest in toddlers 2–4 yrs old; male predominance throughout childhood for encopresis

MANIFESTATIONS

- Dx principally rests w/Hx/physical exam
- Stool withholding common response to painful defecation/difficult toilet training for young child; overflow soiling usually after chronic fecal retention
- Failure to thrive, weight loss, vomiting, localized abdominal pain, severe abdominal distention may indicate underlying organic disease
- Physical examination emphasizes abdominal contents, sacral configuration, anal tone and placement, rectal contents
- Underlying disorders suspected from patulous anus, flat sacrum, ectopic anus, palpable rectal masses, narrow anal canal w/higher retained stool

LABORATORY FEATURES

- *Functional constipation/encopresis:* no abnormal laboratory findings; abdominal radiograph can reveal stool retention; in specific cases, lead level, thyroid tests, abdominal x ray, barium enema, rectal biopsy, ano-rectal manometry obtained for more common differentials

DIFFERENTIAL DIAGNOSIS

- *Drug related:* anticholinergics, barium sulfate, bismuth, iron, opiates, calcium/aluminum agents (antacids)
- *Toxins:* lead ingestion
- Hirschsprung disease
- Hypothyroidism, hypercalcemia, hyperparathyroidism
- Electrolyte abnormalities
- Infant botulism
- Obstructions, eg, sacral teratoma, anterior meningomyelocele, hydrometrocolpos)
- *Intestinal strictures:* IBD, NEC, infectious, congenital
- Anterior displaced anus, anal stricture

TREATMENT

- *Acute simple obstruction:*
  – principal therapy: dietary manipulations
  – for infants: laxative fruits (eg, apricots, prunes, pears); increase water/full-strength juice intake; complex carbohydrate (eg, malt soup extract 1–2 tsp 1–3×/d)
  – for toddlers: limit cow's milk intake, provide adequate fluid intake, bran cereals, muffins; for persistent firm stools, mineral oil/lactulose (1–2 tablespoons/d) used short term
  – older children: bran foods; if required, fiber supplements (fiber tablets 4–6/d) w/additional water
- Voluntary stool withholding:
  – explain withholding behavior to parents (often misinterpret this as excessive straining at stool)
  – toilet training can be abandoned temporarily if aversion has occurred
  – one or two enemas (3 mL/kg 12 hrs apart) to evacuate retained stool
  – forced daily evacuation 10–14 d w/laxative therapy (senna/milk of magnesia, 1–3 tsp/d near bedtime)
  – behavioral conditioning
- Encopresis and megarectum:
  – colonic evacuation: hypertonic phosphate enemas (3 mL/kg) bid until no solid stool (max. of 6); for fecalomas, mineral oil enemas to precede phosphate enemas by 1 hr; administration of balanced polyethylene glycol-electrolyte lavage solution by NG tube for very severe cases
  – daily bowel movements: oral laxative (eg, senna, bisacodyl) to give daily bowel movements (often 2–3 tablets/d)
  – behavioral conditioning: child sits on toilet 5–10 min at same time each day; high-fiber diet +/– lactulose therapy after stimulant laxative withdrawal aids training

PREVENTION

- Rapid initiation of above measures when acute constipation

WHEN TO REFER

- Those who fail to respond or have underlying disease

CONTACT DERMATITIS (ALLERGIC AND IRRITANT)

STEPHEN O. KOVACS AND SUSAN B. MALLORY

BACKGROUND

- *Children <8 yrs of age:* lower threshold to irritants
- Diaper dermatitis most common form of irritant contact dermatitis in infancy; produced by lengthy contact w/urine, feces, detergents, soaps, antiseptics in diapers
- *Children w/preexisting skin disease:* higher propensity for developing irritant contact dermatitis
- Incidence ~10% attending skin clinic
- Eruption site clue to cause
- *Common causes of allergic contact dermatitis:* poison ivy, poison sumac, poison oak
- ~85% of population susceptible to poison ivy allergy after adequate exposure. Other common contact allergens include nickel, cosmetics, dyes, metal, rubber products, industrial chemicals
- Initial sensitization w/o skin manifestation required in susceptible individuals for allergic response
- *Contact dermatitis:* 90% occupational skin disease, most cases involve irritant

CLINICAL MANIFESTATIONS

- Can be acute, subacute, chronic
  - acute dermatitis: erythema, pruritus, stinging, burning vesicles, crusts, scale
  - subacute dermatitis: erythema, scale, fissures, papules, pustules, dryness
  - chronic dermatitis: hyperkeratosis, scales, lichenification, hyperpigmentation, fissures
- Dx irritant contact dermatitis based on Hx contact, negative patch tests to appropriate allergens
- Allergic contact dermatitis sometimes difficult to differentiate from irritant dermatitis; former often more delayed presentation
- Irritant diaper dermatitis usually involves genitalia/buttocks w/sparing creases
- Perianal dermatitis often caused by diarrhea

DIFFERENTIAL DIAGNOSIS

- Psoriasis
- Atopic dermatitis/eczema
- Fungal infection
- Seborrheic dermatitis

TREATMENT

- Avoid irritant/allergen (most successful treatment regimen)
- Patch testing for suspected allergic dermatitis: useful to determine inciting agents. Education in avoidance of allergen important
- Acute dermatitis:
  - extensive: oral corticosteroid therapy: prednisone, 1–2 mg/kg/d ×10–21/d w/gradual taper, Burow's solution cool compress 2–6×/d 20–30 min at a time, antihistamines
  - localized: mid-potency to high-potency topical corticosteroids bid for <2 wks
- *Subacute dermatitis:* low to mid-potency topical corticosteroid bid w/frequent application of moisturizers
- *Chronic dermatitis:* low to mid-potency topical corticosteroids bid w/plastic wrap occlusion overnight, frequent application of moisturizers. If infection occurs, antibiotic w/*Staphylococcus aureus* coverage necessary (erythromycin: 50 mg/kg/d, divided q6h)
- Irritant diaper dermatitis prevented by changing diapers frequently. Treatment involves use of hydrocortisone 1% mixed w/antifungal cream bid. Avoid alcoholic diaper wipes
- Perianal dermatitis treated w/zinc oxide ointment

COMPLICATIONS

- Erythroderma can result; may require hospitalization/more intensive therapy
- Prolonged use of strong topical steroids may result in atrophy or striae

WHEN TO REFER

- Referral for patch testing indicated in refractory cases
- If condition chronic, alternate treatment regimes, including light therapy, may be warranted

CONVERSION DISORDER

J. KENNETH WHITT AND ROBERT A. BASHFORD

BACKGROUND

- Characterized by (1) one or more symptoms or deficits affecting voluntary motor or sensory function that suggest neurologic or other general medical condition; and (2) psychological factors and conflicts that seem important in initiating, exacerbating, maintaining disturbance
- Not intentionally produced or feigned
- Cannot be fully explained by known pathophysiologic mechanisms, direct effects of substance, or as culturally sanctioned behavior/experience; and not better accounted for by another mental disorder
- Symptom or deficit causes clinically significant distress/impairment in social, academic, occupational, other important areas of functioning
- Usually begins during late childhood to early adulthood: rarely in children <5 yrs of age
- Equal numbers of affected prepubertal boys and girls; among adolescents and adults, females predominate, w/reported ratios 2:1–10:1. Prevalence ranges: 11–300/100,000 in general population samples
- Onset of conversion disorder (CD) generally acute and "purely" functional, but may develop following mild illness or injury, w/gradual increase and/or extended maintenance of symptoms modeled by physical illness
- Termed "hysteria" by ancient Greeks, CD nosology evolved from hypothesis that somatic symptom represents symbolic resolution of unconscious psychological conflict. As traumatic event/stressor overwhelms person's capacity for emotional adaptation, affect and painful memories "dissociated" from conscious awareness and "converted" into somatic symptom that symbolizes some aspect of traumatic episode, serving to reduce anxiety and avoid conflict ("primary gain"). Individual may derive other benefits and/or social reinforcements ("secondary gains) from symptom. Many clinicians link conversion symptoms to psychological conflict and secondary gain, but *DSM-IV* removed all inference of unconscious mechanisms and psychodynamics in etiology of CD, requiring only that "psychological factors judged to be associated with symptom or deficit based upon observation and history that initiation or exacerbation of symptom or deficit was preceded by conflicts or other stresses"

MANIFESTATIONS

- Conversion disorder can mimic almost any physical symptom
- Change in motor function can present as weakness/paralysis, impaired coordination/balance, aphonia, tics, difficulty swallowing/sensation of lump in throat, tremors. Pseudoseizures and inability to stand or to walk esp dramatic conversion symptoms, as is coma, intractable coughing, sneezing, hiccuping
- Common alterations of sensory functions include unilateral/bilateral blindness/deafness, restricted visual field (tunnel vision), hallucinations, "stocking-glove" anesthesias/paresthesias
- More complex symptoms may present in persons w/greater medical sophistication. *DSM-IV* does not differentiate sensorimotor from autonomic dysfunction, eg, recurrent vomiting may in some cases meet criteria for CD. Pain may occur alone or in conjunction w/CD symptoms. Absence of physical findings to account for pain or its intensity should technically be categorized under somatoform pain disorder (SPD), although little in literature to date differentiates SPD from CD in children
- Dx made based on positive findings, may include evidence that normal function possible; Hx acute triggering psychosocial stress w/failure to express associated affect; possibly accompanied by preexisting vulnerabilities or co-occurring chronic stresses (eg, learning disabilities, high expectations, illness/death in family member, sexual abuse [esp incest], or previous physical and psychological problems including "growing up fears" about separation and autonomy); primary gains; secondary gains; a model for the symptoms; and, perhaps, a symbolic meaning. Family system conflicts, enmeshment, difficulty w/emotional communication may be evident
- CD symptoms typically do not conform to known anatomic pathways and physiological mechanisms, but instead follow individual's conceptualization of condition. Conversion "anesthesia" of extremity may follow so-called stocking-glove distribution w/uniform (no proximal to distal gradient) loss of all sensory modalities (ie, touch, temperature, pain) sharply demarcated at an anatomic landmark rather than according to dermatomes. CD symptoms often inconsistent; "paralyzed" limb may be moved inadvertently while engaged in routine function, playful activity, when attention directed elsewhere. "Seizures" may vary from convulsion to convulsion, and paroxysmal activity not concurrently evident on EEG

LABORATORY FEATURES

- Although not associated w/specific laboratory results, *diagnosis of CD not Dx of exclusion. Failure to establish a physical illness a necessary, but not sufficient, condition*

DIFFERENTIAL DIAGNOSIS

- *Undiagnosed physical illness:* other mental disorder

MANAGEMENT AND TREATMENT

- Concurrent medical and psychological approach allows family's perspective to evolve (as they disclose psychosocial Hx, acute situational and chronic developmental stress, family dysfunction), rather than feeling "dumped" at the end of a negative medical workup
- Present findings authoritatively, but nonjudgmentally. Legitimize symptom as communication via nonverbal, somatic language, pointing out temporal associations to triggers, as well as other common mechanisms (eg, "butterflies in stomach") by which body signals impact of stress. Explicitly distinguish CD from malingering or "faking"
- Help parents initiate environmental changes, encourage child to directly and appropriately express anxiety and/or communicate desires, and minimize secondary gain from physical symptoms
- Plan active intervention, discouraging unnecessary diagnostic tests and doctor shopping, other than to obtain second opinion. Medical treatment (eg, physical therapy) often allows child to take active role in recovery process, and, in context of increased verbal communication (talking about feelings), provides face-saving way to get "well" and give up symptom
- Many cases require child mental health professional. Referral to child psychiatrist or pediatric/clinical child psychologist may be presented as one component of comprehensive care, w/continuing coordination by and collaboration w/pediatrician/primary care provider

COMPLICATIONS

- Favorable prognosis associated w/acute onset; identified stressful events; brief interval between CD onset and institution of treatment; above-average IQ; family collaboration; good health w/no psychiatric, medical, neurologic disease
- Individual conversion symptoms self-limited, remitting within days/weeks, and do not lead to physical changes or disabilities. However, prolonged conversion symptoms can cause muscle atrophy, demineralization of bones, contractures as result of extended disuse. Delayed or unsuccessful intervention may contribute to entrenchment of secondary gains and failure of adolescent passage—extended dependency on caregivers, difficult school reentry, and/or school absences w/academic failure

PREVENTION

- Provide opportunities for mastery via debriefing following physically and/or emotionally traumatic incidents. Anticipate nodal stress points in child developmental process (eg, help parents facilitate their young adolescents' upcoming physical and emotional separation)

WHEN TO REFER

- Indicated when Hx atypical or otherwise does not provide adequate basis to "rule-in" psychological disorder, if unusual symptoms exist or an absence of rapid resolution once family recognizes and appropriately responds to precipitating situation. Negative results of psychological assessment may indicate need to consider less common physical disorders
- Initiate immediate request for consultation whenever pediatric hospitalization is necessary. Delaying a child psychiatric/psychological evaluation until other workups have been completed communicates to family that considering emotional factors a last resort, not as important as other referrals, and, given short lengths of stay, not a priority

CORNEAL ABRASION

BRUCE T. CARTER

BACKGROUND

- One of most common conditions seen in ER
- Most often associated w/tangential/shearing injuries, contusion to globe, contact lens misuse

MANIFESTATIONS

- Severe pain, foreign body sensation, tearing, photophobia most common presenting symptoms; conjunctival injection frequent presenting sign
  - irregular/distorted corneal light reflex in larger abrasions
  - fluorescein staining of corneal epithelial defect diagnostic, accomplished by moistening fluorescein-impregnated strip w/ophthalmic irrigating solution, touching strip to conjunctiva of lower lid; illumination w/a cobalt blue light demonstrates area stain/epithelial injury
  - slit lamp examination of eye not always necessary but extremely helpful, esp in determining if corneal perforation present
- Linear vertical striae suggest foreign body beneath upper lid: necessitates upper lid eversion for inspection of conjunctival surface; foreign body can be removed w/moistened cotton tip applicator
- Central punctate staining of cornea suggests hard contact lens overwear syndrome secondary to corneal epithelial hypoxia/improper fit
- If blunt trauma Hx to globe, other signs of deeper injury to anterior segment should be excluded (eg, hyphema, lens dislocation, scleral rupture)
- If at time of injury pt was engaged in hammering metal against metal, careful examination of anterior segment with slit lamp followed by x ray of orbit (PA and lateral) to r/o intraocular foreign body indicated

TREATMENT

- Instillation of topical anesthetic if blepharospasm precludes adequate examination. *At no time is topical anesthetic prescribed for pain management*
- Removal of foreign body
- Instillation of mild short-acting cycloplegic agent (1% Cyclogel/2% Homatropine) to relieve ciliary spasm/accompanying discomfort
- Instillation of topical antibiotic ointment in inferior conjunctival cul-de-sac
- Modified pressure patch to immobilize lid. Often difficult to get children <3 yrs of age to leave patch in place for any length of time. Since young child frequently sleeps after such injury, topical antibiotic drops/ointment often sufficient
- Follow-up in 24 hrs w/fluorescein staining to assess epithelial defect/look for signs of infection

COMPLICATIONS

- Bacterial superinfection w/subsequent development of corneal ulcer
- Recurrent erosion syndrome in which epithelial defect subsequently spontaneously reappears accompanied by pain, tearing, photophobia

WHEN TO REFER

- Most pts managed w/o referral
- If signs of significant anterior segment contusion, reduced corrected/pinhole visual acuity
- If concomitant eye infection, eg, conjunctivitis, blepharitis
- Failure of epithelial defect to close after 48 hrs patch therapy
- Development of whitish corneal stromal infiltrate at site of abrasion

JANET L. WALKER

DEFINITIONS

- *Femoral-neck shaft angle:* angle described by lines that run along long axes of femoral neck and its shaft (normal 150° newborn to 126° adult)
- *Coxa vara:* ↓ femoral neck-shaft angle of proximal femur; may be associated w/many orthopedic conditions
- *Congenital coxa vara:* localized dysplasia of unknown etiology resulting in coxa vara. Also known as infantile or developmental

BACKGROUND

- Usually not evidence at birth; first noted when child begins walking
- Prevalence 1:13,000–25,000 live births, M:F ratio: 1:1, no racial predilection
- *Unilateral:* bilateral ratio: 2–3:1
- Case reports support autosomal dominant inheritance; ↑ occurrence in identical/nonidentical twins
- Results from primary defect in enchondral ossification in medial part of femoral neck (unable to withstand normal weight-bearing forces resulting in defective growth
- Histopathology resembles metaphyseal chondrodysplasia Schmid type (a more generalized disease)

CLINICAL FINDINGS

- Painless Trendelenburg lurch (waddling) limp/single leg stance due to mechanical disadvantage of gluteus medius
- Decreased hip abduction
- Femoral segment short, depending on how much varus occurs, resulting in shorter stature if bilateral; positive Galeazzi sign if unilateral
- No telescoping/Ortolani sign

RADIOGRAPHIC FINDINGS

- Decreased neck shaft angle
- Wide, vertically aligned proximal femoral physis
- Irregular metaphyseal ossification
- Shortened femoral neck
- Triangular osseous fragment adjacent to inferior margin of physis, which may be mistaken for fracture
- Delayed but ultimately normal ossification of proximal femoral epiphysis w/osteopenia due to decreased joint reactive forces
- Straight femoral shaft
- More proximal position of greater trochanter may result in false positive interpretation of hip dislocation on neonatal ultrasound

DIFFERENTIAL DIAGNOSIS

- Developmental hip dysplasia w/limp, decreased hip abduction, delayed ossification of proximal femoral epiphysis
- Aiken type A proximal femoral focal deficiency: coxa vara w/femoral shortening, bowing, delayed ossification
- Generalized skeletal dysplasias ie, metaphyseal chondrodysplasia, cleidocranial dysplasia, multiple/spondyloepiphyseal dysplasia, achondroplasia, Morquio disease w/delayed ossification, coxa vara/shortened femoral neck (coxa breva)
- Acquired coxa vara w/coxa breva due to aseptic necrosis of proximal femoral epiphysis due to infection, fracture, Legg-Calve Perthes disease
- Osteomalacia (renal osteodystrophy)/rickets w/coxa vara but normal femoral neck length

NATURAL HISTORY

- Hilgenreiner-epiphyseal angle (HE angle) measures vertical slope that proximal femoral physis makes w/horizontal pelvis
  - HE angle ≥60° likely progressive of deformity
  - HE angle ≤45° likely spontaneous correction of deformity

TREATMENT

- *HE angle <60° w/o progression:* observe w/radiographs, hip abductor muscle strengthening, hip adductor muscle stretching
- *HE angle ≥60° or <60° w/progression:* subtrochanteric osteotomy after 18–24 mos of age to correct HE angle to <45°

COMPLICATIONS

- Persistent limp
- Early osteoarthritis due to abnormal mechanics about hip
- Recurrent deformity after osteotomy requiring repeat surgery

WHEN TO REFER

- Children w/coxa vara should be followed by orthopedic surgeons

BACKGROUND

- Nonpolio human enterovirus
- 23 serotypes numbered 1–24 (type A23 reclassified as echovirus 9)
- Seasonal variation in temperate regions (peak in late summer/autumn), found year round in tropical/subtropical regions
- Primary viral shedding from gastrointestinal tract, predominantly fecal-oral/occasional respiratory secretion transmission, common transmission in swimming/wading pools, rare congenital/neonatal transmission
- Incubation period: 3–6 d
- Attack rates highest in young children/children from low socioeconomic groups
- Coxsackie A viruses less commonly associated w/very severe illnesses (eg, meningitis, encephalitis, myopericarditis, neonatal infection) than Coxsackie B viruses
- IgG necessary for full immune response to virus
- Neonatal disease results from antepartum transmission of Coxsackie A virus to infant followed by delivery prior to maternal antibody response

CLINICAL MANIFESTATIONS

- Protean manifestations (often occur in recognizable clinical syndromes)
- Symptoms age dependent:
  - neonates: fever, rash (macular, maculopapular, rarely petechial/vesicular); very rarely sepsis-like syndrome, pneumonia, hepatitis, meningitis, myocarditis. Note: mothers of neonates w/enteroviral disease often have Hx peripartum illness consistent w/enteroviral infection
  - infants/young children: nonspecific febrile illness, rash (macular, maculopapular, rarely petechial), herpangina, hand-foot-mouth syndrome, pharyngitis, meningitis, gastroenteritis common; less commonly: encephalitis. Possible association w/SIDS

- older children/adults: often asymptomatic, common cold, nonspecific febrile illness, headache, pharyngitis, myalgia, meningitis, gastroenteritis common. Less commonly: pleurodynia, encephalitis, myopericarditis, motor paralysis
  - congenital infection may occur (very rare)
- Illness often biphasic:
  - first phase typically involves only respiratory tract
  - second phase, which presumably follows period of viremia, may involve other sites (eg, meningitis, encephalitis, pleurodynia, myopericarditis)

LABORATORY FEATURES

- Specific virologic Dx rarely needed, but identification of viral infection may allow discontinuation of empiric antimicrobial therapy
- Some Coxsackie A viruses grown/identified in cell culture; many require specialized tissue culture lines, which may not be available routinely
- Specimens should be obtained from oropharynx, urine and stool; Coxsackie A viruses sometimes may be isolated from blood and spinal fluid
- Virus shedding in stool may be prolonged/may not be causally linked to pt's current illness
- In pts w/meningitis, CSF typically shows pleiocytosis w/lymphocyte predominance
  - CSF cell counts/differential occasionally resemble those of bacterial meningitis
  - CSF protein and glucose usually normal (protein may be elevated/glucose depressed if many neutrophils present)
- Enteroviral PCR available from reference/some commercial laboratories
- Virus types identified using specialized antisera/DNA sequencing (research/epidemiologic purposes)

DIFFERENTIAL DIAGNOSIS

- *Neonates:* sepsis, bacterial meningitis, congenital HSV, congenital hepatitis
- *Infants, children, adults:* other enteroviral infections, adenoviral infections, acute EBV infection/mononucleosis, streptococcal pharyngitis/scarletina, bacterial pneumonia, Kawasaki disease, Rocky Mountain spotted fever, ehrlichiosis, bacterial meningitis, leptospirosis

TREATMENT

- *Supportive:* antipyresis, hydration, analgesia for severe stomatitis
- Effective specific antienteroviral Tx available on experimental (compassionate release) basis for pts w/life-threatening enteroviral infections (Pleconaril, ViroPharma, Malvern, PA)
- Use of high-dose immunoglobulin for pts w/overwhelming enterovirus infection controversial, but may ↓ cardiac-related morbidity
- Enteric isolation precautions indicated for hospitalized pts

COMPLICATIONS

- Almost all infections resolve w/o complications
- Agammaglobulinemic pts may develop chronic meningitis

WHEN TO REFER

- Most pts managed w/o referral
- Consultation w/diagnostic virology laboratory needed to ensure appropriate specimen collection if virus culture/PCR required
- Referral indicated when Dx in doubt, for pts w/suspected congenital/neonatal infection, w/immunodeficiencies, w/severe disease (hepatitis, myopericarditis, CNS involvement)

COXSACKIE B VIRUS INFECTIONS

KENNETH ALEXANDER

BACKGROUND

- Non-polio human enterovirus
- 6 serotypes numbered B1–B6
- Epidemics occur in 3–6 yr cycles
- Seasonal variation in temperate regions (peak in late summer/autumn), found year round in tropical/subtropical regions
- Primary viral shedding from gastrointestinal tract, predominantly fecal-oral/occasional respiratory secretion transmission, common transmission in swimming/wading pools, rare congenital/neonatal transmission
- Incubation period 3–6 d
- Attack rates highest in young children/children from low socioeconomic groups
- Coxsackie B viruses more commonly associated w/severe illnesses (eg, meningitis, encephalitis, myopericarditis, neonatal infection) than Coxsackie A viruses
- IgG necessary for full immune response to virus
- Neonatal disease results from antepartum transmission of Coxsackie B virus to infant followed by delivery prior to maternal antibody response

CLINICAL MANIFESTATIONS

- Protean manifestations (often occur in recognizable clinical syndromes)
- Symptoms age dependent:
  – neonates: fever, rash (macular, maculopapular, rarely petechial/vesicular); rarely sepsis-like syndrome, pneumonia, hepatitis, meningitis, myocarditis. Mothers of neonates w/enteroviral disease often have Hx peripartum illness consistent w/enteroviral infection
  – infants/young children: nonspecific febrile illness, rash (macular, maculopapular, rarely petechial), hand-foot-mouth syndrome, pharyngitis, meningitis, gastroenteritis common; less common: hemorrhagic conjunctivitis, encephalitis, orchitis. Possible association w/SIDS

- older children/adults: often asymptomatic, common cold, nonspecific febrile illness, headache, pharyngitis, myalgia, pleurodynia, meningitis, gastroenteritis common; less common: encephalitis, myopericarditis, orchitis, motor paralysis
  – congenital infection may occur (very rare)
- Illness often biphasic:
  – first phase typically involves only the respiratory tract
  – second phase, which presumably follows period of viremia, may involve other sites (eg, meningitis, encephalitis, pleurodynia, myopericarditis)

LABORATORY FEATURES

- Specific virologic Dx rarely needed, but identification of viral infection may allow discontinuation of empiric antimicrobial therapy
- Most Coxsackie B viruses grown/identified in cell culture. Specimens should be obtained from oropharynx, urine and stool; Coxsackie B viruses sometimes isolated from blood. In pts w/Coxsackie B virus meningitis, virus may be isolated from CSF in 50–70% of cases
- Virus shedding in stool may be prolonged/may not be causally linked to pt's current illness
- In pts w/meningitis due to Coxsackie B viruses, CSF typically shows pleiocytosis w/lymphocyte predominance
  – CSF cell counts/differential occasionally resemble those of bacterial meningitis
  – CSF protein and glucose usually normal (protein may be elevated/glucose depressed if many neutrophils present)
- Enteroviral PCR available from reference/some commercial laboratories
- Virus types identified using specialized antisera/DNA sequencing (research/epidemiologic purposes)

DIFFERENTIAL DIAGNOSIS

- *Neonates:* sepsis, bacterial meningitis, congenital HSV, congenital hepatitis
- *Infants, children, adults:* adenoviral infections, acute EBV infection/mononucleosis, streptococcal pharyngitis/scarletina, bacterial pneumonia, Kawasaki disease, Rocky Mountain spotted fever, ehrlichiosis, bacterial meningitis, leptospirosis

TREATMENT

- *Supportive:* antipyresis, hydration, analgesia for severe stomatitis
- Effective specific antienteroviral therapy available on experimental (compassionate release) basis for pts w/life-threatening enteroviral infections (Pleconaril, ViroPharma, Malvern, PA)
- Use of high-dose immunoglobulin for pts w/overwhelming enterovirus infection controversial, but may ↓ cardiac-related morbidity
- Enteric isolation precautions indicated for hospitalized pts

COMPLICATIONS

- Almost all infections resolve w/o complications
- Agammaglobulinemic pts may develop chronic meningitis

WHEN TO REFER

- Most pts can be managed w/o referral
- Consultation w/diagnostic virology laboratory needed to ensure appropriate specimen collection if virus culture/PCR required
- Referral indicated when Dx in doubt, for pts w/suspected congenital/neonatal infection, w/immunodeficiencies, w/severe disease (hepatitis, myopericarditis, CNS involvement)

CRANIOSYNOSTOSIS

DAVID M. McKALIP AND STEVEN K. GUDEMAN

BACKGROUND

- Premature closing of one or more cranial sutures usually resulting in pathognomic cranial deformities based on synostosed suture
- Incidence 0.4/1,000 (sagittal synostosis w/2% familial incidence/coronal 8%)
- Intellectual development almost never impaired except when multiple sutures affected; neurologic complications also rare

CLINICAL MANIFESTATIONS

- Physical findings usually present at birth but may not manifest for several months. Findings include:
  - ridging along fused suture
  - lack of mobility of bones on either side of suture
  - small anterior fontalle of limited value in diagnosing craniosynostosis (fused sutures may still exist in presence of large fontanelle)
- Cranial deformities manifest based on the suture closed

Suture	Calavarial deformity	Notes
Sagittal	Scaphocephaly	A-P elongation ("Boat head")
		Keel-shaped, ridged sagittal suture
		Most common (80% male)
Coronal	Anterior plagiocephaly	Usually unilateral
		May be associated w/orbital/facial deformity
		Compensatory bulge contralateral frontotemporal region
Bilateral coronal	Brachicephaly	A-P shortening
Unilateral lambdoid	Posterior plagiocephaly	May have compensatory bulge in ipsilateral frontal region
Bilateral lambdoid	Turricephaly	Increased height ("Tower head")
		A-P shortening
Metopic	Trigonocephaly	Pointed forehead w/midline ridge
		May have chromosomal abnormality
Multiple	Variable	Tower skull w/orbital and sinus underdevelopment
	Oxycephaly if severe	Most dangerous
		May lead to mental retardation, optic nerve compression
		Increased ICP

- Examine head/face from multiple directions/perspectives (frontal, lateral, occipital, vertex)
- If possible compare findings to old photographs
- Remember certain degree of facial/cranial asymmetry normal

DIFFERENTIAL DIAGNOSIS

- Nonsyndromic (most common)
- Crouzon, Apert, other syndromes (associated w/facial, digital/other abnormalities)
- Underlying cerebral maldevelopment
- Possible overdraining ventricular shunt
- Positional molding (mainly unilateral lambdoid)

RADIOLOGIC FINDINGS

- Skull series:
  - premature suture fusion/sclerosis typical but often not seen if fibrous union only
  - orbital/skull base abnormalities may be present (Harlequin's eye in anterior plagiocephaly)
  - wait ~3 wks postnatally to order
- CT (w/bone windows):
  - normal underlying brain if isolated suture pathology
  - should demonstrate cranial contour, contact neurosurgeon prior to ordering
  - three-dimensional reconstruction of fine-cut CT (bone windows) often helpful

TREATMENT

- Surgical release of sutures/cranial remodeling
- Best performed early (<1 y)
- Potentially complex/extensive surgery w/suboptimal outcome if diagnosed/treated late
- Mainly required for cosmetic reasons, to prevent undue psychological/emotional distress associated w/deformity
- Unilateral lambdoid synostosis w/o severe deformity may be left alone if concealed by hair
- Unilateral posterior plagiocephaly w/no evidence of bony synostosis nearly always positional/should not have operative intervention; treatment may include use of "egg-crate" mattress when lying on affected side/preferential positioning on nonaffected side; banding has very mixed results to date
- Goal of surgery: prevent attraction of unfavorable attention/not to make normal acceptable head more attractive
- Shunt may be needed in rare cases of increased intracranial pressure

COMPLICATIONS

- Rare in cases of single suture fusion
- Increased intracranial pressure, mental retardation, visual abnormalities *possible* if multiple suture craniosynostosis left untreated

WHEN TO REFER

- All cases should be referred to neurosurgeon. Combined management w/plastic oral-maxillofacial surgeon may be required
- Surgery best done at youngest age possible, before progression to severe cranial/facial deformity
- Earliest timing for surgery usually 3–6 wks of age but may delay safely until 3–6 mos

MARTIN H. ULSHEN

BACKGROUND

- Crohn disease: chronic, idiopathic inflammatory disorder involving any region of GI tract from mouth to anus
- Associated w/high morbidity, low mortality
- In childhood, presents most commonly in teens, rarely in infancy, occasionally after first few yrs of life
- Incidence 3–4/100,000 for all ages
- Risk of inflammatory bowel disease (IBD) in family members ~10–20%; if both parents have IBD, child has 1/3 chance of eventually developing IBD
- Prevalence of Crohn disease in whites/blacks 3–10× that of Hispanics/Asians living in US
- *Requirements for Dx:* typical constellation of Sx, elimination of other possible causes, chronicity

CLINICAL MANIFESTATIONS

- Presentation depends on region of bowel involved, degree of inflammation, duration before Dx, presence of complications (eg, fistulae/strictures)
- Distal ileum w/proximal colon (ileocolitis) most commonly involved, followed by small bowel alone. Colon alone occurs in ~10%
- *Most common symptoms:* right lower quadrant/diffuse abdominal pain, diarrhea, blood in stool, anorexia, malaise, weight loss, intermittent fevers, growth retardation (± delayed sexual maturation), arthralgias
- Poor oral intake commonly secondary to associated diarrhea/abdominal pain
- *Most common signs:* tender right lower quadrant mass, perianal skin tags/fistulae, pallor, low weight for height, w/or w/o fall in height velocity
- Extraintestinal manifestations include arthralgias, arthritis, erythema nodosum, pyoderma gangrenosum, digital clubbing, episcleritis, hepatic disorders
- Anemia/arthritis alone rare

LABORATORY FEATURES

- *CBC:* WBC elevated/normal, anemia secondary to iron deficiency or chronic disease common. ESR/platelet count often elevated, but can be normal
- *Chemistries:* serum albumin may be low. Stool alpha-1-antitrypsin may be elevated secondary to enteric protein loss
- Stool for occult blood often positive
- Serum autoantibodies help discriminate from ulcerative colitis

RADIOLOGIC AND ENDOSCOPIC FINDINGS

- *Plain film:* often unremarkable; may demonstrate colonic thumbprinting (ie, edematous, inflamed mucosal folds), air-fluid levels from ileus/obstruction

- *UGI w/small bowel follow-through:*
  – terminal ileum most commonly involved
  – eccentric involvement w/nodular, ulcerated mucosa often w/luminal narrowing
  – can skip areas of bowel
  – aphthous ulcers common
  – transverse ulcers may produce "cobblestone" appearance of mucosa
  – adjacent loops of bowel often separated by thickened bowel wall/mesentery
- *Barium enema:* similar findings can be seen in involved colon, terminal ileum
- Ultrasound/CT scan useful to r/o intra-abdominal abscess
- *Esophagogastroduodenoscopy/colonoscopy:* similar to radiologic findings except subtle mucosal abnormalities more readily apparent than on x ray
  – biopsy confirmation useful, esp to r/o lymphoma

DIFFERENTIAL DIAGNOSIS

- *Infectious enteritis/colitis:* Yersinia enteritis appearance very similar to Crohn disease on contrast studies x rays
  – consider other bacterial enteric pathogens, parasites
  – GI tuberculosis very rare
- *Ulcerative colitis:* concentric uniform involvement w/o skip areas, fistulae/strictures
- Anorexia nervosa
- Periappendiceal abscess
- Foreign body perforating the intestine (eg, swallowed toothpick)
- *Small bowel lymphoma:* on contrast x ray studies, nodularity w/o mucosal ulceration
- Gluten-sensitive enteropathy
- Leukemia
- *Juvenile rheumatoid arthritis:* if joint symptoms first manifestations
- Lymphoid nodular hyperplasia of distal ileum (normal radiologic finding)

TREATMENT

- *Medical:* anti-inflammatory treatment w/prednisone at starting dose 1–2 mg/kg/d in single morning dose most often used w/goal to taper to qod for reduced side effects after one to several months
  – ideally child should taper off prednisone entirely; this frequently not possible
  – 5-aminosalicylate preparations to treat colonic involvement
  – enteric release 5-aminosalicylates to treat/prevent recurrences in small bowel disease
  – other medications include azathioprine (or 6-mercaptopurine), metronidazole, ciprofloxine; in special circumstances, methotrexate/cyclosporine
  – local rectal treatment w/steroid enemas/foam/5-aminosalicylate enemas used for urgency/tenesmus
  – antiinfective therapy for severe, intractable disease

- *Surgical:* reserved for complications; bowel resection does not cure Crohn disease
  – Steroid-dependent/unresponsive localized disease possible indication for resection of localized disease
  – growth failure, by itself, generally not indication for surgery
  – very high risk of recurrence within 5 y, often as soon as 6 mos after bowel resection
- *Nutritional therapy:* oral supplementation to improve nutritional status usually not successful
  – overnight nasogastric/gastrostomy feedings can maintain good intake, adequate weight gain (500–1,000 kcal/night or 50–80 kcal/kg/night for 1 mo out of 4)
  – elemental diets can be used as primary therapy to control active Crohn disease; may be as effective as prednisone treatment, although a much greater effort for pt; more successful w/small bowel than colon disease; early relapse after discontinuing diet common
- *Psychosocial support:* chronic disorder w/concerns about body image, periodic limitations of activity. Crohn's and Colitis Foundation of America (CCFA) very large pt support group

COMPLICATIONS

- *Growth failure:* primarily result of inadequate nutrient intake
- *Stricture:* small bowel/colon
- *Bowel perforation:* can result in peritonitis but more often fistula/abscess
- *Fistula:* perianal region, GI tract, urinary bladder, vagina, scrotum, skin
- *Abscess:* intra-abdominal/liver abscess: persistent fever, discomfort, localized abdominal mass
  – perianal abscess presents as painful perianal mass
- Intractable bleeding
- Short bowel syndrome resulting from repeated bowel resections
- Bile acid/vitamin B_{12} malabsorption from dysfunction or resection of terminal ileum
- Hepatobiliary disease

WHEN TO REFER

- This lifelong Dx difficult to establish; should always be confirmed by gastroenterologist
- Radiologic/endoscopic evaluation of intestinal tract requires experienced interpretation
- Treatment specialized, highly individualized for specific child

BACKGROUND

- Infection w/the fungus *Cryptococcus neoformans,* found worldwide, most commonly in soil contaminated w/bird excreta
- *Mode of acquisition:* inhalation of aerosolized organisms, no person-to-person transmission
- Rare in children
- *Predisposing conditions:* any immunosuppressed pt, but most commonly found in HIV-infected patients w/low CD4 counts; also seen w/organ transplantation, corticosteroid use, lymphoreticular malignancies, sarcoidosis

CLINICAL MANIFESTATIONS

- *Portal of entry:* lung, but may disseminate to involve almost any organ
- *Meningitis:* most frequent, serious complication
- Pulmonary lesions:
  - often asymptomatic w/cryptococcal nodule incidental finding on chest radiograph
  - no typical clinical findings: potential symptoms include fever, headache, weight loss, night sweats, chest pain, productive cough, hemoptysis
- Meningitis:
  - clinical course: often indolent w/waxing and waning symptoms
  - most common clinical manifestations: fever, headache, nausea, vomiting, change in mental status, seizure, cranial nerve involvement, signs of increased intracranial pressure
  - AIDS patients most commonly present w/fever and headache
  - no neurologic findings in 10% pts; meningismus *not* reliable clinical sign

LABORATORY FEATURES

- *Definitive Dx:* only by isolation of cryptococcus from body fluid or tissue
- *Cryptococcal antigen:* 95% sensitive in pts w/meningitis, less reliable in pulmonary disease
- Pulmonary disease:
  - typical chest radiograph: solitary nodule
  - attempt isolation of cryptococcus from sputum, bronchoalveolar lavage, tissue
  - lumbar puncture for all immunocompromised pts w/pulmonary disease
- Meningitis:
  - for *every* pt obtain: CSF opening pressure, culture of large amount of spinal fluid, India ink stain of CSF, serum and CSF cryptococcal antigen
  - *opening pressure:* elevated in >50% pts
  - *CSF culture:* positive 75–90% pts
  - *India ink stain of spinal fluid:* positive at least 50% pts
  - *CT or MRI:* abnormal in 50%, but findings nonspecific

DIFFERENTIAL DIAGNOSIS

Pulmonary cryptococcosis	Cryptococcal meningitis
brucellosis	brucellosis
histoplasmosis	histoplasmosis
tuberculosis	tuberculosis
malignancy	lymphoma or carcinoma
	sarcoidosis
	chronic benign lymphocytic meningitis

TREATMENT

- Pulmonary cryptococcal infection in asymptomatic, immunocompetent pt: usually self-limited, no treatment needed. In symptomatic, immunocompetent pts consider amphotericin B or fluconazole
- Disseminated infection and meningitis:
  - amphotericin B: accepted treatment at dose of 0.5–0.7 mg/kg/d. Side effects include fever, chills, nausea, azotemia. Consider lipid preparations in pts w/renal toxicity. Use of flucytosine w/amphotericin B controversial
  - low-risk pts, fluconazole at high doses may be used as first-line treatment. Optimal dose not known for children
  - treat for minimum of 6 wks from time CSF culture becomes negative
  - HIV-infected pts need chronic, suppressive treatment w/fluconazole (200 mg/d or 3–6 mg/kg/d)

COMPLICATIONS

- Untreated disseminated disease or meningitis fatal
- Risk factors for early death: positive India ink, CSF antigen titers ≥1:32, change in mental status, low CSF white count (<20 cells/μl)
- ≥50% HIV-positive pts w/meningitis relapse, usually in first year

PREVENTION

- Pt isolation not indicated
- Advise immunocompromised pts to avoid areas associated w/bird excreta
- Vaccines in development

WHEN TO REFER

- Immunosuppressed pts w/any form of cryptococcosis
- Immunocompetent pts w/disseminated infection or meningitis

BACKGROUND

- *Definition:* failure of testicular descent from abdomen into scrotum; testis may be found along normal pathway or in ectopic location
- Incidence:
  - preterm: 30.3%
  - full-term: 3.4%
  - 1 yr: 0.8%
  - adult: 0.8%
- 10% bilateral
- 14% have family Hx undescended testicle
- Isolated defect or associated w/congenital, genetic, endocrine, intersex disorder
- If associated w/hypospadias, need to r/o intersex; consider congenital adrenal hyperplasia if bilateral impalpable testes, mixed gonadal dysgenesis if unilateral undescended testicle
- *Histology:* alterations seen by at least 18 mos:
  - smaller seminiferous tubules, fewer spermatogonia, increased peritubular tissue, abnormal Leydig cells
  - changes also noted in contralateral testis

CLINICAL MANIFESTATIONS

- *Physical examination:* location
  - canalicular: between internal and external rings
  - abdominal: proximal to internal ring (impalpable)
  - ectopic: superficial inguinal pouch, perineum, femoral canal, suprapubic area, opposite hemiscrotum
  - absent
  - retractile: gentle traction brings testis to bottom of scrotum
  - gliding: can manipulate to upper scrotum

LABORATORY FEATURES

- *Imaging:* overall accuracy 44%
  - *herniography:* high false positive and false negative results
  - *ultrasound:* can detect canalicular or superficial inguinal pouch testes
  - *CT/MRI:* may detect impalpable testes, expensive, radiation exposure, difficult to perform in young child
  - *angiography/venography:* difficult to perform w/serious potential complications
- *Laparoscopy:* used to evaluate presence/absence of testicular vessels
  - blind ending vessels: confirms intra-abdominal vanishing testis and no further exploration required
  - vessels present: explore
- Hormonal stimulation in bilateral nonpalpable testes/r/o bilateral anorchia
  - measure baseline and poststimulation FSH, testosterone
  - HCG stimulation: 2,000 IU injection q day × 3 d
    - ↑ testosterone: presence of testicular tissue
    - no change in testosterone: bilateral anorchia

DIFFERENTIAL DIAGNOSIS

- Retractile cremasteric reflex most active 1–7 yrs of age
  - document location of testes at birth or during first year of life
  - serial exams if equivocal
- Gliding

TREATMENT

- Most that will descend, will do so within first 3 mos
- Orchiopexy/testicular salvage if possible
- Orchiectomy:
  - unable to salvage testicle
  - older postpubertal male if pt desires
  - certain intersex disorders w/dysgenetic testis

- Hormonal:
  - HCG: stimulation of Leydig cells increases testosterone, promotes testicular descent
    - infant: 250 IU 2×/wk × 5 wks
    - <6 yrs of age: 500 IU 2×/wk × 5 wks
    - >6 yrs of age: 1,000 IU 2×/wk × 5 wks
  - GnRH: replacement of abnormal secretion of hypothalamic GnRH
    - 1.2 mg perinasal spray q day × 4 wks
    - not approved in US

COMPLICATIONS

- Neoplasm:
  - 10% testicular tumors arise in undescended testes
  - 35–48× more likely to undergo malignant degeneration
  - carcinoma in situ 1.7%
  - 20% of tumors in pts w/undescended testes occur in contralateral "normal" testis
    - generally occur at/after puberty
    - seminoma most common then embryonal
    - gonadoblastoma most common w/certain intersex disorders
- *Torsion:* consider in pt w/abdominal pain w/empty ipsilateral scrotum
- *Hernia present:* 90%
- *Infertility:* 25–50% in unilateral; 50–75% in bilateral
  - longer period extrascrotal, greater likelihood

PREVENTION

- Treat as early as possible, not before 6 mos, but at least by 18 mos, to prevent histologic changes, maximize fertility

WHEN TO REFER

- Undescended testicle at birth

CUTANEOUS VASCULAR MALFORMATIONS (PORT-WINE STAINS)

FRANCISCO COLON-FONTANEZ AND LAWRENCE F. EICHENFIELD

BACKGROUND

- Port-wine stain (PWS), also known as nevus flammeus, flat vascular nevi, present at birth
- Occur 0.3–0.6% of newborns
- Composed of mature dilated capillaries in dermis w/o evidence of cellular proliferation
- Grow proportionally w/child w/o proliferative/involutional phase
- Light pink to bright red/purple in color
- Initially smooth, macular, w/advancing age irregularly thickened, w/papules, nodules
- Often on face, unilateral, although may occur in any part of body
- PWS of eyelids (both upper and lower/or lower), bilateral trigeminal lesions, or unilateral PWS involving all three branches of trigeminal nerve may be associated w/glaucoma, central nervous system (CNS) disease
- Only 8–11% PWS involving the trigeminal nerve distribution have associated eye/CNS involvement (Sturge-Weber syndrome)

CLINICAL MANIFESTATIONS

- Isolated cutaneous birthmark
- *Sturge-Weber syndrome (SWS) (encephalotrigeminal angiomatosis):* facial PWS distribution of first branch of trigeminal nerve, associated w/vascular anomalies of ipsilateral leptomeninges, cerebral cortex. Seizures occur in >50% pts, majority starting during first year of life. Mental retardation, hemiparesis, hemiplegia, cortical atrophy, homonymous hemianopsia may occur. Glaucoma present/almost always unilateral (most common w/simultaneous ophthalmic, maxillary trigeminal nerve involvement)
- *Klippel-Trenaunay-Weber syndrome (KTW):* PWS associated w/venous varicosities, hypertrophy (less commonly hypotrophy) of soft tissue, bone, of extremity/trunk associated w/capillary, lymphatic, venous/arteriovenous malformations
- *Cobb syndrome (cutaneomeningospinal angiomatosis):* PWS, angiolipoma/angiokeratoma associated w/spinal cord angioma within 1 or 2 segments of involved dermatome. Symptoms include pain, decreased sensation, weakness, atrophic limb muscles, monoplegia/paraplegia in area supplied by affected spinal cord segment
- *Riley-Smith syndrome (macrocephaly w/unusual cutaneous angiomatosis):* autosomal dominant; includes pts w/KTWS, SWS, cutis marmorata telangiectatica congenita;

macrocephaly w/multiple lipomas/hemangiomas (cavernous); normal CNS function frequently observed
- *Phakomatosis pigmentovascularis:* extensive PWS w/significant oculocutaneous pigmentation (Nevus of Ota), neurologic alterations

DIAGNOSTIC EVALUATION

- SWS:
  - ophthalmologic examination performed soon after birth to r/o glaucoma; repeat exams necessary (glaucoma may develop later)
  - CT: intracranial calcifications, cortical atrophy
  - MRI: more sensitive than CT
  - SPECT/PET: decreased cerebral blood flow/areas of hypometabolism; highly informative in first mos of life for intracranial vascular anomalies
  - by age 20 up to 60% demonstrate typical "railroad track" calcifications (mean age of onset 7 yrs)
  - EEG findings inconsistent early in life/not pathognomonic
- KTWS:
  - Doppler evaluation w/color imaging, ultrasonography (US), MRI helpful
  - evaluation for leg length discrepancy/secondary scoliosis indicated
- Cobb syndrome:
  - cutaneous vascular malformation overlying the spine:US/MRI should be obtained/complete neurologic examination performed

DIFFERENTIAL DIAGNOSIS

- Salmon patch (nevus simplex)
- Hemangioma
- Cutis marmorata telangiectatica congenita:
  - blue violet discoloration of skin in reticulate pattern, at times w/telangiectasia/ulceration
  - vascular pattern does not disappear
  - benign course, ulcerations heal promptly
  - associated anomalies: limb hypoplasia/hyperplasia, bony abnormalities, aplasia cutis congenita, neonatal ascites
- Venous malformations:
  - occur anywhere on body; faint blue patch/soft blue mass
  - slowly enlarge
  - no increase in local heat, no thrill/bruit)
  - episodic thromboses/phleboliths

- MRI best imaging technique
- treatment: sclerotherapy/surgical excision
- Arteriovenous malformations:
  - may occur in cervicofacial region, limb trunk, viscera
  - violaceous overlying skin, local hyperthermia, pulsations, thrill (high flow)
  - may become disfiguring/life-threatening
  - ulceration, bleeding, pain, cardiac failure rare before adolescence
  - diagnostic tests: Doppler ultrasound, MRI, angiography
  - treatment: selective arterial embolization, compression, surgery
- Lymphatic malformation:
  - most lesions present at birth/develop before 2 yrs of age
  - lesions occur anywhere
  - small cutaneous clear vesicles/large soft, translucent masses under normal/bluish skin. No or slow flow on US
  - Dx: US, CT, MRI
  - treatment: surgical excision; regrowth of lesion common

TREATMENT

- PWS:
  - many pts experience psychological trauma if untreated
  - opaque cosmetics: vascular blebs/tissue hypertrophy, seen ~70% pts >45 yrs of age may not be covered by cosmetics such as Dermablend/Covermark
  - pulsed dye laser: treatment of choice; risk of scarring <1%; earlier the treatment, better the results; lateral facial zones respond better than centrofacial areas. Marked lightening/clearing seen after multiple treatments
- KTWS:
  - compression stockings, orthopedic devices, invasive radiological/surgical procedures sometimes required

WHEN TO REFER

- Ophthalmological evaluation 2×/y recommended during first 2 yrs; 1×/y afterward for life in PWS
- Intractable seizures in pts w/SWS
- Pulsed dye laser treatment of PWS. Remember, the earlier the referral, the better the outcome
- KTWS: when leg length discrepancy, refer to orthopedist

CYSTICERCOSIS

MARINA SALVADORI AND JAY S. KEYSTONE

BACKGROUND

- An infection w/larvae of the pork tapeworm, *Taenia solium*
- Humans ingest tapeworm eggs that hatch in the stomach; the emerging larvae migrate to subcutaneous tissues, striated muscle, brain, eyes, other organs, where cysts (cysticerci) form
- Larvae preferentially migrate to the brain
- Pathogenesis related to number of cysts, their location, and host immune response (varies from negligible to intense inflammatory response)
- Infection most frequent during 3rd–4th decade (10% of cases occur in children)
- Worldwide distribution where pigs and humans coexist and poor sanitation
- High prevalence in Mexico, India, South America, northern China, eastern Europe
- Transmission by ingestion of undercooked pork, contaminated food/water, fecal-oral spread from another infected person, auto-infection
- Eating undercooked pork not essential for acquisition of cysticercosis
- Symptoms often appear yrs after infection

CLINICAL MANIFESTATIONS

- *Most common presentation:* seizure in an otherwise healthy child
- Headache, focal neurologic signs, global mental deterioration, hydrocephalus may occur
- Brain cysticerci may be clinically silent
- Children generally have single cyst
- Ocular cysticercosis presents w/scotoma or other visual impairment, w/cysts present in the subretinal area or vitreous

LABORATORY FEATURES

- CT and MRI best tools for Dx
- Serology confirms Dx (enzyme-linked immunotransfer blot assay available through CDC)
- No indication to test CSF for serodiagnosis
- Serology often negative w/solitary brain lesion; sensitivity increases w/multiple and subarachnoid cysts
- Negative serology does not exclude Dx
- Multiple stools should be examined for *T. solium* eggs

DIFFERENTIAL DIAGNOSIS

- Depends on Sx and CT appearance
- Must be differentiated from other space-occupying brain lesions, esp tuberculosis

TREATMENT

- Treatment controversial
- Dying single cysts surrounded by inflammation do not usually require Tx
- Single dead/calcified cysts do not need Tx
- Single lesions w/o surrounding inflammation may be followed or treated
- Multiple cysts require Tx
- Treatment is albendazole, 15 mg/kg/d div 2 doses/d × 2–4 wks, or praziquantel 50 mg/kg/d div 3 doses/d × 15 d
- Steroid administration before and during therapy reduces neurologic symptoms from the inflammatory response associated w/larval death
- Surgery rarely indicated except for ocular and intraventricular cysts
- *T. solium* carriers (eggs in stool, no organ disease) should be treated with single-dose praziquantel, 10 mg/kg

COMPLICATIONS

- Treatment-related cyst destruction may cause intense inflammation/more frequent seizures
- *Other complications:* hydrocephalus, epilepsy, visual loss, focal neurologic deficits, decrease in LOC

PREVENTION

- Thoroughly cook pork
- Wash vegetables well in clean water
- Appropriate disposal of human excrement
- Efforts to improve public sanitation, basic living conditions, personal hygiene
- Handwashing by food handlers before food preparation/after bowel movements

WHEN TO REFER

- Uncertain Dx
- Treatment being considered/surgical intervention contemplated
- Assessment by an infectious diseases expert recommended
- If Dx certain, single, calcified lesions need not be referred

BACKGROUND

- Most frequent life-threatening genetic disease in Caucasians
- 1/3,300 incidence for Caucasian, 1/17,000 for African Americans, 1/9,000 for Hispanic births
- 4% carrier rate; 55% homozygous for ΔF508 gene (over 500 variants w/milder phenotypic expression)
- Defective gene perturbs electrolyte, water transport across epithelial cells in respiratory, GI, genital, sweat glands. Abnormal secretions obstruct secretory processes, resulting in dysfunction, destruction
- Heterozygote "carriers" completely asymptomatic. Survival advantage may be resistance to diarrhea, dehydration as in cholera epidemics in prehistoric and primitive cultures
- Mean survival rates, projected from birth, now >30 yrs

CLINICAL MANIFESTATIONS

- *Meconium ileus* in 20% results in abdominal distention, failure to pass meconium in first 24–36 hrs; meconium plug syndrome?
- *Failure to thrive:* w/or w/o chronic respiratory or GI problems, accounts for majority of early manifestations. Easy to confuse w/common early feeding problems. Voracious appetite characteristic but not always present
- *15% pancreatic sufficient,* lack characteristic steatorrhea. Such pts eventually develop chronic respiratory disease, tend to have milder symptoms, delayed Dx, prolonged survival
- Additional clues to early Dx include salty tasting skin, rectal prolapse, hypochloremic alkalosis, hypoprothrombinemia, hypoproteinemia, respiratory tract colonization w/*Pseudomonas aeruginosa, Staphylococcus aureus,* or *Burkholderia cepacia*
- Digital clubbing common w/advanced respiratory involvement
- Late manifestations that may lead to Dx:
  - sinusitis (100%)
  - obstructive azospermia in males (100%)
  - nasal polyposis (10%)
  - biliary cirrhosis (5%)
  - pancreatitis (rare)
  - diabetic equivalent develops in 20–30% of older pts, beginning during teenage yrs. Usually nonketotic, milder than type I, II diabetes

LABORATORY STUDIES

- Quantitative sweat collection by pilocarpine iontophoresis, analysis of chloride concentration *required* for all suspected cases. Only laboratories approved by ACLS should be used (such as those serving CF centers). Normal range = <40 MM/L Cl⁻; mean abnormal = 100 ± 40 MM/L
- All new or previously untested cases should have genotyping performed to aid in diagnostic classification, family counseling, disease prognostication
- Unusual cases (1% have normal sweat chlorides) may require extensive genotyping or special testing such as nasal electrical potential measurements
- Presence/absence of pancreatic function based on 72 hr stool fat analysis
- Interpretation of testing results should always be delivered by team of CF experts as in CF centers approved by National CF Foundation
- Neonatal Dx based on genotyping from blood "spots" obtained at birth available in some states; prenatal Dx available in most larger medical centers

DIFFERENTIAL DIAGNOSIS

GI/Nutritional
Failure to thrive*
Giardiasis*
Celiac disease
Pyloric stenosis
Cirrhosis of liver
Pancreatitis

Respiratory
Reactive airways
Bronchiectasis
Pneumonia, chronic/recurrent
Pertussis syndrome
Other chronic lower respiratory symptoms
Sinusitis, chronic

Other
Anorexia nervosa*
Infertility

*May present w/falsely elevated sweat chloride.

TREATMENT

- Carefully review, confirm all possible CF manifestations receptive to treatment
- High caloric (100–150 kcal/kg/d) *diet. Do not restrict fatty intake.* Infant formulas useful, not always necessary
- Enzyme replacement (up to 2,000 IU Lipase/kg/meal)
- Multiple vitamin supplement w/2×/d ADEK requirement
- Airway clearance techniques appropriate for age, disease status
- Antibiotics for any signs of lower respiratory infection based on culture, clinical findings
- Monitor bacterial cultures (gag or sputum) and treat all URIs vigorously w/appropriate oral antibiotics
- Treat significant pulmonary exacerbations w/aerosolized and/or IV antibiotics

WHEN TO REFER

- CF center, local physician should follow pt frequently (CF center visits recommended q3mos)
- Care Plan for CF (*Clinical Practice Guidelines for Cystic Fibrosis,* 1997) details all aspects of care for CF centers

CYSTIC HYGROMA

SARAH L. CHAMLIN AND ILONA J. FRIEDEN

BACKGROUND

- *Cystic hygroma:* type of congenital lymphatic malformation
- Dilated and cystlike lymphatic channels
- Due to developmental anomaly of lymphatic embryogenesis
- Present at birth or becomes evident before 2 yrs of age
- Occurs w/equal frequency in males and females; no racial predilection
- Cytogenetic abnormalities relatively common (Turner, Noonan, and trisomy syndromes)
- 75% present in neck, 20% in axillary region, 5% in mediastinum, retroperitoneal, pelvic, groin regions
- 3% of all cystic hygromas associated w/extension to mediastinum

CLINICAL MANIFESTATIONS

- Often diagnosed in utero via ultrasound
- Common presenting complaint of single or multiloculated, painless, soft, fluid-filled mass in posterior triangle of neck
- Most lesions intermittently or continuously enlarge
- Mass most often fluctuant and lobulated, attached to deep tissues and not to skin
- Transilluminates brightly, distinguishing it from other neck masses
- Usually no symptoms unless lesion large enough or located in area that causes dyspnea, dysphagia, pain secondary to compression of vital structures

LABORATORY FEATURES

- Ultrasound can confirm cystic nature of mass
- CT/MRI scan useful to delineate extent of lesion and aid in Dx; required in extensive cases
- *Pathology:* multilocular, multilobular, cystic mass composed of many individual thin-walled cysts varying in size 1 mm–5 cm or more in diameter
- *Chromosomal analysis:* obtained prenatal or postnatal
- Other investigations normal unless pt has infection or hemorrhage of lesion

DIFFERENTIAL DIAGNOSIS

- Deep hemangioma
- Mixed venous-lymphatic malformation
- Branchial cleft cyst
- Thyroglossal duct cyst
- Dermoid cyst
- Cervical meningocele
- Thyroid teratoma
- Lipoma
- Lymphoma

TREATMENT

- *Treatment of choice in well-localized disease:* immediate surgical excision avoiding compromise of vital structures
- Sclerosing agents occasionally used at time of surgery destroy the lining of remaining cysts
- Alternative therapy useful in extensive cases: intralesional sclerotherapy (bleomycin sulfate or OK-432)
- Occasionally, lesions partially or completely regress spontaneously. Treatment should not be delayed in hope of spontaneous regression

COMPLICATIONS

- 2–5% mortality for large neck lesions or lesions extending to mediastinum
- Well-localized excised lesions have ~10% recurrence rate
- Incompletely excised lesions have high recurrence rate
- Bacterial infection common secondary to lymph stasis
- Hemorrhage into mass making it tense, firm, opaque on transillumination
- Dystocia at delivery due to presence of large cystic hygroma
- Respiratory compromise secondary to airway obstruction; esp common in large cervicothoracic lesions
- Postop complications include chylothorax, chylopericardium, seromas, infection, nerve damage

WHEN TO REFER

- Immediate referral to pediatric surgeon or multidisciplinary vascular anomalies clinic indicated for all pts

CYTOMEGALOVIRUS INFECTIONS

GAIL J. DEMMLER

BACKGROUND

- May be primary/recurrent; greater risk for serious disease in primary
- ~1% newborns congenitally infected; 90% asymptomatic at birth
- Commonly transmitted perinatally to newborn/young infant from maternal cervicovaginal secretions, breast milk
- Common acquired infection in toddlers/young children, esp those attending group day care
- Primary CMV infection during pregnancy in 1–4% healthy pregnant women; transmitted to fetus in ~40%
- Recurrent CMV infection during pregnancy <1% healthy pregnant women; rarely produces symptoms in newborn
- Important opportunistic pathogen in immunocompromised, including those with AIDS, recipients of organ/marrow transplants

CLINICAL MANIFESTATIONS

- *Congenital infection:* most asymptomatic; symptoms: small for gestational age, hepatosplenomegaly, petechiae, purpura, microcephaly, chorioretinitis, sensorineural deafness. Sequelae: progressive sensorineural deafness, neurodevelopmental abnormalities, visual impairment
- *Acquired infection:* most asymptomatic; may cause prolonged fever, malaise, pharyngitis, hepatitis, "mononucleosis-like" syndrome; immunocompromised pts may have serious, fatal disease, including progressive retinitis, encephalitis, peripheral radiculoneuropathy, pneumonitis, hepatitis, prolonged fever

LABORATORY

- *Viral culture:* CMV isolated from urine, saliva, blood, cervicovaginal secretions, semen, tissue, respiratory secretions in both primary/recurrent infections. Isolation in first 21 d of life diagnostic of congenital infection
- *Serology:* CMV IgG antibody: recent/past infection; may represent maternal antibody if sample is from newborn; CMV IgM antibody: recent infection; supports congenital infection if sample from newborn
- *Histopathology:* cytomegalic inclusion cells in tissue
- *Viral antigen:* detected in WBCs (CMV antigenemia), respiratory samples, tissue
- *Viral DNA:* detected in blood (CMV DNAemia), plasma, respiratory samples, tissue, urine, CSF by conventional viral probes/PCR-based methods
- *CBC:* atypical lymphocytosis, lymphopenia, neutropenia, hemolytic anemia, thrombocytopenia
- *Hepatitis:* elevated transaminases (usually <500 IU/L); direct hyperbilirubinemia
- *Other:* CT of brain in newborn: linear, periventricular calcifications; auditory brainstem-evoked potentials: unilateral/bilateral senorineural hearing loss

DIFFERENTIAL DIAGNOSIS

- *Other congenital infections:* toxoplasmosis, rubella, herpes simplex virus, syphilis, HIV, lymphocytic choriomeningitis virus
- *Other acquired infections:* Epstein-Barr virus, toxoplasmosis, HIV, hepatitis A, B, C
- *In immunocompromised:* high index of suspicion for other concomitant opportunistic infections
- Metabolic/genetic diseases

TREATMENT

- *No treatment:* asymptomatic pts w/congenital/acquired CMV infection
- *Ganciclovir foscarnet cidofovir:* treatment of serious, life-/sight-threatening CMV disease in immunocompromised. Consultation w/infectious diseases specialist should be considered
- *IVIG, CMV-IVIG:* use of immune globulins to treat CMV disease is controversial
- Experimental treatment protocols for newborns/immunocompromised pts available

PREVENTION

- *Pregnant women:* avoid close and intimate contact w/toddlers/young children likely to be shedding CMV
- IVIG/CMV IVIG used in immunocompromised
- Use of antivirals, such as ganciclovir, to prevent CMV disease controversial
- *CMV vaccine:* live/recombinant vaccines in clinical trials

WHEN TO REFER

- Symptomatic congenital infection
- Infection in immunocompromised host

DACRYOSTENOSIS, DACRYOCYSTITIS, AND RELATED OBSTRUCTIONS

SHARON F. FREEDMAN

BACKGROUND

- *Congenital nasolacrimal duct obstruction* (sometimes called "dacryostenosis")
- Usually results from imperforate membrane at distal end of nasolacrimal duct
  – occurs 2–4% full-term newborn infants; one-third bilateral
  – clinically evident in 1–2 wks of age
  – often in children w/frequent otitis media
  – resolves spontaneously by 6–9 mos of age in most cases
  – predisposes to conjunctivitis, rarely to dacryocystitis/cellulitis
- Other congenital lacrimal system obstructions:
  – atresia (under development/absence) of lacrimal punctae/canaliculi
  – dacryocystocele: dilated lacrimal sac at birth, usually resulting from combination of nasolacrimal duct obstruction/amniotic fluid/mucus trapped in lacrimal sac
- *Acquired lacrimal system obstructions:* may result from trauma to lacrimal system such as canalicular testing from dog bite to eyelids
- *Dacryocystitis:* infection of lacrimal sac; uncommon result of congenital obstruction within nasolacrimal system

CLINICAL MANIFESTATIONS AND DIFFERENTIAL DIAGNOSIS

- Congenital nasolacrimal duct obstruction:
  – clinical features: persistent tearing, chronic low-grade mucoid discharge, matting/crusting of eyelids
  – differential diagnosis: conjunctivitis (red eye, usually acute onset, purulent discharge), congenital lacrimal system anomalies, other causes of tearing: entropion/ectropion (inward/outward turning of eyelids), trichiasis (eyelashes rubbing on cornea), corneal defect, or foreign body under the lid, congenital glaucoma (cornea usually enlarged and cloudy, often very sensitive to light)
- Absent/underdeveloped lacrimal punctae or canaliculi:
  – clinical features: punctae absent/small, ± discharge, eyelid crusting, matting

– differential diagnosis: same as for congenital nasolacrimal duct obstruction
- Dacryocystocele:
  – clinical features: firm bluish mass just below medial canthus (where lower eyelid meets nose), may be accompanied by signs of infection, usually with tearing, ± discharge
  – differential diagnosis: dermoid cyst, hemangioma, encephalocele, other anterior orbital mass
- Acquired lacrimal system obstructions:
  – clinical features: same as for congenital nasolacrimal duct obstruction, but w/evidence of eyelid/facial trauma
  – differential diagnosis: same as for congenital nasolacrimal duct obstruction
- Dacryocystitis:
  – clinical features: pain, redness, swelling over lacrimal sac area, tearing/discharge, ± fever, elevated WBC count, ± accompanying surrounding cellulitis, ± "pointing" of the lacrimal abscess w/fistula formation
  – differential diagnosis: acute ethmoid sinusitis (nasal discharge, x-ray evidence of sinusitis), facial/preseptal cellulitis (lacrimal system normal/patent if irrigated)

DIAGNOSTIC TESTS

- Congenital nasolacrimal duct obstruction:
  – clinical inspection w/penlight for features noted above
  – gentle pressure to area over lacrimal sac; reflux of mucoid or mucopurulent material from lower punctum confirms Dx
- Congenital and acquired lacrimal system obstructions:
  – clinical inspection w/penlight for clinical features described above
- Dacryocystitis:
  – clinical inspection for features noted above
  – Gram stain/culture discharge expressed by gentle compression over lacrimal sac
  – WBC count/differential
  – Blood cultures if febrile/appears acutely ill
  – CT scan of orbits/paranasal sinuses if atypical/severe

TREATMENT AND WHEN TO REFER

- Congenital nasolacrimal duct obstruction:
  – digital lacrimal sac massage 2–4 ×/d (index finger placed by inner corner of eye, stroked gently downward)
  – topical antibiotic drops (eg, gentamicin)/ointment (eg, erythromycin) bid–tid × 1 wk if significant discharge/redness
  – oral antibiotic (amoxicillin/clavulonate) if conjunctivitis/lid erythema persists after topical antibiotic trial
  – warm compresses 2–3 × d to remove eyelid crusting if present
  – *refer* for nasolacrimal duct probing ~1 yr of age (requires brief anesthesia, success 80–90%), sooner if repeated conjunctivitis or one episode of cellulitis/dacryocystitis
- Other congenital and acquired lacrimal system obstructions:
  – *refer* to ophthalmologist as soon as possible
- Dacryocystitis:
  – oral amoxicillin/clavulonate/cefaclor if afebrile, systemically well, available for daily follow-up; otherwise hospitalize, IV antibiotics (eg, cefuroxime, equivalent); monitor clinical response closely; change antibiotics in response to culture results
  – warm compresses over lacrimal sac area
  – *refer*/consult ophthalmology as soon as possible—incision/drainage may be needed acutely; nasolacrimal duct probing needed later when acute infection passes

COMPLICATIONS

- Failure to resolve congenital nasolacrimal duct obstruction by 1–2 yrs of age may lead to permanent obstruction requiring more complex surgery
- Congenital dacryocystocele often progresses to dacryocystitis (within a few wks) if not properly treated
- Failure to recognize/vigorously treat dacryocystitis/orbital cellulitis may lead to life-threatening infection

KENNETH B. ROBERTS

BACKGROUND

- Most frequent in association w/enteritis, esp w/secretory diarrhea because of amount of fluid lost in stool, or when vomiting precludes adequate oral intake to replace losses
- Generally develops over 2–3 d; can be more rapid if losses profuse
- Rehydration usually accomplished orally

CLINICAL MANIFESTATIONS

- *Mild:* thirst, decreased urine output w/increased concentration of solutes, dry mouth, dry eyes
- *Moderate:* tachycardia, sunken fontanelle (in infants)
- *Severe:* hypotension, decreased peripheral perfusion
- Mild/moderate/severe degrees of dehydration generally correspond to 5%/10%/15% of body weight in infants, 3%/5%/7% in adolescents/adults. (Note: 5% = 50 mL/kg; 10% = 100 mL/kg; 15% = 150 mL/kg)
- Degree of dehydration underestimated if sodium concentration >150 mEq/L (hypertonicity pulls fluid from cells, bolstering circulation); severity of dehydration overestimated if sodium concentration <135 mEq/L

LABORATORY FEATURES

- *Renal:* ↑ urine specific gravity; ↑ serum urea nitrogen, creatinine
- *Hemoglobin/hematocrit:* ↑ (hemoconcentration)
- *Acid-base:* ↓ bicarbonate common (↑ lactate from decreased tissue perfusion, bicarbonate losses in diarrhea)
- *Electrolyte:* serum sodium defines whether dehydration isotonic (135–150 mEq/L), hypertonic (>150 mEq/L), hypotonic (<135 mEq/L)

TREATMENT

- *Acute:* if signs of cardiovascular compromise present, 20 mL/kg isotonic fluid (normal saline/Ringer's lactate), infused IV; repeat q30min until BP normal/heart rate approaches normal
- *Rehydration:* deficit should be estimated from clinical examination/from a change in body weights; deficit replaced over several hours, orally if possible, IV if necessary; rehydration fluid: half-normal sodium concentration; most infants who refuse to drink accept small amounts by teaspoon q5–15min
- *Persistent diarrhea:* 10 mL/kg rehydration fluid/each diarrheal stool
- *Maintenance:* child's usual need for fluids approximated from Holliday-Segar formula: 100 mL/kg/d × first 10 kg body weight; 50 mL/kg/d × next 10 kg; 20 mL/kg/d × each additional kg. Maintenance fluids required as well as deficit replacement
- *Refeeding:* begin as soon as possible, esp malnourished infants
- Hypernatremic dehydration represents special case because of fluid shifts from intracellular space to the extracellular space; rehydration given more slowly (an even rate for 48 hrs) to avoid complications of rapid fluid shifts (eg, seizures)

COMPLICATIONS

- Dehydration can progress to state of cardiovascular compromise, shock, death. In most cases, prompt recognition, simple rehydration measures prevent these complications
- If the sodium concentration high/rehydration rapid, cerebral edema/seizures can occur due to fluid shifts from extracellular space into cells

WHEN TO REFER

- Most children can be managed w/o referral
- Referral indicated if dehydration has progressed to shock/fluids need to be administered IV and cannot be delivered in setting in which child being examined

BACKGROUND

- Although mean age of onset typically early childhood, onset in childhood not uncommon
- *Pediatric prevalence:* 0.3% preschoolers; 1.8% prepubertal children; 4.7% 14–16 yr olds
- Rates vary by ascertainment site: 59% pts in psychiatric hospital; 53% pts in educational diagnostic center; 28% pts in psychiatric outpatient clinic
- General distribution even in childhood; incidence in females increases w/puberty; females predominate in adult samples
- Familial Hx important variable in predicting risk:
  - by age 20, as many as 50% offspring of depressed parents report onset of depression
  - proximity to affected relative predicts degree of risk/earlier age of onset
  - offspring of depressed parents at greater risk; also for other types of psychopathology

CLINICAL MANIFESTATIONS

- Dx major depressive disorder (MDD) in children made using same criteria as adults w/minor modifications for different developmental levels
- Syndrome includes alterations of mood, cognition, behavior, physical functioning
- Dx based on following criteria:
  - duration at least 2 wks required: least 5 of following symptoms (either number 1 or 2) must be present: (1) depressed mood, (2) diminished interest/pleasure in activities, (3) significant weight/appetite loss/gain, (4) insomnia/hypersomnia, (5) psychomotor agitation/retardation, (6) fatigue/loss of energy, (7) feelings of worthlessness/excessive guilt, (8) poor concentration/indecisiveness, (9) recurrent thoughts of death, suicidal ideation, attempt/plan
  - significant clinical distress/impairment of functioning
  - symptoms not due to substances/medical condition

Developmental variations:
  - irritability/anger equivalent to dysthymic mood in adults
  - somatic complaints, withdrawal, hopelessness more common
- Children use less lethal means of suicide; probably reflects cognitive immaturity, not decreased severity

DIFFERENTIAL DIAGNOSIS

- Mood disorder due to general medical condition
- Substance-induced mood disorder
- Bipolar disorder
- Post-traumatic stress disorder
- Adjustment disorder w/depressed mood
- Normal bereavement
- Normal sadness

TREATMENT

- Given the multidimensional impact of this disorder, treatment often tailored to specific needs of pt
- *Individual counseling:* presence of impaired peer relationships/poor self-esteem remedied w/1:1 counseling (see behavioral therapy below as well)
- *Education:* psychoeducational interventions (knowledge about disease, course, treatment) help reduce morbidity
- *Family support/counseling:* disorder impacts basic familial functioning (increased discord/dysfunction), family counseling required; disruptive behaviors in children usually treated through family-centered behavioral intervention
- *Behavioral therapy:* cognitive-behavioral therapy (CBT) effective adjunct in management
- *Medications:* antidepressant medications often indicated/effective; selective serotonin reuptake inhibitors (SSRI: fluoxetine, paroxetine, sertraline, fluvoxamine, nefazadone) typically better tolerated than tricyclic antidepressants/appear effective in adolescents; limited data regarding efficacy, dosing, safety in children; consultation warranted

- *Hospitalization:* reserved for situations in which pt at risk; usually brief; functions to stabilize pt to point where treatment safely resumed as outpatient

PROGNOSIS

- Depression typically recurrent
- In adults 50% recover from single episode within 6 mos; 10–20% exhibit more chronic course
- Recurrence in children; 26% by 1 yr; 40% by 2 yrs; 70% by 5 yrs
- Untreated episode in adult has duration of ~6 mos; in children age of onset inversely relates to time to recovery; duration of single untreated episode in children may be longer (9 mos)
- Recovery time in children/adolescents complicated by lesser repertoire of coping responses/resources to ameliorate depression
- Early onset of illness often correlates w/poorer prognosis
- In children/adolescents, clinical course/outcome complicated by *persistent* dysfunction in *all domains:* school performance, peer relationships, family relations, drug abuse/behavioral disorders, suicide ideation/attempts

WHEN TO REFER

- Most pts require referral for mental health services
- Presence of suicidal ideation, regardless of "perceived" seriousness, requires immediate psychiatric consultation
- Consultation also indicated for initiation of antidepressant medications/for failure to respond to initial interventions

BACKGROUND

- Most frequent onset 2–11 yrs of age; peak incidence 3–7 yrs
- *M:F ratio:* 3:2
- ↑ onset in summer; geographic fluctuations in incidence
- *Antecedent illness frequent:* eg, enteroviral, streptococcal infections
- *Indicators of severity:* extensive vascular involvement/tissue infarction; dysphagia; poor secretion handling; persistently elevated muscle enzymes; increased circulating %B cells (CD19+) despite lymphopenia
- *Recovery:* variable; many children asymptomatic/off therapy within 2–4 yrs; 20–30% calcinosis w/associated morbidity; may evolve into overlap syndromes; mortality: 2–7%

CLINICAL MANIFESTATIONS

- Rash (usually sun-exposed areas, associated w/localized edema, Gottron papules): eyelids, malar, shawl area, MCPs/PIPs, elbows, knees, medial aspect of ankles
- Dilated tortuous small blood vessels: eyelid margins (may have thromboses), nailfold capillary vessels, soft palate
- *Muscle weakness:* symmetrical proximal, neck flexor involvement; nasal speech
- Muscle pain 73%, fever 65%, dysphagia 44%, hoarseness 43%, abdominal pain 37%, arthritis 35%, melena 13%, calcinosis 20–30%; hepatosplenomegaly in young children at onset
- Often insidious onset, increasing irritability, loss of strength, decline in self-care
- Acanthosis nigricans if partial body lipodystrophy present
- Raynaud syndrome more frequent in inflammatory myopathy positive for Pm/Scl

LABORATORY FEATURES

- Elevated serum muscle-derived enzymes: creatine phosphokinase (64%), aldolase (75%), lactic acid dehydrogenase (81%), serum aspartate aminotransferase (75%)
- Electromyogram indicative of inflammatory myopathy w/insertional irritability, high amplitude, bizarre frequency (82%)

- *Muscle biopsy reviewed by pathologist experienced in muscle and vascular disease:* pathognomonic perifascicular atrophy, small vessel thrombosis w/capillary dropout; perivascular mononuclear cell infiltrate, macrophage localization in damaged muscle (81%)
- *Inflammatory myopathy focal:* MRI (T2 weighted image) to localize site for EMG, muscle biopsy in mild cases; if MRI negative, yield of other invasive tests low
- *Immunology:* peripheral blood flow cytometry
  – increased circulating %B cells (CD19+), lymphopenia, increased CD4/CD8 ratio
  – immunoglobulins: ↑ IgM early, occasional IgA deficiency; C3/C4, CH50 normal
- *Hematology:* mild anemia, normal platelet count, ESR often normal, ↑ von Willebrand factor antigen
- Antinuclear antibody positive (speckled pattern 80%); may have other myositis-associated antibodies (MSA) such as anti t-RNA synthetase antibody (Jo-1 most common) w/associated progressive lung disease
- Increased cholesterol, triglycerides, insulin, serum glucose associated w/partial lipodystrophy

DIFFERENTIAL DIAGNOSIS

- Inflammatory myopathy associated w/other connective tissue disease: systemic onset juvenile rheumatoid arthritis; mixed connective tissue disease, arthritis
- Polymyositis, infantile polymyositis
- *Endocrine dysfunction:* hypothyroidism; alterations in pituitary, adrenal gland activity
- *Muscular dystrophies:* Becker, Duchenne
- *Acute viral infections:* influenza, hepatitis B
- Metabolic muscle disease

TREATMENT

- Early Dx/aggressive therapy essential to optimal outcome
- Baseline eye exam
- Options include corticosteroids, methotrexate, hydroxy-chloroquine (steroid sparing), IV gamma globulin
  – corticosteroid dosage: IV solumedrol: 30 mg/kg, 1 g max./d. In less severe cases/IV ther-

apy not feasible, po prednisone: 2 mg/kg/d max. div
- *Methotrexate:* 15–20 mg/m²/wk IV/po (cases with moderate–severe vasculitis on muscle biopsy); 1 mg/d folic acid to ameliorate bone marrow suppression
- *Hydroxychloroquin:* 7 mg/kg/d max. if rash does not resolve rapidly
- *For steroid-resistant cases:* IV Cytoxan 500 mg/m² (dose sufficient to drop white count at day 9–11); cyclosporine dose to achieve blood therapeutic range
- *Calcium-sufficient diet / 25-OH vitamin D:* <30 kg, 20 mcg/d on MWF; ≥30 kg, 50 mcg/d on MWF
- *Antacids:* decrease motility, reduce gastric distress

COMPLICATIONS

- *Disease related:* osteopenia, paronychia, calcinosis; GI reflux w/aspiration pneumonia, GI perforation and blood loss; decreased GI motility; partial lipodystrophy
- *Medication related:* steroids: hypertension, growth retardation, weight gain, glaucoma, cataracts, electrolyte imbalance, mood swings; methotrexate: hepatotoxicity, nausea, hair loss; cyclosporine: renal, liver compromise, nausea, infection

WHEN TO REFER

- At Dx for evaluation/therapy by pediatric rheumatologist
(Note: mild-appearing cases [relatively normal muscle enzymes] may have severe muscle disease on muscle biopsy)
- To enter newly diagnosed in NIH Registry, call JDMS Hotline, (773) 880-3333

DERMOID CYST

BACKGROUND

- Rare congenital SubQ cyst; incidence ~1/20,000–1/50,000 live births; equal sex distribution
- 40% recognized at birth; 70% by age 5 yrs; may be undetected until enlargement/ infection occurs
- Most formed during embryonic development when epidermis sequestered/trapped along lines of embryonic fusion

CLINICAL MANIFESTATIONS

- Usually present as discrete slow-growing mass most often on head/neck, usually near midline, often in periorbital area
- Sites of predilection:
  - outer third of eyebrow ("external angle dermoid")
  - midline nose, usually near bridge
  - scalp
  - submental area
  - anterior neck
  - anterior chest wall
  - occipital area
- Typically SubQ "doughy" spherical nodule 0.5–6.0 cm in diameter
- Up to 50% of nasal dermoid cysts have sinus opening w/sebaceous discharge/projecting hairs; may indicate higher risk of intracranial extension

LABORATORY FEATURES

- MRI scan of choice to identify extent of growth/potential intracranial extension
- For neck lesions, $^{99m}Tc/^{123}I$ scintillation scan to identify possible ectopic thyroid tissue
- CT scan, high-resolution ultrasound, fistulography may be required prior to surgical intervention

	Dermoid	Encephalocele	Glioma
Age at detection	Usually infant, child; occasionally adult	Usually infancy	Any age
Appearance	Solid mass, may be associated w/sinus, hair; often 2° infection; does not transilluminate	Blue, soft, compressible; may transilluminate, enlarges w/crying	Red-blue and solid, not compressible; does not transilluminate
Location	25% extend intracranially	Always intracranial involvement	Stalk connects to intracranial space only rarely

Adapted with permission: Paller et al., *Arch Dermatol* 127 (March 1991), p. 365. Copyright 1991, American Medical Association.

DIFFERENTIAL DIAGNOSIS

- Nasal glioma/meningoencephalocele
- In neck distinguish from ectopic thyroid, thyroglossal duct cyst, branchial cleft cyst
- Less common entities to consider include:
  - other benign cysts such as epidermal cysts
    - facial trauma sequelae
    - hemangioma
    - rhabdomyosarcoma/fibrosarcoma

TREATMENT

- Complete surgical excision advisable to prevent:
  - potential infection including meningitis/intracranial abscess
  - bone atrophy/distortion of nose because of progressive growth/2° infection
- Surgical exploration needed to:
  - identify deep tracts that may be adherent to underlying periosteum/septum in nasal cases
  - r/o presence of intracranial connection, esp small fibrous bands that connect to intracranial compartments that may not be detectable on imaging studies

COMPLICATIONS

- Periorbital lesions may displace ocular structures
- Recurrent infection
- Meningitis/intracranial abscess
- Osteomyelitis
- Pressure erosion of bone
- May be accompanied by other anomalies (hemifacial microsomia, hypertelorism, hydrocephalus)

WHEN TO REFER

- Immediately
- *Do not* aspirate/attempt biopsy
- Lesions w/intracranial connections require combined extra/intracranial approach utilizing otolaryngology, neurosurgery, facial plastic surgery

ETIOLOGY

- Craniopharyngioma
- Langerhans cell histiocytosis
- Brain tumor
- Head trauma
- Neurosurgery
- CNS infections: encephalitis, meningitis
- Intraventricular hemorrhage
- AIDS
- Leukemia
- DIDMOAD (Wolfram) syndrome: diabetes insipidus, diabetes mellitus, optic atrophy, deafness
- Familial (autosomal dominant trait)
- Sarcoidosis
- Idiopathic

CLINICAL MANIFESTATIONS

- Polyuria, polydipsia, thirst, chronic dehydration
- Irritability, unexplained fever, vomiting
- Symptoms of associated hormonal deficits
- Growth failure
- Constipation
- Hyperthermia
- Enuresis, nocturia
- Disruptive behavior
- Rash (in histiocytosis)
- Bone lesions (in histiocytosis)
- Development of hydroureter or hydronephrosis

LABORATORY AND RADIOGRAPHIC FEATURES

- Dilute urine
- Hypernatremia
- ↑ Serum osmolality, ↓ urine osmolality, ↑ BUN
- Normal urinalysis
- Normal serum calcium, phosphorus, potassium, creatinine (when hydrated)
- Serum arginine vasopressin (AVP): not needed; results difficult to interpret
- MRI of brain: unenhanced T_1-weighted images do not show normal high signal intensity (bright spot) in neurohypophysis in central diabetes insipidus; "bright spot" may be present in familial form
- Correction of abnormalities w/DDAVP (desmopressin acetate)

DIFFERENTIAL DIAGNOSIS

- Diabetes mellitus
- Chronic renal insufficiency
- Langerhans cell histiocytosis
- Primary polydipsia (eg, psychogenic water drinking)
- Nephrogenic diabetes insipidus
- Hypokalemia
- Hypercalcemia

TREATMENT

- *DDVAP intranasally:* safe/efficacious
  - dosage:
    - older children: start w/5 µg (0.05 mL)–10 µg (0.1 mL) q12h, intranasally
    - younger children: dilute DDAVP: withdraw 0.1 mL DDAVP (10 µg/0.1 mL solution) from vial; dilute 1:10 by adding 0.9 mL normal saline; final DDAVP concentration: 1 µg/0.1 mL solution; for small children, start with 1 µg (0.1 mL diluted DDAVP); ↑ as needed
    - titrate dosage so antidiuresis lasts 10–12 hrs
    - if one spontaneous episode of polyuria does not occur each wk, delay one dose of DDAVP on weekend until polyuria begins
- Alternatives:
  - DDAVP tablets (0.1 mg):
    - little experience in children
    - initial dose: 1/2 tablet bid
    - titrate dose
  - vasopressin tannate in oil, aqueous vasopressin, lysine vasopressin no longer used

COMPLICATIONS

- From underlying disease or condition
- Excessive water intake, resulting in hyponatremia/fluid overload
- Seizure (very unusual)
- Heart failure (very unusual)

WHEN TO REFER TO PEDIATRIC ENDOCRINOLOGIST

- To determine etiology
- For Dx/treatment of other endocrinopathies
- To establish DDAVP dose
- For management DDAVP, fluids, electrolytes during surgery, periods of unconsciousness, other occasions during which fluid intake reduced/IV fluids being administered
- Children w/impaired thirst mechanisms

FAMILIAL NEPHROGENIC DIABETES INSIPIDUS

BACKGROUND

- *Onset:* infancy
- *Sex:* males: severely affected; females: usually mildly affected, rarely severe
- *Inheritance:* x-linked recessive, Xq28 gene locus, long arm X chromosome
- *Associated lesions:* none

CLINICAL MANIFESTATIONS

- Same as for central diabetes insipidus
- Failure to gain weight
- Constipation
- Mental/physical retardation 2° to prolonged dehydration during infancy

LABORATORY FEATURES

- *Similar to central diabetes insipidus:* anterior pituitary function not relevant
- ↑ levels of arginine vasopressin (AVP)
- No response to exogenous vasopressin/ DDAVP administration urine osmolality remains less than serum osmolality

TREATMENT

- None truly effective
- Thiazide diuretics (slight efficacy)
- High dose DDAVP
- Indomethacin/low salt diet

WHEN TO REFER

- As soon as diagnosis suspected

DRUG-INDUCED NEPHROGENIC DIABETES INSIPIDUS

BACKGROUND

- *Causative drugs:* demeclocyline, methoxyflurane anesthesia, lithium, fluoride excess

CLINICAL MANIFESTATIONS, LABORATORY FEATURES, TREATMENT

- Same as familial nephrogenic diabetes insipidus

WHEN TO REFER

- As soon as diagnosis suspected

BACKGROUND

- Also known as juvenile onset or type I diabetes
- *Peak incidence of onset:* 11–14 yrs of age
- *Minor peaks of onset:* 12–24 mos of age, 5–7 yrs of age
- *M:F ratio:* ~1:1
- Caucasians > African Americans > Native Americans > Orientals
- Genetic predisposition but not Mendelian inheritance:
  – HLA B8, DR3 and DR4 antigens ↑ risk
- Child's risk for IDDM if relative has IDDM:
  – 8% if nonidentical sibling, 35% if identical twin
  – 9% if father, 5% if mother
- *Etiology:* autoimmune destruction of pancreatic B cells
- Triggering event unknown (viral, environmental, other)
- ↓ insulin secretory capacity occurs over many mos, yrs

MANIFESTATIONS

- Pathophysiology related to insulin insufficiency:
  – ↑ endogenous glucose, FFA, ketone body production; ↓ glucose, ketone body disposal
  – leads progressively to hyperglycemia, hyperketonemia, glycosuria, ketonuria, osmotic diuresis, polydipsia, polyuria, volume constriction
  – volume constriction leads to ↑ "insulin counterregulatory hormones" (cortisol, GH, epinephrine, glucagon), ↑↑ insulin resistance, and ↑↑ glucose, ketone body, FFA production
  – ↓ fluid intake 2° to nausea and/or vomiting leads to rapid metabolic decompensation, acidosis, loss of body potassium, sodium, water

- Common clinical symptoms:
  – polyuria, polydipsia, fatigue, weight loss, vulvovaginitis in females, candida diaper rash in infants/young children, occasionally as metabolic acidosis and dehydration (diabetic ketoacidosis)

LABORATORY FEATURES

- Hyperglycemia
- Glycosuria
- Ketonemia/ketonuria: mild to severe
- ↓ Blood pH
- Hemoglobin A_1c: ↑
- Increased anti-islet cell antibodies, anti-GAD antibodies, insulin autoantibodies

DIFFERENTIAL DIAGNOSIS

- Type II diabetes mellitus
- Renal glycosuria w/or w/o other renal tubular defects
- Nephrogenic diabetes insipidus

TREATMENT

- Correction of DKA
- Diabetes education: etiology, pathophysiology, insulin action and use, carbohydrate-counting diet, home glucose monitoring, acute and long-term complication of disease, importance of normalizing blood glucose in prevention of complications
  – insulin program:
    ○ short- and intermediate-acting insulin 2×/d
    ○ intensified management w/multiple daily injections of short-acting insulin plus intermediate- or long-acting insulin, or
    ○ insulin pump Tx
  – carbohydrate-counting diet
  – home glucose monitoring 3–5×/d

COMPLICATIONS

- Acute:
  – hypoglycemia: asymptomatic (hypoglycemic unawareness), or hunger, nervousness, tremor, headache, altered sensorium (confusion, combative behavior, change in behavior, coma), seizure
  – hyperglycemia: asymptomatic or headache, feeling funny, thirst, polyuria, polydipsia, fatigue, weight loss, candida infections
- Chronic:
  – microvascular:
    ○ eye: background retinopathy, proliferative retinopathy, vitreous and/or retinal hemorrhage, blindness
    ○ kidney: microalbuninuria, proteinuria, progressive ↓ in GFR, azotemia, ↑ BP
    ○ neural: hand-glove peripheral sensory neuropathy, impotence, autonomic neuropathy (vascular and gastrointestinal), stroke from ↑ BP
  – coronary heart disease
  – peripheral vascular disease
    ○ poor tissue healing
    ○ ↑ risk extremity amputations
  – hyperlipidemia: ↑ LDL and ↓ HDL

PREVENTION

- No effective treatment available to preserve islet mass and prevent destruction of B cell of the islet. Trials under way to evaluate benefit of B cell suppression with exogenous insulin, desensitization w/oral insulin and effects of high-dose nicotinamide
- Intensified management of IDDM to normalize blood glucose concentration decreases long-term risk microvascular disease, peripheral neuropathy, nephropathy 50–70%

WHEN TO REFER

- When Dx diabetes suspected or proven

DIABETIC KETOACIDOSIS

MOREY W. HAYMOND

BACKGROUND

- Found primarily in individuals w/insulin dependent diabetes mellitus (IDDM):
  - occurs: at time of Dx
  - in established IDDM:
    - when insulin injections omitted
    - occasionally w/illness in poorly controlled IDDM
- Insulin insufficiency:
  - ↑ endogenous glucose, FFA, ketone body production, ↓ glucose/ketone body disposal
  - leads progressively to hyperglycemia, hyperketonemia, glycosuria, ketonuria, osmotic diuresis, polydipsia, polyuria, volume constriction
  - volume constriction leads to ↑ "insulin counterregulatory hormones" (cortisol, GH, epinephrine and glucagon), ↑↑ insulin resistance, ↑↑ glucose, ketone body, FFA production. At home pt must maintain fluid/electrolyte balance w/oral hydration
  - ↓ fluid intake 2° to nausea/vomiting: rapid metabolic decompensation, acidosis, potassium/sodium/water losses

MANIFESTATIONS

- History:
  - 2 wk–several month Hx: polyuria, polydipsia, weight loss, fatigue; rarely infection
  - rapid onset of nausea, vomiting, dehydration, heavy breathing; if untreated/severe: vascular collapse, shock; rarely renal vein/cerebral thromboses, death
- Physical examination:
  - breath: ↑ min volume (Kussmaul respiration), acetone (fruity) smell
  - dehydration (difficult to quantify): tachycardia, hypotension/postural changes in pulse, BP, dry mouth, sunken eyes
  - candida infections: vulvovaginitis, diaper rash
  - occasionally altered sensorium (sleepy to coma)

LABORATORY FEATURES

- Glucose > 250 mg/dl (14 mM), anion gap >18–20 mM, pH <7.25, HCO_3^- <12 mEq/L, pCO_2 <30 mmHg, Na+/K+ ↑, ↓, or normal; specific gravity > 1.040 2° to glycosuria/ketonuria, ↑ triglycerides/cholesterol, mild ↑ LFTs, leukocytosis w/left shift
- Chest x ray, cultures (eg, blood, urine, throat) as indicated

DIFFERENTIAL DIAGNOSIS

- Other causes of metabolic acidosis:
  - chemical ingestion (salicylates, ethanol, methanol, ethylene glycol)
  - inborn error in metabolism (organic acidemia including lactic acidosis)
- Other causes of polyuria/polydypsia:
  - central/nephrogenic diabetes insipidus
  - hypercalcemia

TREATMENT

- Volume expansion (first hr): 20 cc/kg lactate Ringer's/NS
- 0.1 units human regular insulin /kg/hr
- Rehydration:
  - 3,000 mL/m^2/24 hrs first 4–24 hrs w/1/2 NS + 20 mEq/L KPO_4 + 20 mEq/L K acetate if renal function/plasma K+ normal
  - when glucose ≤300 mg/dl, add 5% glucose to IV
  - adjust IV fluid rate/content depending on acute tubular necrosis, anuria, hypo-/hyperkalemia, hypo-/hypernatremia
  - follow glucose/electrolytes; use anion gap to monitor correction of ketonemia
  - controversy exists about use of $NaHCO_3$/the rate of decrease in glucose concentration in etiology of cerebral edema
- Oral fluids when alert/$NaHCO_3$ >16 mM (anion gap 14–16 mM); decrease IV fluids appropriately
- Home management:
  - mixed split insulin (1/2 to 1 unit/Kg/day) program using regular or lispro-insulin and NPH unless <5 yrs of age
  - if <5 yrs of age, insulin dosing individualized
    - diabetes education
    - 4×/d home glucose monitoring
    - carbohydrate-counting diet
    - insulin adjustment

COMPLICATIONS

- Cerebral edema in first 24 hrs
- Hyper/hypokalemia
- Hypoglycemia
- Aspiration during altered state of consciousness
- Failure to clear metabolic acidosis
- Renal/cerebral thromboses

WHEN TO REFER

- When DKA suspected/diagnosed

DIAMOND-BLACKFAN ANEMIA

GEORGE R. BUCHANAN

BACKGROUND

- Typically presents during first 2 or 3 mos of life w/severe anemia and absent reticulocyte response
- 10% cases atypical and present w/less severe anemia after 6 mos of age
- Due to congenital absence of erythroid progenitors
- Occurs equally in males and females
- Most cases sporadic, but autosomal dominant inheritance increasingly identified
- Variable clinical course, w/some pts entering spontaneous remission

CLINICAL MANIFESTATIONS

- Pallor, lethargy, feeding difficulties, and other manifestations of severe anemia
- May present at birth w/severe anemia or even hydrops
- Abnormal thumbs, short stature, other congenital anomalies (including Turner syndrome–like phenotype)
- Positive family Hx of anemia or thumb abnormalities in some cases
- Absence of hepatosplenomegaly or lymphadenopathy

LABORATORY FEATURES

- *Anemia:* usually moderate to severe (Hgb 3–7 g/dl); mean corpuscular volume (MCV) usually elevated; reticulocyte count inappropriately low (often zero)
- *WBC count:* usually normal; platelet count normal or high
- Occasional older and atypical pts may have mild leukopenia and thrombocytopenia
- *Peripheral blood smear:* macrocytes, ovalocytes, absence of polychromasia
- *Fetal hemoglobin level:* often increased
- *Bone marrow aspirate:* markedly reduced or absent erythroid progenitors but otherwise normal
- *Other studies:* Parvovirus B19 studies negative, peripheral blood and bone marrow chromosomes normal, RBC adenosine deaminase usually elevated

DIFFERENTIAL DIAGNOSIS

- Transient erythroblastopenia of childhood
- Parvovirus B19 infection, either complicating a congenital hemolytic anemia or in an HIV-infected or otherwise immunocompromised pt
- Fanconi anemia
- Congenital dyserythropoietic anemia or aplastic anemia

TREATMENT

- Corticosteroids:
  – prednisone 2 mg/kg/d div. Reticulocyte count increases within 1 wk w/subsequent sustained rise in Hgb (to normal or near normal) in ~50%
  – after response, prednisone should be switched to qOd and slowly tapered to lowest possible dose that maintains normal or near-normal hemoglobin value
- most pts require low-dose maintenance corticosteroids (2.5–10 mg several times weekly)
- pts requiring continued high daily dosing should be considered candidates for alternative Tx
- Blood transfusions:
  – most pts require transfusion of packed RBCs at Dx
  – one-third pts resistant to corticosteroids and totally transfusion dependent
  – transfusion-dependent pts should be monitored for iron overload and other complications of transfusions; deferoxamine chelation should begin after several yrs
- Bone marrow transplantation:
  – steroid refractory and transfusion-dependent pts should be considered for bone marrow transplantation if a matched sibling donor available
- Other treatment strategies:
  – interleukin-3 and other growth factors rarely effective
  – anti-thymocyte globulin, cyclosporine, other immunosuppressive agents, androgens usually ineffective

COMPLICATIONS

- Growth delay/other complications of corticosteroids in pts dependent on high maintenance doses
- Hemochromatosis, viral infection, and alloimmunization in transfusion-dependent pts
- Small risk of developing malignancy (~15 cases of leukemia and solid tumors reported)

WHEN TO REFER

- All pts should be referred to a pediatric hematologist-oncologist for confirmation Dx and development of management plan
- Pts should be enrolled on the Diamond-Blackfan Registry (coordinated by Mt. Sinai School of Medicine) and parents referred to Diamond-Blackfan Foundation support group

BACKGROUND

- Irritant contact dermatitis affecting children/elderly requiring diapers
- *Caused by combination of factors:* chronic occlusion, maceration, friction/irritation; diarrhea/frequent bowel movements
- *Most frequent complication:* overgrowth of candida albicans
- *Prevention:* frequent diaper changes, gentle cleansing, irritant avoidance, judicious protection of skin

CLINICAL MANIFESTATIONS

- *Early:* convex areas of buttocks, upper thighs, pubis, scrotum, present w/erythematous patches studded by papules, then papulovesicles/erosions
- *Later:* eruption spreads to folds; secondary candidal infection suspected when bright erythema/superficial erosions surrounded by papulopustules in normal skin

LABORATORY FEATURES

- No investigation usually necessary
- Skin scraping/staining w/potassium hydroxide may confirm candida infection, but usually not needed
- If Dx in doubt, selective blood work may help in differential Dx

DIFFERENTIAL DIAGNOSIS

- Other entities considered when refractory to treatment/in immunosuppressed pts
- Candidosis
- Seborrheic dermatitis
- Atopic dermatitis
- Psoriasis
- Allergic contact dermatitis
- Congenital syphilis
- Acrodermatitis enteropathica (zinc deficiency)
- Histiocytosis X
- Biotin deficiency
- Immunosuppression/AIDS when chronic

TREATMENT

- Prevention best approach/not always possible if diarrhea present
- Goals:
  - keep diaper area as clean/dry as possible (frequent changing of diapers, gentle cleansing w/tap water, cautious drying w/towel/hair dryer set at low temperature)
  - limit mixture of urine/feces, which results in ammonia release by fecal enzymes/↑ pH (use of superabsorbent disposable diapers most effective)
- When skin fragilized, avoid soap/commercial wipes; zinc oxide ointment not irritating/induces good protection
- Use antifungal such as topical nystatin/an imidazole after 48 hrs because of candida overgrowth
- Avoid combinations of high-potency steroid creams/antifungals

COMPLICATIONS

- Secondary infection by candida common when eruption >2 d
- Secondary bacterial infection unusual, more frequent when underlying topic dermatitis 2° to *Staphylococcus aureus* overgrowth

WHEN TO REFER

- Referral indicated when doubt about Dx
- Failure to respond to proper Tx

BACKGROUND

- Common adverse reaction to antibiotic treatment occurring in up to 30% of children
- Most likely in children <6 yrs of age
- Occurrence depends on antibiotic dose, antimicrobial spectrum, pharmocokinetic properties of drug, recent hospitalization
- Most cases of unknown cause (enigmatic)
- Some caused by *Clostridium difficile*
- Enigmatic cases usually benign/associated w/disruption of normal colonic flora
- *Most common implicated drugs:* ampicillin, cephalosporins, clindamycin

CLINICAL MANIFESTATIONS

Enigmatic	C. difficile
loose stools	watery diarrhea, cramps, fever
symptoms unusual	progressive; chronic
benign; usually self-limited	may follow hospitalization
sporadic	not dose related
antibiotic dose related	symptoms persist, colitis present
diarrhea abates if antibiotic stopped	*onset:* 72 hrs–6–8 wks
colitis not usually present	
onset within 24 hrs	

LABORATORY FEATURES

- *C. difficile* toxin–induced diarrhea often accompanied by fever; leukocytosis; WBCs, blood, *C. difficile* toxin in stool
- Enigmatic diarrhea accompanied by normal blood count; no blood, WBCs, toxin in stool

DIFFERENTIAL DIAGNOSIS

- Parenteral diarrhea (accompanies infection in ears, respiratory or urinary tract)
- Viral gastroenteritis accompanying same viral infection in another organ
- Bacterial enterocolitis (Salmonella, Shigella, Campylobacter, Yersinia)
- Giardiasis (acute)
- Transient lactase deficiency (postinfectious) and/or carbohydrate intolerance
- Irritable bowel syndrome of infancy/childhood (toddler's diarrhea)
- Too much juice in diet
- Sorbitol-induced diarrhea

TREATMENT

- *Enigmatic diarrhea:* stop/reduce antibiotic dose; disease often improves despite ongoing treatment
- *C. difficile*–induced diarrhea (toxin present in stool):
  - stop antibiotic if possible
  - if diarrhea persists/worsens:
    - metronidazole: 7 mg/kg/dose po q8h × 10–14 d
    - vancomycin: 10 mg/kg/dose po q6h × 10–14 d

COMPLICATIONS

- Some children w/*C. difficile* relapse/require treatment for longer period
- Small percentage of children w/*C. difficile* develop fulminant pseudomembranous enterocolitis
- Rare child progresses to colonic perforation

WHEN TO REFER

- Most pts do not require referral
- Referral may be necessary for those w/multiple relapses
- Referral indicate for fulminant pseudomembranous colitis/impending perforation

DIARRHEA, CHRONIC NONSPECIFIC (CNSD) OR TODDLER'S DIARRHEA

JONATHAN E. TEITELBAUM AND
RONALD E. KLEINMAN

BACKGROUND

- *Most frequent age:* 6 mos–4 yrs; peak incidence 1–3 yrs
- Most frequent cause of prolonged diarrhea w/o failure to thrive in this age group
- May follow gastroenteritis; exacerbated by respiratory infections, teething, immunizations, stress
- Etiology unclear; may be related to ↓ dietary fat (<28% of daily calories), excess carbohydrate (fructose/sorbitol) in diet leading to ↑ osmotic load, excessive fluid intake (>2.5× maintenance requirements), ↑ prostaglandin F_2 alpha leading to disordered intestinal motility w/decreased transit time
- Family Hx bowel-related problems (ie, irritable bowel syndrome/constipation) present in 67%
- 90% symptom free by 39 mos of age
- Many later in life have problems w/irritable bowel syndrome, constipation, headaches

CLINICAL MANIFESTATIONS

- Diarrhea ≥2 wks duration, w/average 3–4 bowel movements/day
- Bowel movements typically in daytime w/first of day larger than subsequent ones; may contain mucus/undigested vegetable matter
- Normal growth/development
- No evidence of malabsorption

LABORATORY FEATURES

- Accurate dietary Hx required to assess fat content/fluid intake
- Stools often have ↑ sodium, bile acids, extractable water content; no value to checking these parameters
- Level of prostaglandin F_2 alpha may be ↑; not of diagnostic value
- If concern about malabsorption, 72-hr fecal fat collection helpful (normal in CNSD)
- If concern about infectious etiology stool culture, stool for ova/parasites should be performed (negative in CNSD)
- Stools may be positive for occult blood, usually related to fissures

DIFFERENTIAL DIAGNOSIS

- Celiac disease
- Allergic enteropathy
- Pancreatic insufficiency (cystic fibrosis, Schwachman-Diamond syndrome)
- Disaccharidase deficiency
- Infectious colitis/enteritis (ie, Salmonella, Shigella, Yersinia, Campylobacter, *E. coli* 0157, *C. difficile,* Giardia, etc)
- Intestinal lymphangiectasia

TREATMENT

- Benign self-limiting condition; parental reassurance often sufficient
- Suboptimal fat intake (<28% caloric intake)/excessive carbohydrate intake (usually in juices) should be corrected (limit fluids other than milk and water to 6 oz/d)
- Fiber additives (eg, psyllium) may have some beneficial effect
- Family stress reduction
- Agents such as diodoquin, aspirin, loperamide not recommended

PREVENTION

- Mainly accomplished through proper nutrition/avoidance of very low-fat, high-carbohydrate diets

WHEN TO REFER

- Most pts managed w/o referral
- Pts not easily determined to have this benign condition (because of age/evidence of malabsorption) should be evaluated by gastroenterologist

BACKGROUND

- *Caused: Corynebacterium diphtheriae*
- Generalized/localized symptoms follow production, elaboration of toxin
- Recent outbreaks in independent states of former Soviet Union; worldwide distribution, endemic in developing countries
- Acquired by contact w/either a carrier/person w/disease, usually transmitted in respiratory droplet
- Peak incidence in autumn/winter
- Majority in unimmunized children <15 yrs of age
- Increased cases w/crowding, limited access to health care
- *Incubation period:* 1–6 d

CLINICAL MANIFESTATIONS

- Sx depend on site of infection, immunization status, systemic distribution of toxin
- Nasal:
  - serosanguineous to mucopurulent nasal discharge w/foul odor
  - lack of systemic signs; occurs most often in infants
- Tonsillar/pharyngeal:
  - insidious, more severe
  - white to gray adherent membrane
  - may be associated w/soft tissue edema of neck, "bull neck"
  - respiratory/circulatory collapse
- Laryngeal:
  - generally reflects downward extension from pharynx
  - occasionally primary involvement; then indistinguishable from croup
  - acute obstruction
- *Cutaneous:* generally ulcerative w/sharply demarcated border/membranous base
- *Conjunctival:* corneal erosions
- *Aural:* otitis externa w/foul-smelling discharge

LABORATORY FEATURES

- Dx should be made on basis of clinical findings; delay in treatment poses serious risk
  - culture of material from beneath membrane/portion of membrane: alert lab
  - direct smear, fluorescent antibody technique, counter immunoelectrophoresis helpful in experienced hands
  - other lab studies of little diagnostic value; electrocardiogram if myocarditis

Differential Diagnosis

Nasal	Tonsillar/pharyngeal	Laryngeal
Common cold	Group A *Streptococcal* pharyngitis	Viral croup
Foreign body	Infectious mononucleosis	Epiglottitis
Sinusitis	Viral tonsillitis	Aspirated foreign body
Congenital syphilis	Herpes simplex infection	Laryngeal masses
	Vincent angina	
	Oral candidiasis	

COMPLICATIONS

- Directly related to 1° disease:
  - 2° to bacterial infection
  - airway obstruction
- 2° to elaborated toxin:
  - myocarditis, may follow mild or severe cases, occurs mostly when antitoxin administration delayed, appears in 2nd week
  - neurologic complications, paralysis of soft palate, ocular paralysis, peripheral neuropathy, usually resolves spontaneously
  - kidney failure

TREATMENT

- Neutralization of toxin (antitoxin):
  - only specific treatment
  - equine origin
  - IV, single dose
  - Dosage on basis of membrane site/size, toxicity degree, illness duration
  - test for sensitivity to horse serum prior to administration
  - dosage:
    - mild nasal/pharyngeal: 40,000 units
    - moderately severe pharyngeal: 80,000 units
    - severe pharyngeal/laryngeal: 120,000 units
    - mixed symptoms, brawny edema, duration >48 hrs: 120,000 units
- Antibiotics:
  - not substitute for antitoxin Tx
  - aqueous procaine penicillin G IM at 300,000 units if <10 kg, 600,000 units if >10 kg qd × 14 d
  - alternative: erythromycin 40 mg/kg/d orally in 4 div doses × 14 d
  - Tx endpoint: 3 consecutive negative cultures at least 24 hrs apart
- Supportive:
  - bed rest
  - pulmonary toilet
  - serial electrocardiograms
  - hydration, nutrition
- If underimmunized, complete series

PREVENTION

- Active immunization on communitywide basis:
  - diphtheria toxoid, usually given in combination w/tetanus toxoid/pertussis antigen (either whole cell/acellular)
  - primary immunization (7–25 Lf/dose): 2, 4, 6 mos
  - booster: 12–18 mos, 4–6 yrs
  - adult-type booster (<2 Lf/dose): q10yrs (w/tetanus toxoid)
- Management of contacts:
  - surveillance/ culture
  - antimicrobial prophylaxis: oral erythromycin 40 mg/kg/d ×7d/benzathine penicillin 600,000–1,200,000 u IM once (same treatment for carriers)
- *Isolation of pt:* strict until 3 negative cultures

WHEN TO REFER

- Most pts w/presumed diphtheria should be referred to pediatric center w/facilities for isolation/respiratory support

BACKGROUND

- After peaking at 5.3 in 1979/1981, divorce rate in US ↓ 4.4 in mid-1990s
- >1 million children experience parental divorce each year
- Mother awarded custody 75–85% settlements; 5–10% custody cases awarded to father; joint custody 15%
- *Children from fatherless homes:* 85% all children exhibiting behavioral disorders, 71% pregnant teenagers, 71% all high school dropouts, 63% youth suicides

MANIFESTATIONS AND COMPLICATIONS

- Degree to which children experiencing divorce manifest problem physical/behavioral symptoms varies significantly
- Factors in adaptation to loss include:
  - ability to attain developmentally appropriate perception of loss
  - adequacy of child's coping mechanisms
  - adequacy of situational support (first two factors dependent on age/level of development)

	Perception of loss	Common manifestations
Birth–2 yrs	Unable to conceptualize loss	Feeding/sleeping problems Irregularity, irritability
2–7 yrs	Loss viewed as reversible Blames self for loss	Developmental regression Attempt to be "perfect child" Play out fantasies of unified family
7–11 yrs	Attempts to identify single cause of loss	Open grieving Feel rejected, withdrawn/act out Place blame on one parent Decline in academic performance
≥12 yrs	Understands multiple facets of cause/outcome of loss	Truancy Substance abuse Sexual experimentation Fearful of own inability to maintain relationship

- Complaints of headaches, stomachaches, sleeping, elimination disturbances common to all ages; may be only manifestations that bring child to attention of health care provider; majority of symptoms represent age-appropriate but often maladaptive coping mechanisms
- Adequacy of situational support frequently significant issue because children often experience abandonment by one parent/diminished support from other parent due to grief/anger over divorce, increased responsibilities for economic support of family

TREATMENT AND RECOMMENDATIONS

- Predivorce:
  - minimize fighting in presence of children
  - tell children about separation/divorce before departure of parent; tell all children at same time
  - reassure children that both parents love them
  - give specific details about visitation plan w/noncustodial parent; best done w/both parents present
  - make clear that divorce is final; if accurate, that every effort has been made to reach reconciliation
- Postdivorce:
  - encourage children to share their feelings; respect all expressed feelings; honestly answer all questions at level appropriate to child's development; expect same questions to be asked multiple times
  - encourage/acknowledge children's positive feelings for both parents; do not speak negatively about ex-spouse to children; allow child-initiated phone calls to noncustodial parent
  - avoid visitation disputes that require children to take sides
  - keep children separate from any ongoing, hostile interactions between parents
  - maintain discipline/consistent limit setting in both households as normally as possible
  - maintain as much of predivorce daily routine as feasible
  - reassure children that divorce not their fault
  - be patient w/children's behavioral/physical problems that develop as part of their coping strategies; be patient w/recurrent reevaluation of divorce by children as they mature through progressive developmental stages
  - notify significant adults in children's life such as schoolteachers, scout leaders, friends' parents about divorce so they can be prepared to be patient/offer additional encouragement
  - parents need to obtain necessary support to help themselves adjust to divorce; otherwise, they will be unable to provide support their children need
- Custody:
  - in absence of abuse, frequent/predicable contact w/both parents provides optimal environment for children to adapt to divorce/continue normal development
  - open hostilities between parents are single most disruptive influence in children's ability to adapt to divorce
  - no hard evidence to support routine placement of children w/mother or w/father, but significant indications that father, in addition to mother, needs to have on ongoing influence w/children for optimal long-term development
  - joint custody is primary legal arrangement that permits both parents to be significant influences in their children's lives after divorce; less formal, but equally effective arrangements can be made between parents when they view parenting as high priority; such arrangements, whether legal/informal, require that both parents respect each other's role/skills. Commitment to effective communication/tolerance for differences between parents essential

WHEN TO REFER

- Mental health services may be needed in following situations:
  - persistence of severe manifestations/complications w/o any improvement beyond 6 mos after divorce
  - continued fighting between parents
  - inadequate situational support

BACKGROUND

- First described in 1865 by John Langdon Down
- Health, longevity, prospects in life have improved w/closure of institutions, better health care, early intervention, educational services, greater inclusion of people w/disabilities in community life
- Phenotype results from excess of genetic material from distal long arm of 21st chromosome
- 95%, nondisjunction causing trisomy 21; 4%, unbalanced translocations; 1%, mosaic genotype

CLINICAL MANIFESTATIONS

- *Phenotypic features:* hypotonia, midface hypoplasia, small external ears, upslanting palpebral fissures, stippling of irides (Brushfield spots), shortened digits, single transverse palmar crease, widened space between first/second toe w/vertical crease
- *Congenital heart defects:* 50%, most commonly (65%) complete atrioventricular canal
- *Obstructive GI defects:* 10%, most commonly duodenal atresia, celiac disease
- *Hearing impairment:* usually conductive, 30–50%
- *Ophthalmologic disorders:* 60% (congenital cataracts, congenital glaucoma, strabismus, refractive errors)
- *Sleep apnea:* as many as 25%
- *Seizure disorders:* 10% w/peaks in early childhood (commonly myoclonic)/adulthood
- *Leukemia:* 1/150
- *Autoimmune disorders:* more common (thyroiditis, diabetes, rheumatoid arthritis, alopecia areata)
- *Joint laxity:* common (atlantoaxial/atlanto-occipital instability on x ray in 15% w/clinical myelopathy in 1%)
- *Short stature/microcephaly:* nearly universal
- *Mild–moderate mental retardation:* in most individuals w/visual processing a strength compared to auditory processing in many
- *Specific expressive language disorder:* 70%
- *Alzheimer-type dementia:* increased frequency/earlier onset (mean age of onset = 52 yrs)

LABORATORY FEATURES

- Karyotype of cultured lymphocytes confirms presence of excess chromosome 21 material as trisomy 21, translocation, mosaicism

TREATMENT

- Medical:
  - provide all usual newborn screening tests/subsequent health promotion including all usual immunizations
  - screen all newborns for congenital heart defects including pediatric cardiologic consultation/echocardiography
  - provide careful audiologic evaluations at 6 mos, 12 mos, annually thereafter
  - provide infant screening for cataracts/glaucoma w/annual pediatric ophthalmologic examinations
  - screen newborns for congenital hypothyroidism followed annually by T4/TSH
  - use Down-syndrome-specific growth charts
  - obtain complete cervical spine x rays including lateral views in neutral, flexion, extension ~ 3 yrs of age (earlier if suspicious Sx occur) to r/o atlantoaxial instability/bony anomalies of cervical spine; if normal repeat q10yrs
  - screen for celiac disease w/endomysial IgA @ age 3 yrs
- Developmental/educational:
  - provide prompt referral for early intervention services
  - promote early emphasis on development of communication skills including use of "total communication" (verbal communication paired w/visual augmentations such as manual sign language)
  - refer to local school district for identification for special education services at age 3
  - advocate for educational placements in regular classroom settings w/necessary supports/modifications
  - consider medical causes for changes in school performance (eg, thyroid disorder, sleep apnea)
  - support vocational/community opportunities aimed at regular employment, highest attainable level of independence
- Family support:
  - convey Dx to both parents promptly/empathetically w/adequate discussion time, access to further information, close follow-up
  - refer family to local/state family support agency for services such as respite care, care coordination, information access, financial supports
  - offer contact w/other parents of children w/Down syndrome/refer to parent-to-parent agency; refer to regional/national Down syndrome advocacy organizations
  - periodically assess adequacy of insurance coverage/eligibility for public programs such as Medicaid, Title V, SSI

PREVENTION

- Cause unknown; no primary preventive measures available
- Prevention/early treatment of medical complications; appropriate educational/family supports promote best outcomes
- Prenatal measurement of maternal serum factors (alpha fetoprotein, estriol, human chorionic gonadotropin) together w/maternal age provide enhanced assessment of risk during pregnancy
- Prenatal Dx by karyotyping of fetal cells offered in pregnancies considered high risk due to maternal age/maternal serum screening results, previous affected pregnancy, family Hx Down syndrome
- Support parents following prenatal Dx Down syndrome w/accurate information, consideration of choices, genetic counseling

WHEN TO REFER

- All individuals should have pediatric cardiologic evaluation including echocardiogram within 1 mo of birth
- Down syndrome clinics/child development clinics may provide assistance w/guidelines for health promotion, psychoeducational/behavioral assessments, access to current information
- Appropriate referrals when medical complications suspected/identified

WILLIAM D. GRAF

BACKGROUND

- *Near drowning:* survival of significant submersion injury for at least 24 hrs
- *Drowning:* second most common cause of death by unintentional injury in pediatric population
- *Bimodal age distribution:* toddlers (peak age 1–2 yrs)/adolescents (18–24 yrs)
- M:F ratio 4:1
- *Freshwater submersion:* disrupts surfactant, may lead to atelectasis/pulmonary edema
- *Saltwater submersion:* can cause alveolar osmotic fluid shift, leading to pulmonary edema
- *Ice water submersion:* severe hypothermia (<31°C) may provide CNS protection
- ~20% near drowning survivors have at least some permanent neurologic disability
- *Submersion time:* exact Hx may be unavailable/unreliable
- *Duration of CPR:* bad outcome associated w/CPR >25 min

CLINICAL MANIFESTATIONS

Estimate of submersion injury severity at initial assessment

	Mild	Moderate	Severe
Vital signs			
Pulse	normal	↓ or ↑	absent
BP	normal	↓ or ↑	absent
Respiration	normal	↓ or ↑	absent
Temperature	>35°C	31–35°C	<31°C
Pulmonary injury			
Auscultation	normal/coarse breaths	rales, wheezes	apnea/rales
Cerebral hypoxic injury			
Mental status	normal/mild disorientation	stupor, agitation/postictal state	coma
Pupillary response	normal	sluggish	absent
Seizures	none	possibly present	none
Motor	normal	↓ or ↑ tone	flaccid

LABORATORY FEATURES

- In mild submersion injury:
  - if pt does not have significant pulmonary/neurologic symptoms at time of initial assessment, use oximetry to monitor O_2 saturation; if oximetry remains normal/pt stable during 4–6 hr observation period then no blood draw/chest x ray necessary
- In moderate–severe submersion injury:
  - most useful tests:
    - blood gas analysis: arterial/capillary blood serve as estimate for degree of acidosis/hypercapnia
    - serum glucose: when measured within 6 hrs of event, normal blood sugar present in mild–moderate submersion injury; hyperglycemia (>300 mg/dL) strongly associated w/ severe submersion injury/bad outcome
    - chest x ray: normal/perihilar infiltrates in mild injury; basilar infiltrates in moderate injury; atelectasis/lobar consolidation in severe submersion injury
  - less useful tests:
    - in severe injury, consider electrolytes, UA, urine drug screen, renal, liver function studies, blood coagulation tests prior to hospital transfer

DIFFERENTIAL DIAGNOSIS

- *Accidental drowning "syndromes" of childhood:* swimming pool, bath tub, hot tub, pond, river, lake, toilet
- *Trauma:* esp head/neck injuries from shallow water diving
- Nonaccidental trauma
- *Intoxication:* ~50% adolescent submersion injuries associated w/ alcohol consumption
- *Seizure:* w/ or w/o prior Hx epilepsy

TREATMENT

- *Initial resuscitation:* evaluate for associated injuries, immobilize neck if indicated; assess vital signs/cardiopulmonary status, begin CPR/intubate if indicated; Heimlich maneuver not indicated unless upper airway obstruction present
- *Hypotension:* as indicated for treatment of shock, obtain venous access/give repeat boluses of fluid (0.9% NS or LR), 20 mL/kg; central line should be placed in ED/ICU setting
- *Metabolic acidosis:* 1 mEq/kg $NaHCO_3$ empirically if clinically indicated
- Monitor for evolving pulmonary edema in moderate/severe submersion injury; in self-ventilating pts, give O_2 3–6 L/min/albuterol nebulization, 0.15 mg/kg prior to transport; endotracheal intubation required in pts w/ unstable airway/apnea
- *Monitor for evolving cerebral edema in moderate/severe submersion injury:* if seizures present, give diazepam 0.5 mg/kg followed by phenytoin (Dilantin) 18 mg/kg IV load over 30 min; ↑ intracranial pressure (ICP) from cerebral edema generally occurs several hours after submersion/should be managed in ICU setting
- *Mild hypothermia:* remove wet clothes, passive rewarming
- *Severe hypothermia:* consider active rewarming in ED/ICU setting
- *Prophylactic antibiotics:* not required for transient postsubmersion fever within 24 hrs of event

COMPLICATIONS

- True aspiration pneumonia (brief fever often develops within 24 hrs of submersion)
- Adult respiratory distress syndrome
- Mild–severe hypoxic encephalopathy/resultant neurologic disability

PREVENTION

- *Public education:* submersion injuries silent (no scream or splash usually heard)
- Fenced pools w/ lockable gates
- Adult supervision of water-related activities at all ages; teach children age 4/older to swim
- Personal flotation devices (PFD) in boats

WHEN TO REFER

- Asymptomatic pts (mild submersion injury, duration of submersion usually <2–3 min) should receive full medical evaluation/be observed for a period of 4–6 hrs; can be managed as outpts if appropriate adult supervision/telephone follow-up available
- Routine hospital admission of all mild submersion injuries not necessary: virtually all pts w/ mild submersion injury have good outcome; postsubmersion pulmonary symptoms, if any, develop 4–6 hrs of event in vast majority of pts
- Symptomatic pts (moderate–severe submersion injury) require initial stabilization, emergent transport/admission to hospital ICU

BACKGROUND

- 6–17% pts admitted to pediatric hospitals experience adverse drug reactions
- 25% less frequent in children than adults >50 yrs old
- *Frequency:* antibiotics > antipyretics/NSAIDs > anticonvulsants
- Morbilliform, urticarial eruptions the most common drug eruptions
- Drugs may exacerbate preexisting cutaneous disorders such as psoriasis
- Drug eruptions may resolve despite continuing offending drug or may progress to more serious eruption
- Most drug eruptions not life threatening, w/no long-term complications
- Complications of more severe cutaneous reactions depend on type, severity of reaction (see table)

APPROACH TO PATIENT WITH SUSPECTED DRUG ERUPTION

- *Analysis of drug exposure:* medication exposure relative to rash onset, previous drug exposure, determination of which drugs commonly cause cutaneous eruptions
- *Cutaneous findings:* morphology of rash, symptoms such as pruritus, skin tenderness
- *Extracutaneous manifestations:* lymphadenopathy, fever, arthralgia, myalgia, respiratory distress, BP alterations, mucous membrane changes
- Laboratory testing:
  - routine: CBC, liver enzymes, UA
  - specific: antinuclear antibodies, rheumatoid factor, complement levels (C3, C4), measures of liver function (prothrombin time, partial thromboplastin time, albumin), skin biopsy
- Consider differential Dx
- Monitor response to drug removal, possibly rechallenge

CATEGORIES (SEE TABLE)

- *Mild:* morbilliform/exanthematous, fixed drug eruption/generalized fixed drug, photosensitivity
- *Severe:* urticaria/angioedema/anaphylaxis, Stevens-Johnson syndrome (SJS)/toxic epidermal necrolysis (TEN), hypersensitivity syndrome, exfoliative dermatitis/erythroderma, vasculitis, serum sickness
- *Other:* pemphigus, linear IgA disease, acute generalized exanthematous pustulosis, pseudoporphyria, erythema nodosum, contact dermatitis (neomycin), acneiform (phenytoin, phenobarbital, corticosteroids), coumadin-induced necrosis, lichenoid eruptions, erythema annulare centrifugum, psoriasiform eruptions, pityriasis rosea-like eruptions, alopecia, hyper/hypopigmentation, lupus erythematosus–like syndrome, dermatomysotitislike reactions, sclerodermalike reactions, ichthyosiform eruptions, acanthosis nigricans–like eruptions, hypertrichosis, nail changes

DIFFERENTIAL DIAGNOSIS

- Often difficult to determine w/100% certainty offending drug. In children, differentiating viral exanthem from drug eruption frequently difficult, commonly not possible on clinical grounds alone. Furthermore, drug eruptions often precipitated by intercurrent viral illness

TREATMENT

- Eliminate all unnecessary drugs, change to chemically dissimilar drugs when possible
- *Minor drug eruptions (exanthematous):* withdraw drug; provide symptomatic treatment w/emollients, mild–moderately potent topical steroids, antihistamines
- *Serious drug eruptions:* see table for category-specific management

PREVENTION

- Thorough drug Hx essential to prevent drug eruptions
- Skin testing (prick, intradermal) may help differentiate those pts at risk for immediate hypersensitivity reactions
- Patch testing useful in evaluating contact dermatitis or fixed drug eruptions
- Photo patch testing utilized to evaluate for photosensitivity reactions
- Relatives of pts w/anticonvulsant hypersensitivity syndrome may be at risk for similar reaction

WHEN TO REFER

- Widespread cutaneous involvement, extracutaneous manifestations, laboratory abnormalities may indicate more serious drug eruption; should prompt referral to specialist for evaluation, treatment
- Pts w/multiple drug allergies/photosensitivity may benefit from further diagnostic evaluation such as skin testing, patch testing, photo patch testing

Characteristics of drug of eruptions

Dx	Onset of Rash After Initiation of Drug
Morbilliform/exanthematous	7–10 d
Urticaria/angioedema/anaphylaxis	Minutes to hours; NSAIDs: 1–7 d, ACE inhibitors: <4 wks
Vasculitis	1–3 wks
Photosensitivity	Phototoxic reactions: 5–20 hrs after exposure; photoallergic: <24 hrs after reexposure
Exfoliative dermatitis/erythroderma	1–3 wks
Fixed drug/generalized fixed drug	10–14 d after first exposure; <48 hrs after second exposure
Hypersensitivity syndrome	2–6 wks
Serum sickness/sickness-like illness	8–14 d; lasts 4–5 d
Stevens-Johnson syndrome (SJS)/toxic epidermal necrolysis (TEN)	1–14 d; Maximal disease expression in 4–5 d

DYSLEXIA (READING DISORDER)

DAVID A. KUBE AND FREDERICK B. PALMER

BACKGROUND

- *Reading disorder ("Dyslexia"):* unexpected difficulty in reading in one who otherwise possesses intelligence, motivation, schooling considered necessary for accurate fluent reading
- ~20–30% of school-age children have difficulty learning to read
- 5–10% of schoolchildren have learning disability in reading
- Recent experience indicates males/females equally affected
- Other learning disabilities include mathematics disorder/disorder of written expression
- Commonly identified in early elementary school, but may present at any age
- Linguistic deficit in phonologic awareness/analysis, independent of general cognitive abilities (IQ), underlying feature in many w/reading disorder
- Differences in temporo-parieto-occipital brain regions between some people w/dyslexia/normal readers
- *Heritable:* dyslexic parents have 23–65% risk of dyslexic child
- *Nongenetic risk factors:* low birth weight, Hx brain injury/anomaly, toxin exposure

CLINICAL MANIFESTATIONS

- Generally suspected only after school failure demonstrated
- *Preschooler:* language delay, poor articulation, difficulty learning letters/other readiness skills
- *Early elementary school age:* poor decoding skill ("sounding out" of unknown/familiar words), halting/dysfluent reading, behavior problems, school avoidance
- *Late elementary school age:* poor academic achievement, poor reading comprehension, slow reading ability, inability to complete work in allotted time, poor social skills, behavior problems
- *Middle school:* school failure, behavior problems, mood disorders
- ADHD type behaviors in ≥25% w/reading disability
- Comorbid depression, oppositional defiant disorder/conduct disorder may cloud picture
- No specific features on physical/neurologic examination diagnostic, although evidence of underlying disorders should be sought (eg, NF1, fetal alcohol syndrome)

LABORATORY FEATURES, COGNITIVE AND ACADEMIC TESTING

- Neuroimaging, EEG, other laboratory procedures not useful in routine evaluation
- Basic hearing/vision screening essential
- School work, report cards, previous testing may give clues to reading/language disorders
- Thorough family Hx (poor reading, special education, tutoring, school failure) essential
- Cognitive (IQ) testing by psychologist experienced in evaluating children necessary to identify overall cognitive potential, deficits in phonologic awareness/analysis, areas of cognitive strengths/weaknesses associated w/reading disorders
- *Educational achievement testing:* identify deficits in reading achievement when compared w/cognitive performance predicted by IQ; suggest strategies for academic intervention

DIFFERENTIAL DIAGNOSIS

- Developmental language disorders
- Mental retardation
- Seizure disorder, particularly absence spells
- Visual/auditory deficits
- Chronic illness/excessive school absence may cause school failure
- *Psychiatric disorders:* mood disorders, oppositional defiant, conduct/attachment disorders, anxiety
- Attention deficit hyperactivity disorder, particularly inattentive-distractible type

TREATMENT

- *Treatment goals:* improvement in learning, treatment of comorbidities, prevention of adverse mental health outcomes, prevention of school dropout
- Standard educational Tx. Interventions must be individualized based on Dx, psychoeducational testing, comorbidities, other child/family needs
- Earlier interventions emphasize remediation, later interventions emphasize accommodation for deficits
- Remediations include individualized, systematic, structured curricula focusing on identified deficits
- Accommodations may include classroom aide, individualized/small group teaching, taped books/reading material, study partners, outside tutoring (esp in summer), adapted testing procedures include oral/untimed examinations
- Individual/family counseling to address issues of self-esteem, appropriate social skills, behavior management, improved parent-child relationships
- Nonacademic activities that enhance individual skills/interests should be encouraged
- Pharmacologic management of ADHD/psychiatric comorbidity may improve classroom performance
- Periodic reevaluations may be needed q2–3 ys to update the educational program

COMPLICATIONS AND PROGNOSIS

- Most children achieve functional literacy
- May have less economic, social, psychological success as adults
- Comorbid conditions likely to worsen long-term prognosis
- School dropout lessens likelihood of successful employment as adult

PREVENTION

- Screen for language development in preschool years/school programs at every school exam
- Recognize that problems in areas of language development, behavior, early school performance lead to early Dx/intervention
- Notify school of suspected reading disability so timely diagnostic/educational services can be provided
- Reading disability must be treated <9 yrs of age; children respond poorly to interventions after that

WHEN TO REFER

- Refer as soon as reading disability suspected, not after child failing
- Complete diagnostic evaluation requires psychoeducational testing by experienced child psychologist/educational specialist
- Evaluation/treatment of severe comorbid mental illness/behavioral problems may require referral
- Refer to community resources (eg, The Learning Disability Association of America) for information, parental support, advocacy, legal assistance

BACKGROUND

- Refers to pain associated w/menses
- 1° dysmenorrhea 75–90% of women who have menses
- 1° dysmenorrhea not associated w/any abnormality of genital tract, in contrast to 2° dysmenorrhea/chronic pelvic pain
- 1° dysmenorrhea results from ovulatory menstrual cycles; pain occurs when secretory endometrium breaks down releasing prostaglandins, which increase nerve sensitivity/intensity of uterine contractions while decreasing uterine blood flow

CLINICAL MANIFESTATIONS

- *1° dysmenorrhea:*
  – onset within 2 yrs onset of menarche
  – pain crampy/colicky, localized to lower abdomen/supra pubic area; may radiate to lower back/inner thighs
  – pain begins hrs before onset of menses, lasts 1–3 d
  – pelvic examination normal
- *2° dysmenorrhea* (menstrual pain associated w/physical abnormality):
  – pain begins days prior to onset of menses
  – pelvic/rectal examination may reveal abnormal bulges, suggesting obstruction
- *Chronic pelvic pain:*
  – suspect if onset occurs ≥2 yrs after menarche
  – pain not clearly associated w/menses

DIFFERENTIAL DIAGNOSIS

- Gynecologic disorders:
  – pregnancy (intrauterine or ectopic)
  – endometriosis
  – ovarian cysts
  – ovulation (Mittelschmerz)
  – torsion of ovary/paraovarian structure
  – pelvic inflammatory disease
  – pelvic adhesions
- Gastrointestinal tract disorders:
  – constipation
  – irritable bowel syndrome
  – appendicitis
  – mesentric adenitis
  – gastroenteritis
  – gallbladder disease
  – lactose intolerance
  – pancreatitis
  – hernia
- Urinary tract disorders:
  – cystitis
  – pyelonephritis
  – renal calculi
- Other:
  – orthopedic problems (lordosis, scoliosis)
  – myofascial pain
  – sexual/physical abuse
  – psychiatric illness/stress

APPROACH

- Hx should include relationship of pain to onset, menses, elucidation of menarche, urinary tract/bowel symptoms, date of last menstrual period, extent of interference w/school/daily activities, sexual Hx for risk of pelvic inflammatory disease/sexually transmitted disease, social Hx/Hx of abuse
- Physical exam includes abdominal exam w/rectal palpation of cervix/ovaries, inspection of genitalia, where possible, pelvic exam
- Laboratory studies performed if chronic pain present/if dysmenorrhea persists after treatment
- Beta-HCG, urinalysis, cervix culture, pelvic ultrasound may be appropriate

TREATMENT

- NSAIDs effective in 75%; approved drugs include:

Drug	Initial dose (mg)	Subsequent dose (mg)
Ibuprofen	—	400 q4–6h
Naproxen	500	250 q6–8h
Naproxen sodium	550	275 q6–8h
Mefenamic acid	500	250 q6h
Ketoprofen	—	50 q6–8h

- If pain control not achieved next line Tx oral contraceptive medication; combination low-dose (<50 mcg) ethinyl estradiol/norgestimate or desogestrel recommended to reduce androgenic side effects; 50% have pain relief within 3 cycles/90% by 6 cycles

WHEN TO REFER

- 1° dysmenorrhea physiologic/should respond to NSAIDs/oral contraceptives
- If pain persists beyond 3 cycles oral contraceptives/if abnormal bulge suggesting Müllerian structural malformation, pts should be referred

BACKGROUND

• Supraventricular tachycardia (SVT), also known as paroxysmal atrial tachycardia (PAT) or paroxysmal supraventricular tachycardia (PSVT)
• Most common symptomatic dysrhythmia in childhood
• Defined as abnormal tachycardia arising above ventricles in either atria or within atrioventricular node
• Occurs in 1/1,700 children and frequently associated w/ congenital heart disease, cardiomyopathy, myocarditis, CHF
• Usually begins in early infancy w/ 80% recurrence rate. Recurrences ↓ in frequency over first year of life; ~ one-third have late recurrences
• *Mortality: 0–1%*

CLINICAL MANIFESTATIONS

	Symptoms	Heart Rate (HR)
Infants	pale, mottled, irritable, CHF	240–300 bpm
Children	dizziness, chest pain, palpitations	200–240 bpm (child) 150–180 bpm (teenager)

• Abnormally fast HR, out of proportion to physical activity (eg, 240 bpm during exercise, 150 bpm during sleep)
• Poorly tolerated when associated w/ accompanying congenital heart disease, cardiomyopathy, myocarditis, CHF

ELECTROCARDIOGRAPHY

• Rhythm extremely regular w/ very little beat-to-beat variation
• P waves usually absent or difficult to see as they may be superimposed on QRS or T wave
• QRS wave usually same as sinus rhythm or occasionally wide and bizarre (SVT w/ aberrant conduction) in which case very difficult to distinguish from ventricular tachycardia

DIFFERENTIAL DIAGNOSIS

• Sinus tachycardia
• Ventricular tachycardia

TREATMENT

• Vagal maneuvers:
  – diving reflex: icebag over bridge of nose in neonates and infants or facial immersion in ice water in older children
  – valsalva maneuver in older, cooperative children
• Antiarrhythmic medications:
  – acute:
    ◦ adenosine, 50–250 mcg/kg rapid IV bolus (may repeat q3min, $T_{1/2}$: 9 sec)
  – chronic:
    ◦ digoxin, 8–12 mcg/kg/d (1–2 div doses)
    ◦ propranolol, 1–4 mg/kg/d (3–4 div doses)
    ◦ flecainide, 115–230 mg/m²/d (2–3 div doses)
    ◦ sotalol, 100–220 mg/m²/d (2–3 div doses)
    ◦ amiodarone, 5 mg/kg/d (double dose load × 1 wk)
• Direct current (DC) cardioversion:
  – 0.5–2 synchronized joules/kg (should be used immediately when pt presents in cardiovascular collapse)

COMPLICATIONS

• CHF and cardiovascular collapse if left untreated
• May deteriorate and convert to ventricular tachycardia and/or ventricular fibrillation
• Sudden death in pts w/ Wolff-Parkinson-White syndrome

WHEN TO REFER

• Most pts managed acutely w/o referral
• Correct Dx should be confirmed before starting chronic antiarrhythmic medication
• If medications other than digoxin and/or beta blockade needed
• Wolff-Parkinson-White syndrome
• Wide QRS tachycardia

BACKGROUND

- Nonpolio human enterovirus
- >30 serotypes (Echovirus 1–9, 11–27, 29–33)
- Peak incidence summer, fall in US; less seasonal variation in tropics
- Children more susceptible to both infection, disease
- ↑ frequency of infection in lower socioeconomic groups, tropical climates
- Incubation period ~3–6 d
- Transmission via fecal-oral or respiratory secretions, also via contaminated food/water
- Perinatal transmission may occur from infected mother

CLINICAL MANIFESTATIONS

- Clinical sequelae depend on virus type, age, immune status of individual
- Infection often asymptomatic
- Neonatal sequelae may include fever, rash (macular, maculopapular, rarely petechial), occasionally sepsislike syndrome, hepatitis, myocarditis, pneumonitis, and/or CNS disease
- Symptomatic disease in children may include fever, malaise, rash, conjunctivitis, and/or upper respiratory symptoms; pneumonitis, diarrhea reported
- CNS sequelae include meningitis, encephalitis, transient paralysis, ataxia, or Guillain-Barré syndrome
- Myocarditis, pericarditis, hepatitis rare sequelae

LABORATORY FEATURES

- CSF in echovirus meningitis: moderate pleocytosis w/predominance of lymphocytes (occasionally neutrophils), protein normal/slightly ↑, glucose normal/slightly ↓
- Viral culture: highest yield from stool or respiratory secretions; dependent on clinical presentation, conjunctiva, CSF, blood, other tissues/fluids may yield virus
- Virus isolated from respiratory secretions or stool provides strong evidence but not proof of disease etiology
- Enterovirus PCR more sensitive than virus culture in CSF, respiratory secretions, urine; should consider for Dx CNS or other severe disease
- Type-specific antibody: available for use in research, epidemiologic studies, not for routine Dx echovirus infections

DIFFERENTIAL DIAGNOSIS

- Dependent on clinical presentation, entities include other enteroviruses, adenovirus, EBV, HSV, mycoplasma, rickettsial agents, *Streptococcus pyogenes,* Kawasaki disease, other pathogens
- Neonatal disease may mimic sepsis, bacterial meningitis

TREATMENT

- Supportive Tx
- Pleconaril (ViroPharma, Inc.) an investigational agent w/efficacy against echoviruses; agent may be available (currently compassionate use protocols) for treatment of life-threatening infections
- IV immunoglobulin may be efficacious in severe enterovirus infections, esp in neonates, immunocompromised pts

COMPLICATIONS

- Most infections resolve w/no complications
- Perinatal echovirus infection may result in liver failure, mortality due to severe liver, cardiac, or CNS disease
- Chronic meningitis associated w/immunodeficiency

PREVENTION

- No vaccine available
- Good handwashing practices may reduce transmission

WHEN TO REFER

- Referral indicated for severe disease manifestations or when Dx uncertain
- Communication w/clinical virology laboratory suggested to ensure appropriate specimen collection, processing

ENCOPRESIS

LAURIE GLADER AND LEONARD RAPPAPORT

BACKGROUND

- Repeated, involuntary fecal soiling not due to medication, organic, anatomic causes, occurring in children ≥4 yrs of age
- Up to 3% general pediatric population affected
- Fecal retention/constipation in 80% of encopretics
- *M:F ratio:* 2.5:1–6:1
- *Frequency:* occasional–multiple times/d, most often in afternoon

ASSESSMENT

- History:
  – soiling details: duration/frequency, associated constipation, 1° vs. 2°, precipitating event, stool quality, child's awareness of soiling, stool-withholding behaviors
  – toilet training Hx/toileting routines
  – associated symptoms, ie, vomiting, abdominal pain/distention, failure to thrive
  – age of child at first stool
  – dietary habits
  – psychologic impact of encopresis, including reactions of family/school
- Physical should emphasize:
  – growth parameters
  – abdominal exam
  – lumbosacral/anal inspection
  – rectal digital inspection (may be omitted if abdominal radiography planned)
  – motor/sensory exam in lower extremities
  – psychological/behavioral assessment

DIAGNOSTIC FEATURES

- *Abdominal radiograph:* useful in assessing presence of retained stool, its extent, whether lower spine normal; useful if rectal exam negative for fecal retention
- *Urine culture:* obtained routinely in females to r/o urinary tract infection
- *Bloodwork:* rarely required. Consider thyroid function studies, electrolytes, calcium if indicated by Hx/physical
- *Anorectal manometry:* reserved for refractory cases; useful in evaluating for Hirschsprung disease, abnormalities of anal pressure/sensation
- *Rectal biopsy:* children with lifelong Hx severe constipation beginning at birth; reveals presence/absence of ganglion cells
- *Barium enema:* rarely useful except in evaluating children w/question of Hirschsprung/corrected anal atresia w/subsequent fecal soiling

DIFFERENTIAL DIAGNOSIS

- Functional constipation/stool retention (95%)
- Neurogenic constipation (Hirschsprung disease, pseudo obstruction, disorders of spinal cord, cerebral palsy, hypotonia)
- Anal lesions (fissures, anterior placement, stenosis/atresia)
- Endocrine/metabolic disorders (hypothyroidism, renal acidosis, diabetes insipidus, hypercalcemia)
- Constipation induced by medication
- Sexual abuse

TREATMENT

- *Education:*
  – involuntary problem, neither fault of parent or child
- *Pharmacotherapy:*
  – laxative disimpaction ("cleanout"):
    ○ significant soiling: 3 day cycle alternating commercial enema, rectal suppository, oral bowel stimulant for 4–5 cycles (12–15 d)

Day 1	sodium biphosphate/phosphate enema (Fleet*) q pm**
Day 2	Bisacodyl rectal suppository (Dulcolax*) bid
Day 3	Bisacodyl oral laxative (Dulcolax) q pm

*<40 lbs use pediatric size; >40 lbs use adult size
**First cycle, use two Fleet enemas

    ○ milder soiling: 2 day cycle alternating oral laxatives, lubricants for 7 cycles (14 d)

Day 1	Senna (Senekot) <50 lbs: 1/2–1 tsp syrup bid >50 lbs: 1–2 tsp syrup bid *or* 1/2–1 tsp granules bid *or* 1–2 tablets bid
Day 2	Mineral oil (cold, mixed w/food, eg, juice, yogurt, chocolate milk) 15 cc/yr of age div bid up to max 240 cc School-age children start w/30 cc bid

  – maintenance laxative regimen:
    ○ may include combination of oral lubricant w/or w/o stimulant
    ○ continue until child develops daily/qOd self-initiated stooling in toilet w/o soiling (several months to year)
    ○ wean slowly, over several wks minimum

- *Behavioral interventions:*
  – structured toileting regimen:
    ○ 2×/d 5–10 min sits after meals
  – treatment diary to record sits, successful bowel movements, soiling, medications
  – sticker chart for successful bowel movements, "extra stars" for accident-free days
  – dietary: abundant intake of fiber: several helpings daily of cereals, fruits, vegetables, other fiber-rich foods
  – fluid intake: 6 glass minimum in addition to daily milk
- *Physician follow-up:*
  – visit after initial cleanout to establish plan
  – regular review of treatment diary/positive reinforcement of child's achievements, initially qOwk, then monthly
  – if encopresis/enuresis coexist, treat encopresis first; if enuresis continues beyond first few mos Tx, evaluate as separate entity

COMPLICATIONS

- *Mineral oil:* avoid in children w/dysphagia/vomiting, those <1 yr of age because of danger of aspiration; anal seepage benign but common/undesirable side effect
- *Senna-based compounds:* associated w/stomach cramping; long-term use (6–12 mos) may make weaning difficult

OUTCOME

- 65% complete, long-lasting remission within 6 mos; 30% substantially improved
- Minor relapses common/often associated w/early laxative cessation; return to original induction plan may be necessary; behavioral modifications including regular toilet sitting of paramount importance for long-term success

WHEN TO REFER

- Continuation of soiling despite compliance w/treatment; referral for rectal manometry indicated
- Coexisting behavioral/psychological problems resistant to standard treatment should be referred for appropriate psychological counseling to be combined w/medical encopresis Tx

BACKGROUND

- 80% have underlying congenital heart disease, artificial valves, grafts, shunts
- Average age early adolescence w/subset found in premature neonates
- Most common pathogens *Staphylococcus aureus,* viridans streptococci
- Historically divided into subacute/acute
- *Subacute:* community acquired or postop; usually have underlying structural heart disease; most common pathogen viridans streptococci
- *Acute:* most often community acquired/may occur postop; most common pathogen *Staphylococcus aureus*
- Early postop (<60 d) usually Staphylococci/Gram stain negative bacilli. Late postop (60 d–1 yr) often viridans streptococci

CLINICAL MANIFESTATIONS

- *Subacute:* indolent course wks to mos, low-grade fever, vague symptomatic complaints, mild embolic phenomenon
- *Acute:* fulminant course, high fever, systemic toxicity, sepsis, major embolic events

LABORATORY EVALUATION

- *Blood culture:* pathogen 90% if not previously treated w/antibiotics; ideally 2–3 cultures obtained at least 1 hr apart if pt stable; repeat q24–48h until sterile for 2 consecutive cultures
- Pathogen susceptibility determined by minimal inhibitory concentration (MIC)/minimal bactericidal concentration (MBC) using tube dilution
- Echocardiography

DIFFERENTIAL DIAGNOSIS

- Bacterial sepsis w/o endocarditis, viremia

TREATMENT

- Medical (see table)
- Surgical for intractable heart failure/recurrent major embolic phenomenon. Consider for >1 wk persistent positive cultures despite appropriate Tx

COMPLICATIONS

- *Cardiac:* CHF, pericarditis, abscess, rupture of chordae
- *Extracardiac:* (20–40% of pts) 2° to septic embolic phenomenon
- *Bone marrow suppression:* (neutropenia) 2° to long-term use of penicillins

PREVENTION

- Repair underlying cardiac defect, reduce likelihood of significant bacteremia in pts at risk
- Use antibiotics in at-risk pts who undergo certain procedures (see chapter: Endocarditis: Prophylaxsis)

WHEN TO REFER

- Children w/suspected/confirmed endocarditis should be co-managed w/pediatric cardiologist

Antimicrobial therapy for infective endocarditis in children

Etiologic Agent	Primary Antibiotics	Duration (wks)	Alternative Antibiotic(s)
Unknown (start of therapy or culture negative)			
Community acquired or late postsurgery	Nafcillin[1]	4–6	Vancomycin[3]
	+ gentamicin[2]	1–2	+ gentamicin
Nosocomial or early (≤60 d) postsurgery	Vancomycin	4–6	Add rifamin[4] if poor or w/o clinical response
Streptococci			
Native value, MIC < 0.1 µg/ml	Penicillin[5]	4	Vancomycin
(Native value)	Penicillin[5]	2–4	+ gentamicin
	+ gentamicin	2	
Native value, MIC ≥ 0.1 µg/ml	Penicillin	4–6	Vancomycin
(includes enterococci)	+ gentamicin	4–6	+ gentamicin
Prosthetic value, graft, or surgical shunt	Penicillin	4–6	Vancomycin
	+ gentamicin	2–6	+ gentamicin
Staphylococci			
Methicillin-susceptible	Nafcillin	4–6	Vancomycin
	+ gentamicin	1–2	+ gentamicin
	± rifampin	2–4	± rifampin
Methicillin-resistant	Vancomycin	4–6	
	+ gentamicin	1–2	
	± rifampin	2–4	
Gram-Negative Bacilli	Use antimicrobial susceptibility patterns	6	
Fungi	Amphotericin B[6]	Minimum 40–50 mg/kg	
	± 5-fluorocytosline[7] or rifampin	total dose	

[1]Nafcillin 150–200 mg/kg/d (max: 12–20 g/d); oxacillin or methicillin may be substituted. [2]Gentamicin 5–7.5 mg/kg/d; tobramycin or amikacin (15–30 mg/kg/d) may be substituted. Must check serum levels. [3]Vancomycin 40–60 mg/kg/d (max: 2 g/d). Must check serum levels. [4]Rifampin 10–20 mg/kg/d in 2 doses PO or IV; use if slow clinical response or staphylococcal infection of a prosthetic valve. [5]Penicillin G 200,000–300,000 U/kg/d (max: 12–24 million U). [6]Amphotericin B 1 mg/kg/d. [7]Fluorocytosine 50–100 mg/kg/d divided q6h. Must check serum levels.

Cardiac Conditions Requiring Prophylaxis*

Endocarditis Prophylaxis Recommended

Prosthetic cardiac valves, including bioprosthetic and homograft valves

Previous bacterial endocarditis, even in the absence of heart disease

Most congenital cardiac malformations

Rheumatic and other acquired valvular dysfunction, even after valvular surgery

Hypertrophic cardiomyopathy

Mitral valve prolapse with valvular regurgitation

Endocarditis Prophylaxis Not Recommended

Isolated secundum atrial septal defect

Surgical repair without residua beyond 6 mos of secundum atrial septal defect, ventricular septal defect, or patent ductus arteriosus

Previous coronary artery bypass graft surgery

Mitral valve prolapse without valvular regurgitation†

Physiologic, functional, or innocent heart murmurs

Previous Kawasaki disease without valvular dysfunction

Cardiac pacemakers and implanted defibrillators

*This table lists selected conditions but is not meant to be all-inclusive.   †Individuals who have a mitral valve prolapse associated with thickening and/or redundancy of the valve leaflets may be at increased risk for bacterial endocarditis, particularly men who are 45 years of age of older.   *Source:* JAMA, Dec. 12, 1990, Vol. 264, No. 22, p. 2920.

Dental or Surgical Procedures*

Endocarditis Prophylaxis Recommended

Dental procedures known to induce gingival or mucosal bleeding, including professional cleaning

Tonsillectomy and/or adenoidectomy

Surgical operations that involve intestinal or respiratory mucosa

Bronchoscopy with a rigid bronchoscope

Sclerotherapy for esophageal varices

Esophageal dilatation

Gallbladder surgery

Cystoscopy

Urethral dilatation

Urethral catheterization if urinary tract infection is present†

Urinary tract surgery if urinary tract infection is present†

Prostatic surgery

Incision or drainage of infected tissue†

Vaginal hysterectomy

Vaginal delivery in the presence of infection†

Endocarditis Prophylaxis Not Recommended‡

Dental procedures not likely to induce gingival bleeding, such as simple adjustment of orthodontic appliances or fillings above the gun line

Injection of local intraoral anesthetic (except intraligamentary infections)

Shedding of primary teeth

Tympanostomy tube insertion

Endotracheal intubation

Bronchoscopy with a flexible bronchoscope, with or without biopsy

Cardiac catheterization

Endoscopy with or without gastrointestinal biopsy

Cesarean section

In the absence of infection for urethral catheterization, dilatation and curettage, uncomplicated vaginal delivery, therapeutic abortion, sterilization procedures, or insertion or removal of intrauterine devices

*This table lists selected procedures but is not meant to be all-inclusive.   †In addition to prophylactic regimen for genitourinary procedures, antibiotic therapy should be directed against the most likely bacteria pathogen.   ‡In patients who have prosthetic heart valves, a previous history of endocarditis, or surgically constructed systemic-pulmonary shunts or conduits, physicians may choose to administer prophylactic antibiotics even for low-risk procedures that involve the lower respiratory, genitourinary, or gastrointestinal tracts   *Source:* JAMA, Dec. 12, 1990, Vol. 264, No. 22, p. 2920.

Recommended Standard Prophylactic Regimenfor Dental, Oral, or Upper Respiratory Tract Procedures in Patients Who Are at Risk*

Drug	Dosing Regimen†
Standard Regimen	
Amoxicillin	3.0 g orally 1 h before procedure; then 1.5 g 6 h after initial dose
Amoxicillin/Penicillin-Allergic Patients	
Erythromycin	Erythromycin ethylsuccinate, 800 mg, or erythromycin stearate, 1.0 g orally 2 h before procedure; then half the dose 6 h after initial dose
or	
Clindamycin	300 mg orally 1 h before procedure and 150 mg 6 h after initial dose

*Includes those with prosthetic heart valves and other high-risk patients.   †Initial pediatric doses are as follows: amoxicillin, 50 mg/kg; erythromycin ethylsuccinate or erythromycin stearate, 20 mg/kg; and clindamycin, 10 mg/kg. Follow-up doses should be one half the initial dose. Total pediatric dose should not exceed total adult dose. The following weight ranges may also be used for the initial pediatric dose of amoxicillin: <15 kg, 750 mg; 15 to 30 kg, 1500 mg; and >30 kg, 3000 mg (full adult dose).   *Source:* JAMA, Dec. 12, 1990, Vol. 264, No. 22, p. 2920.

BACKGROUND

- *Three subtypes:* nocturnal only (nighttime), diurnal only (daytime), or both
- *1° diurnal enuresis:* persistent daytime wetting beyond 4 yrs of age
- *1° nocturnal enuresis:* persistent nighttime wetting beyond 6 yrs of age
- *2° enuresis:* daytime or nighttime wetting following min. 6 mo period of continence
- Incidence varies by age and sex:

Age	Nocturnal†	Diurnal‡
5 yrs	15–20%	5–8%
10 yrs	3–5%	1–2%
15 yrs	1%	<1%

†More common in boys; ‡more common in girls.

- <3% of cases have organic etiology
- Nocturnal enuresis accounts for ~85% of all cases
- *Genetic predisposition:* incidence of neither parent enuretic = 15%, if one parent enuretic = 44%, if both parents enuretic = 77%
- *Multifactorial etiology for nonorganic enuresis:* maturational delay, arousal defect, small functional bladder capacity, antidiuretic hormone deficiency

CLINICAL MANIFESTATIONS

- Generally normal physical examination
- *Detailed voiding Hx:* number of voids per day, daytime wetting (temporal pattern, antecedents), number of wet nights per week, signs of urgency, number of bowel movements per week, history of constipation, fecal soiling, or UTI; if necessary implement 2 wk voiding diary to obtain more complete Hx
- Psychosocial Hx to evaluate parents' attitudes, social, emotional consequences of enuresis, treatment motivation
- Signs of bladder instability or small bladder capacity:
  - daytime frequency, urgency
  - intermittent/weak stream
  - infrequent voiding
  - wetting every night
- Does not awaken spontaneously; difficult to arouse from sleep

LABORATORY FEATURES

- U/A screening in all cases
- Urine culture, sensitivity if UTI suspected
- *Persistent daytime wetting:* renal/bladder ultrasound, voiding cystourethrogram if urethral obstruction/neurogenic bladder suspected
- Urodynamic study to characterize dysfunctional voiding pattern in children w/abnormal imaging studies or who fail to respond to conventional Tx
- Functional bladder capacity measurement (normal capacity in oz is child's age plus 2); parents measure three times at home or performed in office after child drinks 12 oz

DIFFERENTIAL DIAGNOSIS

- UTI
- Constipation
- Diabetes mellitus/insipidus
- Neurogenic bladder
- Urethral obstruction
- Spinal cord abnormality
- Ectopic ureter

TREATMENT

- *No treatment:* generally indicated for children <5 yrs w/no UTI/abnormal physical findings
- Nocturnal enuresis:
  - enuresis alarms: teaches child to awaken to sensation of full bladder; highest cure rate (70%) of available Tx; relapse rate of 30%; however, most respond to second application; requires motivated child (usually at least 7 yrs of age), parents; alarm must be used 2–3 mos; can be used concurrently w/medication in refractory cases, particularly older children; relatively inexpensive
  - desmopressin: synthetic analogue of vasopressin that reduces urine production by ↑ water retention, urine concentration; administered intranasally via spray pump (delivers 10 mcg/spray); starting dosage for all ages 20 mcg hs (2 sprays); increase by 10 mcg/week to max. 40 mcg; avoid excessive fluids to prevent hyponatremia; also available in tablet form; effective in

12–65% of children; relapse rate as high as 95% when discontinued; expensive
  - imipramine: anticholinergic effect that increases bladder capacity and noradrenergic effect that reduces bladder excitability; starting dosage: 6–7 yrs: 10–25 mg hs; 8–12 yrs: 25–50 mg hs; >12 yrs: 50–75 mg hs; overdose can be fatal, advise of need for strict dosage adherence, keep safe from children; effective in 10–60% of children; relapse rate of 90% when discontinued; inexpensive
- Diurnal enuresis (uncomplicated):
  - voiding schedule q2h; positive reinforcement program to increase cooperation if needed
  - exercises to strengthen pelvic floor muscles; augment w/biofeedback training where available; appropriate for children ≥7 yrs
  - oxybutynin: anticholinergic, antispasmodic effect that reduces uninhibited bladder contractions; dosage: 6–12 yrs: 5 mg, bid–tid; side effects include dry mouth, flushing, drowsiness, constipation
  - functional bladder capacity stretching, double voiding technique, selective fluid restriction, postural training can be considered in combination with above, depending on wetting pattern

COMPLICATIONS

- Potential consequences of enuresis include parent-child conflict, behavior problems, low self-esteem; social environment should be supportive, facilitate child's taking responsibility for bladder control w/o resorting to punitive methods

WHEN TO REFER

- Referral indicated when Dx in doubt or organic etiology suspected
- Failure to respond to conventional Tx

EPIDIDYMITIS AND ORCHITIS

JOHN W. BROCK III, AND SAM S. CHANG

BACKGROUND

- *Definition:* inflammatory process involving epididymis/testicle; if involving both called epididymo-orchitis
- Rarely occurs before puberty; if occurs, evaluate genitourinary system to r/o any congenital anomalies (frequently found)
- Essential to determine if pt sexually active; if yes, need to evaluate for STDs
- Difficult to distinguish from torsion
- *Causes/predisposing conditions:* UTIs, chemical irritation, viral illnesses, autoimmune diseases, vasculitides

CLINICAL MANIFESTATIONS

- Usually painful; gradual onset of pain
- May have irritative voiding symptoms such as dysuria, frequency, urgency
- *Differential Dx:* be cognizant of testicular torsion: w/ epididymitis more likely to have fever, irritative voiding symptoms, less likely to have nausea, vomiting; physical exam often similar between the two processes

LABORATORY FINDINGS

- Usually yield little information/on occasion helpful; UA normal in majority of cases
- Urine cultures oftentimes negative in these cases
- If UA suspicious for UTI, Dx epididymitis/orchitis becomes more likely

TREATMENT

- ↓ activity, elevation of scrotum, avoidance of any scrotal trauma, bed rest
- *Antibiotics:* should be effective for urinary pathogens as well as STD pathogens if STD likely
- NSAIDs
- *Key point:* always keep possible Dx torsion in mind; in general, any male < late teens w/ acute scrotal pain/swelling should be presumed to have torsion until proven otherwise/should be referred to urologist immediately

BACKGROUND

- *Epiglottitis/supraglottitis:* bacterial infection of supraglottic area, esp epiglottis, but also arytenoids, aryepiglottic areas
- *Usual cause:* H. influenzae type b, presumably from primary bacteremia
- Significant ↓ incidence due to *H. influenzae* type b immunization
- Other bacterial causes include *S. pneumoniae/S. pyogenes*
- Clinical Dx must be made quickly/calmly; confirmed by direct visualization of epiglottis at bronchoscopy
- *Peak incidence:* 2–6 yrs of age

CLINICAL MANIFESTATIONS

- Prodrome uncommon
- Toxic appearance, rapid onset
- 6–12 hrs fever, irritability, dysphonia, dysphagia
- Pt typically sits forward/drools in "sniffing dog" position w/cautious breathing
- Abrupt onset of inspiratory stridor/hoarseness; barky crouplike cough/aphonia usually *not* present

LABORATORY FEATURES

- *WBC count/differential:* moderate leukocytosis w/left shift
  - microbiology:
    ○ *H. influenzae* type b isolated from blood culture
    ○ *H. influenzae* type b/other bacteria isolated on Gram stain/culture of epiglottis obtained during initial intubation
  - radiographs: should *not* be obtained w/initial evaluation; when radiographs obtained after intubation, an underaerated chest radiograph w/possible cardiomegaly or evidence of pneumonia seen in up to 25%. Lateral neck radiographs show swollen epiglottitis (thumb sign)/distended hypopharynx
  - bronchoscopy: erythematous, edematous supraglottic structures seen; diagnostic of epiglottitis

DIFFERENTIAL DIAGNOSIS

- Viral laryngotracheitis (croup syndrome)
- Bacterial tracheitis
- Foreign body aspiration
- Retropharyngeal abscess, peritonsillar abscess, lingual tonsillitis
- Angioneurotic edema (allergic laryngeal edema)
- Diphtheria

TREATMENT

- Maintenance of adequate airway primary concern/goal of management; minimal stimulation/agitation while arranging evaluation
- When Dx suspected, transported to OR by personnel competent to provide artificial airway if pt develops acute respiratory failure; airway should then be directly visualized, uncuffed, endotracheal tube inserted
- >90% require artificial airway (mean intubation period: 2 d)
- Once airway established, blood/epiglottis cultures obtained
- *IV antibiotics:* third-generation cephalosporin (eg, ceftriaxone, 50–75 mg/kg/d) should be initiated after appropriate cultures
- Most improve after 12–48 hrs; can be extubated during this time if clinical course remains stable; total duration of antibiotics 7–10 d/does not have to be IV if clinical situation stable

PROPHYLAXIS

- Pt should receive rifampin 20 mg/kg/d in one dose (max 600 mg/d) ×4d before discharge to prevent reintroduction of *H. influenzae* type b into household
- Household contacts <4 yrs of age receive rifampin prophylaxis at same dose/schedule

COMPLICATIONS

- Respiratory failure if airway not obtained/maintained during initial presentation
- Small percentage develop pulmonary edema of unknown mechanism
- Rare to have airway sequelae after epiglottitis
- Rare complications include meningitis, cervical adenitis, otitis media, pneumonia, arthritis, pericarditis, epiglottic abscess

WHEN TO REFER

- If epiglottitis suspected, arrange expedient transport to OR for direct visualization of epiglottis by otolaryngologist, anesthesiologist, or others competent to obtain an airway

EPIPHORA (TEARING)

DAVID EDWARD E. HOLCK

BACKGROUND

- Categorized as congenital or acquired
- Congenital nasolacrimal duct obstruction most frequently due to blockage at nasolacrimal duct opening into nose (valve of Hasner)
- 2–4% term infants have symptomatic nasolacrimal duct obstructions after birth
- ~one-third bilateral
- In 80–90% of pts, obstruction spontaneously resolves in first few months of life
- After 12 mos of age spontaneous resolution of obstruction becomes much less likely
- Acquired nasolacrimal obstruction most frequently has blockage in bony nasolacrimal duct; generally do not improve spontaneously

CLINICAL MANIFESTATIONS

- Tearing (may be absent during first few weeks of life; may be intermittent)
- Mucopurulent discharge, crusting on eyelashes
- Lacrimal sac mass (dacryocele, mucocele, amniotocele, tumor)
- Reflux of mucoid or mucopurulent discharge from punctum upon compression of lacrimal sac (dacryocystitis)
- Eyelid swelling and redness
- Prolonged dye disappearance (persistence of drop of 2% fluorescein solution placed in inferior eyelid cul-de-sac after several minutes)

LABORATORY FEATURES

- Generally clinical Dx, unless 2° etiology present
- Ancillary tests include imaging if CNS, orbital, nasal pathology suspected
- Laboratory evaluation for infectious process (CBC, conjunctival, lacrimal sac, and/or blood cultures), CT scan esp if preseptal or associated orbital cellulitis observed

DIFFERENTIAL DIAGNOSIS

- Nasolacrimal duct obstruction at valve of Hasner
- Congenital atresia of puncta, canalicular system, lacrimal fistula
- Lacrimal sac mass, obstruction (mucocele, amniotocele), inflammation, infection (dacryocystitis)
- 2° epiphora:
  – corneal abnormality (abrasion, foreign body, recurrent erosion, infection)
  – uveitis
  – eyelash abnormality (trichiasis, entropion, ectropion, cyst, foreign body)
  – conjunctival abnormality (laceration, foreign body, tear abnormality, dry eye syndrome, conjunctivitis)
  – congenital glaucoma

TREATMENT

- Treat any 2° cause of tearing if present
- Treat active infection w/ topical and oral antibiotics
- For congenital nasolacrimal duct obstruction that does not resolve spontaneously after few months of observation, digital massage of lacrimal sac 2–4 ×/d (important to teach parents correct method to massage sac posterior to anterior lacrimal crest along inner corner of eye!)
- Warm compresses and topical ophthalmic antibiotic ointment may be helpful for mucopurulent discharge and lid hygiene
- If still no improvement by 12 mos of age, refer for probing of nasolacrimal system w/ or w/o infracturing the inferior turbinate to enlarge distal opening
- Some ophthalmologists routinely probe at 6–12 mos, as delaying probing beyond 12 mos associated w/ decreased success rate
- Earlier probing indicated for acute dacryocystitis, chronic mucopurulent discharge, or inability of pt to follow up
- If probing ineffective, can be repeated alone or w/ silicone stent intubation of nasolacrimal system (some ophthalmologists recommend silicone intubation if pt >18–24 mos old at first intervention)
- Dacryocystorhinostomy rarely indicated in infants w/ congenital obstruction. In acquired nasolacrimal duct obstruction, dacryocystorhinostomy (surgical drainage bypass surgery) may be necessary
- For acquired nasolacrimal duct obstruction, treat infection w/ topical and oral antibiotics and refer for definitive care—often surgical

COMPLICATIONS

- *Of no treatment:* permanent obstruction of nasolacrimal duct requiring dacryocystorhinostomy, progression of local infection to periorbital or orbital cellulitis
- *Of surgery:* persistent epiphora, recurrent obstruction, infection, canalicular obstruction, canalicular slitting from silicone tubes

WHEN TO REFER

- As soon as possible if acute infection arises
- 6–12 mos if symptomatic epiphora persists despite adequate lacrimal sac massage

MARK J. MENDELSOHN

BACKGROUND

- Occurs commonly in children 2–10 yrs; 30%, one nosebleed by 5 yrs; 56%, 6–10 yrs
- Rare in infancy/infrequent after puberty
- Occurs most commonly in fall/winter when upper respiratory infections (URIs) most common/environmental humidity low
- Most often 2° to irritation/excoriation of anterior septum in Kiesselbach's plexus/Little's area

PATHOPHYSIOLOGY

- 90% nosebleeds anterior; 10% posterior
- Mucosa covering Kiesselbach's plexus thin/friable
- Usually 2° local trauma/inflammation (infection, allergies)

CLINICAL MANIFESTATIONS

- Usually occurs w/o warning
- *Anterior nosebleeds:* blood exits from anterior portion of nose
- *Posterior nosebleeds:* bleeding from nasopharynx, mouth, nose
  - usually heavier/more difficult to control
- Children w/bleeding disorders may have other features:
  - prolonged bleeding (>10 min)
  - multiple bruises/easily bruisability
  - family Hx prolonged bleeding/easy bruising
- Usually unilateral in children
- Can present w/melena/hematemesis if blood swallowed

HISTORY

- Nose picking
- Trauma
- Recent infection/allergies
- Dry conditions
- Medication use
- Length of bleeding
- Measures to stop bleeding
- Recurrent bleeding/bruising

PHYSICAL EXAMINATION

- Assess hemodynamic status
- Check for petechiae, purpura, lymphadenopathy, hepatosplenomegaly
- Observe for telangiectasias
- Look for foreign bodies, nasal polyps, intranasal masses

LABORATORY

- Rarely indicated
- Check Hct if significant blood loss evident
- If clinical setting suggests systemic disease/severe bleed consider CBC, platelet count, coagulation studies, cross match
- Imaging studies rarely indicated

DIFFERENTIAL DIAGNOSIS

- Local causes:
  - inflammatory:
    - allergy
    - infection
    - rhinitis sicca (dry mucosa becomes very friable)
    - rhinitis medicamentosus (2° to pseudoephedrine, cocaine abuse)
  - trauma:
    - nose picking
    - foreign body
    - nasal fracture
    - surgery (sinus procedures)
  - anatomic:
    - septal deviation
    - unilateral choanal atresia
    - meningocele
  - inhalants:
    - tobacco
    - cocaine
    - cannabis
    - toxic fumes
  - tumors:
    - polyp
    - angiofibroma
    - rhabdomyosarcoma
- Bleeding disorders:
  - factor VIII, IX deficiency
  - Von Willebrand disease
  - Glanzmann thrombasthenia
  - idiopathic thrombocytopenic purpura/other causes of thrombocytopenia
- Blood vessel disorders:
  - hereditary hemorrhagic telangiectasia (Osler-Weber-Rendu)
  - vitamin C deficiency
- Drugs:
  - aspirin
  - warfarin, heparin
  - chloramphenicol
  - antineoplastic agents
- Neoplasms:
  - leukemia
  - lymphoma
- Idiopathic disorders:
  - Wegener granulomatosis
  - lethal midline granuloma
  - marrow or liver failure
  - malabsorption

TREATMENT

- No treatment: majority stop by time present to office
- Local care: application of petroleum jelly/antibiotic ointment inside involved nares 2×/d; discourage nose picking; direct pressure applied to nares 5–10 min, sit upright, lean forward slightly
- Active bleeding: if local measures ineffective, consider placing cotton pledget soaked in 0.25% Neo-Synephrine in anterior nares; topical anesthesia w/4% Xylocaine; cauterization w/silver nitrate stick; ointment or gel foam applied; anterior or posterior packing

COMPLICATIONS

- Small number require transfusion
- Sinusitis from anterior/posterior nasal packs

WHEN TO REFER

- Active bleeding unresponsive to above
- Embolization (rarely)

ERYTHEMA MULTIFORME

WILLIAM L. WESTON

BACKGROUND

- Very uncommon in childhood
- Infants have been described
- No prodrome
- 50%: preceding herpes labialis/rarely, herpes progenitalis by 3–14 d
- 30%, no history of HSV, yet HSV demonstrated in EM skin lesions

MANIFESTATIONS

- Abrupt onset of itching/burning skin lesions; almost all appear within 24 hrs
- *Primary lesion:* round, red papule fixed at same site ×7d or more
- ~ 20% of red papules evolve into "target" lesions: concentric zones of color change, w/central dusky/purple zone and outer red zone. Central zone may blister/crust after several days
- >100 lesions on upper arms, hands, neck, legs
- Discrete oral erosions in 50%, few in number (mildly symptomatic)
- Recurrences occur up to 6 ×/y
- Fever, lymphadenopathy, organomegaly absent

LABORATORY FEATURES

- *Skin biopsy:* keratinocyte necrosis/mononuclear leukocytes and T lymphocytes, perivascular infiltrate w/exocytosis into epidermis. Histology excludes lupus erythematosus/vasculitis compatible w/EM

Differences between erythema multiforme and urticaria

Urticaria	EM
Central zone is normal skin	Central zone damaged skin (dusky, bullous, crusted)
Lesions move within hours	Lesions "fixed" for at least 7 d
Associated w/swelling of hands and feet (angioedema)	No edema
New lesions appear daily	All lesions appear within first 72 hrs

DIFFERENTIAL DIAGNOSIS

- Large areas of urticaria often misdiagnosed as EM
- Polymorphous light eruption
- Systemic lupus erythematosus
- Urticarial vasculitis
- No trials support use of oral steroids; some have prolonged/overlapping episodes if given oral steroids

TREATMENT

- Symptomatic treatment often suffices; oral antihistamines ×3–4d reduce stinging/burning of skin; oral antacids for oral ulcers
- In children on oral steroids, advisable to discontinue steroids, despite likelihood of EM flare

COMPLICATIONS

- Usually heals w/o sequelae
- Some macular pigmentation may remain in previous skin sites

PREVENTION

- Prophylaxis w/acyclovir (10 mg/kg/d) may prevent frequent recurrences of EM

WHEN TO REFER

- Most children can be managed w/o referral
- If EM associated w/systemic Sx, has prolonged (>3 wk) course, refer to dermatologist

SIMON S. RABINOWITZ

BACKGROUND

- 50,000 caustic ingestions reported in 1997; peak incidence <3 yrs of age; adolescent ingestions usually suicide attempts
- ↓ alkali in cleansers/widespread use of childproof containers has ↓ esophageal strictures
- Difficult to predict significant esophageal burn/endoscopic evaluation needed
- Prevention of accidental ingestions part of routine anticipatory guidance: *keep all caustic materials out of reach of small children/never place in juice, soda containers*
- *Farm children at higher risk:* more caustic agents, more accessible containers

CLINICAL MANIFESTATIONS

- No specific symptoms predict which esophageal injury will require intervention
- *Oropharyngeal burns:* not sensitive/specific
- *Other symptoms:* emesis, dysphagia, drooling, abdominal/chest pain, refusal to drink, fever, respiratory compromise
- Tablets, granules worse than liquids
- Caustic agents:
  - alkali substances w/pH >7: minimal immediate symptoms lead to greater ingestions; examples: lye (sodium hydroxide) in Liquid Plumber, Drano, Clinitest tablets, oven cleaners; weaker sodium phosphate/carbonate found in dishwashing, laundry detergents, other cleaners
  - acidic substances w/pH <7: bitter taste limits accidental ingestion: eschar formation protects esophagus; examples: Mister Plumber (sulfuric acid), toilet bowl cleaners (hydrochloric acid/sodium bisulfate), metal cleaners (hydrofluoric acid), swimming pool cleaners (sodium hypochlorite), disk batteries
  - household bleach (dilute sodium hypochlorite)/ammonia used to clean windows rarely cause injury
  - others: hot Mexican peppers, medications: doxycycline, other antibiotics (tetracycline, clindamycin, ampicillin, erythromycin), potassium chloride, ferrous sulfate, aspirin, NSAIDs, ascorbic acid

LABORATORY FEATURES

- Plain films of chest/abdomen: only if esophageal perforation, mediastinitis, pneumonitis, peritonitis, suspected
- Early upper endoscopy (6–48h, usually 12–24 h) identifies children w/significant esophageal burn
- Endoscopy sometimes controversial; indications: multiple symptoms, oropharyngeal burns, ingestion of strong acid (pH <3)/alkali (pH >11.5), attempted suicide findings: 1° burn: mild erythema/edema of mucosa; 2° burn: exudate, erosions, ulceration to submucosa; 3° burn: deeper ulceration, can progress to full thickness injury, most ominous w/circumferential necrosis

DIFFERENTIAL DIAGNOSIS

- W/clear Hx caustic ingestion, no differential
- Rarely, disk battery ingestion presents w/respiratory symptoms

TREATMENT

- Send child to ER w/container that held caustic substance; if not original container, description of chemical composition of material ingested
- *Emesis can reinjure esophagus:* avoid
- *Observe in ER w/clear fluids, then discharge:* asymptomatic children w/o clinical findings/true caustic ingestions
- *Pts requiring endoscopy:* NPO w/IV fluids/antibiotics; intubate if clinically indicated
- 1°/no injury: as per asymptomatic pt
- 2°/3°: (possible perforation/stricture)
  - initial: NPO, on IV antibiotics, w/parenteral nutrition × 7–21 d; H$_2$ blockers to prevent acid reflux; steroids (prednisolone 2 mg/kg/d IV then 2.5 mg/kg/d prednisone po × 21 d followed by taper over 14–21 d) controversial; gastrostomy, strings, and/or stents sometimes placed for nutrition, future dilation, to maintain lumen
  - after 21 d: greatest risk for perforation has passed. Barium swallow; dilate identified stricture; if unsuccessful esophageal replacement; otherwise, as asymptomatic pt, taper steroids

COMPLICATIONS

- *Early:* respiratory problems, hematemesis, perforation, mediastinitis, peritonitis
- *Late:* esophageal stricture/replacement
- *Very late (40 yrs):* 1,000-fold ↑ risk squamous cell carcinoma; fistulas to trachea/alveoli

WHEN TO REFER

- Whenever Hx, physical exam, ingested material suggests injury

BACKGROUND

- Ewing sarcoma (ES) family of tumors include Ewing sarcoma of bone, soft tissue, peripheral primitive neuroectodermal tumor
- Second most common pediatric bone tumor after osteosarcoma
- ES occurs more commonly in second decade of life rather than first
- Vast majority of pts w/ES Caucasian (96%), 1.8% African American/2.2% other races
- In 90–95% of ES cases chromosomal analysis by RT-PCR demonstrates an (11;22) translocation/in 5–10% of cases (21;22) translocation; translocations create chimeric genes EWS-FLI1 and EWS-ERG, respectively, expressed as novel fusion transcripts
- Detection of these fusion genes valuable tool in molecular Dx of ES
- Studies indicate 50–70% of pts w/localized disease have long-term disease-free survival in contrast to 20–30% for pts who present w/metastatic disease

CLINICAL MANIFESTATIONS

- *Sites of presentation:* 53% in extremities/47% axial (pelvis > chest wall > spine/paravertebral region > head/neck)
- Vast majority present w/pain at tumor site
- *Also common:* palpable mass, pathologic fractures, fevers
- Sites of metastases include lung, bone, bone marrow; less commonly liver, lymph nodes, CNS

LABORATORY EVALUATION/ DIAGNOSTIC IMAGING

- Plain film (diaphyseal destruction) can help differentiate ES from osteosarcoma, which generally involves epiphysis
- MRI of 1° site
- CT of chest for pulmonary metastases
- Bone scan for bone metastases
- Bilateral bone marrow aspirates/biopsies to assess for bone marrow involvement
- LDH

DIFFERENTIAL DIAGNOSIS

If ES presents as bone tumor	If ES presents as soft tissue tumor
Osteomyelitis	Rhabdomyosarcoma
Eosinophilic granuloma	Undifferentiated sarcoma
Osteosarcoma	Non-Hodgkin lymphoma
1° lymphoma of bone	
Malignant fibrous histiocytoma	
Metastases from nonbone tumor (ie, neuroblastoma)	
Other benign bone tumors	

TREATMENT

- Tx for ES inherently multimodal approach; requires elimination of tumor at its presenting site achieved through local control measures such as surgery, radiation/sites of micrometastatic, metastatic disease accomplished w/chemotherapy; most important prognostic variable in ES: presence/absence of detectable metastatic disease at Dx; other factors associated w/worse outcome: tumor size of >100 cc, older age at Dx, pelvic 1°, poor response to chemotherapy, elevated LDH; recent studies also suggest structure of EWS-FLI1 fusion transcript also has prognostic significance
- *Surgery:* effective for local control; preferred over radiation Tx for dispensable bones such as fibula, scapula, rib, small lesions of hands/feet; also appropriate for younger pts in whom radiation Tx may cause major growth problems/functional deficits; limb-sparing surgery can be used; surgical debulking can be used in conjunction w/radiation Tx
- *Radiation:* used for tumors that cannot be resected w/o major morbidity (large central axis lesions, in pts whose tumors have been excised but w/inadequate margins); may also be used to treat pulmonary metastases
- *Chemotherapy:* adjunctive chemotherapy used in all cases of ES to prevent recurrence due to micrometastases; if treated solely w/local Tx, 80% of pts experience recurrence because of presence of micrometastases at Dx; chemotherapy can also be used preop to shrink large tumor/make surgery more feasible
- Drugs most often used include vincristine, actinomycin, cyclophosphamide, doxorubicin, ifosfamide, etoposide

WHEN TO REFER

- Once a mass is confirmed to be present, it is very important to refer pts to tertiary care center prior to biopsy. The biopsy should be done in a center where diagnostic techniques such as cytogenetics and electron microscopy are available.
- Additionally, a poorly placed biopsy may compromise the definitive surgical procedure. A team approach that includes the skills of the general pediatrician, pediatric surgeon, pediatric oncologist, radiation oncologist, rehabilitation specialists, social workers is imperative to ensure pts achieve optimal survival/quality of life. For progress to be made in treating these pts, Tx should be delivered in the context of a clinical protocol. All eligible children should be enrolled on well-designed clinical trials

BACKGROUND

- Abnormally low position of upper eyelid w/eye looking straight ahead
- Unilateral or bilateral
- Categorized by age of onset (congenital/acquired) and etiology (pseudoptosis, neurogenic, myogenic, aponeurotic, mechanical)
- Congenital ptosis generally noted at birth/remains stable
- Usually not inherited
- Approximately two-thirds unilateral
- Associated w/strabismus/anisometropia:
  – up to one-third have ocular motility disturbances (superior rectus muscle weakness)
  – up to 12% may anisometropia (differing refractive error between two eyes); may be severe enough to induce amblyopia
- Rarely severe enough to cause occlusional amblyopia
- Normal eyelid retractor replaced by fibrous connective tissue
- Often results in decrease in normal eyelid excursion/lag in downgaze
- Severity of fibrous replacement dictates severity of ptosis
- Seen in blepharophimosis syndrome (6% of cases of congenital ptosis):
  – autosomal dominant/sporadic; ptosis, epicanthus inversus, blepharophimosis (shortened horizontal eyelid dimensions)

CLINICAL MANIFESTATIONS/EXAMINATION

- *Range of ptosis:* mild–severe
- *Range of eyelid function:* good–poor
- Often present w/faint–absent eyelid crease
- Often shows eyelid lag in downgaze
- If bilateral, compensatory brow/chin elevated head position
- Need to r/o causes of 2° ptosis
- Need complete eye examination (visual acuity testing critical, pupillary evaluation, extraocular motility, anterior segment/fundus examination, evaluation of eye protective mechanisms—tear production, Bell phenomenon)

LABORATORY FEATURES

- Generally a clinical Dx, unless 2° ptosis suspected
- Ancillary tests include neuroimaging if CNS/orbital pathology suspected
- Laboratory evaluation if thought to be 2°

DIFFERENTIAL DIAGNOSIS

- Pseudoptosis:
  – strabismus: hypotropia
  – opposite eyelid retraction: thyroid eye disease
  – blepharospasm/hemifacial spasm
  – orbital volume loss
  – chronic ocular surface disease
  – uveitis
- Neurogenic ptosis:
  – third nerve palsy
  – Horner syndrome (ptosis, miosis, anhydrosis, w/or w/o lighter colored irides, esp congenital Horner)
  – misdirected third nerve fibers: Marcus Gunn Jaw-wink (unilateral ptosis that elevates intermittently w/mastication)
  – trauma
- Myogenic ptosis:
  – congenital (developmental dystrophy)
  – progressive external ophthalmoplegia, myotonic dystrophy, oculopharyngeal dystrophy
  – trauma
  – myasthenia gravis
  – toxic myopathy
  – acquired myopathy
- Aponeurotic ptosis: aponeurotic detachment, dehiscence, redundancy

- Mechanical ptosis:
  – eyelid/orbital tumors
  – eyelid edema, infection, hematoma
  – conjunctival scarring
  – eyelid skin diseases
  – brow ptosis, dermatochalasis

TREATMENT

- Treat any refractive error/amblyopia first
- Dictated by etiology/degree of ptosis
- If 2°, treat underlying cause
- Observe if vision unaffected/cosmetic deformity minor
- *Surgical treatment warranted for visually significant ptosis:* amblyopia (correct as soon as possible), superior visual field loss, cosmetically significant ptosis (correct before social interaction/school, etc)
- Surgery based on amount of levator muscle function, degree of ptosis, corneal protective mechanisms
- Some surgeons recommend bilateral surgery, even on unilateral ptosis, for better symmetry, cosmesis

COMPLICATIONS

- Amblyopia, psychosocial difficulties from cosmetic deformity
- Failure to diagnose 2° cause of ptosis
- *Of surgery:* under-/overcorrection of ptosis, eyelid contour deformities, poor eyelid crease formation, conjunctival prolapse, infection, scar formation, poor eyelid closure, lagophthalmos, exposure keratopathy, ectropion (out-turning of eyelid), entropion (in-turning of eyelid)

WHEN TO REFER

- As soon as possible if any question regarding visual acuity, amblyopia, strabismus
- If ptosis cosmetically significant, but not affecting visual development (refer prior to entering school, day care)

FEMORAL TORSION (ANTEVERSION/RETROVERSION)

ALAN R. GURD

BACKGROUND

- When femur in neutral position, w/knee facing forward, femoral neck directed medially and forward toward acetabulum of hip joint. Forward angle of neck 10–15° in adults and known as "anteversion angle." If angle >15°, then increased femoral anteversion; if <10%, femoral retroversion
- Most children born w/anteversion angle ≥35°

CLINICAL MANIFESTATIONS

- Children frequently present to pediatrician w/feet that point inward (in-toeing). In pts 3 yrs of age–skeletal maturity, usual cause internal (medial) femoral torsion. In most cases phenomenon of toeing in normal compensation of hip joint and femur to increased femoral neck anteversion
- For normal articulation between femoral head and acetabulum to occur, degree of anteversion must be decreased. This happens when femur internally rotates (femoral torsion). Clinically, these individuals not only toe in but also "knee in." Many have up to 90° of medial rotation of hip w/minimal external rotation when hip tested in full extension
- Conversely, children presenting "toeing out" usually have decreased anteversion angle (retroversion) and compensate by externally (laterally) rotating the leg (external femoral torsion)

DIFFERENTIAL DIAGNOSIS

- Medial femoral torsion may be result of abnormal muscular activity such as in cerebral palsy or in a bony deformity such as acetabular dysplasia. These must be clinically or radiologically excluded
- Toeing in at different ages may have different causes. Prior to walking cause usually in foot such as metatarsus adductus. Between 1–3 yrs of age most children have internal (medial) tibial torsion

Age	Toeing in
0–1 yr	Metatarsus adductus, hallux varus
1–3 yrs	Internal tibial torsion
age 3–maturity	Internal femoral torsion

TREATMENT

- Normally no treatment necessary; ~90% spontaneously correct, often by 9 yrs of age, and sometimes not until prepubertal growth spurt. Few pts, <1%, require corrective derotational femoral osteotomies, occasionally for appearance, but usually for patellar malalignment problems
- Wearing adjusted shoes not been shown to help

WHEN TO REFER

- Orthopedic opinion should be sought if child, after 10 yrs of age, continues to toe in, and examination has virtually no hip external rotation, or if persistent knee pain or patellar subluxation occurs

BACKGROUND

- Incidence (estimates):
  - alcohol: 3–5/1,000 live births have effects; fewer have syndrome
  - cocaine: up to 10–40% rate of fetal exposure; fewer have sequelae
  - heroin: 1–2/1,000 live births exposed, many w/symptoms
- Incidence varies w/regional variation in substance use

CLINICAL MANIFESTATIONS

- Exposure to each increases risk for prematurity, being small for gestational age, stillbirth, spontaneous abortion, low APGARs, behavioral state abnormalities (NBAS: Neonatal Behavioral Assessment Scale), neonatal abstinence syndrome, small head circumference
- Teratogenic:
  - alcohol: fetal alcohol syndrome (FAS) or alcohol-related birth defects (ARBD) w/anomalies of face (short palpebral fissures, smooth philtrum, thin upper lip), heart (VSD, others), CNS (including lower cell number), extremities (joint positioning, small distal phalanges)
  - cocaine: porencephaly, cerebral infarction, urogenital anomalies, intestinal atresias, limb-reduction defects
  - heroin: nonspecific
- Neurobehavioral:
  - alcohol: sleep disturbances, NBAS abnormalities, withdrawal rare
  - cocaine: seizures, cerebral hemorrhage, abnormal EEGs, hypertonicity, tremors, dystonia, NBAS abnormalities
  - heroin: neonatal abstinence syndrome w/hyperactivity, irritability, tremors, hypertonicity, exaggerated primitive reflexes, autonomic disturbances of tachypnea, diaphoresis, vomiting, and diarrhea, which may lead to weight loss; appears in first 72 hrs or 2–3 wks later

LABORATORY

- Toxicology screening:
  - techniques
    - blood: alcohol screen may be indicated if mother positive at delivery; otherwise low sensitivity
    - urine: alcohol, high false negatives due to hepatic metabolism; cocaine/heroin, metabolites presence reflects recent maternal use (1–7 d)
    - meconium: cocaine metabolites reflect fetal exposure at last 2 trimesters; heroin less sensitive than cocaine (positive in up to 67% exposed)
    - hair: cocaine and heroin metabolites reflect exposure in final trimester
  - who to screen: maternal history of poor/late prenatal care, unexplained preterm delivery, chemical dependency, previous drug-exposed infant, placental abruption, other risk-taking behavior; infant w/neurobehavioral or teratogenic sequelae
  - screen for all substances; high frequency of polydrug exposure
- Other:
  - based on clinical Sx (glucose for SGA, tremors; Hct for placental abruption)
  - monitor for maternal STDs

TREATMENT

- *No treatment;* indicated for asymptomatic exposed infants w/normal physical examination, neonatal course
- *Environmental modulation:* indicated for mild neurobehavioral changes; includes swaddling, cuddling, hands to midline, pacifier, reduced lighting/noise
- *Non-narcotic medication:* indicated for significant neurobehavioral changes of narcotic withdrawal; phenobarbital 5–8 mg/kg/d, tapered over 2 wks
- *Narcotic medication:* indicated for non-neurologic withdrawal symptoms (diarrhea, vomiting, tachypnea) affecting growth; paregoric 0.4% opium solution: 2 drops/kg/dose q4–6h or laudanum 10% solution: 2 drops/kg/dose q4–6h; both weaned over 4–6 d after infant asymptomatic
- *All medication titrated to avoid heavy sedation*
- *Maternal support/rehabilitation:* referral to chemical dependency treatment program based on assessment of level of addiction

COMPLICATIONS

- Neurologic:
  - alcohol: low IQ, hypotonia, poor coordination, ADHD
  - cocaine: mixed findings, visual motor deficits reported
  - heroin: mild cognitive, motor delays potentiated by environment
- Growth:
  - alcohol: infants w/FAS and some w/ARBD have marked postnatal deficiency
  - cocaine/heroin: occasional postnatal deficit
- Outcome highly influenced by environmental factors

WHEN TO REFER

- Child protective service involvement indicated in all cases (mandatory in some states)
- Subspecialty consultation for identified/suspected teratogenic effects
- Early intervention for infants demonstrating delays

BACKGROUND

- Neutrophils (or granulocytes) are phagocytic WBCs primarily responsible for containing and clearing invasive bacteria and fungi. Neutropenia defined as profound ↓ in number of circulating neutrophils, leaving pt vulnerable to infections. In children, neutropenia usually consequence of cytotoxic cancer chemotherapy, which causes ↓ in WBC count for few days–several weeks. Leukemia, aplastic anemia, or drug-induced dyscrasias may also cause neutropenia
- Critical reduction in neutrophil count to <500/mm³ identified as major risk factor for invasive bacterial infections. Duration of neutropenia also determines infection risk, w/ most fungal infections occurring after 10–14 d neutropenia. Bacterial infections cause >80% of infections associated w/ first fevers. Usually due to endogenous GI and skin flora that colonize pt. Fever may be only sign of severe infection in neutropenic pt. Prompt initiation of empirical broad-spectrum antibiotics essential for all neutropenic pts who develop fever. Empirical antibiotics given at onset of fever (instituted at least 24–48 hrs prior to availability of culture results)

CLINICAL MANIFESTATIONS

- Fever alone, even in absence of objective physical findings, may be only indication of underlying infection in granulocytopenic host. Sx inflammation may be lacking in absence of neutrophil responses: no pus formation to create abscesses, no pyuria associated w/ UTI and no infiltrate on chest x ray to signify pneumonia
- Fever itself may be absent, and localized pain or sudden hypotension or hypoxia may be presenting features of serious infection. Hypotension or presence of pulmonary infiltrate on chest x ray may suggest gram-negative bacteremia and/or pneumonia. Tenderness and mild erythema around catheter exit site or esophageal pain may indicate site of infection
- In most cases not possible to distinguish bacteremic pts from those w/ sterile blood cultures when they initially present w/ neutropenic fever
- Thorough Hx of febrile illness and physical examination may point to site of infection. Pay special attention to oropharynx (herpes simplex, thrush, or gingivitis), chest and abdominal examinations for localizing signs of infection, and to perianal region where mild tenderness and/or erythema may indicate deep soft tissue infection. Continued daily evaluations during course of fever and neutropenia critical to detect signs of evolving infectious complications

LABORATORY FEATURES

- Neutropenia defined by absolute neutrophil count (ANC) <500/mm³ or a count expected to fall below this level in next 48 hrs. ANC calculated by multiplying total WBC count by percentage of polymorphonuclear cells plus band forms. Fever may be defined as single temperature ≥38.3 or two temperatures ≥38.0 in 12 hr period. These criteria define which pts should receive empirical antibiotic Tx
- Prior to institution of antibiotics, send specimens of blood, urine, and any possible infected site for culture. In ~50–70% cases of febrile neutropenia, no microbiologic Dx made (cultures remain sterile). However, ~10–20% pts have bacteremia. Gram-positive bloodstream infections predominate, w/ coagulase-negative staphylococci being most common. Enteric bacteria such as *E. coli, Klebsiella,* and *Enterobacter* now most common gram-negatives causing bacteremia. *P. aeruginosa* a rare finding

TREATMENT

- Empirical antibiotic regimen must have broad spectrum against array of gram-positive and gram-negative bacteria. Potent activity against gram-negative bacteria (particularly against *Pseudomonoas aeruginosa*) considered mandatory due to rapidly lethal effects of gram-negative bacteremia during neutropenia. Combinations of extended-spectrum penicillins (e.g. piperacillin or ticarcillin) plus an aminoglycoside (e.g. gentamicin or amikacin) have traditionally been efficacious. Same efficacy can be achieved w/ antibiotic monotherapy such as ceftazidime, imipenem/cilastatin, and meropenem used alone or w/ aminoglycoside. Some centers employ ceftriaxone w/ aminoglycoside, both given on once-daily basis, for "low-risk" pts anticipated to have short duration of neutropenia (eg, <1 wk) and who have no medical comorbidity. Notably, vancomycin not necessary component in initial regimen, unless high incidence of life-threatening gram-positive infections exist in population seen at a particular center
- Modifications of initial regimen should be made according to microbiologic culture results as well as on basis of changes in physical exam. For example, if gram-positive catheter infection documented or if skin/soft tissue infection noted, vancomycin should be started
- Finding of herpes simplex in mouth or evolution of perirectal tenderness should prompt initiation of acyclovir or metronidazole, respectively

- Empirical Tx usually continued until ANC >500/mm³ or until course Tx completed for documented infection
- Persistent or recrudescent fever after 5–7 d broad-spectrum antibiotic Tx requires empirical addition of antifungal agent, usually daily amphotericin B, until counts recover

COMPLICATIONS

- Progressive or breakthrough bacterial infection, due to resistant organisms, and development of deep fungal infection, particularly due to *Aspergillus sp.*, are two complications of prolonged neutropenia (generally ≥7 d). Lung a common site for these severe infections
- Right lower quadrant abdominal pain suggests typhlitis, severe inflammatory bacterial disease of cecum, sometimes requiring emergent surgery
- Hepatosplenic candidiasis often causes persistent fever as counts recover
- Cytomegalovirus pneumonitis or gastroenteritis occur almost exclusively in allogeneic marrow transplant pts
- *Clostridium difficile*–associated diarrhea a common consequence of antibiotic Tx for fever and neutropenia. *C. difficile* infection often presents with fever, diarrhea, abdominal cramps

PREVENTION

- Prophylactic antibiotics, particularly fluoroquinolones (ciprofloxacin and norfloxacin) shown to decrease incidence of serious gram-negative infections when started before onset of neutropenia. Should be used very sparingly and reserved for pts undergoing intensive chemotherapy such as induction Tx for leukemia or bone marrow transplantation
- GM-CSF and G-CSF are cytokine growth factors that stimulate neutrophil precursor growth and differentiation. When started immediately after chemotherapy, they can shorten overall duration of neutropenia and decrease incidence of fever and infection during neutropenia. However, these expensive agents should only be used w/ intensive chemotherapy

WHEN TO REFER

- Children given chemotherapy for cancer should be under care of pediatric oncologist familiar w/ effects of cytotoxic Tx, specifically neutropenia and its consequences
- Those neutropenic due to underlying disease should also be under care of pediatric hematologist or oncologist
- In cases of prolonged neutropenia or severe infection, advice of infectious disease physician should be sought

FEVER WITHOUT A SOURCE (<2 MOS OF AGE)

CAROL A. McCARTHY AND KEITH R. POWELL

BACKGROUND

- Viral etiologies for fever most common; frequently seen viruses: influenza/respiratory syncytial virus (winter), enteroviruses (summer); other common viruses include rotavirus, herpes simplex, parainfluenza
- Bacterial process found in 5–10% of nontoxic-appearing infants evaluated for possible sepsis; common bacteria include *Streptococcus agalactiae, Streptococcus pneumoniae, Neisseria meningitidis, Hemophilus influenzae, Listeria monocytogenes, Escherichia coli, Enterococcus, Enterobacteriaceae*
- Numerous other possible pathogens (ie, *Treponema pallidum, Mycobacterium tuberculosis, Bordetella pertussis, Candida albicans*)
- Criteria have been developed to identify infants *unlikely* to have a serious bacterial infection

Rochester low-risk criteria for young, febrile infant

- Infant nontoxic appearing
- Infant has been previously healthy:
  – born at term (≥37 wks gestation)
  – no previous antimicrobial Tx
  – not treated for unexplained hyperbilirubinemia
  – no previous hospitalization
  – no chronic/underlying illness
- Infant has no evidence of skin, soft tissue, bone, joint, ear infection
- Infant has the following laboratory values:
  – WBC 5,000–15,000/mm^3
  – absolute band form count <1,500/mm^3
  – ≤10 WBC per HPF (×40) on microscopic examination of spun urine sediment
  – ≤5 WBC per HPF (×40) on microscopic examination of a stool (if diarrhea)

CLINICAL MANIFESTATIONS

- Initial assessment to determine need for immediate laboratory testing/treatment
- Complete Hx/physical examination important
- Rectal temperatures most accurate; temperature ≥38° C considered ↑
- Social Hx often helpful when considering disposition of infant; infants may be well appearing but still have serious bacterial infection

LABORATORY FEATURES

- Usual evaluation for possible sepsis includes CBC w/differential (CBC), UA, CSF evaluation, bacterial cultures of blood, urine, CSF
- In selected, well-appearing infants, initial laboratory evaluation may be limited to CBC, UA, bacterial cultures of blood/urine
- Chest roentgenogram recommended in infants w/respiratory symptoms
- For infants w/diarrhea, stool smear for WBC; if >5 WBC/HPF, stool for culture
- Cultures of selected sites as indicated (ie, bone, joint, skin)
- Viral studies may be useful; available testing includes rapid testing (RSV, influenza, rotavirus), viral culture, PCR (HSV, enterovirus)
- Bacterial antigen testing may be useful in infants who have been on recent antibiotics

TREATMENT

- Following young, febrile infants should be hospitalized:
  – all ill-appearing infants/infants who need Tx such as O$_2$, fluids
  – infants w/, at high risk for serious bacterial infection
  – when close follow-up questionable (ie, caregiver is unable to monitor infant closely, lack of transportation/telephone, no identified 1° care provider)
  – discharged infants should be seen again within 24 hrs/laboratories followed; caregiver must have easy access to physician if problems/questions arise
- Guidelines for use of antimicrobial agents:
  – complete testing (evaluation of blood, urine, CSF) if antimicrobials given
  – antimicrobials commonly used are ceftriaxone/cefotaxime; add ampicillin if *L. monocytogenes, Enterococcus* considerations
  – if pneumococcal meningitis suspected, cetriaxone plus vancomycin recommended pending susceptibility test results
  – antiviral Tx should be considered in certain settings (ie, acyclovir for suspected HSV, ribavirin for ill infants w/RSV)
  – close observation w/o antimicrobial Tx preferred for low-risk infants

COMPLICATIONS

- Close monitoring of all young, febrile infants essential
- Antimicrobial Tx should be discontinued if bacterial cultures no growth/bacterial process unlikely; most reported complications 2° to IV Tx

PREVENTION

- Parents of young infants should be counseled regarding limiting potential infectious exposures (ie, avoidance of individuals w/cold symptoms, fevers, vesicular skin lesions)

WHEN TO REFER

- Referral to infectious disease specialist should be considered if infant has unusual/severe infection, meningitis, HSV disease

BACKGROUND

• 5–20% febrile children <5 yrs of age do not have localizing signs
• Fever w/o localizing signs (FWLS) arbitrarily defined here as fever of relatively brief duration (<5–7 d). Fever that persists >7–10 d referred to as fever of unknown origin (FUO) and not discussed here
• FWLS most common in children 6–24 mos of age
• ~5% children w/ FWLS have occult bacteremia

CLINICAL MANIFESTATIONS

• *Hx:* duration and height of fever, ill contacts, day-care attendance, immunosuppression, appetite/activity levels
• *Physical examination:* height of fever, hydration status, toxic appearance, behavior (eg, alert, playful), absence of localizing signs of infection
• Hx, physical examination alone do not reliably differentiate children w/ occult bacteremia from those w/o
• Most cases FWLS resolve w/o identification of specific etiology
• Focal (eg, otitis media, pharyngitis) or nonfocal (eg, varicella, roseola) process may become apparent as cause of fever

INCIDENCE RATE OF OCCULT BACTEREMIA IN CHILDREN W/ FWLS

• No racial, geographic, socioeconomic predisposition to development of occult bacteremia
• Incidence rate increases as degree of fever increases:
  – 1% risk w/ temperature <38.9°C
  – 5% risk w/ temperature 38.9°–40.5°C
  – 12% risk w/ temperature >40.5°C

PATHOGENS ASSOCIATED W/ OCCULT BACTEREMIA

• *Streptococcus pneumoniae* is organism implicated most frequently in cases of occult bacteremia
• *Haemophilus influenzae* type b, *Neisseria meningitidis,* Salmonella other important causes of occult bacteremia
• After exposure to pathogen and colonization, host either eliminates pathogen w/o developing illness, becomes carrier, or develops local or systemic infection

LABORATORY FINDINGS

• Diagnostic laboratory studies should be considered in child 6–24 mos w/ FWLS and temperature >39.4°C (100°F)
• Bacteremia suspected in child w/ FWLS and WBC count >15,000/μL

• Bacteremia also suspected in child w/ toxic appearance or focal infection (eg, septic arthritis, facial cellulitis) commonly associated w/ bacteremia
• Lumbar puncture performed if any concern for meningitis exists, esp in young infants who often fail to manifest obvious meningeal signs
• UA, urine culture indicated in female infant w/ FWLS to exclude "occult" UTI
• Chest roentgenogram not indicated routinely for all children w/ FWLS, but considered for young infants and pts w/ high fever, signs of toxicity, or markedly ↑ WBC count

MANAGEMENT

• Expectant antibiotic Tx justified for child w/ FWLS, high fever, WBC count >15,000/μL
• Expectant antibiotic Tx also indicated for febrile children who appear seriously ill, those w/ underlying disease predisposing to serious bacterial infection (eg, immunodeficiency states, sickle-cell disease)
• Expectant antibiotic Tx directed against common bacterial pathogens, esp *S. pneumoniae* and *H. influenzae* type b
• Careful follow-up essential, and child reevaluated immediately if clinical condition deteriorates, or if blood culture yields pathogen

BACKGROUND

- *Etiologic agent:* human parvovirus B19 (small, nonenveloped, single-stranded DNA virus)
- B19 causes number of clinically distinct syndromes
- *Pathogenesis:* B19 infects and lyses erythroid precursor cells, leading to transient arrest of erythropoiesis. Clinically results in reticulocytopenia and ↓ serum Hgb
- Infection most common in school-age children (ages 5–15) but can occur at any age in susceptible individuals; 2° attack rate for susceptible household contacts ~50%
- Community and school outbreaks occur; asymptomatic infections common
- Transmission by close contact, presumably through respiratory secretions
- Period of infectivity varies among different clinical syndromes:
  - pts w/ erythema infectiosum (fifth disease) only infectious *before* rash appears; rash related to immunologic response
  - Pts w/ transient aplastic crisis infectious when they present

CLINICAL MANIFESTATIONS

- *Erythema infectiosum (EI; also called "fifth disease"):* benign rash illness of childhood and most common clinical manifestation of B19 infection. Mild prodromal phase of low-grade fever and nonspecific symptoms such as headache, URI symptoms, etc, followed by characteristic rash: begins as intense red facial flushing giving child a "slapped-cheek" appearance; spreads to trunk and extremities as more diffuse macular erythema. As rash progresses, central clearing occurs giving distinctive reticular or lacy character, esp on extremities. Rash may persist for >1 wk and may recur in response to various stimuli such as sunlight, exercise, warm bath
- *Transient aplastic crisis (TAC):* commonly associated w/ sickle-cell disease but can occur w/ B19 infection in any pt w/ chronic hemolysis. Pts present w/ fever, malaise, Sx profound anemia (pallor, tachycardia, etc). Rash rarely present
- *Arthropathy:* arthritis and arthralgias can occur as complication of fifth disease or may present as only clinical manifestation of B19 infection. More common in older adolescents and adults than in children. Joints most often affected: hands, wrists, knees, ankles. Joint symptoms self-limited and majority resolve within 2–4 wks
- *Chronic anemia:* persistent infection manifesting as chronic anemia can occur in pts w/ impaired humoral immunity from variety of causes such as cytotoxic chemotherapy, congenital immunodeficiency states, AIDS

LABORATORY FEATURES

- EI diagnosed primarily on clinical grounds by recognition of typical rash
- Routine laboratory studies in EI nonspecific
- Pts w/ TAC reticulocytopenic (often undetectable) and profoundly anemic w/ Hgb levels as low as 2–3 g/dL
- *Specific serology:* B19 IgM best marker of acute/recent infection. IgG seroconversion on paired sera also used to confirm recent infection
- Serologic tests not widely available and rarely necessary for Dx EI
- In immunocompromised pts, serologic Dx unreliable and methods to detect viral DNA (eg, polymerase chain reaction, DNA hybridization, etc) necessary for Dx
- Viral cultures not available

DIFFERENTIAL DIAGNOSIS

- *EI:* rubella, measles, enteroviral infections, drug reactions
- *Arthropathy w/ or w/o rash:* JRA, SLE, other connective tissue disorders, postviral syndromes

TREATMENT

- No Tx necessary for EI; symptomatic care, reassurance only
- Children w/ TAC usually require hospitalization for transfusion and supportive care until hematologic status stable
- IV immunoglobulin (IVIG) used successfully in immunocompromised children w/ chronic anemia from B19 infection (in addition to transfusion)

COMPLICATIONS

- *Most common complication of EI:* arthritis that may persist after rash resolves
- Rare reports of B19 as cause of thrombocytopenic purpura and aseptic meningitis after EI

PREVENTION

- Hand washing and control of respiratory secretions recommended in group settings and during outbreaks
- Exclusion of children w/ EI from school or day care not indicated; no longer infectious once rash appears

WHEN TO REFER

- EI, accompanying arthralgias managed w/o referral once Dx established
- Arthritis persisting after rash of EI has resolved may warrant referral for exclusion of other rheumatologic conditions
- Pts presenting w/ TAC may require referral for intensive care during transfusion if cardiovascular status unstable due to profound anemia
- Immunocompromised pts w/ chronic anemia likely require referral for bone marrow exam and specific viral studies prior to initiation of IVIG Tx

BACKGROUND

- Nematodes of superfamily Filaroides cause worldwide disease in tropical/subtropical regions between latitudes 45° N/25° S
- Most cases found in Africa, Asia, Pacific, northeastern part of South America

ONCHOCERCIASIS (RIVER BLINDNESS)

BACKGROUND

- *Onchocerca volvulus* causative agent; males measure 2–5 cm, females 30–70 cm
- Spread by flies of family Simuliidae
- Endemic in equatorial Africa, Central, South America, distribution parallels vector distribution
- Estimates of 20–40 million pts have disease
- Blindness most serious complication
- Fly feeds on tissues containing microfilaria; develop in thoracic muscles in 1 wk, migrate to mouth parts, into human skin on subsequent feeding

CLINICAL MANIFESTATIONS

- Pruritus common
- Exanthem frequently appear initially on legs, spreads to rest of body
- Rash subsides but itching persists, leading to chronic lichenification
- Hyper-, hypo- or depigmentation follows, along w/scars/skin atrophy
- Nodules containing microfilaria 3–35 mm, which may calcify (onchocercomata)
- Nodules mostly on scalp in Central America/upper parts of trunk, in pelvic areas and thighs in African patients
- Microfilaria may be found in eyes, leading to keratitis, retinal pigmentation, scarring, blindness; in endemic areas 5–10% may suffer blindness

DIAGNOSIS

- Dx clinically evident; must be differentiated from other causes of pruritus
- Examination of skin snips/biopsy material for microfilaria
- Nodules may be excised for study of adult worms/microfilaria
- ELISA/immunofluorescent test positive, 60–90%

TREATMENT

- Surgical removal of nodules
- Diethyl carbamazine kills microfilaria given as follows:
  - 1 mg/kg/d × first 3 d
  - 2 mg/kg/d next 4 d
  - 4 mg/kg/d × 2nd, 3rd wks
- Herxheimer reaction may occur; care should be taken if eye involvement for fear of producing blindness; prednisone, 40 mg/d may alleviate this reaction
- Suramin kills adult worm/seldom used because of side effects

LOIASIS

BACKGROUND

- Loa loa causative agent
- *Vector:* blood-sucking fly of genus Chrysops/transmits infection from person to person
- Larvae enter skin at puncture wound as fly is feeding; after 1 yr adult worms appear in skin/conjunctiva

CLINICAL MANIFESTATIONS

- May be symptomless/parasthesias may be felt by movement of worm
- In eye there may be irritation/worm may be seen crossing conjunctiva
- Swellings may appear w/movement of parasite usually lasts for few days/may be painful (Calabar/Cameroon swellings)

DIAGNOSIS

- Clinical picture/sighting of parasite diagnostic
- Eosinophilia/demonstrating microfilaria in daytime blood smear
- Immunofluorescent antibody, ELISA useful

TREATMENT

- Diethylcarbamazine used cautiously as in onchocerciasis
- Prednisone, 40 mg/d starting 1 d before treatment may ↓ untoward reactions

LYMPHATIC FILARIASIS

BACKGROUND

- *Wuchereria bancrofti, Brugia malayi, B. timori* causative agents
- Diseases produced by different genera noted above not distinguishable, although *W. bancrofti* more widespread
- Occur between latitudes 40° N/30° S
- Transmitted by various anthropophilic mosquitoes from person to person
- Larvae migrate to lymphatics, mature; females discharge microfilaria cyclically usually at night
- Antibody/cell-mediated immunity normal in uninfected individuals in endemic areas; infected show depressed immunity
- Adult worms lodged in lymphatics

CLINICAL MANIFESTATIONS

- Initially short febrile periods occur w/swelling in extremities/scrotum
- Headache, nausea, photophobia, muscle pain accompany initial symptoms
- Lymphangitis very common
- Orchitis/epididymitis may be painful
- Lymph node enlargement esp inguinal/femoral areas; abscesses may form
- Lymphatic obstruction/elephantiasis follows

DIAGNOSIS

- Hx lymphangitis in residents of endemic areas
- Demonstration of microfilaria in blood/lymph
- Indirect immunofluorescent/ELISA tests positive in high percentage

TREATMENT

- Diethylcarbamazine as in treatment of onchocerciasis/used until microfilaria disappear; not effective against adult worm

SUBUNGUAL HEMATOMA

- *Causes:* blow to finger by heavy object such as hammer
- *Treatment:* decompression w/ end of hot paper clip over center of damaged area of nail

CRUSHED NAIL INJURY

- *Causes:* nail crushed by object such as car door, house door, or flywheel of exercise bike
- Usually associated w/ partial fingertip amputation
- Treatment:
  - repair nail bed (matrix) w/ fine absorbable suture
  - replace nail for 3 wks as splint for remodeling of new nail
  - use ice bag, analgesics, antibiotics

FINGERTIP AMPUTATION

- *Causes:* usually associated w/ crushed nail injury
- Treatment:
  - no surgical repair necessary in young children
  - use petrolatum gauze dressing until fingertip and new nail remodels or regrows
  - flap coverage elected when distal phalangeal skeleton protruding from wound

MALLOT FINGER INJURY

- Rupture of terminal extensor tendon or avulsion of epiphysis of distal phalanx
- Occurs mostly in sport activities of older children
- *Treatment:* splint in full extension of dip joint ×5–6 wks w/o interruption

FLEXOR TENDON INJURY

- *Causes:* tendon severed by sharp object such as knife or broken glass
- Dx for young child depends on loss of position of rest (cascade of increasing digital flexion)
- Treatment:
  - clean wound. Splint or cast in flexion and refer to hand surgeon for surgical repair
  - always splint ×3 wks in suspicious case of partial laceration of flexor in finger

DISLOCATION OF DIP JOINT

- Often result of sports participation and misdiagnosed as sprain. Wise to take x rays
- Treatment:
  - early case: simple reduction w/ traction and splint in flexion ×3 wks
  - old unreduced dislocation: needs open reduction

DISLOCATION OF PIP JOINT

- Very common injury in sports
- Treatment:
  - simple reduction w/ traction
  - splint in flexion position ×2 wks
  - at 2 wks, perform active flexion exercises w/ extension block
  - splint ×2 more wks before returning to sports activities
- *Common complication:* flexion contracture from prolonged immobilization

DISLOCATION OF MCP JOINT

- Index finger most often affected
- Treatment:
  - irreducible by manipulation and requires open reduction in most cases
  - refer to orthopedic surgeon immediately

JAMMED FINGER OR SPRAINED FINGER

- Most common injury from participation in sports
- Result of collateral ligament injury
- Treatment:
  - immobilize by using aluminum splint or by strapping injured finger to adjacent digit
  - after 2 wks, implement active exercise program
  - resume sport activity after 3 wks

DISTAL PHALANX FRACTURES

- Most often open fracture from crush injury of fingertips
- Salter I, II fractures regarded as pediatric mallot injuries
- Longitudinal fractures may be unappreciated on standard x ray unless proximal nail retracted distally or entire nail removed

- *Treatment:* fracture site should be debrided and irrigated before reduction
- Osteomyelitis common complication in unrecognized open fracture

PROXIMAL AND MIDDLE PHALANX FRACTURES

- Most displaced and/or angulated subcondylar fractures
- Recurrent reduction essential to restoring digital flexion
- Physeal injuries most common at proximal phalangeal level—esp abduction injury of little finger (so-called extra-octave fracture)
- *Treatment:* closed treatment sufficient; remodeling potential in young children

BURN INJURY

- Hand one of most common burn sites in children
- Treatment:
  - first aid—cold/water immersion
  - blister should be aspirated or debrided to remove fluid
  - prevent infection w/ administration of antibiotics, topical cream of silver sulfadiazine
  - refer to hand surgeon for elective treatment

FROSTBITE INJURY

- Physeal injury common and results in epiphyseal arrest or destruction
- Nail abnormalities often associated w/ distal phalangeal physeal arrest
- *Treatment:* rewarm at 110°F

FLATFEET (FLEXIBLE PES PLANOVALGUS)

THERESA L. DISE

BACKGROUND

- Talar, navicular, medial cuneiform bones of foot have abnormal relationship in weight-bearing position
- Up to age 3 yrs, normal foot universally appears "flat"
- In-toeing commonly associated posture to keep child in balance
- Most commonly congenital/familial
- Three categories: mild—on weight-bearing arch lower than usual but still seen; moderate—entire sole of foot rests on floor; severe—talar head comes out below/anterior to medial malleolus

CLINICAL MANIFESTATIONS

- Usually brought to physician's attention by parents who notice "flat" foot
- Painless/asymptomatic
- Associated in-toeing
- *Shoe examination necessary:* worn down medially on inner side, instead of normal wear on lateral edge of shoe

LABORATORY FEATURES

- Routine radiographs not necessary in mild/moderate flatfoot; w/severe flatfeet, lateral views of weight-bearing foot obtained; loss of normal straight line relationship of talus, navicular, cuneiform bones seen

DIFFERENTIAL DIAGNOSIS

- Acquired flatfoot 2° to muscle/nerve disorders
- Shortened heel cord
- Tarsal coalition

TREATMENT

- *No treatment:* mild/moderate flexible flatfoot
- *Removable, longitudinal arch supports / orthopedic evaluation:* severe flatfoot
- *Orthopedic evaluation:* rigid flatfoot

WHEN TO REFER

- *>3 yrs of age plus any of the following:* pain present, "severe" designation, abnormal shoe wear, arch of foot not restored when pt rises on tiptoe, foot not supple, longitudinal arch absent when foot non–weight bearing

CALCANEOVALGUS FOOT

BACKGROUND

- Foot maintained in dorsiflexed/everted position ("banana-shaped" foot)
- *Incidence:* 1/1,000
- More common in girls, firstborn, breech position
- Most common newborn foot deformity
- Felt to be 2° to intrauterine positioning

CLINICAL MANIFESTATIONS

- Foot acutely dorsiflexed, sometimes in contact w/anterior shin
- Plantar flexion limited to neutral position
- Heel valgus may be ↑ (viewed from behind foot)
- Heel cord abnormally long
- Usually foot supple; can be brought into some plantar flexion/supination
- Always examine hips to exclude associated abnormalities

LABORATORY FEATURES

- Routine radiographs not indicated, unless Dx in doubt

DIFFERENTIAL DIAGNOSIS

- Congenital vertical talus (rocker-bottom foot) associated w/arthrogryposis, neuromuscular diseases, chromosomal abnormalities

TREATMENT

- Daily passive stretching/taught to parents; rarely, casting to hasten resolution; natural Hx: complete correction in 3–6 mos

COMPLICATIONS

- Predisposition to flexible pes planovalgus (flatfoot)

BACKGROUND

- *Folic acid:* water-soluble, heat-/photo-labile vitamin found in high concentrations in liver, kidney, orange juice, fresh greens, cereal, bread
- Absorption by carrier-mediated transport occurs in proximal third of small intestine, supplemented by enterohepatic circulation
- Acts as coenzyme in cellular single carbon metabolism/essential for synthesis of purines, pyrimidines, some methyl groups
- *Recommended intake:* 200/µg/d provides 3 mo supply for healthy individual
- *Inadequate intake:* primary cause of folic acid deficiency/prevalent among pts living in poverty, w/ chronic malnutrition states/infections, including HIV
- Malabsorption/↑ demand, destruction/excretion also contributes to deficits
- Highest risk populations for deficiency include infants, pregnant/breast-feeding mothers, elderly
- Infants:
  - neonatal cord blood/breast milk maintain adequate folate levels even w/ maternal deficits
  - premature infants require supplementation
  - hemolysis 2° vitamin E deficiency/other high RBC turnover states such as sickle-cell anemia ↑ demand
  - diarrhea associated w/ ↓ absorption
- Children and adults:
  - most common cause of deficiency: malabsorption (sprue, Whipple syndrome, HIV)
  - 2° causes include ↑ demand states: sickle-cell anemia, hereditary spherocytosis, other hemolytic anemias
  - other causes: alcohol abuse, medications (trimethoprim-sulfamethoxazole, pyramethamine, anticonvulsants, oral contraceptives, methotrexate, hypothyroidism, rare diseases such as homocystinurea/inborn errors of folate metabolism

CLINICAL MANIFESTATIONS

- *Neural tube defects:* anencephaly, sphingomyelocele, spina bifida; mechanism possibly due to ↑ demand in early gestation (first 12 wks); incidence ↑ 8 fold by multiple gestations, adolescent pregnancies, minimal time between conceptions; may be associated w/ ↑ homocysteine levels/↑ methionine load
- *Infants:* irritability, poor weight gain, chronic diarrhea
- Vascular disease including strokes, coronary artery disease, MI, other thrombotic diseases such as deep vein thrombosis/arterial thrombosis may be associated w/ folic acid deficiency
- Cervical/colon cancer may be associated w/ folic aid deficiency
- Developmental delay, seizures, microcephaly common presentations in rare inborn errors of folate metabolism such as methylene tetrahydrofolate reductase deficiency

LABORATORY FEATURES

- Macrocytosis w/ or w/o anemia
- *Low serum folate:* <3 ng/mL (nL 4–20 ng/mL) within 2 wks of folate removal from diet
- *Low erythrocyte folate:* <150 ng/mL (nL 200–800 ng/mL) within 3 mos folate removal from diet
- Erythrocyte folate level more accurate indicator of folate status than serum level
- Plasma homocysteine levels ↑ in >80% pts w/ folate deficiency
- Normal serum B_{12} levels
- Sometimes coexist w/ iron deficiency
- *Premature neonates:* deficiency manifests as thrombocytopenia and neutropenia w/ anemia masked by RBC transfusions
- *Chemistries:* ↑ LDH, ↑ bilrubin
- *Peripheral blood film:* large neutrophils w/ hypersegmentation, large RBCs
- *Bone marrow aspirate:* asynchronous maturation of RBC nucleus/cytoplasm

DIFFERENTIAL DIAGNOSIS

- B_{12} deficiency
- *Malignant disease:* lymphoma, leukemia, myeloma, polycythemia rubra vera, carcinoma
- *Dyserythropoiesis:* pernicious anemia, sideroblastic anemia, paroxysmal nocturnal hemoglobinuria, asplastic anemia, myelodysplastic syndrome
- *Macrocytosis:* normal newborn, reticulocytosis, ↑ Hgb F, trisomy 21, valproate
- Defects in metabolism of homocysteine/methylmalonic acid

TREATMENT

- Exclude B_{12} deficiency
- *Dietary deficiency:* correct diet
- *Malabsorption:* supplement w/ 100 µg/kg/5–15 mg folic acid per day
- *Neural tube prophylaxis:* preconceptual to at least 1 mo of gestation receive 0.4 mg/d; Hx neural tube defect, supplement w/ 4–5 mg/d
- *Hyperhomocysteinemia:* supplementation w/ folate lowers levels but clinical impact of supplementation under investigation
- *Vascular disease:* folate supplementation investigational

COMPLICATIONS

- Potential to delay Dx of pernicious anemia (B_{12}/cobalamin deficiency) allowing for progression of neurologic damage esp if treating w/ folate at doses >5 mg/d
- Transfusion of RBC/platelets
- Developmental delay/neurologic deficits from inborn errors of folate metabolism

WHEN TO REFER

- Association of folate deficiency w/ developmental delay, seizures, failure to thrive/neurologic complications (for evaluation of inborn errors of metabolism such as homocystinuria, methylene-tetrahydrofolate reductase deficiency)
- Pancytopenia

BACKGROUND

- *Pathogen:* predominantly *Staphylococcus aureus*
- *Provocative factors:* moist environment, maceration, poor hygiene, application of occlusive emollient, drainage from adjacent wound or abscess
- Children w/ Down syndrome prone to folliculitis on trunk and proximal extremities

CLINICAL MANIFESTATIONS

- Discrete, dome-shaped pustules, sometimes w/ erythematous base
- Located at ostium of pilosebaceous canals, usually on scalp, buttocks, or extremities
- Asymptomatic to mildly tender
- Heals w/o scarring
- Clinical variants:
  - HIV-infected pts: confluent erythematous patches w/ satellite pustules in intertriginous areas, violaceous plaques composed of superficial follicular pustules in scalp, axillae, or groin
  - sycosis barbae: deeper, more severe, recurrent, inflammatory form involving entire depth of follicle. Erythematous, follicular papules and pustules develop on chin, upper lip, angle of jaw, primarily in young black males. Papules may coalesce into plaques; healing may occur w/ scarring. Affected individuals frequently *S. aureus* nasal carriers

LABORATORY FEATURES

- Pathogen identified by Gram stain and culture of purulent material from follicular orifice

DIFFERENTIAL DIAGNOSIS

- Folliculitis due to other organisms:
  - yeast:
    - Dx made by potassium hydroxide examination of scrapings from lesion
    - *Candida:* satellite follicular papules and/or pustules surrounding patches of intertrigo, particularly in pts on longterm corticosteroid or antibiotic Tx
    - *Malassezia furfur:* pruritic, 2–3 mm, erythematous, perifollicular papules and papulopustules on back, chest, extremities, particularly in pts w/ diabetes mellitis, or on long-term systemic corticosteroids or antibiotics
  - gram-negative folliculitis:
    - occurs primarily in pts w/ acne vulgaris who have received long-term Tx w/ broad-spectrum systemic antibiotics
    - Dx established by culture of infected follicles
    - superficial pustular form due to *Klebsiella* spp., *Enterobacter* spp., *Escherichia coli,* or *Pseudomonas aeruginosa.* Occurs around nose, spreads to cheeks, chin
    - deeper, nodular form due to *Proteus* spp. Occurs on face and trunk
    - hot tub folliculitis due to *P. aeruginosa,* predominantly serotype O-11. Pruritic papules and pustules or deeply erythematous to violaceous nodules develop 8–48 hrs after exposure, most dense in areas covered by bathing suit. Pts occasionally develop fever, malaise, lymphadenopathy
- Acne (vulgaris, chloracne, drug induced)
- Dermatophyte infection (tinea)
- Eosinophilic pustular folliculitis
- Folliculitis decalvans
- Folliculitis keloidalis
- Follicular mucinosis
- Miliaria

TREATMENT

- Identify, eliminate predisposing factors (eg, avoid tight-fitting clothes, use of occlusive emollients)
- Mild cases:
  - topical antibiotic cleansers (ie, chlorhexidine or hexachlorophene). Avoid in individuals w/ atopic dermatitis
  - topical mupirocin 3×/d
- Severe, widespread cases:
  - penicillinase-resistant systemic antibiotics ×7–10 d (see Impetigo)
    - dicloxacillin, 12.5–50 mg/kg/d div 4 daily doses
    - cephalexin, 25–50 mg/kg/d div 2–4 daily doses
    - erythromycin (ethylsuccinate, 25–50 mg/kg/d div 3–4 daily doses) or clindamycin (15 mg/kg/d div 3–4 daily doses) in penicillin-allergic pts
- Chronic recurrent folliculitis (in addition to above measures):
  - daily application of benzoyl peroxide lotion or gel, and/or
  - mild keratolytic, nonocclusive emolliant containing alpha-hydroxy acid

COMPLICATIONS

- Extension to deeper tissues
- Abscess formation

WHEN TO REFER

- Chronic recurrent or recalcitrant folliculitis:
  - skin biopsy, including Gram stain and culture may be necessary to identify causative organism

BACKGROUND

- Multiple mechanisms may lead to symptoms after foods. Possible mechanisms include:
  - IgE-mediated food allergy: antigen-specific IgE bound to mast cells recognizes food and signals mediator release w/ resulting symptoms. Term *allergy* implies immune reaction
  - pharmacologic food intolerance: pharmacologically active chemicals in food induce symptoms in those w/ abnormally low threshold for substance (eg, caffeine)
  - food-induced enterocolitis syndrome
  - toxin-induced food reactions: foods contaminated by bacterial or fungal toxins induce symptoms specific to toxin
  - metabolic food intolerance: congenital metabolic disorders place pts at risk of symptoms from particular foods (eg, diarrhea after milk in lactase deficiency)
  - celiac disease: sensitivity to gluten of unknown mechanism causes typical enteropathy
  - cellular and antibody-mediated immune responses have been postulated in diseases such as milk protein sensitivity and celiac disease, but proof for these mechanisms not strong
- Other syndromes that might be food related (but are less well documented) include:
  - some cases of allergic eosinophilic gastroenteritis
  - some cases of pulmonary hemosiderosis (Heiner syndrome)
  - some instances of migraine
- Claims of psychiatric, behavioral, learning disorders related to foods unsubstantiated or, at best, very poorly substantiated

CLINICAL MANIFESTATIONS

- IgE-mediated reaction to single, acute exposure to food may cause cutaneous, cardiovascular, respiratory, GI symptoms:
  - cutaneous: erythema, hives, angioedema, eczema
  - respiratory: rhinorrhea, sneezing, airway edema, laryngeal edema, wheezing
  - cardiovascular: hypotension, cardiac arrhythmia
  - GI: cramping, vomiting, diarrhea
  - isolated cutaneous reactions common
  - isolated involvement of cardiovascular system after acute exposure uncommon
- *Chronic* exposure to offending food in IgE-mediated allergy may aggravate atopic dermatitis and occasionally asthma. IgE-mediated food allergy probably very rarely involved in isolated GI disease, rhinitis, or recurrent ear infections
- Mimics of IgE-mediated sensitivity:
  - any of other mechanisms listed above may mimic IgE-mediated food allergy
  - hives, erythema, hypotension follow ingestion of spoiled tuna or other fish that contain large quantities of histamine (scombroid fish poisoning). Preformed histamine in fish, rather than allergic reaction, cause of symptoms

COMMON ALLERGENS

- *Infants:* egg, cow's milk, peanuts
- Reactions may occur on first oral exposure due to in utero exposure. In milk protein sensitivity (usually not IgE-mediated), up to 30% of affected infants also intolerant of soy
- *Older children and adolescents:* peanuts, tree nuts, seafoods

GENERAL PRECAUTIONS IN FOOD ALLERGY

- Take care to recognize IgE-mediated reactions. In very sensitive, even small exposures may lead to catastrophic anaphylaxis
  - systemic symptoms within 1–2 hrs of ingestion of common allergen should lead to caution about reexposure
  - children most at risk of fatal or near fatal reactions are the peanut sensitive who also have asthma
  - seek advice if question about significance of presumed reaction

TREATMENT

- Avoidance only effective Tx for food allergy. Other Tx vary from controversial to dangerous
- Avoidance requires extensive family education to recognize allergens in prepared foods
- Alternate caregivers must also understand avoidance measures
- Provide epinephrine injector for those who have had significant, systemic reactions. Family must understand indications for and use of epinephrine
- Medic-Alert tags may be needed for older children who spend time away from family caretakers

WHEN TO REFER

- Confusion over nature of possible food reaction
- Need for further family education

FOREIGN BODIES OF THE EAR, NOSE, AND ESOPHAGUS

AMELIA F. DRAKE

BACKGROUND

• Children naturally have curiosity about body orifices and may be exploratory in nature w/ regard to foreign bodies
• Most frequently found 1–4 yrs of age, but can occur at any age (ie, insect in ear)

CLINICAL MANIFESTATIONS

• Ear:
  – foreign bodies of ear may present w/ pain and drainage from superimposed external otitis
  – may be asymptomatic and discovered on routine exam. Removal not considered urgent or emergent
  – if foreign body insect, topical lidocaine can be helpful in removal by killing bug, anesthetizing TM
• Nose:
  – usually present either w/ nasal obstruction or evidence of sinusitis (ie, purulent nasal secretions 2° to obstruction of sinus ostea)
  – 2° polypoid mucosal changes can make visualization difficult
• Esophagus:
  – presentation may be subtle w/ difficulty w/ solid feedings in young child
  – dysphagia may occur in older child as well
  – in infant and toddler, compression anteriorly of posterior membranous trachea can cause stridor, airway compromise

LABORATORY FEATURES

• Foreign bodies of ear and nose usually visible on physical examination; however, esophageal foreign bodies may be subtle and require radiographic imaging for discovery or confirmation
• Esophageal foreign body may be radio-opaque, as in coin trapped in cricopharyngeus muscle in proximal esophagus
• Blood work usually not helpful
• Barium swallow may be helpful in outlining esophageal foreign body that has been in place for prolonged period of time
• Consider audiologic evaluation for complaints of ↓ in hearing

DIFFERENTIAL DIAGNOSIS

• Ear:
  – cerumen
  – osteoma
  – keratoma of ear canal
• Nose:
  – nasal polyps
  – papilloma
• Esophagus:
  – stricture
  – esophagitis

TREATMENT

• Ear:
  – office removal: certain instruments make process easier. Cupped foreign body suction helps, as on occasion do alligator forceps
• Nose:
  – topical decongestant nose drops help decongest nose w/ nasal foreign bodies, allowing easier removal. Sinusitis, when present, treated medically w/ antibiotics

– removal not considered urgent unless foreign body suspected to be watch battery, which can corrode and cause soft tissue damage, including septal perforation
• Esophagus:
  – treatment of foreign body should be individualized
  – consider repeat chest x ray to r/o migration
  – esophageal foreign bodies may require trip to OR and removal under general anesthesia w/ protection of airway so foreign body not aspirated

COMPLICATIONS

• Complications w/ nasal foreign bodies include sinusitis 2° to obstruction, erosion through surrounding tissue or septum if foreign body is watch battery
• Complications w/ esophageal foreign body include migration, erosion, pseudo diverticulum, airway compromise

WHEN TO REFER

• One atraumatic attempt to remove foreign body of ear or nose appropriate; however, if repeated attempts necessary, refer pt to otolaryngologist because of limited pt tolerance
• Although radiographically guided removal has become popular, esophageal foreign body ideally removed in controlled setting w/ protection of airway to avoid aspiration of foreign body during removal

BACKGROUND

- Occurs commonly, usually self-limited because lacrimation drains the foreign body (FB) from conjunctival surface. For example, eyelashes, fine pebbles strike eye, only to wash away
- *FB of cornea:* 25% of serious ocular injuries
- FB symptoms mimic those of corneal abrasions, so in pediatric population where Hx often unclear, first r/o FB, then evaluate for possible abrasion
- *Always* obtain visual acuity for any type ocular injury, even if involves asking whether child can see clock hands, numbers, figures on opposite wall
- *FBs to eye best categorized by anatomy:* conjunctival, corneal, intraocular, orbital

CONJUNCTIVAL FBS

- Typically include tiny pebbles, airborne grasses, fine twigs, broken toy pieces, eyelashes, contact lenses
- *Symptoms* vary from localized FB sensation to none. Pain usually minimal, unless cornea scratched. Eventually, tissue irritation causes redness, tearing
- Dx by Hx object on eye, clinical observation of FB. Upper lid eversion often difficult to perform, esp in noncooperative pt. Use cotton applicator as fulcrum to evert lid. Make decisive flip of lid when holding lashes firmly. Children resist repeating maneuver. Once lid folded upward on itself, apply pressure on lashes against upper orbital rim to maintain conjunctival exposure; provides examiner w/free hand to remove FB
- *Adjuncts to assist in this maneuver:* have pt look down, resulting in less pressure applied on pain-sensitive cornea; apply topical anesthetic drop only if absolutely necessary. When anesthetic *not* used, pt can relate to examiner that he or she feels better after removal of FB; no further treatment needed. However, if associated corneal abrasion, pain will be masked by anesthetic; examiner will not know whether to evaluate cornea w/fluorescein. In children sometimes necessary to use topical anesthetic drop simply to perform examination
- *Treatment:* removal of FB. Any fine object will suffice. Items include fine forceps, a 22–23 gauge needle tip, spud, irrigation jet from syringe, cotton applicator. Sweep applicator in upper fornix (cul-de-sac), facilitated w/petrolatum gel on applicator. No antibiotic needed for these superficial FBs

CORNEAL FBS

- Unlike conjunctival mucosal membrane, cornea highly sensitive to touch, pain (trigeminal innervation)
- Symptoms:
  - FB sensation
  - pain: often severe. Pain localized (pt tells you where FB located). However, lightweight FB, such as popcorn kernel, might elicit minimal pain, but eventually causes discomfort, redness, tearing. In children, Dx may be delayed until these occur
  - lacrimation: reflexive, to protect irritated eye
  - bulbar injection, often diffuse, but might be greater toward affected side of cornea
  - blepharospasm: lids squeeze shut. In children might require total anesthetic in order to obtain examination
  - photophobia
- *Note:* all these findings can apply for corneal abrasion. Thus when Hx vague, consider both diagnostic possibilities. Or both, if FB also scratched cornea

DIAGNOSIS

- Hx of FB
- Observation of FB
- Magnification often helpful (loupes, slit lamp, ophthalmoscope w/+15 diopter black focus setting)
- Children not always good historians, so physical examination important; might need topical anesthetic, papoose board, assistant to hold head

TREATMENT

- First, assess visual ability, using objects to recognize if Snellen chart is unintelligible to child. Topical anesthesia is now definitely needed for FB removal. Try irrigation first, using syringe. Potentially dangerous trick is to *screw on* 21–23 gauge needle to a Luer lock syringe. Cut the needle at plastic base, leaving 1–2 mm bore through which saline can be injected w/force. *Never* use this needle on a plastic syringe; it can shoot out like an arrow and perforate eye. An imbedded FB not removable by jet stream probably will not slide off w/cotton applicator tip. Cotton merely creates larger abrasion
- *Turn to metallic tip:* spud, 21–23 gauge needle edge, forceps. Approach eye *tangentially* to scrape off FB. Pointing needle at eye incurs risk of pt leaning forward, perforating eye
- After FB removed, treat residual abrasion w/topical antibiotic, patch. Best antibiotic choices cover gram-positive organisms w/some broad-spectrum (erythromycin, sulfacetamide, neomycin, tobramycin)

COMPLICATIONS

- Iron leaches into corneal stroma, is toxic to epithelial cells. Ferrous ions cause stromal edema, eventual tissue necrosis. Thorough removal required, usually w/high-speed dental drill–like burr. Thus referral to ophthalmologist needed

INTRAOCULAR FBS

- Virtually all cases require referral to ophthalmologist
- *Signs:* hyphema, irregular pupil (corneal laceration), vitreous hemorrhage, prolapsed uvea (dark spot over sclera), late-onset cataract, possible ↓ vision, pain not necessarily prominent
- Iron and copper toxic to eye, *must* be removed. Iron (and nickel) can be removed by scleral incision, magnet extraction. Copper requires vitreoretinal surgical procedure
- Inert FBs may remain in eye, as long as not in visual axis. Include glass, lead, plastics, stones, plaster, rubber, silver, porcelain, highly alloyed steels. Aluminum, copper alloys (bronze, brass) eventually oxidize, produce chronic, low-grade inflammation. Thus these latter are best removed
- Wood, vegetable matter inflammatory; need excision from eye

ORBITAL FBS

- Uncommon event, but often due to BB pellets
- Usually severe trauma to tissues to allow FB to penetrate behind eye. Thus r/o posterior extension to CNS (by neurologic workup, radiologic studies)
- *Iron, copper, organic matter incite cellulitic reaction:* orbital edema, proptosis, myositic pain on EOM movements, possible impairment of vision, papilledema
- Inert objects may remain in orbit w/o structural harm
- Refer to ophthalmologist

PREVENTION

- Always wear goggles w/workbench activities involving metal-on-metal hammering, grinding
- Wear goggles in woodwork, metal classes
- Wear protective eyewear in dangerous sports, such as hockey
- Extra caution when around shotguns, BB guns, working under car, etc

FOREIGN BODIES OF THE LUNG

MICHELLE S. HOWENSTINE

BACKGROUND

- *Definition:* accidental inhalation of foreign material into respiratory tract
- *Incidence:* highest 1–2 yrs of age
- Items most commonly aspirated by young children:
  - small, round, or cylindrical objects: seeds, peanuts, popcorn, grapes, beads
  - hard or tough foods: carrots, frozen foods
  - compressible, bulky foods: hot dogs, bread, skinned meats
- *Older children aspirate items habitually chewed:* grasses, seeds, small toy parts
- *Mortality:* 500 deaths/y children <5 yrs of age in US

CLINICAL MANIFESTATIONS

- Most aspirated foreign bodies immediately expelled by violent cough
- Symptoms of acute foreign body vary according to degree of airway obstruction and location in airway; vary from abrupt severe respiratory distress (occluded larynx) to dry cough (bronchial lesion)
- Chronically retained vegetable material causes arachidic bronchitis w/ progressive cough, fever, airway inflammation

Location of Aspirated Foreign Bodies	Sx
Larynx	acute dyspnea
	stridor
	croupy cough
	drooling
	hoarseness
Trachea	dyspnea
	stridor or wheezing
	cough
	ausculated "slap or thud"
Bronchus	mild dyspnea
	unilateral wheeze or chest movement
	cough

LABORATORY FEATURES

- *Radiographic studies:* helpful for Dx and often localization of foreign body
  - plain films: localization of radiopaque foreign body; atelectasis seen in long-standing obstruction
  - fluoroscopy or expiratory films: a "ball-valve" or partially obstructed lesion causes obstructive overinflation of affected side causing incomplete exhalation and shift of heart to unaffected side
  - chest CT scan: bronchiectasis and possible obstructed airway observed in chronic lesions

DIFFERENTIAL DIAGNOSIS

- Pneumonia
- Asthma
- Croup

TREATMENT

- Basic airway resuscitation should be initiated if airway totally occluded
- Rigid endoscopy w/ ventilating bronchoscope indicated for adequate airway visualization and removal of foreign body
- Avoid use of chest physiotherapy or aerosol bronchodilators prior to foreign body removal
- *Antibiotics:* indicated for 2° infection
- *glucocorticosteroids:* may be helpful for airway swelling
- *Thoracotomy:* rarely necessary for failed extraction or severe disease

COMPLICATIONS

- Fatal airway obstruction can occur if foreign body in larynx or trachea not recognized and appropriately treated
- Complications following rigid bronchoscopy include airway swelling, pneumothorax, or retained foreign material
- Chronic foreign body retention can lead to atelectasis, bronchiectasis, empyema, pulmonary abscess

PREVENTION

- Avoidance of small, round, firm foods or foods easily compressible to children <4 yrs of age
- Supervision of child's environment and removal of objects easily propelled into respiratory tract
- Parental education regarding basic airway rescue

WHEN TO REFER

- Pts w/ recognized foreign body of lung require referral to specialist trained in rigid bronchoscopy
- Pts w/ respiratory symptoms unresponsive to conventional Tx may require referral to pulmonary specialist for evaluation of possible retained foreign body

BACKGROUND

• Long bones in children consist of *diaphysis* (shaft), *metaphysis* (flared bone near end), *epiphysis* (2° ossification center at end of bone). Growth cartilage at end of bone between metaphysis and epiphysis called *physis*

• By 14–15 yrs of age entire distal tibial epiphysis ossified. Physis closed by 16–18 yrs of age

• Ankle and foot fractures 10.3% of all childhood fractures

• Growth plate (physis) biomechanically weak; fails before ligaments at ankle. Distal tibial and fibular physeal fractures 25–38% of all physeal fractures. Most result from sports injuries. Peak occurrence of injury 8–14 yrs of age. Special subgroup of ankle fractures that disrupt articular surface occur near skeletal maturity; called triplane and Tilleaux fractures

• Tarsal bone fractures rare in younger children due to elasticity of bones. Calcaneus, talus, navicular, cuboid fractures occur in descending order. Metatarsal fractures common; 5.9% of all fractures in childhood. Phalangeal fractures rare in younger children; common in older children. Toe dislocations rare

• Ligamentous injuries (Lis Franc) to foot rare and associated w/ high-energy trauma in older children

• Stress fractures have been reported for metatarsals, calcaneus, cuboid in descending order

CLINICAL MANIFESTATIONS

• Swelling and point tenderness
• *Mechanisms of ankle injuries:* twisting injuries or falls
• Foot fractures 2° to direct crushing trauma or high-energy falls onto foot
• Stress fractures associated w/ sudden ↑ activity level

LABORATORY/X-RAY FEATURES

• Perpendicular x-ray views (AP and lateral); oblique views helpful
• Technetium bone scan for occult fractures
• CT for complex ankle fractures (ie, triplane)

DIFFERENTIAL DIAGNOSIS

• Normal ossification centers of foot
• Köhler disease (osteochondrosis of navicular)
• Freiberg disease (osteochondrosis of second metatarsal head)
• Ligamentous injuries (sprains); unusual in children w/ open growth plates
• Overuse injuries: calcaneal apophysitis, plantar fasciitis, Achilles tendonitis, retrocalcaneal bursitis
• Osteomyelitis, septic arthritis
• Juvenile rheumatoid arthritis
• Neoplasms: Ewing sarcoma, leukemia, osteosarcoma, soft tissue sarcomas, osteoid osteoma

TREATMENT

• Splinting and immobilization as initial treatment; crutches and protected weight bearing
• Cast immobilization of nondisplaced fractures once swelling subsides
• Repeat radiographs 10–14 d for occult fractures

COMPLICATIONS

• Compartment syndrome following crush injuries to foot. Emergent fasciotomy required
• Growth arrest of distal tibia. Significant in child w/ >2 yrs of growth remaining
• Degenerative arthritis from malunited articular fractures of ankle or tarsal bones
• Malunion in markedly angulated fractures in children >10 who have limited remodeling potential

WHEN TO REFER

• Nondisplaced or minimally displaced fractures can be managed w/o referral by cast immobilization after swelling ↓
• All displaced fractures of ankle
• All fractures that disrupt joint surface
• Any open (compound) fracture
• Displaced first metatarsal fractures
• Displaced tarsal fractures
• Any fracture w/ massive soft tissue swelling

BACKGROUND

• Clavicle serves as only bony connection between shoulder girdle and trunk. Mechanism of injury in active child generally as follows:

   – medially directed blow, generally due to fall on shoulder, transmitted to clavicle

   – force applied on outstretched hand, elbow, or shoulder

• Fractured clavicle very common injury in children; >60% clavicle fractures seen in children <10 yrs of age

• 90% fractured clavicles occur along shaft

• Fractured clavicle also can occur at birth. 5/1,000 vertex deliveries; 160/1,000 breech deliveries. Clavicular fractures frequently occur in breech deliveries when difficulty delivering extended arms and shoulder occurs

CLINICAL MANIFESTATIONS

• *In newborn or very young child:* pseudoparalysis of arm on affected side

• Pain when arm moved on affected side

• Tenderness in region of injury. Bruising along clavicle and surrounding tissues

• In severely comminuted fracture, tenting of skin or break of skin

X-RAY FINDINGS

• X-ray examination generally confirms presence or absence of fracture and location of fragments. Fractures may be nondisplaced (greenstick fractures)

DISPLACED FRACTURES

• Overriding of bony ends occur when fracture displaced; also seen w/ comminuted fractures

• Fractures at outer end of clavicle generally show little displacement. When skin open, fracture becomes open or compound fracture

DIFFERENTIAL DIAGNOSIS

• Congenital pseudoarthrosis of clavicle and cleidocranial dysostosis considered when no definite Hx trauma and deformity in clavicle exists. Child abuse considered when other suspected signs such as bruising over body present

• W/ pseudoparalysis of arm, brachial plexus injury may have occurred, esp in newborn

TREATMENT

• *Infant, young children:* greenstick fracture. Injury most common and fracture expected to heal w/o any significant complication. No special treatment needed and child will resume motion of arm and activity when pain gone. Figure-of-eight strap used to support and maintain comfort

• *Older children:* strapping w/ shoulder in extended position using figure-of-eight splint generally helps maintain reduction and comfort. Shoulders held upward and back; splint needs constant adjustment so support maintained

• *Severely overriding fractures:* may need reduction using local anesthesia. Following reduction shoulder held upward and backward and figure-of-eight splint applied

• *Epiphyseal fracture of proximal end of clavicle:* more common in older children and can be maintained in reduction by splint

• *Comminuted fracture:* tenting skin may require open reduction. Rarely, internal fixation by metallic plating indicated

SECONDARY COMPLICATION

• Venous occlusion, vascular lacerations, injury to subclavian artery and vein rarely reported

• Neurovascular injuries rare

• Malunion w/ shortening generally not problem. Angular deformities rare because of remodeling. Nonunions also rare and may be possibly associated w/ congenital pseudoarthrosis of clavicle

• Mass after fracture healing may be present for up to 2 yrs and mistaken for bone tumor

WHEN TO REFER

• Most pts managed w/o referral

• If skin tenting or eroded, fracture would be open fracture; would require debridement, reduction, and maintenance of reduction

• Referral also indicated for serious complications when Dx in doubt or if fracture fails to respond to treatment

BACKGROUND

- Most commonly seen in boys 5–10 yrs of age
- Elbow fractures most often occur w/ fall on outstretched hand
- Types of common elbow fractures:
  - distal humerus: supracondylar fractures, lateral condyle fractures, medial epicondyle fractures
  - proximal radius/ulna: radial neck fractures, olecranon fractures, Monteggia fractures (proximal ulna fracture w/ radial head fracture or dislocation)

CLINICAL MANIFESTATIONS

- In nondisplaced fractures, point tenderness only seen w/ minimal swelling
- In angulated/displaced fractures, elbow tender and swollen
- In severely displaced supracondylar fractures, hyperextension deformity of elbow often seen w/ skin puckering and ecchymosis anteriorly. Pulse may be diminished or absent. Nerve injury seen in 7%

- Nerve lesion signs:
  - median: loss of thumb abduction, numbness of volar index fingertip
  - ulnar: loss of finger abduction, numbness of volar small fingertip
  - radial: loss of wrist extension, numbness of thumb/index finger web space

X-RAY FEATURES

Humerus

- *Supracondylar fractures:* on lateral x ray nondisplaced fractures diagnosed by presence of fat pad sign, which is lucency seen posterior to olecranon fossa. Mildly angulated fractures present when center of capitellum displaced posterior to line drawn along anterior border of humeral shaft. Severely displaced fractures resemble elbow dislocations w/ marked posterior displacement of distal fragment on lateral x ray
- *Lateral condyle fractures:* nondisplaced fractures difficult to see. Fat pad sign may be positive. Most of fracture line hidden in growth plate except for portion in edge of lateral metaphysis
- *Medial epicondyle fracture:* difficult to see in young pts because epicondyle relatively unossified. Comparison x rays of normal elbow usually helpful

Radius/Ulna

- *Radial neck fractures:* nondisplaced fractures may have fat pad sign
- *Olecranon fractures:* seen best on lateral x rays
- *Monteggia fractures:* subtle subluxation of radial head associated w/ ulnar fractures easy to overlook. Assess w/ line drawn down radial shaft, which should intersect middle of capitellum if joint normal

DIFFERENTIAL DIAGNOSIS

- Nursemaid's elbow
- Elbow dislocations
- Congenital deformity of elbow
- Septic arthritis
- Juvenile rheumatoid arthritis

TREATMENT

Nondisplaced fractures	Long arm cast for 4 wks
Angulated supracondylar fractures, radial neck fractures, Monteggia fracture/dislocations	Closed reduction. Supracondylar fractures placed in hyperflexion cast; other fractures placed in 90° long arm cast for 3–4 wks
Displaced supracondylar fractures, lateral condyle fractures, medial epicondyle fractures	Closed reduction and percutaneous pin fixation w/ casting 3–4 wks. Open reduction needed for irreducible fractures
Open fractures	IV antibiotics in ER, surgical debridement/reduction w/ pin fixation as soon as possible, cast 3–4 wks
Rehabilitation	Physical Tx usually not needed

COMPLICATIONS

- Nerve injury
- Arterial injury
- Volkmann ischemic contracture
- Loss of elbow motion
- Cubitus varus of elbow (gunstock deformity)
- Infection

WHEN TO REFER

- Nondisplaced fractures treated w/ cast w/o referral. Exception is nondisplaced lateral condyle fracture of humerus, which tends to displace spontaneously in cast and should be referred

- All angulated, displaced, or open fractures referred. Document pulse and neurologic examination, apply posterior plaster splint w/ elbow flexed to 90° for temporary immobilization for most fractures, but splint supracondylar fractures in only 45° flexion to avoid vascular problems

BACKGROUND

- Fractures of forearm and wrist 40% all childhood skeletal injuries
- Fractures may be classified by location, type of deformity, displacement
- 80% of fractures in distal third of radius and ulna
- Large majority fall into 1 of 3 categories:
  – minimally angulated *and* nondisplaced: includes torus, hairline, greenstick, complete fractures in anatomic or nearly anatomic position
  – angulated or rotated *and* nondisplaced (hinged): includes greenstick, complete fractures that have deformity
  – angulated or rotated *and* displaced: includes severe fractures, most open injuries
- Pitfalls, problems requiring special consideration include growth plate injuries, plastic deformation w/o cortical disruption, associated dislocations. Latter two conditions may be difficult to recognize
- Younger children have better prognosis because of greater potential for remodeling
- Remodeling can be dramatic, esp in distal fractures

CLINICAL MANIFESTATIONS

- Amount of swelling usually reflects severity of injury. Minor swelling may be difficult to detect, but point tenderness can identify site of injury
- Moderate swelling may obscure deformity. If obvious deformity noted immediately following injury and prior to onset of swelling, reduction often indicated
- Plastic deformation w/o obvious fracture can occur. More likely in younger children. Arm appears bowed. Range of motion may be limited, esp pronation-supination
- Tenderness or swelling in wrist or elbow may indicate joint disruption in addition to fracture

RADIOGRAPHS

- Anteroposterior and lateral radiographs that include elbow and wrist obtained in most cases

DIFFERENTIAL DIAGNOSIS

- Hx minor trauma often obtained in cases of tumor or infection. Consider possibility of osteomyelitis or malignancy when Dx fracture obscure

TREATMENT

- Minimally angulated *and* nondisplaced: These stable fractures only require protection. Removable velcro-fastening splints often adequate. Fiberglass splints for small children or cast protection for older children may be indicated
- Angulated or rotated *and* nondisplaced (hinged): Angulation >15° for distal fractures or 10° for shaft fractures usually necessitates reduction. Greenstick shaft fractures w/ angulation may have deceptive rotational component to deformity. Apex volar greenstick fractures require reduction in pronation (palm down). Apex dorsal greenstick fractures require reduction in supination (palm up). Pain control for reduction may be achieved w/ conscious sedation or anesthetic block
- Angulated or rotated *and* displaced: Reduction may be difficult, requiring >1 attempt or requiring surgical reduction and fixation in severe cases. More prolonged anesthesia often necessary

COMPLICATIONS

- Growth disturbance occurs in ~5% distal radius growth plate injuries
- Malunion w/ angulation of 10–20° may be observed for 6 mos in all children. Angulation up to 30° in distal radius may be observed in children <10 yrs of age. If deformity persists w/ loss of motion beyond 6 mos, osteotomy for realignment usually indicated

WHEN TO REFER

- Minimal fractures, esp in younger children, can be managed w/o referral
- Hinged fractures (angulated or rotated and nondisplaced) in younger children can usually be straightened on first attempt under sedation or anesthetic block. Referral advised if treating physician inexperienced w/ performing fracture reductions
- Displaced fractures may be difficult to reduce. Referral to specialist recommended
- Refer fractures w/ joint disruption, neurovascular compromise, or open wounds

FRACTURES, HIP (APOPHYSITIS/HIP POINTER), FEMORAL NECK, AND FEMUR

S. TERRY CANALE, WILLIAM C. WARNER, AND JAMES H. BEATY

HIP POINTER

- Contusions over prominence of iliac crest can irritate attachments of abdominal and thigh muscles, causing pain
- *Treatment:* rest, anti-inflammatory medications, topical modalities such as heat; athletes who continue sports activities w/ hip pointer injury have persistent pain and limited function; recovery can be prolonged

APOPHYSITIS/APOPHYSEAL AVULSION FRACTURE

MECHANISM

- Overuse, microtrauma (apophysitis)
- Sudden violent, forceful contraction w/o external trauma
- Sudden excessive passive muscle lengthening

DIAGNOSIS

- No clear Hx trauma
- Significant pain, localized tenderness
- Limited ROM

TREAMENT

- Controversial
- Most advocate nonsurgical treatment, although some recommend open reduction and internal fixation for displacement >2 cm

HIP FRACTURES

BACKGROUND

- Uncommon: <1% of all fractures in children
- High-energy trauma: look for associated injuries!

CLASSIFICATION

- *Type I:* transepiphyseal separation
- *Type II:* transvervical, most common; usually displaced
- *Type III:* cervicotrochanteric; displacement can occur late
- *Type IV:* fewest complications, rapid union

COMPLICATIONS

- Avascular necrosis (~40–50%)
- Coxa vara (20%)
- Nonunion: rare
- Premature physeal closure; pins across physis = 80% will close

Treatment of hip fractures in children

Type I: w/ or w/o dislocation	Closed reduction + cannulated screw; if closed reduction unsuccessful, open reduction + internal fixation
Type II	Closed or open reduction + internal fixation
Type III	
Displaced	Closed or open reduction + internal fixation
Undisplaced	Abduction spica cast; observe closely for displacement; pin if necessary
Type IV	Traction + abduction spica cast; occasionally internal fixation for polytrauma, irreducible fracture

FEMORAL SHAFT FRACTURES

BACKGROUND

- *Mechanism of injury:* high-energy trauma (automobile-related accidents, falls); child abuse in young children (<3 yrs of age)
- General treatment considerations include chronologic age, bone age, size of the child, cause of injury, isolated injury vs. polytrauma, socioeconomic factors

COMPLICATIONS

- Delayed union and nonunion
  - rare, in children 1–6 yrs of age: continue cast immobilization if healing progressing; in children >6 yrs of age bone grafting, w/ plate-and-screw fixation may be performed; however, interlocking intramedullary nailing w/ bone grafting preferred, esp in children >10–12 yrs of age

- Leg-length discrepancy
  - most common complication; usually not significant, most pts unaware of discrepancy
  - in children 2–10 yrs old, overgrowth more likely; in those ≥10 yrs old, shortening more likely
  - max. acceptable shortening in cast, 2–3 cm depending on age of child
- Torsional deformities
  - usually asymptomatic, rarely require treatment

Treatment options for femoral shaft fractures in children

Age	Closed Head Injury Multiple Trauma	Closed Fracture	Open Fracture*	Age	Closed Head Injury Multiple Trauma	Closed Fracture	Open Fracture*
0–2 yrs	No	Skin traction Spica cast	External fixation 90/90 femoral traction	6–11 yrs	No	Femoral traction Spica cast External fixation Flexible IM nail	External fixation Flexible IM nail Compression plate
	Yes	External fixation Spica cast	External fixation		Yes	External fixation Flexible IM nail Compression plate	External fixation Flexible IM nail Compression plate
2–5 yrs	No	Spica cast Traction, delayed spica cast	External fixation 90/90 femoral traction Flexible IM nail Compression plate	12 yrs or older	No	Locked IM nail External fixation Compression plate Femoral traction, cast	Locked IM nail External fixation
	Yes	External fixation	External fixation 90/90 femoral traction		Yes	Locked IM nail External fixation Compression plate	Locked IM nail External fixation

*Open fractures also require debridement, appropriate IV antibiotic Tx, tetanus vaccine.

DISTAL FEMORAL PHYSEAL FRACTURES

CLASSIFICATION: SALTER-HARRIS

- *Types I, II:* most common, older children, frequently displaced, physeal arrest common
- *Types III, IV:* infrequent
- *Type V:* compression fracture, premature physeal closure, rare

TREATMENT

- *Types, I, II:*
  - gentle closed reduction: "90% traction, 10% manipulation"
  - redisplacement may occur

  - perfect anatomic reduction not required; <5° varus-valgus angulation necessary
  - unstable fracture may require percutaneous cross-wire fixationn
  - type II w/ large metaphyseal spike: percutaneous transverse cannulated screw in metaphyseal fragment
  - open reduction for irreducible fracture or vascular injury
- *Types III, IV*
  - require anatomic reduction
  - open reduction plus internal fixation indicated when closed reduction cannot be obtained
  - 2 mm or less displacement generally acceptable
  - younger child, more rigid criteria

COMPLICATIONS

- *Types I, II:* growth arrest w/ length/angulation problems
- *Growth disturbance, types III, IV:* nonanatomic reduction, insecure fixation

WHEN TO REFER

- Depending on physician's level of skill, availability of equipment and personnel, most physeal fractures, fractures that require open reduction and internal fixation probably best treated by pediatric orthopedist
- Malunion or nonunion and length or angular deformities should be evaluated by specialist

BACKGROUND

- Epiphyseal injuries can occur from direct trauma at any age
- Because growth plates around knee are largest and fastest growing in body, any effect on growth may be large
- Fractures around knee can result from variety of mechanisms
- Distal femoral metaphyseal fracture can occur at any age as result of fall or direct blow
- Distal femoral physeal separation may result from varus, valgus, or hyperextension moments around knee; such injuries common in football
- Patellar fractures may occur as result of direct blow, as in dashboard injury, or as result of sudden extension force as in landing from jump. Patellar osteochondral fracture can result from direct blow or patellar dislocation
- Fractures into knee joint result from direct trauma or twisting forces about knee
- Tibial eminence avulsion may occur from sudden severe force such as twisting or hyperextension across knee, which would rupture anterior cruciate ligament in adults. Classically injury occurs as 8–12 yr old child falls from bike w/ knee in hyperextension
- Proximal tibial metaphyseal injuries occur 1½–6 yrs of age as result of valgus or hyperextension force
- Intraarticular fractures occur generally in adolescence
- Tibial tubercle avulsion results from sudden quadriceps contraction as in initiating or landing from jump

CLINICAL MANIFESTATIONS

- Hx usually includes direct blow or fall, although twisting knee common mechanism of sports injury
- Deformity, inability to bear weight, loss of motion, or swelling seen
- Specific examination for perfusion and nerve function should be performed in severe fracture and dislocations. Popliteal artery, peroneal nerve, tibial nerve at risk at knee

- Hx patellar dislocation may suggest presence of associated intraarticular fracture
- Tense hemarthrosis suggests intraarticular injury
- Varus and valgus instability must be tested; may result from ligamentous disruption or epiphyseal separation

LABORATORY FEATURES

- Plain radiographs mainstay of Dx, and should include, at least, A-P and lateral views. Notch and patellar sunrise views if intraarticular fracture suspected
- Oblique radiographs if fracture strongly suspected but not seen on routine radiographs
- Stress radiographs if varus-valgus instability to discriminate between ligamentous instability and epiphyseal separation
- Bone scan useful to locate occult fracture
- MRI can reveal associated meniscus injury, ligament rupture, subchondral fracture, bone bruises
- Occasionally, CT scanning needed to better delineate intraarticular fracture, usually as preop consideration

DIFFERENTIAL DIAGNOSIS

- Collateral ligament injury
- Cruciate ligament injury
- Meniscal tear
- Osgood-Schlatter disease
- Rupture of quadriceps or patellar tendon
- Hip pathology w/ referred pain
- Bone or joint acute infection

TREATMENT

- Metaphyseal fractures of distal femur or proximal tibia must be reduced, if displaced, and immobilized 4–6 wks
- Epiphyseal separation of distal femur or proximal tibia must be reduced and immobilized or pinned if unstable. Healing occurs 4–6 wks
- Intraarticular fractures must be anatomically reduced and fixed to restore smooth

joint surface and physeal alignment. Undisplaced fractures must be immobilized and followed radiographically to watch for late displacement and nonunion
- Fractures of patella or tibial tubercle often require surgical repair to restore extensor mechanism continuity
- Tibial eminence avulsion fracture can often be reduced by fully extending knee in cast. If reduction does not occur, surgical repair required

COMPLICATIONS

- Epiphyseal fractures and physeal separations may cause growth derangement resulting in slowing or angular growth in spite of adequate treatment
- Any articular fracture may lead to degenerative joint disease
- Tibial eminence fracture, if malunited, may result in permanent loss of full knee extension
- Proximal tibial fractures often grow into valgus in spite of adequate treatment. Parents must be warned of possibility

PREVENTION

- Because children active and adventurous, not possible to prevent all fractures about knee
- Children should always wear seat belts when riding in automobiles
- Discourage use of motorbikes, ATVs, trampolines

WHEN TO REFER

- If Dx unclear
- Displaced or intraarticular fractures
- Fractures w/ gross deformity or loss of knee motion
- Fracture associated w/ loss of perfusion or nerve function

BACKGROUND

- Epiphyseal or metaphyseal in location
- *Rare:* <1% of all children's fractures
- *Adolescent:* most common age group due to sports and higher energy trauma (epiphyseal)
- *Newborn:* second most common due to birth trauma (epiphyseal)
- *5–12 yrs of age:* more often metaphyseal
- 80% humeral growth at proximal epiphysis
- Anatomy:
  - ossification of proximal humeral epiphysis occurs by 6 mos of age
  - greater tuberosity ossification center appears 7 mos–3 yrs of age
  - lesser tuberosity ossification center appears 2½ yrs–5 yrs of age
  - tuberosity ossification centers unite together 5–7 yrs of age
  - epiphyseal closure 14–17 yrs (girls), 16–18 yrs (boys)

CLINICAL MANIFESTATIONS

- Mechanism of injury:
  - neonate: traumatic delivery w/arm hyperextension or excessive rotation
  - older child: fall on outstretched arm or direct blow to posterolateral shoulder
  - child abuse
- Clinical presentation:
  - neonate:
    - pseudoparalysis of arm
    - arm held extended and externally rotated at side
    - palpation elicits pain and spontaneous movement of arm
    - no crepitus
    - occasionally fever
    - swelling
  - older child:
    - Hx of trauma
    - pain, swelling, ecchymosis
    - deformity consistent w/ amount of displacement, angulation, shortening
  - associated neurovascular injury rare

LABORATORY FEATURES: X RAY

- *Neonate:* usually not helpful due to nonossification of proximal humeral epiphysis; other imaging techniques may be helpful:
  - arthrography
  - ultrasound
- *Child >6 mos of age:* plain x rays w/ two views at 90° to each other should be diagnostic:
  - AP of shoulder
  - axillary or transcapular lateral
  - x-ray uninjured shoulder for comparison when needed

DIFFERENTIAL DIAGNOSIS

- Neonate:
  - clavicle fracture
  - brachial plexus palsy
  - infection
  - dislocation
  - child abuse
- Older child:
  - dislocation
  - pathologic fracture through benign lesion (cyst, fibrous cortical defect, eosinophilic granuloma) or malignancy (lymphoma, leukemia, osteosarcoma, Ewing sarcoma)
  - child abuse

TREATMENT

- Closed manipulation for significantly displaced or angulated fracture:
  - 70% epiphyseal fractures nondisplaced or minimally displaced
  - significant displacement:
    - 100% of width of shaft if <5 yrs of age
    - >50% of width of shaft if 5–12 yrs
    - >one-third of width of shaft in adolescents
  - significant angulation:
    - >70° 1–5 yrs of age
    - >40–45° 5–12 yrs of age
    - >25° in adolescents
- Percutaneous pinning for unstable fractures

- *Open reduction for irreducible fractures:* rare
- Immobilization:
  - infant: sling and swathe for 2 wks
  - older child: sling and swathe or velpeau dressing for 4 wks

COMPLICATIONS

- Neurovascular injury uncommon
- Nonunion virtually unknown
- Malunion w/ shortening or angulation usually well tolerated
- Shoulder stiffness uncommon
- Growth disturbance rare
- *Loss of reduction:* treat w/ rereduction

PREVENTION

- *"Play it safe":* playground and bicycle safety

WHEN TO REFER

- Any neurovascular compromise
- Any angulation or displacement more than minimal
- Any other fractures in same extremity

FRACTURES, TIBIAL (TODDLER'S)

DAVID M. HEILBRONNER

BACKGROUND

- Occurs in pts 9 mos–3 yrs of age
- Majority occur in distal tibia. Fractures may be found in proximal tibia, femur, pelvis, foot
- Hx trauma, injury variable. Many times no specific Hx obtained
- Fractures from birth trauma, high-energy trauma, child abuse excluded from this Dx
- Onset to presentation: immediate–2 wks
- Full recovery: 3–4 wks

CLINICAL MANIFESTATIONS

- Acute onset of limp, failure to bear weight on leg, irritability in otherwise healthy-appearing child
- Localized swelling or erythema unusual
- Localized pain over fracture may be severe to palpation or surprisingly mild

PHYSICAL EXAMINATION

- Begins w/ palpation of normal leg and moves to involved leg to attempt to localize site of discomfort. Starting w/ involved leg may stimulate child to cry, making localization almost impossible
- May be subtle skin temperature changes between normal and involved limbs acting as further aid to localization

RADIOGRAPHIC FINDINGS

- Helpful to attempt to localize site of discomfort in order to minimize number of x rays obtained. Try to avoid "babygram"
- On radiology request specify "toddler's fracture" as possible Dx to assist radiologist
- AP, lateral, and internal rotation oblique films generally most helpful
- Wide range of radiographic findings:
  - no obvious fracture on initial x ray
  - obvious fracture, usually oblique or spiral of tibia. Fibula usually intact
  - soft tissue swelling and edema
  - subperiosteal new bone, esp if symptoms have been present >1 wk
  - fracture becomes apparent 10–14 d on repeat films when original x ray was "normal"
- Many cases present w/ no obvious bony finding on radiograph; close look for soft tissue swelling on x ray helpful to assist in early Dx

DIFFERENTIAL DIAGNOSIS

- In decreasing order of likelihood
  - soft tissue trauma
  - toxic synovitis
  - septic arthritis
  - osteomyelitis
  - neoplasm

TREATMENT

- If symptoms acute, x ray positive, or high index of suspicion, casting appropriate. Allow child to weight bear as tolerated
- Short or long leg cast depending on level of fracture
- Few reported pelvis fractures have been isolated pubic rami fractures and require only symptomatic limitation of activities
- If Dx made later than 10–14 d, immobilization often not needed if child relatively comfortable and walking
- If any concern fracture might be present, safest rule of thumb in this and any pediatric fracture: treat it as such to avoid problems. In this case simple splint would be appropriate w/ follow-up in 5–7 d w/ repeat x ray to look for any periosteal change or appearance of fracture line

WHEN TO REFER

- If Dx in doubt
- If uncomfortable casting small children
- If pain seems inappropriate to severity of injury
- If fever associated w/ pain
- If rapid improvement not seen
- If any question or suspicion of child abuse, immediate notification of appropriate agency mandatory

FREIBERG DISEASE

ANDREW A. FREIBERG

BACKGROUND

- *Freiberg disease:* type of osteochondrosis that affects distal end of metatarsus, the metatarsal head. Disease most commonly occurs in second metatarsal head in adolescents, more commonly in girls. Pathogenesis most likely ischemic necrosis or result of repetitive microtrauma

CLINICAL MANIFESTATIONS

- *Most common complaints:* foot pain and limited motion
- Symptoms aggravated by physical activities such as sports and often relieved by rest
- *Physical exam findings:* increased warmth and tenderness about metatarsal-phalangeal joint
- Limited metatarsal-phalangeal joint motion often occurs because of pain

LABORATORY FEATURES

- Radiographs typically show flattening and/or collapse of metatarsal head
- Bone scan often demonstrates increased uptake before radiographic changes of flattening or collapse seen
- Foot may be painful 3–6 mos before plain radiographic changes seen
- MRI also can be used for early Dx

DIFFERENTIAL DIAGNOSIS

- Fracture from trauma
- Stress fracture
- Rheumatoid arthritis
- Metatarsal-phalangeal joint synovitis
- Epiphyseal dysplasia

TREATMENT

- Initially treated w/ metatarsal bar or short leg walking cast or w/ stiff postop shoe
- Short trial of NSAIDs can help w/symptoms
- If persistent pain, disability occur, surgery considered

COMPLICATIONS

- Persistent pain and stiffness

PREVENTION

- None known

WHEN TO REFER

- Metatarsalgia that does not respond within 6 wks to alterations of activity and trial of shoe modification (metatarsal bar or cast shoe)
- Cases w/ involvement >1 metatarsal

BACKGROUND

- Follicular cutaneous abscesses
- Usually originate from a preceding folliculitis; may arise initially as nodular abscess
- *Sites of predilection:* hair-bearing areas on face, neck, axillae, buttocks, groin
- *Pathogen: Staphylococcus aureus,* particularly phage type 80/81
- *Predisposing conditions:* warm, humid environment; obesity; hyperhidrosis; maceration; friction; preexisting dermatitis; treatment w/ corticosteroids or cytotoxic agents
- More common in males than females
- More common in individuals w/ low serum iron, diabetes mellitus, malnutrition, HIV infection, other immunodeficiency states, particularly those involving defects in neutrophil function. Most affected individuals, however, do not have identifiable immune deficiency
- Recurrence often associated w/ carriage of *S. aureus* in nares, axillae, perineum, under fingernails, or sustained close contact w/ carrier

CLINICAL MANIFESTATIONS

- Furuncle:
  – deep-seated, tender, erythematous, perifollicular papule, evolves into fluctuant nodule
  – influx of neutrophils, followed by vessel thrombosis, suppuration, central tissue necrosis leads to rupture, discharge of central core of necrotic tissue, follicle destruction, scarring
  – pain may be intense if lesion situated in area where skin relatively fixed, such as external auditory canal or over nasal cartilage
  – constitutional symptom usually absent
- Carbuncle:
  –infection of group of contiguous follicles, w/ multiple drainage points, inflammatory changes in surrounding connective tissue
  – suppuration delayed, inflammation extends more deeply into subcutaneous tissue, compared to furuncle

– may be accompanied by fever, chills, malaise

LABORATORY FEATURES

- *Leukocytosis:* carbuncle or extensive furunculosis
- Gram stain and culture of pus indicated because other bacteria or fungi may occasionally cause furuncles or carbuncles

DIFFERENTIAL DIAGNOSIS

- Acne conglobata
- Hidradenitis suppurativa
- Dissecting cellulitis of scalp (perifolliculitis capitis)
- Tinea barbae
- Infected epidermal cyst
- Scrofuloderma
- Actinomycosis
- Cat scratch disease
- Granuloma inguinale
- Lymphogranuloma venereum
- Botryomycosis

TREATMENT

- Frequent application of warm, moist compress to facilitate drainage. May suffice for simple furunculosis
- Surgical drainage for large, localized, pointed lesions
  – avoid incision or squeezing of lesions in external auditory canal or central face
- Avoid application of moist dressings after drainage has occurred; resultant maceration may enhance local spread. Apply topical antibiotic (bacitracin, mupirocin); cover draining lesions w/ sterile gauze
- Oral penicillinase-resistant systemic antibiotics 7–10 d for carbuncles, large or multiple furuncles, all lesions located on central face, those associated w/ constitutional signs or local cellulitis:
  – dicloxacillin, 12.5–50 mg/kg/d div 4 daily doses

– cephalexin, 25–50 mg/kg/d div 2–4 daily doses
  – erythromycin (ethylsuccinate, 25–50 mg/kg/d div 3–4 daily doses) or clindamycin (15 mg/kg/d div 3–4 daily doses) in penicillin-allergic pts. Emergence of erythromycin resistance among phage type 80/81 isolates of *S. aureus* has limited utility of erythromycin
- Recurrent furunculosis:
  – wear loose, lightweight, porous clothing
  – launder all bed linens, towels, clothing in *hot* water
  – close attention to personal hygiene; use of chlorhexidine, povidone-iodine, or hexachlorophene, particularly in groin, axillae, hands
  – careful search for, treatment/elimination of predisposing factors or systemic process (eg, anemia)
  – carriage state of pt and close contacts can be eliminated temporarily by application of mupirocin formulated in white petrolatum and lanolin 2–4 ×/d × 5 d to anterior nares, or administration of rifampin concurrently w/ penicillinase-resistant systemic antibiotic
  – consider prophylactic low-dose oral penicillinase-resistant penicillin or clindamycin

COMPLICATIONS

- Cellulitis
- Bacteremia, leading to osteomyelitis, endocarditis, brain abscess
- Cavernous sinus thrombosis associated w/ severe lesions on upper lip or cheek
- Scarring

WHEN TO REFER

- Severe, recurrent, or recalcitrant lesions

BACKGROUND

- Red cell rendered vulnerable to oxidative attack by lack of glucose 6 phosphate dehydrogenase (G6PD); acute or chronic hemolytic anemia occurs on exposure to oxidant stress

  – sex-linked recessive males affected; females heterozygous for G6PD deficiency affected if X chromosome inactivation happens to lead to red cells w/low G6PD levels

  – Caucasians have virtually complete lack of enzyme; most vulnerable to sudden severe anemia. Blacks have exaggerated loss of activity over time, but less at risk for life-threatening anemia

CLINICAL PRESENTATION (3 SYNDROMES)

- Neonatal jaundice:
  – not present at birth
  – onset after day 2 or 3 of life
  – anemia absent or mild
  – wide range of severity (not all pts w/G6PD deficiency have neonatal jaundice)
  – actual "oxidant stress" or trigger often not identified
  – treatment of jaundice most important
- Acute hemolytic episode:
  – response to oxidant stress: fava beans, viral or bacterial infection, medications (see table), mothballs, etc
  – mild fever, nausea, mild to moderate abdominal pain
  – dark urine/jaundice appear simultaneously
  – appearance of pallor, tachycardia
  – occasional splenomegaly, hepatomegaly
  – in severe deficiency may lead to shock, congestive heart failure
  – usually self-limited; Hgb level returns toward normal by 3–6 wks if transfusion not required
- Chronic nonspherocytic hemolytic anemia (rare):
  – difficult to diagnose, not dramatic, episodic
  – chronic anemia ranges from mild to transfusion dependent
  – may or may not have Hx neonatal hyperbilirubinemia
  – morphology not characteristic
  – hemoglobinuria rare
  – splenomegaly common

– when suspected, verified by determination of the exact G6PD variant of pt's red cells

LABORATORY FEATURES

- Neonatal presentation:
  – probably 2 presentations: (1) exaggeration of physiologic jaundice, (2) oxidant hemolysis. Can have indirect hyperbilirubinemia w/little evidence of hemolysis. When actual hemolysis detected:
    - indirect hyperbilirubinemia
    - mild anemia
    - "oxidant damage" appearance of red cells: bite cells, blister cells, fragments
- Acute hemolysis:
  – anemia may be extremely severe (Hgb as low as 2.5 g/dl has been seen)
  – red cell morphology striking: spherocytes, blister cells, bite cells, fragments, polychromasia
  – supravital staining reveals precipitates of hemoglobin on red cell membranes (Heinz bodies) in some, but not all cases
  – hemoglobinuria (positive test for blood in urine, but no red cells)
  – indirect hyperbilirubinemia
  – WBC moderately elevated (secondary to stress)
- Chronic nonnspherocytic hemolytic anemia:
  – anemia mild to severe requiring transfusion
  – MCV elevated (chronic reticulocytosis)
  – increased reticulocytes
  – gallstones or indirect hyperbilirubinemia may be reason for investigation
  – indirect hyperbilirubinemia when hemolysis significant
  – decreased haptoglobin
  – increased lactic acid dehydrogenase
  – specific G6PD genetic variants associated w/syndrome

DIFFERENTIAL DIAGNOSIS

- Neonatal:
  – hemolytic disease of the newborn
  – congenital hemolytic anemia
  – oxidant hemolysis of the newborn (not secondary to G6PD deficiency)
  – physiologic jaundice
- Acute hemolysis w/hemoglobinuria and chronic nonspecific hemolytic anemia:
  – autoimmune hemolytic anemia

– previously undiagnosed chronic hemolytic anemia (membrane or enzyme defect)
  – unstable hemoglobin
  – Wilson disease
  – very rare: malaria, paroxysmal cold hemoglobinuria, paroxysmal nocturnal hemoglobinuria

TREATMENT

- Neonatal jaundice:
  – follow guidelines for neonatal jaundice to prevent bilirubin toxicity
  – transfusion almost never required
  – instruct parents on future guidelines to avoid oxidant stress
- Acute hemolytic episode:
  – remove oxidant if possible (medications, foods)
  – transfuse for severe anemia. Since there is rapid reticulocyte response, *do not* transfuse in preventative fashion
  – guidelines for transfusion: (clinical status of pt more important factor) If Hgb <7, transfuse; Hgb, <9 and hemoglobinuria, transfuse; if Hgb 7–9 and urine clear, watch
  – if new Dx, instruct pt in avoidance of oxidants, early recognition of attacks from known or unknown (eg, infections) oxidant stresses
- Chronic nonspherocytic anemia:
  – transfuse as needed
  – consider splenectomy, esp > age 5 for transfusion-dependent, or for the severely anemic who do not require transfusions (Hgb usually >6)
  – folic acid supplements
  – genetic counseling

COMPLICATIONS

- Neonatal jaundice can lead to bilirubin toxicity syndromes
- Acute and chronic hemolysis can lead to cardiac collapse, heart failure, death if anemia not appropriately treated in time

WHEN TO REFER

- When pts require transfusion
- If Dx in doubt
- When sophisticated diagnostic techniques required (detection of G6PD variant)
- For education and genetic counseling

Medications to be avoided in G6PD deficiency

(This is a list of relatively common medications, not exhaustive)

Analgesics
Aspirin
Phenacetin
Tylenol OK

Sulfonamides and sulfones
  (*All* commonly used)
Sulfonamide antibiotics, including trimethoprim-
  sulfomethoxazole
Azulfidine
Dapsone

Other antibiotics
Nitrofurans: nitrofurantoin, furazolidone,
  nitrofurazone
Nalidixic acid
Chloromphenical
P-Aminosalicyclic acid

Antihelminthics
B Naphthol
Stibophen
Niridazole

Antimalarials
Primaquine
Pamaquine
When critical, chloroquine can be used under
  careful surveillance

Miscellaneous
Vitamin K analogues (1 mg menaphthone can be
  given to neonates)
Mothballs

BACKGROUND

- Autosomal recessive metabolic disorder w/ frequency ~1/70,000 births
- Classical galactosemia caused by mutation of enzyme, galactose-1-phosphate uridyl transferase, resulting in total inability to metabolize galactose, found (w/ glucose) in disaccharide, lactose
- Symptoms begin in neonatal period, soon after introduction of lactose-containing feeds (breast milk, milk-based formula) and accumulation of galactose
- Symptoms may develop before results from newborn screening reported. Not all states screen for galactosemia as part of newborn screening panel
- Newborn screening results may include false positives for newborns who have diminished (but not absent) enzyme activity and/or galactose accumulation but do not exhibit clinical manifestations of galactosemia
- W/o treatment (galactose elimination), neonatal mortality high often due to 2° *E. coli* sepsis

CLINICAL MANIFESTATIONS

- Failure to thrive
- Vomiting, often w/o diarrhea
- Jaundice and/or hepatomegaly
- Ascites
- Cataracts observed by slit lamp, w/ delayed treatment
- Increased intracranial pressure and cerebral edema
- Renal tubular dysfunction
- Sepsis

LABORATORY FEATURES

- *UA:* galactosuria w/o glucosuria: positive reducing substances (Clinitest, Benedict's reagent w/ negative glucose-specific dipstik (Clinistix, glucose oxidase test). Proteinuria and aminoaciduria also may be present
- *Hgb:* may see drop of several grams followed by rapid reticulocytosis in absence of bleeding prior to removing galactose from diet
- *Liver function:* ↑ bilirubin, w/ conjugated > unconjugated; hypoprothrombinemia
- Gram-negative sepsis
- Elevated whole blood galactose plus galactose-1-PO_4
- No significant RBC galactose-1-PO_4 uridyl transferase activity detectable
- *Note:* Do not delay treatment, but take heparinized whole blood sample for confirmatory assays *prior* to restricting galactose or initiating transfusions. If prior exchange transfusion, this should be noted, along w/ date, on pt information sent w/ sample. Contact regional genetics laboratory to receive instruction on sample size, preparation, delivery

DIFFERENTIAL DIAGNOSIS

- *E. coli* sepsis w/o galactosemia
- Significant liver disease or prematurity
- Galactokinase deficiency (very rare) or UDP glucose-4-epimerase deficiency
- Milder galactosemia variants that have partial enzymatic activity

TREATMENT

- Even if galactosemia only a possibility, galactose should be immediately removed from diet by replacing current formula/breast milk w/ soy-based formula or casein hydrolysate from which lactose removed
- Establish fluid and electrolyte balance
- If sepsis suspected, treat w/ broad-spectrum antibiotics until bacteriologic reports available
- Evaluate need for phototherapy or exchange transfusion
- Restrict galactose for life in classical galactosemia (individuals w/ no enzyme activity)
- Restrict galactose until 1 yr of age and challenge w/ galactose load in galactosemia variants (individuals w/ partial enzyme activity)

COMPLICATIONS

- Acute illness of neonate can be reversed w/ elimination of galactose from diet; however, 30–90% chance of one or more of following long-term complications:
  - learning disabilities
  - articulation (speech) disorders
  - small stature, delayed puberty
  - cataracts, esp w/ delayed treatment or poor compliance
  - ovarian failure and infertility in females
  - shyness
  - calcium deficiency, if not supplemented

WHEN TO REFER

- Referral to genetics center w/ galactosemia clinic to help coordinate special services that may be necessary: developmental evaluation, ophthalmology, speech Tx, endocrinology, metabolic, nutrition, genetic counseling; and to provide laboratory resources for periodic monitoring of galactose and galactose-1-PO_4

BACKGROUND

- Most common tumor of hand, wrist, knee
- M:F ratio: 1:3
- Wrist/hand ganglion cysts occur between second and fourth decades; popliteal cysts occur during first and second decades
- Etiology unknown; hypotheses include trauma, mucoid degeneration of collagen tissue, joint herniation
- Filled w/ clear gelatinous fluid w/ one-way valve duct to adjacent joint or tendon synovial sheath
- In children, popliteal cysts insignificant and resolve spontaneously within several months or even years, unlike popliteal cysts in adults, which usually signify intraarticular knee derangement

CLINICAL MANIFESTATIONS

- Size may fluctuate over time
- Usually painless unless bumped
- At knee, may cause pain w/ prolonged standing w/ knee extended
- Wrist ganglion cysts usually occur on dorsal aspect between extensor pollicus longus and extensor digitorum communis, on volar aspect adjacent to radial artery
- Popliteal cysts occur distal to popliteal crease, between gastrocnemius and semimembranous muscles
- May occur in other areas, including dorsolateral aspect of foot and ankle, metacarpophalangeal joints, other joints and tendon sheaths
- Firm cystic consistency; fairly mobile
- Large cysts may transilluminate
- Not pulsatile
- No bruit

DIAGNOSTIC STUDIES

- Radiographs unremarkable, but should be done to r/o other conditions
- MRI indicated only when Dx in doubt, when location not typical, or pt needs assurance to confirm Dx. At knee, may be indicated to r/o intraarticular pathology

DIFFERENTIAL DIAGNOSIS

- At wrist/hand:
  - radial artery aneurysm: pulsatile or bruit
  - metacarpal boss: hard, attached to bone
  - extensor digitorum brevis manus muscle
  - giant cell tumor of tendon sheath
  - chronic tenosynovitis of extensor tendons: swelling diffuse
  - synovial cell sarcoma: radiograph may be abnormal
  - neural tumor
- At knee:
  - lymph node
  - varicose vein
  - aneurysm
  - synovial cell sarcoma
  - osteosarcoma

TREATMENT

- Family may want no treatment after assured cyst benign
- Wrist ganglion cysts require removal if symptomatic
- Aspiration w/ or w/o injection of corticosteroid ineffective at wrist and knee; sometimes effective at metacarpophalangeal joints
- Injection of sclerosing agent and direct blow to cyst contraindicated
- Knee cysts rarely require surgical excision because of spontaneous resolution within months or even years

COMPLICATIONS

- *Extremely rare except as result of surgical treatment:* hypertrophic incisional scar; wrist stiffness; recurrence; injury to posterior tibial artery or nerve, radial artery, or sensory branch of radial nerve
- Recurrence usually due to incomplete excision

PREVENTION

- None

WHEN TO REFER

- *If Dx in doubt:* atypical location or consistency
- Abnormal radiograph
- MRI does not show fluid-filled cyst
- Pulsatile
- Bruit
- Persistent pain
- Persistent increase in size
- Excessive pt anxiety

GASTROENTERITIS, BACTERIAL

JAY A. HOCHMAN AND MITCHELL B. COHEN

BACKGROUND

- Bacterial enteropathogens account for ≤10% of acute childhood diarrhea, but infection can result in severe disease/serious complications
- Children have ↑ susceptibility to many bacterial pathogens w/higher age-specific attack rates for *Salmonella* sp., *Campylobacter* sp., *Aeromonas* sp., and *E. coli O157:H7*
- *Risk factors for infection:* immature immune systems, day-care center exposure, disruption of normal enteric flora by antibiotics, travel to areas of endemic infection
- Fecal-oral contamination most common route of infection acquisition; however, water/food-borne transmission route when larger inocula required (eg, *V. cholera, Salmonella* sp.)

Organism	Foods Associated with Infection
Campylobacter	Raw milk
E. coli O157:H7	Hamburgers
Salmonella	Eggs, poultry
V. cholerae	Shellfish, fish

CLINICAL MANIFESTATIONS

- Not always easy to differentiate from viral gastroenteritis, which usually causes watery diarrhea. *Suggestive of inflammatory diarrhea* (bacterial colitis): fever, tenesmus, bloody diarrhea, fecal leukocytes, severe abdominal pain
- *Organisms that cause inflammatory diarrhea:* *Campylobacter* sp., *C. difficile*, *E. coli O157:H7, Salmonella* sp., *Shigella* sp.
- *Organisms that cause secretory (watery) diarrhea:* *V. cholerae,* enterotoxigenic *E. coli, Bacillus cereus, Clostridium perfringens, Staphylococcus aureus*
- *Persistent diarrhea* (>10 d duration): more common w/parasitic infections, inflammatory bowel disease; however, *C. difficile, Plesiomonas* sp., *Aeromonas* sp., *Salmonella* sp., *Yersinia* sp. can cause persistent diarrhea

LABORATORY FEATURES

- Stool culture diagnostic. *Campylobacter sp, Salmonella* sp., *Shigella* sp., *E. coli O157:H7* most frequently cultured etiologies of bacterial enteritis. *E. coli O157:H7* may be most common pathogen identified when pt has bloody diarrhea
- Stool culture *should be obtained* in cases of bloody diarrhea, in pts w/underlying medical problems, in cases of community outbreaks, in persons requiring hospitalization due to diarrhea
- Stool culture *not recommended* for uncomplicated acute watery diarrhea, and in pts who develop diarrhea after being hospitalized ≥3 d
- *Fecal leukocytes* and heme-positive stools characteristic of inflammatory diarrhea, but not always present w/bacterial gastroenteritis. Also, can be seen in noninfectious colitis (eg, inflammatory bowel disease)
- Many laboratories require notification in order to use appropriate culture media for certain pathogens; specific examples include *E. coli O157:H7, Yersinia* sp., *V. cholerae*
- *C. difficile toxin assay* also must be requested, should be considered in hospitalized pts, in pts w/recent antibiotic exposure. Assay must be cautiously interpreted in infants (<12 mos) who have ~40% colonization rate without evidence of disease

DIFFERENTIAL DIAGNOSIS

- Viral gastroenteritis
- Inflammatory bowel disease
- Appendicitis
- Celiac disease
- Henoch-Schönlein purpura
- Irritable bowel syndrome
- Disaccharidase intolerance
- Immunodeficiency
- Allergic colitis
- Hirschsprung's enterocolitis
- Necrotizing enterocolitis
- Drug-induced diarrhea
- Factitious diarrhea

TREATMENT

- Assure adequate hydration. If dehydration mild–moderate in severity, hydrate w/oral rehydration solutions. When severe dehydration present, IV fluid replacement may be necessary
- Antidiarrheal agents for symptomatic relief *not recommended;* furthermore, opiate derivatives, including loperamide, diphenoxylate-atropine, contraindicated in severe bacterial gastroenteritis, because may exacerbate toxigenic illness
- Antimicrobial Tx may not be required by time stool culture result obtained if pt asymptomatic; symptomatic pts should be treated w/appropriate antibiotic (see table)

COMPLICATIONS

Organism	Complications
Campylobacter sp.	Reactive arthritis, mesenteric adenitis, toxic megacolon, Guillain-Barré syndrome
Clostridium difficile	Toxic megacolon
E. coli O157:H7	Hemolytic-uremic syndrome
Salmonella sp.	Bacteremia, reactive arthritis, osteomyelitis
Shigella sp.	Seizures, toxic megacolon, hemolytic-uremic syndrome, reactive arthritis

WHEN TO REFER

- Most pts managed w/o referral
- If stool culture and *C. difficile* toxin assay negative, persistent symptoms (≥10 d) warrant additional evaluation including consideration of sigmoidoscopy/colonoscopy

Antibiotic Selection in Infectious Diarrhea

Enteropathogen	Antibiotic
Aeromonas sp.	ampicillin, trimethoprim-sulfamethoxazole, or quinolone
Campylobacter sp.	erythromycin
V. cholerae	tetracycline, trimethoprim-sulfamethoxazole, or quinolone
C. difficile	metronidazole or vancomycin
Salmonella sp.*	ampicillin, amoxicillin, trimethoprim/sulfamethoxazole, or quinolone
Shigella sp.	ampicillin, trimethoprim/sulfamethoxazole, or quinolone

*Only in situations other than uncomplicated gastroenteritis, ie, in documented or suspected extraintestinal infection including sepsis, in pts who have undergone splenectomy, in an infant, or in immunocompromised host

BACKGROUND

• In US, Canada, Europe parasites most likely associated w/ diarrhea include protozoa *Giardia lamblia*, *Cryptosporidium*, *Entamoeba histolytica*. Infrequent or rare protozoal causes are *Cyclospora*, *Balantidium coli*, *Isospora belli*, perhaps *Blastocystis hominis* (debatable), and helminths, *Strongyloides stercoralis*, *Hymenelepsis nana*, *Trichinella spiralis*, *Capillaria philippinensis*
• Less common in children ≤6 mos of age
• Common children ≥6 mos of age who attend day-care centers or in institutions, have Hx travel to tropical or lesser developed areas, or have drunk fresh natural water while camping in wilderness areas, and in immunodeficient hosts
• Infections commonly "asymptomatic," esp in day-care settings
• Most infections mainly affect small intestine except for *E. histolytica*, which affects colon

CLINICAL MANIFESTATIONS

• Symptomatic infection associated w/ acute diarrhea; less commonly w/ persistent or chronic diarrhea (≥2 wks duration) w/ or w/o failure to thrive
• All parasites can cause acute onset, watery diarrhea (most common), w/ some mucus, colicky abdominal pain w/ or w/o vomiting; are usually afebrile but fever can occur; dehydration not typical but does occur. Most often diarrhea self-limited to 5–10 d, but in <10% of cases may continue to persistent diarrhea, w/ weight loss, growth retardation
• Bloody diarrhea found w/ *E. histolytica* and *Balantidium coli*
• Persistent diarrhea more common w/ *Crysptosporidium*, *G. Lamblia*, *Strongyloides*, *C. philippinensis*

• Pulmonary symptoms uncommon but can occur w/ *Strongyloides* (Loffler-like pneumonitis), *E. histolytica*, *Cryptosporidium*
• Muscle pain w/ *Trichinella*
• Itching w/ or w/o skin eruptions can occur (rarely) w/ *Strongyloides*, *Giardia*

LABORATORY FEATURES

• *Most frequently used (but relatively less sensitive) diagnostic tool for identifying parasites:* microscopic stool examination for presence of cysts, trophozoites, eggs, larvae. Two or 3 separate specimens should be examined
• Sampling upper small intestine contents by string test, endoscopy, or biopsy followed by microscopy ↑ diagnostic yield, esp for *strongyloides*. Proctoscopy w/ scrapings or biopsy increases yield for *E. histolytica* and *Balantidium coli* when stools negative by microscopy
• Stool ELISA, immunofluorescence, or counterimmunoelectrophoreses tests for *G. lamblia*, *Cryptosporidium*, and *E. histolytica* substantially increase diagnostic yield
• Presence or absence of WBCs, or blood in stools usually not helpful
• In more chronic cases, anemia can occur
• *WBC count and differential:* normal, except eosinophilia can occur w/ *Strongyloides*, *Trichinella*, *Isospora*
• Specific serologic antibody testing available but usually does not differentiate between current vs. past infections

DIFFERENTIAL DIAGNOSIS

• Other infectious causes of acute diarrhea (eg, viral, bacterial)
• Other causes of persistent or chronic diarrhea w/ or w/o growth failure (eg, cow milk allergy, celiac disease, inflammatory bowel disease, lactose intolerance)

TREATMENT

• No treatment indicated for asymptomatic carriers of *G. lamblia*
• See table

COMPLICATIONS

• *Strongyloides*: "hyperinfection" syndrome rare, involves larval dissemination to all organs w/ severe sepsislike symptoms, esp in immunocompromised hosts
• Persistent diarrhea, malabsorption (or failure to thrive) syndromes uncommon in developed countries but do occur; also protein-losing enteropathy
• *E. histolytica*: liver (rare lung) abscess, toxic megacolon, bowel perforation

PREVENTION

• Hygienic measures to prevent fecal-oral transmission (eg, handwashing)
• Filter, boil (3 min), or iodine-treat drinking water in wilderness areas

WHEN TO REFER

• Most pts managed w/o referral
• Recurrent infections
• Referral indicated if treatment fails, suggesting that parasite an "innocent bystander" not related to pt symptoms, or an underlying condition present (eg, immunodeficiency, or alternative medications needed)
• If serious complications develop (eg, amebic liver abscess, intestinal perforation, failure to thrive)

Protozoa	Recommended Tx
G. lamblia	metronidazole (15 mg/kg/d, max 750 mg/d × 7–10 d) most effective, but not officially approved for this use in US (also in US pediatric syrup not available); furazolidone (5 mg/kg/d × 7 d, max 400 mg/day). Also quinacrine, tinidazole (but not available in US)
B. coli	metronidazole, tetracycline
B. hominis	metronidazole
E. histolytica	diodohydroxquin (10 mg/kg/d, max 650 mg/d) × 20 d for noninvasive disease. For severe cases and/or invasive disease, metronidazole
Cyclospora	trimethopim: sulfamethoxazole (usual pediatric dose according to weight)
Isosporo belli	trimethopim: sulfamethoxazole
Cryptosporidium	No definitive Tx currently available, but agents are being tested

Helminths	Recommended Tx
Strongyloides	thiabendazole (25 mg/kg/d, max 1.5 g) × 3 d (uncomplicated infection) to 5–15 d (complicated infection)
T. spiralis	thiabendazole
H. nana	praziquantel, 25 mg/kg × 1 dose; niclosamide (<34 kg: 1g followed by 0.5 g/d × 6 d; >34 kg: 1.5 g followed by 1 g/d × 6 d)
C. philippinensis	mebendazole, 100 mg × 1 dose; albendazole, 40 mg × 1 dose (>2 yrs of age)

J. MARC RHOADS

BACKGROUND

- Diarrheal morbidity 3–5 billion episodes annually in children, worldwide
- Associated w/ 12% hospitalizations of American children <4 yrs of age
- *Etiologic agents producing diarrhea w/ dehydration in babies:* ~65% unknown, ~25% viral, ~9% bacterial, ~1% parasitic
- *Peak season:* November–April. Transmission fecal to oral (? aerosol for rotavirus)
- Of major viruses, rotavirus causes 50% of severe episodes
- Viruses associated w/ diarrhea in infants:
  – rotavirus
  – Norwalk agent
  – enteric adenovirus (types 40, 41)
  – calicivirus
  – astrovirus
  – cytomegalovirus
  – coronavirus

PATHOPHYSIOLOGY

- Virus invades enterocytes on villi, resulting in cell death, villus sloughing
- Crypt cells proliferate to regenerate villi, initially w/ low disaccharidase activity and reduced active transport. Therefore, diarrhea malabsorptive (not secretory)
- Site of infection small bowel for all viruses except CMV, which invades colon in immunocompromised. "Gastroenteritis" misnomer because stomach spared. In CMV colitis, diarrhea similar to dysentery, w/ blood and mucus in stool
- Rotaviral N5P (a nonstructural protein produces chloride secretion by intracellular Ca^{++} signaling

CLINICAL MANIFESTATIONS

- Incubation usually <48 h. Initially vomiting occurs in 90–100% cases rotavirus enteritis, perhaps less in most other viral enteridites. Subsequently, diarrhea lasts ~5 d. Fever: 80%
- Norwalk enteritis differs; produces vomiting in 85% but diarrhea in <50%
- *Dehydration:* usually isotonic, occurs in 10% rotavirus-infected children, probably less in other viral infections
- Diaper rash due to carbohydrate malabsorption, w/ resulting increased fermentation to fatty acids in colon

LABORATORY FEATURES

- Blood work typically shows metabolic acidosis w/ HCO_3 ~15 mEq/L, BUN ~18
- Stool Na 30–40 mEq/L, K ~45 mEq/L (vs. normal stools w/ Na ~10, K ~35 mEq/L and vs. secretory diarrhea, w/ Na ~75, K ~20 mEq/L)

Differential Diagnosis

Fecal Exam	Appearance	Hemoccult	Fecal Leukocytes	Stool-Reducing Substances
Bacterial colitis	mucoid	+	+	−
Viral enteritis	watery	−	−	+

- Rotavirus detected by ELISA assay, latex agglutination, or PCR. For conventional ELISA, fecal blood can produce false positive test. Other viruses detectable by electronic microscopy (expensive), or molecular tests not presently commercially available

TREATMENT OF INFANT VIRAL DIARRHEA

- Oral rehydration solutions (ORS):
  – efficacy based in glucose-coupled Na^+ absorption in virus-infected bowel
  – all commercially available, solutions in US (Pedialyte, Rehydralyte, Ricelyte, Resol) adequate; some available in packets cheaper (Cerealyte, WHO packets). "Sports" solutions (Gatorade) have low Na:glucose ratio, but acceptable in those >3 yrs of age
  – new hypo-osmolar ORS (~240 mOsmolar) preferable in 2 published trials
- Refeeding:
  – only 6–12 hrs oral rehydration necessary under most circumstances. Early refeeding of regular diet, esp "meat and potatoes," advised
  – subsequently, regular diet plus ORS to replace ongoing losses after rehydration
  – lactose can be resumed in ~80% infants; if not tolerated, formulas which contain corn syrup solids indicated
- New approaches:
  – oral immunoglobulins (IVIG): 300 mg/kg, one dose. Shortens diarrheal symptoms by 2 d and rotavirus excretion by 3 d. Expensive
  – lactic acid bacteria ("probiotics") (*Lactobacilli casei GG, L. reuterii*). Shown in several European studies to ↓ duration of diarrhea and number of stools 40–50%. Not yet commercially available in US
  – drugs: no indication. Mineral clays (attapulgite, smectite) available OTC, safe, improve fecal consistency. Should not be substitute for ORS

COMPLICATIONS

- Dehydration (10% rotavirus-infected infants)
- Chronic diarrhea (esp infants <3 mos of age)
- *Rare complications reported w/ rotavirus enteritis:* protein-losing enteropathy w/ edema, hypoglycemia, hemorrhagic shock and encelopathy, seizures, encephalitis, intussusception, methemoglobinemia, Reye syndrome, acholic stools

PREVENTION

- Breast feeding has shown beneficial effect in most studies
- *Vaccine:* US rotavirus vaccine efficacy testing recently found that tetravalent vaccine produced ~90% seroconversion rate and ~55% protection from diarrhea. Cost-effectiveness analysis predicts vaccine would save money and decrease hospitalizations in US, but vaccine results disappointing in developing countries
- *Complications:* Vaccine recently recalled because of possible association with increased rate of intussusception.

WHEN TO REFER

- Diarrhea persisting >2 wks in infants (excluding toddlers w/ high fruit juice intake)
- No weight gain in infants <6 mos of age after ~10 d elemental diet (may require NG feeding)

GASTROESOPHAGEAL REFLUX

SUSAN R. ORENSTEIN

BACKGROUND

- *Two age-related forms:* infantile, childhood (latter similar to adult form)

- *Epidemiology:* of all infants, 50% regurgitate ≥2×/d; 20% of parents consider it problem; 7% seek medical attention; 5% resolve w/minimal Tx, no testing; ~2% (or more, currently) receive phar- macotherapy; ~0.4% require fundoplication. Of older children, 0.4–5% manifest reflux disease 1–18 yrs of age. More frequent in children w/neu- rologic or respiratory disease

CLINICAL MANIFESTATIONS

	Infantile	Childhood
Age	<12 mos	>12 mos
Peak incidence	2–4 mos	Random?
Course	Resolve by 8–18 mos (~90%)	Chronic, relapsing (~50%)
Sex	Slight male preponderance	Slight male preponderance
Symptoms	Regurgitation: vomiting, poor weight gain	Esophagitis: heartburn, chest pain, epigastric pain, odynophagia, *dysphagia, hematemesis, anemia, regurgitation*
	Esophagitis: crying, poor intake, *hematemesis, anemia, dysphagia*	
	Airway reflexes or aspiration: apnea, choking, stridor, *bronchospasm, aspiration pneumonia*	Airway reflexes or aspiration: asthma exacerbation, *hoarseness, stridor*
	Neurobehavioral: arching, *Sandifer's syndrome*	Neurobehavioral: *Sandifer's syndrome*

Uncommon symptoms italicized.

DIFFERENTIAL DIAGNOSIS

- Regurgitation, vomiting:
  - central vomiting center: drugs, toxins, meta-bolic disease
  - supramedullary receptors: overfeeding, air feeding, baby bouncing, ↑ ICP
  - peripheral receptors:
    - pharyngeal: gag reflex (eg, postnasal drip)
    - other esophageal: structural (eg, stric-ture, stenosis), functional (eg, achalasia)
    - gastric: peptic ulcer disease, dysmotility, obstruction (eg, pyloric stenosis)
    - intestinal: infection, nutrient intolerance (eg, cow, soy, eosinophilic gastroenteropathy), ob-struction (eg, web, volvulus, intussusception, Hirschsprung)
    - other: urinary infection, sepsis, pancre-atitis, peritonitis, hepatobiliary, pregnancy, psy-chogenic (bulimia, rumination, etc)
- Esophagitis symptoms:
  - infants: many causes of nonspecific irritabil-ity in infants: "colic", parent-infant dysfunction, nutrient intolerance, otitis, etc
  - older children: inflammatory, motor abnor-malities of upper GI tract: peptic ulcer disease, 1° esophageal dysmotility, etc
- Airway symptoms:
  - apnea: apnea of prematurity, pertussis or other URI, sepsis, seizure, other neurologic dis-ease, metabolic disease, Munchausen-by-proxy, etc
    - other respiratory symptoms:
      - extrinsic compression (eg, vascular ring)
      - intrinsic obstruction (eg, malformation, foreign body, cyst, tumor)
      - airways reactive to other stimuli (eg, al-lergens, infection)
      - infection, inflammation, cystic fibrosis, pertussis, asthma, other ·
      - aspiration during swallowing, rather than during reflux
- Neurologic symptoms:
  - seizures
  - dystonic reactions
  - vestibular disorders
  - pertussis

EVALUATION

- *Regurgitation, vomiting:* requires *GI radiogra-phy,* to r/o malrotation, other anatomic/obstruc-tive causes, not to "diagnose reflux." CBC w/dif-ferential (for eosinophilia), IgE w/food RASTs useful to screen for allergic causes

- *Esophagitis symptoms: endoscopy and esophageal biopsies* (or *blind suction esophageal biopsy* in infants w/o hematemesis). CBC to screen for anemia; rectal exam to screen for esophageal bleeding. Dysphagia in absence of esophagitis requires *barium esophagram*
- *Airway symptoms: esophageal biopsies* can di-agnose esophagitis, provide presumptive evidence for causation of respiratory symptoms, prompt Tx. *24 hour pH probe* documents abnormal quan-tity of reflux; occasionally temporal linkage of symptoms w/esophageal acidification. *Linked pH probe w/pneumogram* (including nasal airflow channel) identifies abnormal reflux, reflux-linked bradycardia/apnea. *Modified Bernstein test* (esophageal acid infusion) more rigorously shows esophageal acidification causes symptoms. *Gas-troesophageal scintigraphy* shows aspiration
- *Neurobehavioral symptoms: esophageal biop-sies* function as for airway symptoms
- *Trial of therapy—all symptoms: formula thicken-ing* (see later) improves infant regurgitation, weight. Avoidance of supine, seated *positions* in infants, *smoke exposure,* also useful. If thickening unsuccess-ful, or if crying/feeding refusal, suspect formula aller-gy, rice cereal–thickened *elemental formula* (Pregesta-mil, Alimentum) ×2 wks. *Antacid* doses can test whether crying/chest pain due to esophagitis
- Pharmacotherapy prior to investigation debat-ed. Trial of Tx may be cost effective for all except airway symptoms. (Improvement in airway symp-toms requires prolonged, aggressive Tx; therapeu-tic trial inefficient diagnostically, may delay Dx.) Empiric Tx *requires* prior careful consideration of differential Dx. Prokinetic should not be used in vomiting child w/o prior radiography to prove ab-sence of partial/intermittent obstruction. If no clear benefit within few wks or resolution in 2–3 mos, stop empiric Tx, except in markedly improv-ing infants, who might be continued several months more until resolution, if carefully followed

TREATMENT

- *Basic:*

	Infant	Child
	Rice cereal (1T rice/oz formula = >30 cal/oz)	Avoid carbonated, acid drinks
	Avoid seated, supine position	Treat obesity
		Fast before bed
	Avoid tocacco smoke exposure	Elevate head of bed
		Avoid tobacco smoke exposure

- *Prokinetic:* use in most pediatric reflux dis-ease—first step in pharmacotherapy
  - cisapride, 0.2 mg/kg/dose qid:
    - advantages: no extrapyramidal effects; no respiratory effects
    - concurrent use of -azole or -mycin antibi-otics may produce lethal arrhythmias
  - alternatives: metoclopramide, 0.1 mg/kg/dose qid; bethanechol
- *Acid-suppressing:* use in addition to prokinetic when esophagitis present
  - cimetidine, 10 mg/kg/dose qid:
    - advantages: generic availability reduces cost; qid dosing mimics prokinetic dosing
  - alternatives: ranitidine, etc (less frequent dosing offset by greater expense); omeprazole, etc (more potent; more expensive; long-term risks un-known)
- *Surgical:* in life-threatening or complicated re-flux, or w/gastrostomy or hiatal hernia
  - Nissen fundoplication:
    - advantages: usually eliminates reflux
    - disadvantages: immediate surgical risks. Later "gas bloat," dumping, retching. May become incompetent after months to years, esp if retching occurs
  - alternatives: gastrojejunostomy feedings (allow acid reflux). Incomplete-wrap fundoplica-tions (not better than pharmacotherapy). Chronic pharmacotherapy

COMPLICATIONS

- Hematemesis, stricture, Barrett esophagus, adenocarcinoma

WHEN TO REFER

- When specialized testing required (endoscopy, biopsy, pH probe, etc)
- When pharmacotherapy unsuccessful/cannot be withdrawn within 2 mos
- When complications suspected/surgical Tx (fundoplication) contemplated

GREGORY A. MENCIO

BACKGROUND

• *Most common causes of angular malalignment:* physiologic knock knees (valgus)/bow legs (varus): differentiation: facilitated by understanding natural Hx of tibio-femoral angle development:
 – maximum lateral bowing (genu varum 10–15°): birth
 – maximum valgus angulation (10–15°): 20–22 mos
 – resolution to physiologic valgus (7–9°): by age 7–8 yrs
• Pathologic genu varum/valgum: angulation > mean + 2 SDs
• Classification:
 – apparent deformity: fat thighs (valgus); rotational malalignment
 – physiologic malalignment: knock knees; bow legs
 – pathologic deformity:
  ○ idiopathic: tibia vara (Blount "disease"); unresolved physiologic valgus
  ○ post-traumatic: malunion; asymmetric physeal arrest; proximal metaphyseal tibial fracture (usually valgus deformity)
  ○ metabolic: rickets (varus more common); renal osteodystrophy (valgus most common)
  ○ infectious (osteomyelitis)
  ○ neuromuscular disorders: cerebral palsy; spina bifida
  ○ generalized disorders: inflammatory arthritis; osteochondrodysplasia; osteogenesis imperfecta
• *Most common cause pathologic genu varum:* tibia vara (Blount disease) (growth disturbance of posteromedial juxtaphyseal region proximal tibia)
• Trauma most common cause pathologic genu valgum

CLINICAL MANIFESTATIONS

• Bow legs/knock knees:
 – usually bilateral/symmetric; stature normal
 – gestational, birth, developmental Hx normal
 – growth pattern, dietary Hx normal
 – resolving deformity
• Genu varum/valgum:
 – often unilateral
 – deformity progressive
 – may have Hx trauma, infection, dietary deficiency, systemic illness

• Physical examination:
 – pathologic angular deformity: typically > 90th weight (tibia vara, idiopathic genu valgum)/lower percentiles (< 25th) of height (osteochondrodysplasias, metabolic causes)
 – infant fat masks varus/accentuates valgus malalignment
 – internal tibial torsion often accompanies/accentuates genu varum appearance
 – external tibial torsion/pes planus ("flatfoot") causes excessive valgus loading of the knee/potentiates genu valgum development
 – combination femoral anteversion/external tibial torsion can create genu valgus ("pseudovalgus") appearance
 – angulation assessed by tibiofemoral angle/linear measurement of intermalleolar (valgus)/intercondylar (varus) distance goniometric measurement

RADIOGRAPHIC FEATURES

• Indications for x rays:
 – children w/ short stature (< 25th centile)
 – asymmetric involvement
 – progressive deformity:
  ○ varus angulation >25°, pt >24 mos old
  ○ valgus angulation >15–20°, intermalleolar distance >8 cm, pt > 4 yrs old
• *Lower extremity standing AP radiograph* (hips, knees, ankles): angular alignment measurement/evaluation of osseous, physeal pathology
• *Proximal tibial metaphyseal-diaphyseal angle (MDA) measurement:* differentiation between extreme physiologic genu varum/early Blount disease (MDA rarely >11° in physiologic varus)
• Tibiofemoral angle *(anatomic axis)* good way to track deformity progression
• Measurement of hip, knee, ankle joint orientation relative to weight-bearing axis of extremity *(mechanical axis)* more accurate way to determine site/severity of deformity when considering surgical intervention
• Location of deformity (metaphyseal, diaphyseal, juxtaarticular) varies w/ underlying etiology:
 – idiopathic varus (tibia vara) deformity typically located in proximal metaphyseal/juxtaarticular region of tibia
 – idiopathic valgus usually caused by deformity in distal femur
 – other pathologic causes of angular malalignment may affect any region of tibia/femur in focal (post-traumatic, infectious)/generalized (rickets, osteochondrodystrophies) pattern

TREATMENT

• *Options:* no treatment, medical management, bracing, surgery (hemiepiphysiodesis/osteotomy)
• *No treatment:* children w/ angular malalignment due to physiologic bow legs/knock knees
• Brace treatment effective for young children w/ lesser degrees of angular deformity due to tibia vara/idiopathic genu valgum (indications for orthotic management nebulous/pt compliance generally poor)
• Indications for surgical treatment:
 – varus deformity (TFA) >25° progressive/unresolving, age >24 mos
 – valgus deformity (TFA) >15°, intermalleolar distance >10 cm, age >10 yrs
 – residual deformity following infection/trauma
 – residual deformity associated w/ metabolic disorders
• Surgical treatment options:
 – partial epiphysiodesis (permanent)
 – hemiepiphyseal stapling (potentially reversible)
  ○ both procedures create growth arrest in physis opposite apex of angular deformity
  ○ correction predicated on growth of contralateral half of physis/est 1°/mm linear growth
  ○ stapling preferable when skeletal growth not predictable (ie, in metabolic disorders)
 – osteotomy:
  ○ most common correction method
  ○ performed at any age/only option after skeletal maturity

WHEN TO REFER

• Most children managed w/o referral
• Investigation for underlying systemic/metabolic disorders performed for children w/ short stature (< 25th centile) and angular deformity
• Referral indicated:
 – asymmetric involvement
 – progressive/persistent deformity
  ○ varus >25°, age >18 mos
  ○ valgus >15°, intermalleolar distance >8 cm, age >4 yrs

BACKGROUND

- Very common in infants and children
- Highest incidence in children 1–3 yrs of age
- Most commonly infectious process
- Viral etiology most frequent including Herpes simplex virus (HSV) and Coxsackie virus, other enteroviruses
- Most cases self-limiting; in immunocompromised pts, cases may be severe
- Other causes include bacteria, fungal, trauma, autoimmune disorders, vitamin deficiencies, immune dysfunctions

CLINICAL MANIFESTATIONS

- Painful erosions, ulcers, blisters affecting buccal, gingival, labial, lingual mucosa
- Gums may become mildly swollen, red, ulcerated, bleed easily
- Many w/fever, refusal to eat, irritability, fetid odor, increased salivation, cervical adenopathy
- W/viral etiology, oral lesions often persist well after resolution of constitutional symptoms

LABORATORY/DIAGNOSTICS

- Normal CBC or virally suppressed values most common finding
- Positive Tzanck preparation in HSV infections
- If Dx necessary for immunocompromised pt, rapid EIA antigen detection for HSV available (Kodak SureCell Herpes Kit, Rochester, NY, w/specificity 100%, sensitivity 82–95%)
- Biopsy to r/o pemphigus in complicated, protracted cases
- Gram stain or culture can show spirochete, fusobacteria in necrotizing stomatitis

DIFFERENTIAL DIAGNOSIS

- *Vincent infection (acute necrotizing ulcerative gingivostomatitis, or ANUG): bacterial involving spirochetes and/or fusobacteria*
- Aphthous stomatitis (probable autoimmune mechanism)
- Thrush (candidiasis)
- Chemical burns (alkali, acid, or heat)
- Trauma
- Erythema multiforme or Stevens-Johnson
- *Neutrophilic disorders:* cyclic neutropenia or leukocyte adhesion disorders
- Crohn disease
- Behçet disease
- Systemic lupus erythematous (SLE)
- Pemphigus
- Reiter disease
- Vitamin C deficiency

TREATMENT

- Most often gingivostomatitis self-limiting, needs only symptomatic Tx, close attention to hydration status
- Cool fluids, popsicles, avoidance of acidic, salty/spicy foods most helpful
- Acetaminophen po
- For aphthous ulcers, treatment w/Aphthasol (amlexanox oral paste): apply to erosions qid at first notice of symptoms; continue until ulcers healed (up to 10 d)
- For aphthous ulcers, use topical steroids qid, eg, triamcinolone acetonide 0.1% in Orabase gel
- Other pain relief concoctions include viscous lidocaine 2%, diphenhydramine, liquid antacid compounded in 1:1:1 ratio. Use in children old enough *not* to swallow the solution. It may be swabbed directly to sores/used as "swish and spit" q3–4h as needed for pain
- For ANUG, penicillin or erythromycin in age/weight appropriate doses ×5–7 d used as well as mouth/gum debridement, application 10% carbamide peroxide in anhydrous glycerol qid, or 3% hydrogen peroxide diluted one-half w/warm water rinsing mouth q2–3h
- For cyclic neutropenia, G-CSF has been found to have good clinical response w/resolution of recurrent stomatitis
- For oral candidiasis, nystatin suspension 200,000 units applied topically or swished qid usually efficacious
- Candidiasis can also be treated w/Diflucan (flucanazole) suspension (10 mg/ml or 40 mg/ml) at dosage of 6 mg/kg qd for day 1, followed by 3 mg/kg qd for up to 2 wks. Drug cannot be used concomitantly w/cisapride; for some pts, GI side effects intolerable
- For recurrent HSV gingivostomatitis, some studies support use of oral acyclovir (15 mg/kg 5×/d × 7d) if Tx can be initiated within first 48 hrs of symptoms

COMPLICATIONS

- *Most common:* refusal to eat/drink w/resulting dehydration. Small percentage of children require IV rehydration
- ANUG can be severe, requiring extensive debridement, gingivectomy
- Other complications have more to do w/underlying 1° process, eg, collagen vascular diseases/autoimmune problems/neutrophil dysfunctions
- Intraoral burns, trauma can leave scars

PREVENTION

- Because most common causes of gingivostomatitis are viral infections, prevention best maintained by strict hand washing, no direct contact w/lesions, no sharing of cups, utensils, etc

WHEN TO REFER

- Refractory, persistent episodes, those cases w/complications/Hx consistent w/systemic disorders

CLASSIFICATION

- Congenital (1°) glaucoma
- 2° glaucomas of childhood:
  - associated w/ocular abnormalities:
    - ○ anterior segment dysgenesis (Axenfeld-Rieger syndrome)
    - ○ aniridia (iris and foveal hypoplasia, nystagmus)
    - ○ aphakia (after congenital cataract extraction)
    - ○ tumors (eg, retinoblastoma)
    - ○ uveitis (eg, juvenile rheumatoid arthritis)
  - associated w/systemic syndromes, eg:
    - ○ Sturge-Weber syndrome
    - ○ neurofibromatosis
    - ○ Marfan syndrome

BACKGROUND

- *Incidence of congenital glaucoma:* 1/10,000 births
- *Inheritance:* usually sporadic, occasionally autosomal recessive
- Typical age of onset:
  - congenital glaucoma: birth–early infancy
  - 2° glaucoma: birth–age 10
- Usually bilateral (two-thirds of cases), but can have asymmetric involvement
- *Etiology of congenital glaucoma:* 1° maldevelopment of trabecular meshwork

CLINICAL MANIFESTATIONS

- Typically noted by primary care physician:
  - corneal enlargement (< age 2)
  - corneal clouding
  - excessive tearing
  - light sensitivity
  - blepharospasm
  - enlarged cup-to-disc ratio of optic nerve (may be reversible)
- Typically noted by ophthalmologist:
  - corneal (Haab) striae
  - ↑ intraocular pressure
  - ↑ axial length of eye
  - myopia w/or w/o astigmatism

DIFFERENTIAL DIAGNOSIS OF SIGNS

- *Corneal enlargement (buphthalmos):* 1° megalocornea
- *Corneal clouding:* keratitis, corneal dystrophy, storage disease, birth trauma
- *Excessive tearing:* nasolacrimal duct obstruction, iritis
- *Light sensitivity:* corneal disease or abrasion, iritis

TREATMENT

- Always in concert w/an ophthalmologist
- Medical treatment:
  - useful as temporizing measure until surgery in congenital glaucoma
  - often the preferred treatment in 2° types of childhood glaucoma
- Surgical treatment:
  - generally preferred to medical Tx in cases of congenital glaucoma
  - types of surgery:
    - ○ goniotomy: incision through trabecular meshwork from internal approach
    - ○ trabeculotomy: incision through trabecular meshwork from external approach
    - ○ trabeculectomy: creation of filtering bleb through sclera
    - ○ Seton (Ahmed, Molteno, Baerveldt) implant: placement in anterior chamber of tube connected to external reservoir
    - ○ cyclodestructive procedures: destruction of ciliary body to reduce aqueous production using laser/cryotherapy
  - success rate of goniotomy/trabeculotomy in congenital glaucoma 80–90% w/one/more procedures

Medication Class	Examples	Ocular/Local Side Effects	Systemic Side Effects
Beta-adrenergic antagonists	Timolol (Timoptic)	Ocular irritation	Depression, behavioral changes
	Betaxalol (Betoptic)	Visual disturbances	Arrhythmias, bradycardia
			Bronchospasm, dyspnea
			Masked hypoglycemia (diabetics)
			Dizziness
Carbonic anhydrase inhibitors	Dorzolamide (Trusopt)	Ocular irritation	Bitter taste
	Brinzolamide (Azopt)	Corneal changes	Headache, nausea, fatigue
		Blurred vision	Skin rash
Oral carbonic anhydrase inhibitors	Acetazolamide (Diamox)	Transient myopia	Taste alteration
	Methazolamide (Neptazane)		Parasthesias in extremities
			Nausea, vomiting, diarrhea
			Fatigue
			Renal calculi
			Stevens-Johnson syndrome
			Aplastic anemia
Prostaglandin analogue	Latanoprost (Xalatan)	Increased iris pigmentation	Muscle/joint/back pain
		Excessive eyelash growth	
Alpha-adrenergic agonist	Apraclonidine (Iopidine)	Redness	Bradycardia, heart palpitations
		Pupillary dilation	
Adrenergic agonist	Dipivefrin (Propine)	Conjunctivitis	Tachycardia, arrhythmias
		Conjunctival deposits	Hypertension
Cholinergic agonist	Pilocarpine (IsoptoCarpine, Pilocar)	Induced myopia	Headache
		Pupillary constriction	
		Retinal tears and detachment	

COMPLICATIONS

- Loss of vision
- Progressive corneal enlargement
- Nystagmus
- High myopia
- Anisometropia (difference in refractive error between eyes)
- Amblyopia

WHEN TO REFER

- All pts suspected of glaucoma should be referred to ophthalmologist w/experience in treatment of glaucoma in children

DEFINITION

• Inflammatory diseases of kidney; inflammation in most cases immunologically mediated/initially starts in glomerulus but frequently progresses to involve other components (tubules, interstitium, blood vessels) of renal parenchyma; clinically divided into acute/chronic

ACUTE GN

• Refers both to onset/duration; thus sudden onset/short duration
• Almost all cases due to poststreptococcal GN; poststrept GN develops in susceptible individuals following infection w/only few strains of streptococci (nephritogenic strains)
• *Common sites of infection:* respiratory tract (most often pharyngitis)/skin (impetigo); latent period between strept infection/onset of GN usually ~10 d w/pharyngitis/3 wks w/impetigo

CLINICAL MANIFESTATIONS

• Primarily disease of school-age children w/no predilection for males/females
• Typically sudden onset of painless gross hematuria (tea- or cola-colored urine), edema, hypertension, acute renal failure; important to note that gross hematuria always occurs after latent period/not at time of infection
• Hypertension may produce hypertensive encephalopathy w/headache, nosebleeds, seizures; some may present in pulmonary edema
• Not all pts exposed to nephritogenic streptococci develop clinical GN

LABORATORY FINDINGS

• *UA:* pathognomonic triad of GN, ie, hematuria, proteinuria, abnormal casts; RBC, WBC, granular casts may all be present; RBC generally show dysmorphism (as opposed to normal morphology seen in nonglomerular hematuria); degree of proteinuria variable but urine w/gross hematuria tests 4+ on dipstick test
• Evidence of recent strept infection, ie, positive culture for group A strept from throat/impetigo lesions; positive serologic tests for streptococcal antibodies such as steptozyme, high ASO anti-DNase B anti-hyaluronidase, rising titers of these antibodies in serum
• Low serum C3 complement level
• Serum chemistries may show normal BUN, creatinine/various grades of renal failure ranging from mild–severe (in some cases w/rapidly progressive form of poststrept GN)
• Nephrotic syndrome is rare (7%)

DIAGNOSIS

• Dx suspected in pt who presents w/above clinical/laboratory findings; strengthened if clinical course of progressive resolution of renal failure, hypertension, urinary findings in few days/normalization of serum C3 complement in 8–10 wks
• Renal biopsy not needed in most cases

DIFFERENTIAL DIAGNOSIS

• All other chronic GN can present w/gross hematuria, edema, hypertension, renal failure; many pts w/chronic GN may be asymptomatic/may develop gross hematuria flare-up of underlying chronic GN w/intercurrent illness including streptococcal infection; one differentiating feature: in chronic GN the gross hematuria occurs during infection (pharyngitis)/not after latent period when infection has cleared as in poststrept GN; typical example: IgA nephropathy where recurrent episodes of gross hematuria occur at time when pt has pharyngitis
• If serum complement does not become normal in 10 wks, suspect chronic GN

MANAGEMENT

• Hospitalize all pts w/hypertension, renal failure, hypertensive encephalopathy, pulmonary edema; pts w/hypertension may be treated prior to transport to hospital w/hydralizine 0.02 mg/kg IM or nefidipine 0.1 mg/kg orally; liquid contents of nefidipine capsule can be drawn into syringe/given orally
• Other pts may be managed as outpts/must be seen qd because hypertension/renal failure may develop quickly
• If culture positive for Streptococci, pt should be treated w/antibiotics (penicillin/erythromycin in pts allergic to penicillin) × 10 d

COURSE

• *Course:* progressive improvement of all clinical features; renal failure, hypertension, gross hematuria, edema resolve in few days, but microscopic hematuria/proteinuria resolve over weeks to months/in some cases microscopic hematuria can persist up to 2 yrs; in most cases proteinuria resolves before microhematuria; complete recovery occurs in >95% of cases

WHEN TO REFER TO NEPHROLOGIST

• All hospitalized pts
• When Dx not supported by clinical/laboratory features, clinical course
• Serum complement does not become normal in 10 wks

CHRONIC GLOMERULONEPHRITIS

CLASSIFICATION

• *Primary/idiopathic:* etiology not known; based on characteristic histopathology, following major entities have been recognized:
  – IgA nephropathy
  – membranoproliferative GN (MPGN)
  – membranous nephropathy
  – focal proliferative GN
  – diffuse proliferative GN
  – rapidly progressive GN
• *Secondary:* some knowledge of etiology exists; following major groups recognized:
  – associated w/*multisystem disease:* systemic lupus erythematosus (SLE), Henoch-Schönlein purpura (HSP), other collagen vascu-

lar diseases such as polyarteritis nodosa/other vasculitides associated w/antineutrophil antibodies (ANCA) (Wagner granulomatosis, etc), Goodpasture syndrome
  – associated w/*chronic infections:* hepatitis B/C, HIV, congenital syphilis, subacute bacterial endocarditis, ventriculoatrial shunts for hydrocephalus (shunt nephritis), parasitic (malaria, schistosomiasis, filaria, etc)
  – associated w/certain *drugs* (captopril, penicillamine, gold salts, "street heroin," etc)
  – *hereditary* GN (Alport syndrome, familial hematuria)

CLINICAL MANIFESTATIONS

• Asymptomatic (hypertension, microhematuria, proteinuria detected by chance)
• Edema
• Gross hematuria
• Hypertension
• Similar to acute GN
• Features of chronic renal failure (anemia, renal osteodystrophy, growth failure)
• Features of conditions associated w/2° GN (SLE, HSP, etc)
• Family Hx chronic renal failure/nerve deafness (Alport syndrome)

LABORATORY FINDINGS

• Abnormal UA (hematuria, proteinuria, abnormal casts in sediment)
• Abnormal quantitative proteinuria (protein/creatinine ratio >0.2 on spot urine)
• Abnormal serum chemistries (↑ BUN/creatinine, metabolic acidosis, high phosphorus, low calcium, low total proteins/albumin, high cholesterol, lipids)
• Normal/low serum C3 complement (SLE, MPGN, hepatitis B, SBE shunt nephritis); positive serologic tests: anti-nuclear antibody (SLE), hepatitis B surface antigen (hepatitis B), serology for syphilis (congenital syphilis), antiglomerular basement antibody (Goodpasture syndrome), ANCA (certain vasculitides)

DIAGNOSIS

• Dx suspected from above clinical findings but usually requires renal biopsy; important that renal biopsy performed in an institution where expertise exists in pediatric nephrology/renal pathology including light, immunofluorescence, electron microscopy

MANAGEMENT

• Management of chronic GN complex/best left to nephrologist; usually involves use of immunosuppressive drugs (corticosteroids, cyclophosphamide, chlorambucil, azathioprine, cyclosporine), antihypertensive drugs, diuretics; may also require use of 1,25 dihydroxy vitamin D_3, phosphate binders, alkali supplements, potassium-lowering agents, recombinant erythropoietin, dietary changes; some cases may need dialysis/plasmaphoresis (Goodpasture syndrome)

WHEN TO REFER

• All pts referred to pediatric nephrologist

BACKGROUND

• Infections caused by *Neisseria gonorrhoeae* uncommon in children and common in sexually active adolescents and adults. Acquired by sexual contact and, if found in children, sexual abuse evaluation must be performed

CLINICAL MANIFESTATIONS

• Asymptomatic or symptomatic
• Most commonly, endocervicitis in adolescent females, vaginitis in female children, urethritis in males
• Pelvic inflammatory disease
• Bacteremia w/ nonerythematous or hemorrhagic papular skin lesions, esp on hands
• Arthritis and tendonitis
• Pharyngitis and proctitis (often asymptomatic)
• Perihepatitis
• Conjunctivitis
• Meningitis and endocarditis (rare)

LABORATORY EVALUATION

• Cultures and rapid tests:
– children: swab vagina (not endocervix), urethra (males), pharynx, rectum for culture. *Do not* do rapid test such as DNA probe or enzyme immunoassay test
– adolescents and adults: swab endocervix, urethra (males), pharynx, and/or rectum depending on Hx for culture or do rapid test
• Culturing technique:
– streak swab on warm selective media such as modified Thayer-Martin agar or selective carrying media and incubate at 37% in CO_2 jar or in 5–10% CO_2
– have culture evaluated by laboratory. Use at least two confirmatory bacteriologic tests using different principles (ie, biochemical, enzyme substrate, or serology)

when identifying strains from children. Also, in children, save strain for further identification if necessary

DIFFERENTIAL DIAGNOSIS

• Other causes of vaginitis and urethritis such as:
– *Chlamydia trachomatis*
– *Ureaplasma urealyticum*
– *Trichomonas vaginalis*
– group A streptococcus
– bacterial vaginosis
– *Candida* spp.
– chemical vaginitis
– *Herpes simplex* virus

TREATMENT

• Children <9 yrs of age and <45 kg:
– nondisseminated infections: vulvovaginitis, urethritis, proctitis, or pharyngitis:
  ○ ceftriaxone, 125 mg once, given IV or IM. For IM injection, use lidocaine 1% as diluent because injection painful
– disseminated infections such as ophthalmia, peritonitis, bacteremia, arthritis, meningitis, and endocarditis:
  ○ ceftriaxone, 50 mg/kg/d (max 1 g) in 1 dose/d IV or IM × 7–14 d. For meningitis, treat × 10–14 d. For endocarditis, treat at least 28 d
• Older children, adolescents, adults:
– nondisseminated infections such as asymptomatic and symptomatic vaginitis, proctitis, urethritis, or pharyngitis should be treated w/ any of these choices:
  ○ ceftriaxone, 125 mg IM in single dose (lidocaine 1% may be used as diluent to prevent pain)
    ○ cefixime, 400 mg po as single dose
    ○ ciprofloxacin, 500 mg po as single dose
    ○ ofloxacin, 400 mg po as single dose

• Other considerations:
– also treat possibility of coexisting *Chlamydia trachomatis* infection w/ doxycycline, 100 mg/dose bid × 7 d or azithromycin, 1 g po in single dose
– use ceftriaxone or ciprofloxacin for gonococcal pharyngitis
– in pregnant women, use ceftriaxone
– spectinomycin, 2 g IM in single dose may be used in pts allergic to penicillin who do not have gonococcal pharyngitis
– disseminated infections such as bacteremia, arthritis, tenosynovitis, hepatitis should be treated with one of following regimens:
  ○ for disseminated infections other than meningitis or endocarditis, treat w/ one of following until patient improving for 24–45 h: ceftriaxone, 1 g IV q8h, cefotaxime, 1 g IV q8h, ceftizoxime, 1 g IV q8h, spectinomycin, 2 g IM q12h
  ○ if allergic to above antibiotics then switch to finish 7–10 d of total Tx w/ one of following: cefixime, 400 mg/dose po bid, ciprofloxacin, 500 mg/dose po bid
  ○ for meningitis and endocarditis, get expert help
• Prophylaxis for adolescents who have been sexually assaulted:
– ceftriaxone, 125 mg IM once plus metronidazole, 2 g po once *plus* doxycycline, 100 mg po bid × 7 d or azithromycin, 1g po once. Don't use doxycycline if pregnant
– other considerations:
  ○ contacts must be identified, evaluated, reported, treated
• Prevention:
– abstinence or condoms

BACKGROUND

• Grief reaction in child and in family normal expected emotional response to sudden loss or separation, or to repeated and chronic painful or traumatic experience

• Children grieve in their own special way depending on developmental and cognitive level and cultural or religious background of family. Younger children have more somatic complaints; older children are more emotional

• Grief may take place over considerable amount of time and usually revisited or reawakened by child at each stage of development through adolescence

• Grief 2° to loss affects whole family and aspects of community esp peer relationships of grieving child in school, clubs, other social/religious groups

• High level of family cohesion and adaptability (esp parents) related to better outcomes in children

• If not addressed well, grief reactions can lead to significant clinical depression

• Family rituals (cultural and religious) very important in management of grief work

• Children can and should attend all rituals including funerals if child wishes to attend and family supports exist

CLINICAL MANIFESTATIONS

• *Young children:* tantrums, crying, protesting, subdued withdrawal, quiet, fussy, resistant to authority, problems w/ appetite, sleep disturbances, regression (bed-wetting), headache, stomachache, musculoskeletal complaints

• *School age:* depression, indifference, markedly angry, denial or avoidance, guilty, some somatic symptoms of headache, stomachache. Poor school performance

• *Adolescents:* more intense feelings of anger, depression, guilt, poor school performance, risk-taking behavior (sexual acting out, substance abuse)

DIFFERENTIAL DIAGNOSIS

• Depression
• Post-traumatic stress disorder

TREATMENT BY PRIMARY CARE PEDIATRICIAN

• The physician must:
 – come to grips with his or her emotional response to death and loss and be careful not to withdraw from families or become overly involved

 – help maintain faith in capacity of child and family to cope and adapt successfully

 – understand personal meaning of loss to child and family

 – be available, be there, emotionally for child and family

 – offer realistic information (genetic information in case of neonatal death), support and nurturing; know community resources

 – understand that surviving siblings need special attention

WHEN TO REFER

• If pediatrician feels uncomfortable managing grief and mourning process

• In children and adolescents when following are *severe* (clinical judgment) or *prolonged* (>6–12 mos):
 –regressive behaviors: bed-wetting, thumb sucking, continued irritability
 – separation anxiety
 – eating or sleeping problems
 – school behavior problems, poor grades
 – lack of interest in social life
 – suicidal ideation
 – somatic complaints: headache, stomachache, chest pain

Children's understanding of death

	Age	Response
Preschool	0–2	• Separation anxiety
		• Response to changes in emotions of caregivers
	3–5	• Death reversible and temporary
		• Death is punishment (I caused the death) or wish fulfillment
		• Death is catching
		• Children become angry at parents who cannot control events
School age	6–13	• Death permanent, real, final, universal (will not happen to me)
		• Understands body physiology such as heart and lung functioning
Adolescence	14–21	• Understands existential issues of death and dying (can happen to me)
		• Exaggerated denial of death and thus engages in risk-taking behaviors: sexual acting out, substance abuse

BACKGROUND

- *Growing pains:* chronic, recurrent, night-time leg aches and pains in children
- 15–30% of grade school–age children may complain of pain that disturbs sleep
- Most frequent 4–8 yrs of age
- Males and females affected
- Benign condition that eventually resolves w/o sequelae

CLINICAL MANIFESTATIONS

- *Onset insidious:* no associated trauma or systemic illness
- *Invariably chronic:* usually present several weeks to few months prior to visit to pediatrician
- *Episodes occur several times per week:* often related to strenuous physical activity preceding day
- Pain prevents sleep at bedtime or interrupts within first few hours of sleep
- *Location of pain bilateral:* most often generalized along anterolateral leg or in calf muscles
- *Transient:* each episode relieved by simple measures
- *Pain does not persist into next day:* child resumes normal active physical play w/o limp
- *Physical examination normal:* specifically, lower extremity alignment, ROM, neurologic, vascular status all unremarkable
- Resolution of episodic pain occurs slowly, several mos–2 yrs
- Pts grow up to have normal legs

LABORATORY FEATURES

- Laboratory values normal
- CBC and ESR should be checked because differential does include leukemia
- Radiographs normal; should be obtained only selectively

DIFFERENTIAL DIAGNOSIS

- For pt w/ typical Hx, normal physical examination, childhood leukemia requires consideration
- Deviations from typical Hx must be carefully evaluated. Examples that bring to bear their own important differential may include following: limp, acute pain, pain during daily activity, well-localized or unilateral pain, joint swelling, progressive deformity. None typical for "growing pains"

TREATMENT

- No permanent cure
- Episodes of pain respond well to simple measures
- Parental massage or rubbing of painful limbs
- Stretching of involved muscles
- Local application of heating pad
- Distraction techniques such as extra story or cup of hot chocolate work well for younger children

COMPLICATIONS

- None. Ultimately benign, self-limited condition

PREVENTION

- Regular, routine stretching of quadriceps, hamstrings, gastrocnemius before bed
- Theoretically, pain relief due to increasing local blood flow in affected muscles
- Child's physical activity may end abruptly in evening. Stretching may act as athlete's cooldown
- Parental effort required for stretching may be welcome trade for uninterrupted sleep

WHEN TO REFER

- Whenever Dx in doubt

GROWTH HORMONE DEFICIENCY

RAYMOND L. HINTZ AND E. KIRK NEELY

BACKGROUND

- Growth hormone deficiency (GHD) may be isolated defect or component of hypopituitarism; may be congenital or acquired due to hypothalamic-pituitary lesion; but usually idiopathic
- Growth hormone released by pituitary in pulses, esp during sleep; thus random serum sample will not accurately reflect GH secretion rate
- Growth effects of GH mediated by insulinlike growth factor (IGF) I, present in serum at relatively constant levels
- *Initial diagnostic concern in evaluating short stature:* differentiate pathologic process from two common normal variants of growth: familial short stature and constitutional delay of growth and puberty
- Many children w/ short stature have marginal growth velocities and borderline tests of growth hormone status; thus may be categorized as having partial GHD

CLINICAL MANIFESTATIONS

- Profound, worsening short stature
- Poor growth velocity; differentiates true hormonal deficiency from normal variants of growth
- Growth failure may not be evident until 2–3 yrs of age, when GH becomes essential for growth
- Delayed skeletal maturation; but seen in many conditions
- Normal body proportions
- Frontal bossing, mild obesity
- Hypoglycemia in infancy
- Manifestations of other pituitary hormone deficiencies

LABORATORY FEATURES

- Low serum IGF-I
- Low IGF binding protein 3, also regulated by GH, best test in young children

- Maximal serum growth hormone <7 ng/mL on two stimulation tests (insulin, arginine, L-dopa, clonidine, glucagon), but GH testing imprecise and abandoned by some endocrinologists
- All pts w/ clinical and laboratory evidence of GHD should have hypothalamic-pituitary MRI to r/o anatomic abnormality or tumor
- All pts w/ GHD screened for other pituitary deficiencies

DIFFERENTIAL DIAGNOSIS

- Familial short stature
- Constitutional delay of growth and puberty
- Hypothyroidism
- Turner syndrome
- Intrauterine growth retardation, including Russell-Silver syndrome
- Skeletal dysplasias
- Other syndromes (Prader-Willi, Noonan, Down), pseudohypoparathyroidism, etc
- *Chronic illness:* malnutrition and malabsorption, inflammatory bowel disease, cystic fibrosis, renal failure, renal tubular acidosis
- *Growth hormone insensitivity:* very rare

TREATMENT

- 0.025–0.05 mg/kg/d recombinant human GH by daily SubQ injection, given until growth velocity slows at end of puberty
- Pts achieve genetic target height only if Tx begins early in childhood
- Growth velocity increases immediately—often 3–4 cm/y pretreatment–10–12 cm/y—but response may gradually decline in subsequent years
- Growth response greatest in those w/ classic GHD (stimulated serum GH <3 ng/mL) and w/ lowest pretreatment growth rates
- Ongoing controversy over efficacy and benefit of hGH in partial growth hormone deficiency or "normal variant short stature" w/ borderline IGF levels

- hGH Tx also FDA approved for Turner syndrome, chronic renal failure prior to transplant, adult GHD'

COMPLICATIONS OF TREATMENT

- Diminished insulin sensitivity—common but subclinical, rarely diabetes
- Slipped capital femoral epiphysis (SCFE), monitor for leg pain—rare
- Cerebral hypertension (psuedomotor cerebri), monitor for headache—rare

PREVENTION

- No prevention, but growth should be monitored regularly throughout childhood and adolescence
- All pts w/ midline defects, such as septooptic dysplasia, or who have had brain tumor, chemotherapy, or cranial irradiation should be routinely screened for pituitary deficiencies

WHEN TO REFER

- If height is < –2 SDs and inconsistent w/ parental heights, or if growth rate clearly subnormal
- Appropriate screening for endocrine abnormalities includes serum IGF-I and/or IGFBP-3, thyroid levels, bone age (in older children), karyotype in females, but refer if abnormalities found
- Teenagers w/ delayed puberty, who always appear to have declining growth velocities, should be referred if no sign of puberty by 13 yrs of age in females, 14 yrs of age in boys

BACKGROUND

• Most common cause of acute, generalized weakness affecting ~5/1,000,000/yr. Extremely rare in infants <1 yr of age
• 60% have Hx preceding infection, respiratory or GI (including association recently noted w/ *Campylobacter jejuni*)
• Median time to *improvement* 17 d, to *walk* 37 d, to *asymptomatic* 66 d
• *Better prognosis in children than adults:* 73% completely recover by 6 mos, <5% permanently disabled. Both recurrence, death rare
• Risk factors for more severe course:
  – severe axonal changes in EMG w/ low amplitude or absent compound muscle action potentials and/or changes of acute denervation
  – prolonged ventilation (>1 mo)
  – fulminant onset to severe weakness
  – cranial nerve dysfunction
• *Mechanism:* immune-mediated inflammatory injury to peripheral nerve and root thought to be provoked by preceding immunologic stimulus such as infection or vaccination

CLINICAL MANIFESTATIONS

• Sensory:
  – painful paresthesias in fingers and toes often initial symptom
  – despite severity of symptoms, little or no objective sensory signs on physical exam
• Weakness:
  – often ascending from legs to arms
  – symmetric
  – 50% may be proximal greater than distal pattern, rest equal, or distal more than proximal pattern
  – progresses 1–4 wks, then plateaus (<2 wks in 80%) before slowly resolving over weeks or months
  – bifacial weakness common; other bulbar musculature (eye movements) and sphincters (urinary retention) rarely affected
• Reflexes:
  – absent deep tendon reflexes (may only be depressed early)
• Autonomic dysfunction:
  – instability of BP and arrhythmias

LABORATORY FEATURES

• *CSF:* protein ↑ w/ <10 cells (albuminocytologic dissociation). Protein may not be ↑ first week
• *Nerve conduction studies:* evidence of conduction block and prolonged late responses; slowing of NCVs may occur after 2–3 wks

DIFFERENTIAL DIAGNOSIS

• Common mistake early on to overlook possibility of *any* neurologic disorder

Disorder	Red Flag
Spinal cord lesion	Sensory level
	Bladder dysfunction
	Babinski sign
Myasthenia gravis	Fatigable weakness
	Eye movement and lid weakness
HIV, Lyme disease, sarcoidosis	>10 cells in CSF
Toxic neuropathy	Hx drug or heavy metal exposure
Tick paralysis	Attached tick
Poliomyelitis	Asymmetric
	Painful
	Fever

TREATMENT

• May be withheld in milder cases (~25%) and child followed carefully
• Should be initiated in all children at point ability to walk lost
• Mildest cases can be observed as outpts, but most should be admitted if seen early in course to be watched closely for progression to life-threatening stage
• *Steroids:* no benefit; may worsen outcome
• *Plasma exchange:* proven effective in shortening time to recovery and ameliorating severity of nadir in strength when pts treated in first 2 wks of illness. Technically difficult to perform in children <3 yrs of age
• *IV immunoglobulin (IVIG):* proven effective when given first 2 wks in dose of 0.4 g/kg/d × 5 d. Cost similar to plasma exchange and logistically simpler. May have higher rate of relapse

COMPLICATIONS

• Respiratory failure 14–25%
• Autonomic dysfunction w/ arrhythmias, hypertension, hypotension, or GI motility disorders in 25%
• Adverse reactions to IVIG in <5%

WHEN TO REFER

• Most children would benefit from confirmatory neurologic consultation including nerve conduction studies

HALLUX VALGUS

SARA C. McINTIRE

BACKGROUND

- *Definition:* lateral deviation of great toe at metatarsophalangeal joint
- More common in girls than in boys and may result from congenital deformity in which first metatarsal has abnormal degree of medial deviation (metatarsus primus varus)
- *Bunion:* prominence of medial aspect of head of first metatarsal

CLINICAL MANIFESTATIONS

- In infants, space between first and second toes appears widened
- Older children and adolescents w/ bunions present w/ foot pain, concerns over cosmetic appearance of feet, difficulty finding shoes that fit comfortably
- Pertinent physical findings include pronation of foot on standing, abduction of great toe at metatarsophalangeal joint, pain, thickening over medial prominence of head of first metatarsal

RADIOGRAPHIC FEATURES

- Standing anteroposterior (AP) and lateral views of feet required. Axial calcaneal views and AP standing views of ankle indicated if extreme valgus

TREATMENT

- *Nonoperative:* nonoperative methods will not correct deformity. Athletic-type shoes and use of foot orthosis may be helpful in alleviating bunion pain
- *Operative:* surgery indicated for painful bunions and for progressive, cosmetically unacceptable hallux valgus. Most commonly used technique: proximal metatarsal osteotomy

COMPLICATIONS

- W/o surgery, progressive deformity, pain, difficulty obtaining comfortable footwear occur in many pts
- W/ surgery, recurrent deformity, instability of metatarsophalangeal joint may occur afterward

WHEN TO REFER

- Referral to orthopedic surgeon indicated when operative correction a consideration

DEFINITIONS

- *Common migraine:* recurrent headaches, often bilateral/poorly localized, w/o aura; most common headache of children; pain often bifrontal/can occur anywhere over cranium
- *Classic migraine:* aura; headache unilateral/well localized; unusual < age 8
- *Complicated migraine:* pain dwarfed by severity of neurologic symptoms; acute confusional states, memory loss, florid brain stem symptoms; may result in stroke (rare)
- *Cluster headaches:* severe, frequently repeated, retro periorbital throbbing pain accompanied by excessive tearing, nasal secretions, other florid autonomic signs; very rare in children

BACKGROUND

- Rare < age 4
- By age 7 affects ~4% of schoolchildren
- By age 14 affects ~10–15% of children
- <age 12 males predominate
- During/after puberty ~two-thirds affected pts female

PATHOPHYSIOLOGY

- Etiology unknown
- Vascular changes now thought to be 2° to abnormalities in neuronal discharge in forebrain/brain stem
- Selected pathways modulated by serotonin primarily affected

CLINICAL MANIFESTATIONS

- Dx based on Hx that fulfills generally accepted criteria/absence of any interim neurologic signs that could be related to headache
- Prensky and Sommer:
  - multiple isolated attacks of cephalgia
  - 3 of 6 of following criteria:
    - aura
    - unilateral pain
    - throbbing/pounding pain
    - nausea, vomiting/abdominal pain
    - relief by brief period of sleep
    - family Hx migraine
- The International Classification:
  - common:
    - 5 separate attacks of >2 hrs
    - no other Sx of neurologic illness
    - two of following criteria: unilateral location, pulsating quality, aggravation by routine physical activity, intensity inhibits usual activities
    - one of following criteria: nausea and/or vomiting, photo- *and* phonophobia
  - classic (aura):
    - at least 2 attacks
    - three of following criteria: ≥1 symptom(s) of fully reversible cerebral/brain stem ischemia, ≥ 4 min to develop, does not last >60 min, headache begins during aura or within 1 hr after aura ends

DIFFERENTIAL DIAGNOSIS

- Common migraine:
  - tension headache
  - sinusitis
  - ocular disorders (usually mild/limited to area about eye)
  - temporomandibular joint disease (temporal; spread to other areas questionable)
  - intracranial mass lesions (often well localized, of recent onset progressive increase in intensity)
  - postconcussive syndromes

LABORATORY STUDIES (INDICATIONS)

- EEG:
  - unusual auras often w/altered mental function
  - unusual movements
- Neuroimaging:
  - onset of headaches in last 6 mos w/↑ frequency/intensity
  - onset soon after episode of head trauma
  - presence of concurrent partial seizures
  - aura persists well into the headache/lasts beyond it
  - first attack of complicated migraine
  - interim neurologic signs may/may not be related to headache
- Lumbar puncture:
  - usually preceded by scan
  - acute headache w/fever, meningismus, abnormal behaviors/neurologic signs

REFERRAL TO SPECIALIST

- Suspicion of another neurologic disorder
- Failure to respond to medication
- Headaches ↑ frequency/severity
- Severely significant associated emotional disorder

REFERRAL TO ER

- Child whose Dx established, intractable, incapacitating pain unresponsive to medication at home
- Intense first headache w/no clear-cut Dx

HOSPITALIZATION OF KNOWN MIGRAINEURS

- Intractable pain requiring prolonged/repeated IV Tx
- Dehydration
- Persistent neurologic signs
- Marked, continuing change in mentation, if accompanied by fever
- Initial/unexpected acute severe headache w/findings on Hx/physical examination that make Dx suspect

ARTHUR L. PRENSKY

ACUTE ATTACKS

- Drug Tx more likely effective if used before headache becomes severe; may necessitate taking medication at school
- If not specifically contraindicated, OTC preparations used initially
- Addicting analgesics not given to pts w/>6 headaches/mo; reduce frequency by preventative Tx
- Commonly used drugs (see Table 1)
- Emergency care of severe, intractable headaches:
  – hydroxazine, 1 mg/kg up to 25 kg, then 25–100 mg depending on weight/tolerance; meperidine hydrochloride, 1.0–1.5 mg/kg up to 25 mg, then 25–75 mg, depending on weight/tolerance; allergic reactions, hypotension, sedation common side effects

  – Toradol IV up to 30 mg (children > 12 yrs)
  – chlorpromazine, 0.1–0.2 mg/kg IV/prochlorperazine, 0.2 mg/kg IV up to max. 10 mg; dyskinetic/dystonic movements; sedation, confusion, dizziness may occur
  – dihydroergotamine, 0.02 mg/kg IV up to 1 mg; may repeat in 2–4 hrs/then q8h for up to 3 d; pts usually pretreated w/metaclopramide, 0.2 mg/kg IV up to 10 mg; initial dose 20% of final calculated dose given first to test tolerance; if symptoms refractory, 1–4 mg dexamethasone/5–10 mg diazepam can be given IV after 24 hrs; treatment reserved for children >12 yrs
  – Sumatriptan (> age 12) up to 6 mg SubQ (~0.01 mg/kg). Not to be repeated

PREVENTATIVE MEASURES

- Once started, must be taken daily, on regular schedule, regardless of change in frequency of headaches
- If effective should be continued ≥ 6 mos/until end of school year (whichever longer)/withdraw slowly; restart if headaches occur/↑ in frequency
- Commonly used drugs (see Table 2)
- Behavioral Tx:
  – biofeedback/relaxation, cognitive Tx
  – up to 70% show moderate improvement
  – requires multiple sessions (5–12 wks)
  – requires daily practice at home
  – costs may be prohibitive/often not covered by insurance

Table 1

Generic	Trade	Dosage	Most Common Side Effects
Acetaminophen	Tylenol, 80 mg chewable, 125 mg/5 cc, 325 mg, 500 mg tabs	10–20 mg/kg, up to1000 mg; repeat in 2/more hrs prn up to 4×/d	Gastric upset. Overdosage may cause liver damage. Hypersensitivity reactions rare
Ibuprofen	Advil, 200 mg tabs; Motrin, 300–800 mg tabs	20 mg/kg up to 800 mg/may be repeated in 2–4 hrs; no more than 3 doses/24 hrs	Nausea, dizziness, epigastric pain, rash, tinnitus
Naproxen sodium	Aleve,[1] 200 mg tabs, caplets; Anaprox, 275 mg tabs	1 tab at onset of headache. May be repeated in 8–12 hrs; no more than 3 tabs/24 hrs; children >age 14 who have taken Aleve in the past w/no reactions may try 2 tabs at onset of headache	Nausea, epigastric pain, ulcers, rash, allergic reactions, dizziness, vertigo, edema
Butalbital, 50 mg; acetaminophen, 325 mg; caffeine, 40 mg/tab	Fioricet[2]	*Age 6–12:* 1 tab @ onset of headache; repeat in 1 hr if needed. *Limit:* 4 tabs in 24 hrs. *Age 12–18:* 2 tabs at onset of headache	Drowsiness, dizziness, vomiting, rare allergic reactions. Frequent use can result in withdrawal headaches
Isometheptene mucate, 65 mg; dichlorphenazone, 100 mg; acetaminophen, 325 mg/cap	Midrin[2,3]	*Age 6–12:* 1 cap at onset of headache. Repeat in 2 hrs prn. *Age 12–18:* Take 2 caps at onset of headache; repeat ×1 prn.	Drowsiness, dizziness, rare allergic reactions may interact w/tricyclic antidepressants/↑ levels
Oxycodone, 5 mg; acetaminophen, 325 mg/tab	Percocet[4]	*Age 12–18:* 1–2 tabs at onset of headache; 1 tab in 2 hrs if needed; no more than 4 tabs/d	Sedation, dizziness, nausea; may enhance levels of tricyclic antidepressants; dependence w/frequent use
Butorphanol tartrate; 1 mg/metered spray	Stadol[5]	1 spray in 1 nostril (1 mg); may be repeated in 1 hr if needed; no more than 3 doses in 24 hrs; restrict to children age ≥14	Hypotension, syncope, confusion, anxiety, sweating, rash; dependence w/frequent use
Ergots, ergotamine tartrate + 100 mg caffeine	Ergostat/others,[4] 1/2 mg tabs/2 mg suppositories; Cafergot,[4] 1 mg; Ergot in tabs, 2 mg; Ergot in suppositories	*Age 6–12:* 1 mg at onset of headache/0.5 mg q30min thereafter until 4 mg ingested/vomiting, headache subsides. *Age 12–18:* 1–2 mg at onset/1 mg q half hour thereafter as above; total dose 6 mg. Suppositories: 2 mg at onset of headache; repeat once in 1 hr if needed	Nausea/vomiting; paresthesia, allergic reactions w/prolonged/frequent use can result in constrictive blood vessel changes
Dihydroergotamine mesylate	D.H.E. 45,[4] 1 mg/mL IM injection	1 mg at onset of headache/repeated twice if needed at 1 hr intervals; no more than 3 mg/24 hrs; use in children >age 12	Nausea, vomiting, numbness, tingling, tachycardia, weakness
Sumatriptan	Imitrex,[5,6] 25/50 mg tabs/ metered 6 mg SubQ injectable doses; nasal spray, 5–20 mg	Injectable form should rarely be used in children/only if physician present to measure dose of 0.1 mg/kg; *Tabs: Age 12–18:* take 25/50 mg at onset of headache/repeat in 1 hr if needed; total dose should not exceed 100 mg/24 hrs; nasal spray in one nostril/can be repeated ×1 in 2 hrs	Nausea, abdominal, rarely chest pain; flushing, tingling/burning of scalp, neck, throat, face, sometimes arms; dizziness; should not be used if hypertension, heart disease, active seizure disorder Hx
Naratriptan	Amerge [5,6]	1–2.5 mg; repeat in 4 hrs if needed; do not exceed 5 mg/d	
Zolmitriptan	Zomig[5,6]	2.5–5 mg; repeat in 2 hrs if needed; do not exceed 10 mg/d	
Rizatriptan	Maxalt[5,6]	5–10 mg; repeat in 2 hrs if needed; do not exceed 10 mg/d	

Table 2

Generic	Trade	Dosage	Most Common Side Effects
Amitriptyline HCl (trycicylics)	Elavil,[1] 10, 25, 50 mg tabs	1–2 mg/kg/d taken at night	Sedation, dry mouth, urine retention, syncope, lowering of seizure threshold
Propranolol (beta blockers)	Inderal[2] tabs, 10, 20, 40 mg. LA, 60, 80 mg caps	1–2 mg/kg/d < age 12; tabs used/medication given in 3 div doses; >12, many children tolerate 60/80 mg spansule hs	Not to be given to pts w/asthma, heart disease, strong family Hx depression; dizziness, postural hypotension, sedation, depression; agranulocytosis (rare)
Cyproheptadine HCT	Periactin, 2 mg in 5 Ml, 4 mg tabs	*2–6 yrs:* 2 mg tid; *7–14 yrs:* 4 mg tid; *>age 14:* up to 24 mg/d as tolerated in 3 div doses	Sedation, confusion, dizziness, hypotension, syncope, dry mouth, urticaria
Phenytoin	Dilantin, 50 mg tabs; 30, 100 mg capsules; 125 mg/ 5 cc suspension	4–8 mg/kg/d in 2 doses depending on serum levels	Coarsefacies, enlarged gums, hirsutism, acne, rash, hyperactivity, sedation, ataxia. *Rare:* fever, joint pain, agranulocytosis
Valproate (divalproex sodium)	Depakote, Depakene 250 g/ 5 cc (125, 250 mg tabs; 125 mg sprinkles)	15 mg/kg/d in 3 div doses, ↑ slowly up to 60 mg/kg/d depending on tolerance/serum levels	Drowsiness, nausea, vomiting; increased appetite. Hepatic necrosis, pancreatitis, thrombocytopenia, bleeding, agranulocytosis
Verapamil Hcl	Calan,[3] 40 mg tabs	*>Age 6:* 2 mg/kg/d in 3 div doses, ↑ slowly prn to 5 mg/kg/d	Not to be used w/beta blockers/in pts w/Hx heart failure, arrhythmias
Nifedipine	Procardia,[3] 10 mg tabs	*Age 6–12:* 1 tab bid; ↑ slowly prn up to 2 tabs tid; *Age 12–18:* 1 tab tid; ↑ slowly prn to 3 tabs tid	Constipation/diarrhea, dizziness, hypotension, syncope, flushing, jitteriness

[1]Not to be given < age 12 w/o advice of physician.
[2]Safety/effectiveness < age 12 not established.
[3]Never prescribe to children < age 2.

[4]Safety/effectiveness in children not established.
[5]Not recommended for pts < age 18.
[6]Avoid with hemiplegic or basilar migraine or active epileptic disorder

HEADACHE, OTHER THAN MIGRAINE, MANAGEMENT

ELISE E. LABBÉ

BACKGROUND

- Focus here on muscle contraction or tension headache, most frequent headache disorder other than migraine
- Most frequently reported after onset of puberty
- Before puberty M:F ratio 1:1; after puberty, girls predominate
- Commonly follows psychosocial stressors related to school performance, social functions, family problems
- Female gender and young age best predictors of chronicity
- *Recovery:* w/o intervention many children experience reduced symptoms of relief during summer; some experience several years of no headache but 60% experience chronic headache problems as adults
- *Mortality:* 0%

CLINICAL MANIFESTATIONS

- Frequent, sometimes daily headaches; not as severe as migraine headaches
- Bandlike, constant dull aching pain
- Bilateral or back of head or neck pain
- No relief after rest
- Responds to massage
- Physical findings minimal; may include tenderness over cervical muscles and occipital scalp or frontalis tenderness

LABORATORY FEATURES

- Normal laboratory findings
- Absence of permanent structural change

DIFFERENTIAL DIAGNOSIS

- Migraine headache
- Mixed headache
- Brain tumor
- Neurologic disorder
- Postconcussive reaction
- Sinus
- Variety of other diseases
- Depression and/or anxiety disorder

TREATMENT

- Reassurance to parents and child that no significant medical problem
- Medical treatment rarely needed or indicated but may include symptomatic treatment w/ pain medication, and rarely local anesthetic blocks or sedative-hypnotic medication w/ muscle relaxant properties
- Stress management training
- Electromyographic biofeedback
- Progressive muscle relaxation training
- Family counseling

COMPLICATIONS

- Difficulties exist in obtaining reliable accounts of symptoms from younger children. Use of pain diary for several weeks can be helpful in making Dx

WHEN TO REFER

- If child does not respond to reassurance, refer for psychological counseling

BACKGROUND

- *Definition:* failure of electrical activities to reach ventricle from atria. Atrial and ventricular activities completely independent
- *On electrocardiogram* P waves regular (P-P interval regular) and reflect normal heart rate. Ventricular rate (QRS complexes) slow w/regular R-R interval. P-R interval varies from beat to beat. In congenital complete heart block (CCHB) QRS complexes narrow; however, in acquired heart block QRS complexes usually wide

CONGENITAL HEART BLOCK

- Dx is clinically suspected when fetal heart rate slow. Dx could be confirmed by fetal echocardiography
- Etiology:
  - most common cause systemic lupus erythematosus (both chemically or clinically manifested) in mother of infant w/CCHB. Maternal SSA and SSB IgG antibodies can cross placenta >16 wks gestational age and can damage AV node of fetus. Not all fetuses of mother w/these antibodies develop CCHB; only HLA type specific fetuses affected
  - other immunologic maternal conditions, ie, Sjögren syndrome and other connective tissue diseases also can cause CCHB
  - anatomic abnormalities, ie, agenesis of AV node, tumor in AV node, fibrous discontinuity between AV node and His bundle tissue
- Clinical presentations:

  - CCHB well tolerated in utero. Usually neonates remain asymptomatic, rarely in heart failure. Some of neonates may have associated congenital heart defects (CHD), ie, corrected transposition of great arteries, patent ductus arteriosus, etc
- Treatment:
  - indication for pacemaker therapy in neonates w/CCHB:
    - ○ ventricular rate <55 bpm
    - ○ congestive heart failure from associated CHD
    - ○ significantly enlarged heart size on chest x ray
    - ○ prolonged QTc interval and ventricular arrhythmia
  - indication for pacemaker therapy in older children w/CCHB:
    - ○ syncopal attack (Stokes-Adams attack)
    - ○ very low ventricular rate, usually ~40 bpm
    - ○ ventricular arrhythmia
    - ○ ↓ in exercise tolerance and failure to thrive

ACQUIRED

- Etiology:
  - myocarditis, postcardiac surgery, drugs, ie, digitalis, other antiarrhythmic medications. Metabolic, ie, hypo- and hyperkalemia, hypomagnesemia, cardiac tumor, ie, rhabdomyoma
- Treatment:
  - medications: temporary benefit until pacemaker in place

  - ○ atropine: 0.01–0.04 mg/kg, max. 1 mg IV bolus, may repeat few times
  - ○ isoproterenol: children 0.1–1.5 mcg/kg/min, IV drip
  - ○ epinephrine: 0.1–1 mcg/kg/min IV drip; titrate infusion rate to have desired effect
  - *temporary pacing:* transvenous, or epicardial temporary pacing wire (for postsurgical heart block)
  - *permanent pacing:* indicated if heart block does not disappear in 10–14 d

LABORATORY TESTS

- Fetal echocardiogram when suspected in utero: electrocardiogram after birth
- Two-dimensional and Doppler echocardiogram after birth to r/o associated congenital heart defects and evaluate myocardial functions, and neonatal intensive care monitoring as needed
- Exercise test or electrophysiology tests *not* needed

WHEN TO REFER

- Most infants and children w/heart block followed by pediatrician or family practitioner w/infrequent evaluation by pediatric cardiologist
- Pts w/permanent pacemaker must have periodic transtelephonic EKG follow-up

HEAT STROKE AND HEMORRHAGIC SHOCK AND ENCEPHALOPATHY SYNDROME (HSES)

DAVID JARDINE

BACKGROUND

- Heat stroke and HSES appear to be same illness, but affect pts of different ages
- Heat stroke occurs in children and adults; HSES almost always refers to heat stroke during infancy
- Heat stroke usually follows severe environmental heat stress or overexertion in warm environment
- HSES often occurs when infant sleeping, probably because of inadequate heat transfer to environment

Clinical Criteria	Laboratory Criteria
Seizures	↓ Hct
Encephalopathy (coma)	↓ platelet count
Shock	↑ BUN
Diarrhea (1–2 stools)	↑ creatinine (occasionally)
Hepatomegaly at 48 hrs	Metabolic acidosis
Hemorrhage (infrequently)	Prolonged PT and PTT
High fever (often absent @ diagnosis)	↑ D-dimer
	↑ CPK at 24 hrs
	↑ ALT and AST at 48 hrs

CLINICAL CRITERIA

- Disease bears strong similarity to sepsis in infant; often misdiagnosed as sepsis
- Constant features (must be present to make Dx):
  - *encephalopathy:* seizures, usually coma, often respiratory arrest
  - *shock:* requires large fluid volume and vasopressors
- Variable features:
  - *hepatomegaly:* although the liver may not be enlarged on admission, progressive hepatomegaly common during first 72 hrs
  - *fever:* often absent. Although hyperthermia may be important in pathogenesis of illness, elevated temperature often falls to normal by time child hospitalized
  - *diarrhea:* often occurs shortly after admission. Usually profuse and watery. Resolves quickly
  - *clinically apparent hemorrhage:* may not be present. Despite name of illness, clinically evident hemorrhage present in only minority of pts
  - *age:* almost always <10 mos for HSES. Heat stroke may occur at any age

LABORATORY CRITERIA

- *No single diagnostic test for HSES,* although disease has well-defined clinical and laboratory characteristics
- Dx of illness depends on the presence of characteristic pattern of changes in several routine laboratory tests
- Also important to exclude infectious diseases
- Laboratory tests:
  - *CBC w/platelets:* repeat q24h for first 5 d
    - characteristic findings:
      - ○ progressive anemia over first 48 hrs (HCT may fall by 10 points)
      - ○ progressive thrombocytopenia (often falling to <100,000)
      - ○ little or no evidence of intravascular hemolysis (few RBC fragments)
  - *BUN and creatinine:* obtain on admission and when clinically indicated. Often elevated at time of admission and return to normal over first 72 hrs
  - *blood gas* (arterial or central venous): obtain on admission and when clinically indicated. Almost always reveal metabolic acidosis. Among pts who survive, returns to normal within first 3–4 d
  - *coagulation studies:* repeat q24h for first 5 d. Characteristic findings those of DIC but w/o extensive RBC fragmentation:
    - ○ PT and PTT (prolonged)
    - ○ D-dimer (elevated)
    - ○ fibrinogen (decreased)
  - *AST and ALT* (formerly SGOT, SGPT): repeat q24h for first 5 d. Often nearly normal on admission, but rapidly rise to abnormal levels
  - *CPK:* repeat q24h for first 5 d. Often nearly normal on admission, but rapidly rises to abnormal levels
  - *negative blood and CSF cultures for bacteria:* negative herpes simplex virus diagnostic tests (florescent antibody stain of mucosal cells or culture of lesions). Viral pathogens known to cause mild febrile illnesses (eg, rotavirus) are frequently identified in HSES

TREATMENT

- All Tx supportive:
  - *active cooling rarely necessary.* If rectal temperature >41.5°C on admission, rapid cooling best achieved by spraying skin w/ cool water and fanning pt to accelerate evaporative heat loss. More drastic measures such as packing pt in ice or gastric lavage w/ iced normal saline solution rarely necessary
    - *hypotension or shock:*
      - ○ hypovolemia common problem and should be corrected by infusion of isotonic fluids. Central venous pressure monitoring may aid in determining when central vascular volume restored to normal
      - ○ some pts may remain in shock even after restoration of normal central vascular volume. Dopamine or epinephrine may be necessary to increase cardiac contractility and restore normal BP
  - *seizures* should be treated w/ appropriate doses of anticonvulsants. Continued anticonvulsant Tx may not be necessary if pt does not show evidence of permanent neurologic injury after recovery from illness
  - *antibiotics* should be administered until bacterial cultures negative
  - *respiratory failure* sufficiently severe to require mechanical ventilation commonly caused by severe neurologic impairment during first few days of illness. Because parenchymal lung disease usually not present, high levels of oxygen, airway pressure often unnecessary

DIFFERENTIAL DIAGNOSIS

- Body temperature must be elevated at time injury occurs. By time pt reaches medical care, body temperature may be normal, although sequelae of hyperthermic injury continue to be problem
- In order children, antecedents of heat stroke (environmental heat stress and overexertion in warm environment) almost always identified, so may be no need for differential Dx. When hyperthermic injury not clearly identified, differential Dx should include:
  - *bacterial sepsis:* esp in infants, symptoms of HSES almost identical to bacterial sepsis
  - *accidental drug intoxication:* until hematologic values and liver function tests show characteristic changes (at least 24 h), this cause of hypotension and seizures must be considered
  - *metabolic illness:* abrupt onset of seizures, coma, hypotension may suggest manifestations of metabolic illness. Can be excluded by following diagnostic tests listed above. Serum ammonia levels normal except when severe liver failure accompanies heat stroke and HSES. Extensive evaluation for metabolic illnesses usually not warranted

BACKGROUND

- *Helicobacter pylori (H. pylori):* gram-negative, motile spiral organism producing urease
- *H. pylori colonization:* associated w/ antral gastritis and duodenal ulcers, and to lesser extent gastric ulceration
Incidence: risk of developing *H. pylori* ~1%/yr. Later-born children have higher rates colonization at earlier age
- Prevalence:
  - developed countries: *H. pylori* infection rare in first decade of life
  - poor sanitation or crowded living conditions associated w/ higher rates colonization

CLINICAL MANIFESTATIONS

- *1° ulceration (H. pylori associated):* rare <10 yrs of age; associated w/ epigastric abdominal pain, vomiting, nocturnal awakening
- *2° ulceration not associated w/ H. pylori:* usually young very ill pts, present w/ massive GI blood loss or perforation
- *1° gastritis (H. pylori associated):* asymptomatic but may be associated w/ iron deficiency anemia
- *2° gastritis (eg, associated w/ NSAIDs, stress, infection) not associated w/ H. pylori:* nonspecific symptoms of abdominal pain and GI blood loss
- *H. pylori:* not associated w/ recurrent abdominal pain (RAP) syndrome
- *Rare disorders associated w/ H. pylori:* gastric non-Hodgkin lymphoma and mucosa associated lymphoid tissue (MALT) lymphomas
- Possible relationship w/ gastric adenocarcinoma

LABORATORY FEATURES

- *Endoscopy:* nodularity of gastric mucosa, histology demonstrates spiral-shaped organisms on surface of mucosa. Identification enhanced by silver or Giemsa staining (98% sensitivity and specificity). Biopsies placed in urea medium produce color change if *H. pylori* present (sensitivity, 95%; specificity, 98%)
- *Urease breath test:* noninvasive. Isotopic urea administered orally, degraded in stomach, and released urea detected in breath (sensitivity and specificity: 95%)
- *Serology:* IgG antibodies, IgA antibodies (sensitivity, 45–99%; specificity, 95%)

DIFFERENTIAL DIAGNOSIS

- Esophagitis
- *Biliary tract disorders:* gallstones, anatomic abnormalities
- Functional abdominal pain (FAP)
- *Genitourinary abnormalities:* renal stones, ureteropelvic junction obstruction
- Pancreatitis

TREATMENT

- *H. pylori primary gastritis and ulcer disease:* combination of acid blocker, antibiotic, and/or bismuth subsalicylate. Typical regimens:
  - Clarithromycin 500 mg tid (adult dose) plus omeprazole 20 mg per day (adult dose) or lansoprazole 30 mg per day (adult dose) × 14 days
  - Amoxicillin 1000 mg tid (adult dose) plus metronidazole 500 mg bid (adult dose), omeprazole 20 mg per day (adult dose), or lansoprazole 30 mg per day (adult dose) × 14 days
  - *non–H. pylori gastritis or ulcer disease:*
    ○ histamine receptor antagonists (cimetidine: 20 mg/kg/24 h div qid [max dose 300 mg bid]; ranitidine: 2–4 mg/kg/24 h div bid [max dose 150 mg bid]; famotidine: 1 mg/kg/24 h div bid [max. dose 20 mg bid])
    ○ coating agents: (sucralfate: children <6 yrs old: 0.5 g qid; >6 yrs old: 1 g qid)

COMPLICATIONS

- *H. pylori–associated gastritis and ulcer:* high recurrence rate if acid blockers alone used w/o antibiotics

PREVENTION

- Improvement in sanitary conditions
- *H. pylori* vaccine under development

WHEN TO REFER

- If acid blockade fails to resolve symptoms

BACKGROUND

- *Definition:* benign proliferative tumor of vascular endothelium
- 10% of infants affected
- 20% at birth, all by 4–5 wks
- M:F ratio: 1:3–4
- ↑ incidence in premature infants
- Familial incidence same as general population

CLINICAL MANIFESTATIONS

- Begins as subtle telangiectatic macule or red papule
- Develops superficial "strawberry" mark and/or blue or skin-colored deep component
- 85% w/ single lesion; rarely widespread lesions
- 40% head and neck
- Variable size and growth; most rapid growth within 2–4 mos
- Regression starts 6–12 mos of age
- 25% resolve at 2 yrs, 50% at 4–5 yrs, 75% at 6–7 yrs, 95% at 10–12 yrs
- 50% w/ permanent skin changes

LABORATORY FEATURES

- Usually normal
- In Kassabach-Merritt syndrome ↓ platelets, prolonged PT, PTT
- Rarely anemia from chronic bleeding esp w/ GI lesions

DIFFERENTIAL DIAGNOSIS

- Port-wine stain (vascular malformation) present at birth, no growth, no resolution
- Pyogenic granuloma
- *"Blueberry muffin" lesions:* extramedullary hematopoiesis
- Hemangioendothelioma
- Lymphangioma
- Nasal glioma
- Other 1° or metastatic cutaneous tumors

TREATMENT

- *Most lesions:* observation, careful measurements, photographs, reassurance
- Life-threatening, eye-threatening hemangiomas:
  – prednisone/prednisolene, 3–5 mg/kg/d div bid, pulsed dye laser (for superficial component), compression when possible
  – alpha interferon
  – in rare cases: CO_2 laser, ND-YAG laser, surgical ablation
  – may need blood, platelet, plasma support
  – evaluation, treatment for visceral lesions as indicated
- Rapidly growing lesions on face, diaper area, other strategic sites:
  – pulsed dye laser
  – systemic steroids for impending complications
- Ulcerated hemangiomas:
  – tap water compresses
  – topical antibiotics
  – pulsed dye laser
  – oral antibiotics as needed to cover staphylococci, streptococci

COMPLICATIONS

- Kassabach-Merritt syndrome
- High output cardiac failure
- Rapidly growing mass compressing or obstructing eye, nose, external ear canal, urethra, anus, airway
- Visceral lesions in CNS, liver, bowel, lungs, kidneys
- Associated anomalies when located over lumbosacral spine, large lesions on face, scalp, midchest
- Ulceration, infection leading to sepsis, bleeding

WHEN TO REFER

- Most pts can be managed w/o referral
- Pts w/ eye-threatening or life-threatening lesions
- Pts w/ rapidly growing lesions at strategic sites for possible early laser
- Pts w/ ulceration and infection
- Parents who need further reassurance esp to avoid unnecessary aggressive Tx

BACKGROUND

- Most important step in evaluation of hematuria and/or proteinuria: careful performance of UA, particularly examination of sediment from spun urine
- For pts w/hematuria, morphology of RBCs in urinary sediment directs course of evaluation. Finding >25% dysmorphic RBCs strongly suggests bleeding from glomerulus (acute or chronic glomerulonephritis). RBC casts in sediment and proteinuria by dipstick (in urine not grossly bloody) consistent w/nephritis
- Parts of physical examination most pertinent to evaluation include BP, presence/absence of edema, careful examination of flank, abdomen for tenderness or presence of mass, examination of external genitalia

NEPHRITIS

- Poststreptococcal acute glomerulonephritis often diagnosed/managed w/o performance of renal biopsy; forms of chronic nephritis require referral for renal biopsy for Dx, management

DIFFERENTIAL DIAGNOSIS (CHRONIC NEPHRITIS)

- IgA nephropathy
- Henoch-Schönlein purpura
- Membranoproliferative glomerulonephritis
- Hereditary nephritis (Alport disease)
- Interstitial nephritis
- Rapidly progressive (crescentic, antineutrophil cytoplasmic antibody)
- Systemic lupus erythematosus
- Membranous (hepatitis B–associated or idiopathic)

GROSS (MACROSCOPIC) HEMATURIA)

- Eumorphic RBCs w/o RBC casts. Some proteinuria may be caused by lysis of RBCs
- Ultrasound of kidneys, bladder may help localize bleeding

DIFFERENTIAL DIAGNOSIS

- UTI
- Kidney stones
- *Injury:* unsuspected hydronephrosis may predispose to bleeding w/injury
- Sickle-cell disease or trait
- *Wilms tumor:* abdominal mass usually present; younger children
- *Rhabdomyosarcoma of bladder:* always w/significant voiding symptoms

ISOLATED (ASYMPTOMATIC) MICROSCOPIC HEMATURIA

- Defined by >5 RBC per high-powered field in spun sediment of urine, absence of proteinuria
- Present in 1% of schoolchildren
- Should be demonstrated on three occasions before proceeding w/workup

DIFFERENTIAL DIAGNOSIS

- *Hypercalciuria:* in some regions occurs in 30% of children w/isolated hematuria—may predispose to renal stone formation
- Sickle-cell disease or trait
- *Thin glomerular basement membrane disease:* other affected family members w/hematuria but w/o Hx renal insufficiency have good prognosis
- *Alport disease (hereditary nephritis):* usually x-linked dominant inheritance; isolated hematuria in younger affected males or in affected females
- *IgA nephropathy and other forms of chronic glomerulonephritis:* only isolated hematuria in mild cases or early in course of disease
- Idiopathic

DIAGNOSTIC EVALUATION

- UA (dipstick, microscopic examination) repeated 3×
- Ultrasound of kidneys, bladder
- Urinary calcium quantitation (either 24 hr collection or spot urinary calcium to urinary creatinine ratio, >0.20 is ↑)
- Sickle-cell screen (if status not known) for African American children

WHEN TO REFER

- Development of significant proteinuria (>1+ by dipstick in concentrated, specific gravity >1.018, urine)
- Persistence for >1 yr

PROTEINURIA WITH NEPHROTIC SYNDROME

- If proteinuria found to be associated w/edema and/or chemical evidence for nephrotic syndrome (depressed serum albumin, increased serum cholesterol concentration), then child either has nephrosis or chronic glomerulonephritis w/nephrotic syndrome

ISOLATED PROTEINURIA

- Transient proteinuria commonly occurs w/fever, dehydration, CHF, exercise, seizure
- Repeat dipstick for protein 2/3× before proceeding w/evaluation if transient proteinuria suspected

INITIAL EVALUATION

- Significant proteinuria defined by urinary protein excretion >4 mm/m^2/h or spot urine protein to creatinine ratio >0.2 for older children, >0.5 for infants
- Serum creatinine, albumin, cholesterol concentrations should be obtained and should be normal
- Orthostatic proteinuria benign condition defined by normal protein excretion during recumbency w/proteinuria rarely >1 g/m^2/d
  – obtain 3 recumbent, 3 upright (active) random urine samples and test for protein; only upright samples positive
  – obtained timed collection split into recumbent (overnight) and upright collections; only upright should have significant protein excretion; total protein excretion rarely >1 g/m^2/d
- If proteinuria fixed (not orthostatic), renal ultrasound examination should be performed to exclude renal parenchymal lesion such as chronic pyelonephritis
- Fixed proteinuria may indicate glomerular disease such as focal segmental glomerular sclerosis, diffuse mesangial proliferation w/o immune complex deposits, or chronic glomerulonephritis

WHEN TO REFER

- Steroid-resistant nephrotic syndrome
- Fixed proteinuria >500 mg/m^2/d (renal biopsy indicated for fixed proteinuria >1 g/d)

HEMOLYTIC-UREMIC SYNDROME

JERRY M. BERGSTEIN

BACKGROUND

- Most common cause of acute renal failure in young children, generally <4 yrs of age
- Commonly associated w/ diarrheal illness during warmer months
- Frequently follows gastroenteritis caused by enteropathogenic strain of *Escherichia coli* (0157:H7, others) derived from intestinal tract of domesticated animals
- Transmitted by undercooked meat, esp hamburger, unpasteurized milk, contaminated apple cider, contaminated swimming pools
- Also associated w/ other bacterial (*Shigella, Campylobacter, S. pneumoniae*) and viral (coxsackie, ECHO, influenza, varicella, HIV, Epstein-Barr) infections
- Can be associated w/ certain drugs: cisplatin, mitomycin, cyclosporin, oral contraceptives

CLINICAL MANIFESTATIONS

- Onset usually preceded by prodrome of gastroenteritis: fever, vomiting, abdominal pain, diarrhea (may be bloody)
- Occasionally preceded by upper respiratory infection; may be no prodrome
- 2–10 d after onset of prodrome, sudden onset of pallor, irritability, weakness, lethargy, oliguria
- Examination may reveal dehydration, edema, petechiae, jaundice, hepatosplenomegaly, marked irritability

LABORATORY FEATURES

- *Microangiopathic hemolytic anemia:* Hgb in range of 5–9 g/dL w/ helmet, burr, fragmented RBCs in blood film
- *Evidence of intravascular hemolysis:* ↑ plasma hemoglobin, ↓ haptoglobin
- ↑ reticulocyte count
- *Leukocytosis:* WBC count may rise to 30,000/mm^3 w/ 80–90% neutrophils
- *Thrombocytopenia:* 10,000–100,000/mm^3
- UA shows low-grade hematuria, proteinuria
- Partial thromboplastin and prothrombin times normal unless vitamin K deficient
- Elevated BUN, creatinine
- Stool culture may be positive for pathogenic organism

DIFFERENTIAL DIAGNOSIS

- Other causes of acute renal failure, esp those associated w/ microangiopathic state (lupus, malignant hypertension, bilateral renal vein thrombosis)
- Ulcerative colitis
- Appendicitis

COMPLICATIONS

- Anemia
- Acute renal failure
- Hypertension
- *CNS:* irritability, seizures, coma
- *Colitis:* melena, prolapse, perforation
- *Pancreatitis:* diabetes mellitus
- Rhabdomyolysis

TREATMENT

- Correction of dehydration
- Blood transfusion for Hgb <7 g/dL: 10 mL/kg of packed RBCs
- Early peritoneal dialysis for impending renal failure

PREVENTION

- Thorough cooking of hamburger and processed meats; use of pasteurized milk, apple cider

PROGNOSIS

- W/ aggressive management of acute renal failure, >90% pts survive acute phase; majority recover normal renal function
- Long-term follow-up required for late development of hypertension or renal insufficiency

WHEN TO REFER

- *Impending renal failure:* BUN >60 mg/dL, creatinine >2 mg/dL, or urine output <400 mL/m^2/d
- Hyperkalemia
- Fluid overload
- CHF
- Severe hypertension
- Seizures, coma
- Bowel perforation

BACKGROUND

- X-linked recessive disorder due to abnormality in factor VIII protein
- Factor VIII gene located at Xq28; 50% severely affected pts have gene inversion; DNA probes readily available for carrier and prenatal testing
- Severity proportionate to factor VIII level and consistent within families (severe, <1%; moderate, 1–5%; mild, 6–30%)
- Female carriers can be symptomatic if factor VIII level <30% as result of Lyonization of normal X chromosomes

CLINICAL MANIFESTATIONS

- Apparently spontaneous bruising, esp during toddler years
- Excessive bruising or bleeding after relatively minor trauma
- Deep hematomas, hemarthroses, muscle bleeds. *No petichiae.*
- Only 50% bleed at circumcision
- Mucous membrane bleeding unusual
- Mild cases can be asymptomatic until major surgery or trauma
- Crippling anthropathy if replacement Tx delayed or inadequate
- Intracranial hemorrhage major cause of death in HIV negative pts

LABORATORY FEATURES

- Prolonged APTT. Normal PT, thrombin time, bleeding time (usually)
- APTT corrects w/addition of normal plasma
- Low factor VIII level by specific assay
- Normal von Willebrand factor level
- Factor VIII deficiency diagnosable in neonate
- Carrier testing by specific DNA probes or DNA polymorphism

DIFFERENTIAL DIAGNOSIS

- Child abuse
- Hemophilia B (clinically indistinguishable)
- Von Willebrand disease
- Other inherited and acquired coagulation deficiencies
- Ehlers-Danlos syndrome and other inherited collagen disorders

TREATMENT

- Multidisciplinary management planning, genetic counseling, etc, at comprehensive hemophilia center including education in recognizing bleeds that require treatment, training in home infusion, etc.
- Annual comprehensive evaluations for moderately–severely affected
- Routine immunizations by *SubQ* route
- Ongoing dental prophylaxis and treatment
- Avoid contact sports: direct pt to swimming, golf, etc. Other noncontact sports "as tolerated"

SPECIFIC THERAPY

- Products to elevate factor VIII level:
  - *factor VIII concentrates* (plasma derived or recombinant). Recombinant preferable in newly diagnosed
    - one factor VIII unit/kg increases factor VIII level by 2%. For minor bleeds, use 10–15 units/kg; for major bleeds (eg, hemarthrosis), 20 units/kg; for life-threatening bleeds, 50 units/kg
    - factor VIII in vivo half-life ~ 12 hrs. Depending on clinical situation, treatment may have to be repeated q8–12h
  - *DDAVP* only effective in mild–moderate cases: IV, SubQ, or intranasal (Stimate)
    - 0.3 mics/kg IV or SubQ; 150–300 mics intranasal bleed (150 if wt <50 kg, 300 if wt >50 kg)
    - in vivo increment in factor VIII should be documented to evaluate role of DDAVP in treatment plan
    - tachyphylaxis and fluid retention preclude repeating doses in <24–48 hrs
- "On demand" vs. prophylactic replacement Tx:
  - prophylaxis recommended for all newly diagnosed, severely affected pts starting at age 18–24 mos and in selected cases for pts w/recurrent CNS or target joint bleeds. Dosage schedule 25–40 units/kg 3 ×/wk aimed at keeping nadir >~3%. May require venous access device
  - give replacement treatment at earliest sign of significant bleed (eg, hemarthrosis, head injury, etc)
- Special clinical situations:
  - to cover surgical procedures:
    - facility must have assays and factor VIII supply readily available on site
    - screen for inhibitor
    - infuse 50 factor VIII units/kg. Check factor VIII level: if >~80%, start continuous infusion (1 unit/kg/hr maintains ~25%, 2 units/kg ~ 50% etc)
    - maintain factor VIII level >30–50% × 7–10 d
  - dental extractions:
    - elevate factor VIII level to ~50%
    - Amicar (epsilon aminocaproic acid) 100 mg/kg *or* Cykloprapon (tranexamic acid) 25 mg/kg IV or PO prior to procedure and q6–8h × 7–10 d
  - inhibitors:
    - refer
    - treatment options include activated prothrombin complex concentrates, higher doses of factor VIII for low-titre inhibitors, porcine factor VIII, recombinant factor VIIa, immunomodulation, or plasmapheresis

COMPLICATIONS

- Musculoskeletal deformities
- Neurologic deficit (CNS and peripheral nerve)
- *Inhibitors:* develop in up to 20% of severely affected pts. Suspect if suboptimal clinical or laboratory response to replacement Tx

WHEN TO REFER

- At Dx
- For periodic multidisciplinary evaluation (usually yearly for severely affected pts)
- Major surgery
- If inhibitor suspected or documented
- Prenatal testing
- Delivery of proven or probable affected fetus
- Carrier testing

BACKGROUND

- X-linked recessive disorder due to abnormality in factor IX protein; one-sixth as common as hemophilia A
- Factor IX gene located at ×q26–27; DNA probes readily available for carrier and prenatal testing
- Severity proportionate to factor IX level and consistent within families (severe, <1%; moderate, 1–5%, mild, 6–30%)
- Rare subtype (Hemophilia B Leiden) improves after puberty
- Female carriers can be symptomatic if factor IX level <30% as result of Lyonization of normal X chromosomes

CLINICAL MANIFESTATIONS

- Apparently spontaneous bruising, esp during toddler years
- Excessive bruising or bleeding after relatively minor trauma
- Deep hematomas, hemarthroses, muscle bleeds. *No petechie.*
- Only 50% bleed at circumcision
- Mucous membrane bleeding unusual
- Mild cases can be asymptomatic until major surgery or trauma
- Crippling anthropathy if replacement Tx delayed or inadequate
- Intracranial hemorrhage major cause of death in HIV negative pts
- Inhibitors can be associated with anaphylaxis

LABORATORY FEATURES

- Prolonged APTT. Normal PT, thrombin time and bleeding time (usually)
- APTT corrects w/addition of normal plasma
- Low factor IX level by specific assay
- Normal levels of other vitamin K–dependent factors
- Dx often difficult in newborns because of low levels of vitamin K–dependent factors and transplacental passage of factor IX
- Carrier testing by specific DNA probes

DIFFERENTIAL DIAGNOSIS

- Child abuse
- Hemophilia A (clinically indistinguishable)
- Other inherited and acquired coagulation deficiencies
- Ehlers-Danlos syndrome and other inherited collagen disorders

TREATMENT

- Multidisciplinary management planning, genetic counseling, etc, at comprehensive hemophilia center including education in recognizing bleeds that require treatment, training in home infusion, etc
- Annual comprehensive evaluation for moderate–severely affected pts
- Routine immunizations by *SubQ* route
- Ongoing dental prophylaxis and treatment
- Avoid contact sports: direct pt to swimming, golf, etc. Other noncontact sports "as tolerated"

SPECIFIC THERAPY

- Products to elevate factor IX level:
  - *factor IX concentrates:* plasma derived or recombinant DNA products; both considered to be free of infectious complications
    - 1 factor unit/kg increases factor IX level by ~1%. For minor bleeds, use 10–15 units/kg; for major bleeds (eg, hemarthrosis), 20 units/kg; for life-threatening bleeds, 50 units/kg
    - factor IX in vivo half-life ~24 hrs. Depending on clinical situation, treatment may have to be repeated q8–12h because of biphasic in vivo clearance (rapid initial drop in level)
- "On demand" vs. prophylactic replacement Tx:
  - prophylaxis recommended for all newly diagnosed, severely affected pts starting at age 18–24 mos and in selected cases for pts w/recurrent CNS or target joint bleeds. Dosage schedule 25–40 units/kg 2–3 ×/wk aimed at keeping nadir >~3%. May require venous access device
  - give replacement treatment at earliest sign of significant bleed (eg, hemarthrosis, head injury, etc)

COMPLICATIONS

- Same as for hemophilia A

WHEN TO REFER

- Same as for hemophilia A

HEMORRHOIDS

LESLI A. TAYLOR

BACKGROUND

- Internal and external variety:
  - internal hemorrhoids: varicose dilatation of tributaries of superior rectal vein in left lateral, right anterolateral, right posterolateral positions
  - external hemorrhoids: anal tag or sentinal pile found w/ anal fissure
- Internal hemorrhoids rare in children unless associated w/ portal hypertension. Portal hypertension usually due to extrahepatic portal vein thrombosis due to cystic fibrosis

CLINICAL MANIFESTATIONS

- Swelling
- Itching
- Painless, bright red bleeding w/ defecation
- Prolapse
- Strangulation

LABORATORY FEATURES

- No laboratory studies required

DIFFERENTIAL DIAGNOSIS

- Symptoms may mimic
  - Ulcer or fissure
  - Fistula
  - Inflammatory bowel disease
  - Condyloma acuminatum
  - Rectal prolapse

TREATMENT

- Hemorrhoids w/o complications:
  - local hygiene
  - excision rarely indicated
  - internal hemorrhoids can be banded if symptomatic
- Bleeding hemorrhoids:
  - control portal hypertension; hemorrhoidectomy may aggravate portal hypertension
- Thrombosed hemorrhoids:
  - incision, evacuation of clot

COMPLICATIONS

- Prolapse
- Bleeding
- Incarceration

WHEN TO REFER

- Refer to surgeon if symptomatic

BACKGROUND

- One of most common vasculitis syndromes of childhood
- Known by several names including anaphylactoid purpura and Schönlein-Henoch purpura
- *Peak incidence:* 2–12 yrs of age
- Children more often affected than adults; boys more frequently than girls
- Frequently follows upper respiratory infections but etiology unknown
- Extent of renal involvement best predictor of long-term renal outcome

CLINICAL MANIFESTATIONS

- *Dermatologic:* palpable purpura ranging from petechial to ecchymotic size, characteristically located on lower extremities, buttock, and/or at pressure points, but may occur anywhere; initially may appear urticarial or maculopapular; rash usually precedes other manifestations. SubQ edema most frequently occurs on dorsum of hands and feet, forehead, scalp, periorbital
- *Musculoskeletal:* periarticular swelling or arthritis of large joints, most often knee or ankle
- *GI:* mild colicky abdominal pain, nausea, vomiting, occult GI bleeding frequent; small percentage w/ hematemesis, intussusception, bowel infarct
- *Renal:* glomerulonephritis characterized by varying degrees hematuria and/or proteinuria; hypertension may occur
- *Other:* less common manifestations include orchitis, CNS or pulmonary Sx, parotitis

LABORATORY FEATURES

- No distinct or pathognomonic diagnostic laboratory studies
- *Platelet count:* normal or ↑
- *Coagulation studies:* normal
- *Hgb/Hct:* usually normal, if ↓, suspect GI blood loss
- *WBC count:* normal or ↑
- *Stool examination:* may be positive for blood
- *Serum IgA level:* ↑
- *Serology:* antinuclear antibody negative, rheumatoid factor negative
- *Skin biopsy:* characteristically demonstrates leukocytoclastic vasculitis and IgA deposition in vessel walls
- *Additional diagnostic studies:* ultrasound study often more useful than barium enema for detection of ileoileal intussusception; ultrasound study and technetium 99m radionuclide scan assist in differentiation between orchitis and testicular torsion

DIFFERENTIAL DIAGNOSIS

- Acute poststreptococcal glomerulonephritis
- Drug hypersensitivity
- Hemolytic uremic syndrome
- Hemorrhagic diathesis (eg, clotting factor abnormalities)
- Idiopathic thrombocytopenia purpura
- Infantile acute hemorrhagic edema
- Intraabdominal emergencies
- Scrotal/testicular abnormalities (eg, orchitis, torsion)
- Septicemia
- Systemic lupus erythematosus
- Other vasculitic syndromes (eg, hypersensitivity vasculitis, polyarteritis nodosa)

TREATMENT

- *General supportive:* adequate nutrition and hydration, frequent observation and examination
- *Pain control:* analgesics, such as acetaminophen, can be used for mild to moderate pain of subcutaneous edema and arthritis. NSAIDs may be used for pain relief or arthritis, but should be used w/ caution because of risk of exacerbation of renal insufficiency, GI symptoms and bleeding
- *Corticosteroids:* controversy exists concerning use of corticosteroids in treatment of GI or renal disease. Prednisone generally used for moderately severe abdominal pain at dose of 1–2 mg/kg/d × 1 wk, followed by 2 wk taper
- *Other Tx* (eg, pulse steroids, immunosuppressive agents, IV gammaglobulin, fish oil diet) less well proven and considered for more extensive or severe disease w/ consultation of specialists

COMPLICATIONS

- ~50% have recurrences of rash and GI symptoms
- Intussusception and acute, massive GI bleeding occurs in <5%
- Estimates of <5% patients w/ significant long-term renal disease
- Complications of pregnancy (eg, proteinuria, hypertension) may occur more frequently in women who have had HSP in childhood

WHEN TO REFER

- Pts w/ significant abdominal pain, hematuria and proteinuria, broader or more severe organ system involvement than expected, Dx in doubt, frequent recurrences or disease becomes chronic

BACKGROUND

Adult seropositivity in US	33%
Age preference	
US	10–40 yrs
Developing countries	<5 yrs
Primary mode of transmission	Fecal-oral
Risk factors	Poverty
	Day care
	House/sexual contacts
	Male homosexuality
	Drug use (injecting and nonjecting)
	International travel

CLINICAL MANIFESTATIONS

Similarities

- Many infections asymptomatic
- Typical manifestations include malaise, weakness, anorexia, nausea, vomiting, diarrhea, abdominal discomfort, dysphoria; may be followed 3–10 d later by icteric stage w/ acholic stools, dark urine, jaundice

Incubation period	15–50 d
Onset	Abrupt
Infectivity	Virus in feces
Carrier state	No
Symptom duration	1–12 wks
Extrahepatic signs:	
• Arthritis and rash	Rare
• Other (polyarteritis nodosa, glomerulonephritis)	No
Clinical severity:	
• Asymptomatic/mild	Most children; few adults
• Jaundice	<3 yrs: <5%
	4–6 yrs: 10%
	Adult: 75%
• Fever	30–40%, preicteric
Chronic hepatitis	Rare
Confers ↑ risk of hepatocellular carcinoma?	No
Acute case fatality	0.3%

LABORATORY FEATURES

- Serum aminotransferases (aspartate aminotransferase, or AST, and alanine aminotransferase, or ALT) levels become abnormal during late incubation, peak early in icteric phase (often exceeding 8 × normal), then fall abruptly to remain slightly abnormal for several weeks after jaundice and symptoms resolve
- Bilirubin elevation in icteric hepatitis shows equal rises in direct and indirect fractions
- Cholestatic liver enzymes, such as alkaline phosphatase, gamma-glutamyl-transferase, 5′-nucleotidase, mildly ↑ (1–3 × normal)
- Serologic Dx:

	Infection			
	Acute	Chronic	Past	Vaccination
Anti-HAV				
IgM	+	NA	–	–
IgG	–	NA	+	+

HAV = hepatitis A virus; NA = not applicable

- Virus excretion

Feces	Late incubation and early prodrome
Blood	Transient

DIFFERENTIAL DIAGNOSIS

- Infectious hepatitis (Epstein-Barr virus, cytomegalovirus, herpes simplex virus, varicella-zoster virus, enterovirus, adenovirus, rubella, rubeola, toxoplasmosis, leptospirosis, Q fever)
- Autoimmune chronic active hepatitis
- Drug- or chemical-induced hepatitis
- Metabolic errors (Wilson disease, alpha-1-antitrypsin deficiency, cystic fibrosis, galactosemia, tyrosinemia)

PREVENTION AND TREATMENT

Pre-exposure prophylaxis

- *Vaccines:* inactivated virus vaccines available in US
  - licensed vaccines:
    ○ VAQTA (Merck & Co.)
    ○ Havrix (SmithKline Beecham)
  - usage:
    ○ persons >2 yrs old
    ○ one primary dose ≥2 wks before exposure and booster 6–18 mos later (interval differs by age and vaccine)
  - indications:
    ○ travelers to endemic areas
    ○ children living in areas where the rates of hepatitis A are at least 2× the national average (i.e., ≥20 cases per 100,000 population), which includes some Native American communities
    ○ persons with occupational exposure
    ○ recipients of clotting factor concentrates
    ○ male homosexuals
    ○ injecting and noninjecting illegal drug users
    ○ persons exposed to an outbreak experiencing hepatitis A
- *Immune serum globulin (ISG):*
  - usage:
    ○ children <2 yrs old
    ○ age >2 yrs when immediate protection needed (may give ISG concomitantly w/ vaccine at separate site and w/ separate syringe)
  - dosage:
    ○ 0.02 mL/kg IM if exposure for <3 mos
    ○ 0.06 mL/kg IM q5mos for prolonged exposure

Post-exposure prophylaxis w/ ISG

- *Usage:*
  - administer within 2 wks of exposure (0.02 mL/kg IM)
- *Indications:*
  - household or sexual contacts of index case
  - food handlers working at an establishment where another food handler was diagnosed with hepatitis A
  - see *AAP Redbook* recommendations for management of infections related to use of day-care facilities

BACKGROUND

Adult seropositivity in US 5%

Age preference
- US — Adults
- Developing countries — Perinatal

Primary mode of transmission — Blood/body fluids

Risk factors
- Injecting drug use
- Multiple sex partners
- Male homosexuality
- Custodial care
- Health care worker
- Immigrant
- House/sexual contact
- Transfusion
- Dialysis

CLINICAL MANIFESTATIONS

- Many infections asymptomatic
- Typical manifestations include malaise, weakness, anorexia, nausea, vomiting, diarrhea, abdominal discomfort, dysphoria; may be followed 3–10 d later by icteric stage w/ acholic stools, dark urine, jaundice

Incubation period	45–160 d
Onset	Insidious or abrupt
Infectivity	Viremia
Carrier state	Overall 5–10%:
	◆ adults: 2–5%
	◆ 1–5 yrs: 20–30%
	◆ Infants: 70–90%
Symptom duration	≥1–8 mos
Extrahepatic signs:	
• Arthritis and rash	Occasional
• Other (polyarteritis nodosa, glomerulonephritis)	Yes
Clinical severity:	
• Asymptomatic/mild	Most
• Jaundice	Children: <10%
	Adults: 0–50%
• Fever	Occasional
Chronic hepatitis	3–7%
Confers ↑ risk of hepatocellular carcinoma?	Yes
Acute case fatality	1.4%

- Serum aminotransferases (aspartate aminotransferase, or AST, and alanine aminotransferase, or ALT) levels become abnormal during late incubation, peak early in icteric phase (often exceeding 8 × normal), then fall abruptly to remain slightly abnormal for several weeks after jaundice and symptoms resolve
- Bilirubin elevation in icteric hepatitis shows equal rises in direct and indirect fractions
- Cholestatic liver enzymes, such as alkaline phosphatase, gamma-glutamyl-transferase, 5′-nucleotidase, mildly ↑ (1–3 × normal)
- Serologic Dx:

	Infection			
	Acute	Chronic	Past	Vaccination
HBs	+	+	–	–
Anti-HBc				
IgM	+	+	–	–
IgG*	+	+	+	–
Anti-HBs	–	–	+	+

*Establishes Dx during window after HBs clears, before anti-HBs appears.

HBs = hepatitis B surface antigen; HBc = hepatitis B core antigen; HBV = hepatitis B virus; NA = not applicable

- Virus excretion
  - Feces — Often >2 mos
  - Blood — Late incubation→ may persist for years

DIFFERENTIAL DIAGNOSIS

- Infectious hepatitis (Epstein-Barr virus, cytomegalovirus, herpes simplex virus, varicella-zoster virus, enterovirus, adenovirus, rubella, rubeola, toxoplasmosis, leptospirosis, Q fever)
- Autoimmune chronic active hepatitis
- Drug- or chemical-induced hepatitis
- Metabolic errors (Wilson disease, alpha-1-antitrypsin deficiency, cystic fibrosis, galactosemia, tyrosinemia)

PREVENTION

Pre-exposure prophylaxis w/ recombinant subunit vaccines
- *Licensed vaccines:*
  - Recombivax HB (Merck & Co.)
  - Energix-B (SmithKline Beecham)
- *Usage:*
  - infants born to HBs-negative mothers (3 doses): 0–2 mos, 1–2 mos later, 6–18 mos
  - vaccinate all others at 0, 1, 6 mos
  - vaccinate premature infants at hospital discharge if weight >2000 g or wait until routine immunizations initiated at 2 mos

- test for anti-HBs 1–6 mos after last dose of vaccine to detect persons w/ nonprotective antibody levels (<10 mLU/mL) who require additional vaccine to achieve or maintain immunity or who may need HBIG after exposure (eg, perinatally exposed infants, HIV-infected persons, hemodialysis pts)
- *Dosage:*
  - dose varies by product and indication
- *Indications:*
  - all infants
  - high-risk children, adolescents, adults (see above)
  - vaccination of all children, adolescents encouraged

Post-exposure prophylaxis w/ vaccine and HBIG
- *Newborns:* if mother HBs positive, give HBIG 0.5 mL IM within 12 hrs of birth. If mother's HBs unknown, vaccinate infant; give infant HBIG within 1 wk if mother found HBs positive
- *Infant <12 mos w/ acute infection in caregiver:* HBIG 0.5 mL IM
- *Sexual contact or blood exposure to infected household contact:* HBIG 0.06 mL/kg IM within 14 d of last contact
- For accidental percutaneous or permucosal exposure to blood, individualize management based on vaccination status of index case and HBs status of contact

TREATMENT

- *Drugs:*
  - interferon alfa
  - lamivudine
- *Usage:*
  - adults and children w/ chronic hepatitis B infection
- *Outcome:*
  - 25–55% pts improve; 5–10% relapse after Tx discontinued

WHEN TO REFER

- Persistently elevated serum transaminase concentrations (>2× normal)
- Elevated α-fetoprotein concentration
- Abnormal abdominal ultrasound

HEPATITIS C VIRUS

KAREN L. KOTLOFF

BACKGROUND

Adult seropositivity in US	2%
Age preference	
US	Adults
Developing countries	Adults
Primary mode of transmission	Blood borne
Risk factors	Injecting drug use
	Transfusion
	Hemodialysis
	House/sexual contact

CLINICAL MANIFESTATIONS

Similarities

- Many infections asymptomatic
- Typical manifestations include malaise, weakness, anorexia, nausea, vomiting, diarrhea, abdominal discomfort, dysphoria; may be followed 3–10 d later by icteric stage w/ acholic stools, dark urine, jaundice

Incubation period	40–90 d
Onset	Insidious
Infectivity	Viremia
Carrier state	>60%
Symptom duration	Chronic, fluctuating
Extrahepatic signs:	
Arthritis and rash	Occasional
Other (polyarteritis nodosa, glomerulonephritis)	Yes
Clinical severity:	
Asymptomatic/mild	Most
Jaundice	25%
Fever	Uncommon
Chronic hepatitis	> 60%
Confers ↑ risk of hepatocellular carcinoma?	Yes
Acute case fatality	Unknown, but rare

LABORATORY FEATURES

- Serum aminotransferases (aspartate aminotransferase, or AST, and alanine aminotransferase, or ALT) levels become abnormal during late incubation, peak early in icteric phase (often exceeding 8 × normal), then fall abruptly to remain slightly abnormal for several weeks after jaundice and symptoms resolve
- Bilirubin elevation in icteric hepatitis shows equal rises in direct and indirect fractions
- Cholestatic liver enzymes, such as alkaline phosphatase, gamma-glutamyl-transferase, 5′-nucleotidase, mildly ↑ (1–3 × normal)
- Serologic Dx:

	Infection			
	Acute	Chronic	Past	Vaccination
Anti-HCV	+	+	+	NA

HCV = hepatitis C virus; NA = not applicable

- Virus excretion

Feces	Unlikely
Blood	> 60% chronic, fluctuating

DIFFERENTIAL DIAGNOSIS

- Infectious hepatitis (Epstein-Barr virus, cytomegalovirus, herpes simplex virus, varicella-zoster virus, enterovirus, adenovirus, rubella, rubeola, toxoplasmosis, leptospirosis, Q fever)
- Autoimmune chronic active hepatitis
- Drug- or chemical-induced hepatitis
- Metabolic errors (Wilson disease, alpha-1-antitrypsin deficiency, cystic fibrosis, galactosemia, tyrosinemia)

PREVENTION AND TREATMENT

Pre-exposure prophylaxis

- None. No evidence ISG beneficial

Post-exposure prophylaxis

- None. No evidence ISG beneficial

TREATMENT

- *Drug:*
  - interferon alfa monotherapy
  - combination interferon–alfa-2b plus ribavirin
- *Usage:*
  - adults and children w/ chronic hepatitis C hepatitis
  - not approved for children (available by clinical protocol)
  - not indicated in advanced liver disease
- *Outcome:*
  - with monotherapy, 40% pts improve; relapse common when Tx discontinued
  - may be more favorable with combination therapy

COMPLICATIONS

- Fulminant hepatic necrosis
- Aplastic anemia
- Polyarteritis nodosa
- Glomerulonephritis
- Cryoglobulinemia
- Cirrhosis
- Hepatocellular carcinoma

WHEN TO REFER

- Most pts managed w/o referral
- Referral indicated for serious complications, when Dx in doubt, or if disease becomes chronic (>6 mos w/ hepatitis B antigenemia or w/ HCV seropositivity associated w/ abnormal ALT)

BACKGROUND

• Frequent sporadic cases and occasional outbreaks reported in parts of Asia, Africa, Mexico
• Most outbreaks associated w/ fecally contaminated drinking water
• Most US cases occur after travel to hepatitis E virus (HEV)-endemic regions; rare cases have no Hx travel outside US
• *Average incubation period:* 40 d (range: 15–60 d)
• *Recovery:* generally within 3 wks (range: 1–6 wks)
• No evidence of chronic infection

Non A–E hepatitis
• <5% pts w/signs/symptoms of acute viral hepatitis in US do not have serologic markers of hepatitis A, B, C, D, E virus infections
• Hepatitis G virus (also called hepatitis GB virus C) has been isolated from pts w/ non A–E hepatitis, but no epidemiologic/experimental evidence exists to implicate virus as cause of acute or chronic hepatitis

CLINICAL MANIFESTATIONS

• Sx of all types of viral hepatitis similar
• *Common:* anorexia, abdominal pain, dark urine, fever, headache, hepatomegaly, jaundice, malaise, nausea/vomiting, pruritis
• *Uncommon:* arthralgia, diarrhea, urticarial rash
• Many pts have asymptomatic or mild anicteric infection; illness severity ↑ w/ ↑ age

LABORATORY FEATURES

• Liver chemistries (serum):
  – total bilirubin: levels usually <10 mg/dL, but very high levels (>30 mg/dL) reported
  – aminotransferases: levels variable, generally >10 × upper limit of normal. Alanine aminotransferase (ALT) levels usually higher than aspartate aminotransferase (AST), and fall more slowly
  – alkaline phosphatase: elevation usually <2–3 × normal; higher levels occasionally occur in pts w/ cholestatic hepatitis
  – lactic acid dehydrogenase and gamma-glutamyltranspeptidase: ↑ but offer no additional useful diagnostic information
  – albumin and globulin: concentrations usually normal
• Diagnostic tests:
  – none commercially available
  – serologic assays for antibody to HEV available in research laboratories; HEV RNA can be identified in stool and serum by polymerase chain reaction (PCR)
  – PCR tests for HGV (GBV-C) RNA available in research laboratories, but not clinically useful

DIFFERENTIAL DIAGNOSIS

• Alcoholic liver disease
• Drug- or toxin-induced hepatitis
• Ischemic liver necrosis
• Other viruses (eg, cytomegalovirus, Epstein-Barr virus, varicella-zoster virus, herpes simplex virus, adenovirus, paramyxovirus, enteroviruses [coxsackieviruses, echoviruses], parvovirus B19, rubella virus, hemorrhagic fever viruses, human herpes virus 6, yellow fever)
• Reye syndrome
• Wilson disease

TREATMENT

• No specific Tx exists; treatment supportive
• Most pts managed at home
• Hospitalization indicated for pts who cannot receive adequate care at home, or who have evidence of severe hepatitis
• Pts can usually return to normal activity when jaundice resolves and ALT levels are <2 × upper limit of normal

COMPLICATIONS

• Fulminant hepatic failure should be suspected in pts who develop hepatic encephalopathy, fluid retention, oliguria, impaired clotting
• *Incidence of fatal fulminant hepatic failure in pts w/ hepatitis E:* overall, 1–3%; pregnant women, 5–25%

PREVENTION

• No vaccine or other immunoprophylaxis available
• Assure safe drinking water supplies
• Travelers to HEV-endemic areas should avoid drinking water (and beverages w/ ice) of unknown purity, uncooked shellfish, uncooked fruit/vegetables not peeled or prepared by traveler

WHEN TO REFER

• Most pts managed w/o referral
• Referral indicated if pt develops Sx of hepatic encephalopathy (eg, agitation, confusion, coma), fluid retention, oliguria, impaired clotting (eg, prolonged prothrombin time)

All material in this chapter is in the public domain, with the exception of any borrowed figures or tables.

EMBRYOLOGY

- Testicular descent at 28 wks gestation accompanied by diverticulum of peritoneal sac called *processus vaginalis*
- Failure of processus vaginalis to involute results in hernia formation
- Left testicle descends earlier than right, leading to predominance right-sided hernias

INCIDENCE

- 10–20/1,000 live births
- *M:F ratio:* 4:1–10:1
- *Site:* 60% right, 30% left, 10% bilateral

DIFFERENTIAL DIAGNOSIS

- Hydrocele
- Undescended testicle
- Testicular tumor
- Lymphadenopathy

ASSOCIATED CONDITIONS

- *Prematurity:* hernia preset in 7% infants <36 wks gestation and 30% infants weighing <1,000 g at birth
- Higher incidence in cystic fibrosis, genitourinary anomalies, ascites, ventriculoperitoneal shunts, abdominal wall defects, connective tissue disorders

CLINICAL MANIFESTATIONS

- Groin mass aggravated by valsalva maneuvers; resolves spontaneously w/ relaxation
- Pain usually mild in absence of incarceration
- Incarceration presents w/ firm, painful, erythematous groin mass and evidence of bowel obstruction

COMPLICATIONS OF HERNIA

- Contents of hernia sac may become trapped (incarceration) leading to vascular occlusion and necrosis (strangulation)
- *Incarceration:* 12–15% children overall; 30% infants <1 yr of age; 70% incarceration episodes occur within first year of life. Risk of incarceration slightly higher in females
- 80% incarcerated inguinal hernias reduced nonoperatively
- Evidence of strangulation indication for emergent surgery

SURGERY

- Congenital hernias indirect hernias. Repair requires dissection of cord structures and high ligation of sac. Formal repair of floor of inguinal canal rarely required

Contralateral exploration

- Exploration of asymptomatic contralateral side controversial
- Contralateral patent processus vaginalis present 60–90% infants <2–3 mos of age but only 40% children >12 mos of age
- Incidence of contralateral hernias higher in premature infants, females, those that present w/ left inguinal hernia
- Contralateral hernias develop 20–40% of pts w/ unilateral repair as child
- Most pediatric surgeons recommend routine contralateral groin exploration in children <1 yr of age, esp if infant was premature
- Some advocate exploration of both sides in older males and all females

Surgical complications (1–2% elective cases)

- Wound infection
- Recurrence
- Damage to ileoinguinal nerve
- Damage to vas deferens
- Testicular infarction
- Surgical complications 20 × higher w/ incarcerated hernias

Timing of repair

Age/Presentation	Repair Timing
Strangulation	Emergent
Incarcerated (reduced nonoperatively)	24–48 hrs after reduced
<2–3 mos old	7–10 d
>3 mos	1–3 wks

- Infants <60 wks gestation (prenatal age + postnatal age) require postop monitoring for apnea

VIDYA SHARMA

BACKGROUND

- Large DNA-containing viruses
- *Two distinct types:* type 1 (HSV-1), type 2 (HSV-2)
- HSV-1 usually but not exclusively occurs on face and skin above waist
- HSV-2 most common cause of neonatal disease and genital disease in adults
- *Neonatal HSV:* usually HSV-2, but 15–20% HSV-1. Transmission occurs during birth or postnatally from mouth, hands of parents or nursery personnel
- Postnatal infection w/ HSV-1 from direct contact w/ infected oral secretions. Occurs earlier in children of lower socioeconomic status and in day-care centers
- Prevalence of HSV-2 ↑ at time of puberty and early adolescence in association w/ sexual activity

CLINICAL MANIFESTATIONS

Neonatal

- *Systemic infection:* involves multiple organs: liver and CNS
- Localized CNS disease
- Localized infection of skin, eyes, mucous membranes. Vesicles seen on skin, keratitis in eye

Postnatal

- *Gingivostomatitis:* most common manifestation of primary HSV infection. Presents w/ fever, vesicles on tongue, lips, gingiva, anterior palate; gum friable, ulcerated, bleeding
- *Vulvovaginitis:* may occur in young children either as sexual abuse or handling w/ contaminated hands. HSV-1, HSV-2 infection of genital tract clinically indistinguishable. Presents as vesicles, pustules progressing to ulcers w/ or w/o crusts
- *1° skin infections: Herpetic whitlow:* painful, swollen, erythematous terminal phalanx w/ vesicles. *Herpes gladiatorum:* grouped vesicles seen in wrestlers on trunk or extremities
- *Eye:* blepharitis, conjunctivitis, keratitis w/ minute vesicles (better seen w/ topical fluorescin dye)

LABORATORY FEATURES

- *Tzanck preparation:* from base of lesion. Rapid, nonspecific test reveals multinucleated giant cells w/ occasional intranuclear inclusions
- *Fluorescin antibody test:* rapid, specific
- Culture of vesicular fluid for HSV
- HSV DNA may be detected by polymerize chain reaction (PCR) in CSF

DIFFERENTIAL DIAGNOSIS

- Chicken pox
- Hand, foot, mouth disease
- Herpangiana
- Impetigo
- Blistering diseases of newborn

TREATMENT

- *Symptomatic and supportive:* fluids, pain medication
- Acylovir (may be given either IV or orally) IV 30 mg/kg/d in 3 div doses. Oral dose 80 mg/kg/d in 4 div doses

COMPLICATIONS

- Immunocompromised children have more severe disease and need early treatment
- Children w/ preexisting skin disease (ie, eczema, burns) have unusually severe HSV infections and need treatment
- Erythema multiforme may be seen as allergic response to HSV infection. Presents as macular, urticarial skin eruption lasting 2–3 wks. Tx symptomatic

PREVENTION

- Hand washing
- Avoid direct contact w/ infected secretions
- Antiseptics, soap, hot water, chlorine ↓ risk of spread of virus in institutional settings

WHEN TO REFER

- Most pts can be managed w/o referral
- Referral indicated for newborns, premature newborn w/ systemic infection
- Some children w/ gingivostomatitis may need admission for IV rehydration

HIP DYSPLASIA, DEVELOPMENTAL

JOHN E. HANDELSMAN

BACKGROUND

- *Teratologic dislocations:* 5%
  - intrauterine dislocations associated w/abnormalities such as spina bifida, arthrogryposis, lumbar sacral agenesis
  - hips dislocated, severely dysplastic
- *Typical dislocations:* 95%
  - dislocation perinatal or early postnatal event
  - no significant associated abnormalities (but sometimes metatarsus adductus and torticollis)
  - hip morphology normal or dysplasia very mild
- Incidence in neonates:
  - dislocation 1.3/1,000
  - dislocatable 1.2/1,000
  - unstable or subluxable in further 9.2/1,000
- *Etiology:* combination of genetic and environmental factors
  - high in Caucasians and North American Indians
  - ligamentous laxity
  - maternal hormones at time of delivery
  - breech lie
  - interuterine attitude (preponderance of left hip dislocations)

DIAGNOSIS

- Physical examination key to Dx
- Hip instability never obvious; must be sought
- Clinical examination for DDH:
  - shortening of femur in flexion (Galleazzi sign)
  - shortening of limb in extension
  - skin fold irregularity (unreliable)
  - abduction in flexion: performed w/thumb on medial condyle and finger on greater trochanter. Unilateral or bilateral limitation. Reduction of dislocation w/*palpable* clunk is positive Ortolani sign. Becomes negative when hip no longer reducible
  - Barlow provocative test: dislocates reduced but unstable hip. Performed by flexing and adducting hip, pushing femur gently downward and outward, then abducting in flexion. Hip that dislocates reduces w/Ortolani "clunk"
  - palpation of hip joint: hollow just below mid femoral point and greater tronchanteric buttock bulge. High pointing femoral shaft
  - the "clicking" hip: most are innoxious. May be suction noises from hip or knee joint or tendon snapping over greater trochanter. Caution: follow clinically at 3 mos and w/x ray at 6 mos to avoid missing occasional dysplastic hip
- Imaging techniques:
  - x rays: unhelpful until capital epiphyses appear in cartilaginous femoral heads at 4–6 mos. Then provide excellent measurement of dysplasia. Acetabular index should be 24° or less and capital epiphyses equal on each side
  - sonography: outlines cartilage and can detect early dysplasia. Best when performed w/Barlow provocative maneuver during exam
  - danger: both x ray and sonography show hip joint in moment in time. Hip seen reduced on imaging may be dislocated immediately thereafter

TREATMENT

- Position of abduction in flexion critical in first few days of life to maintain reduction while ligaments tighten. Do not swaddle legs!
- Forceful reduction after first 2 wks of life may stretch vessels to epiphysis and cause avascular necrosis
- Accepted methods:
  - Pavlik harness for first 3 mos. Infant may "kick" dislocated hip into socket during that time
  - if succeed, use Camp or similar abduction brace at nap and nighttime thereafter until dysplasia, as seen on x rays at 6 mo intervals, resolved
  - if fail, move to overhead traction for 2 wks then reduction under anesthesia, w/or w/o adductor tenotomy and hip spica for 8–12 wks. Then Camp abduction brace. Occasionally soft tissue interposition necessitates surgery

WHEN TO REFER

- Once Dx is made

MESSAGE

- Early treatment = normal hip; delay = disaster

BACKGROUND

- *Definition:* dysmotility syndrome caused by lack of ganglion cells in submucosal and myenteric plexuses of distal bowel. Aganglionic bowel fails to relax normally, resulting in defective peristalsis, intestinal obstruction
- 75% cases limited to rectum or rectosigmoid; 5–8% involve entire colon and, in some cases, portion of distal small bowel as well. Aganglionosis of entire small and large bowel occurs rarely
- *Incidence:* ~1/5,000 live births. Boys predominate 4:1
- Incidence ↑ in Waardenburg syndrome, cartilage-hair hypoplasia syndrome, multiple endocrine neoplasia syndrome type 2, trisomy 18 and trisomy 21. Some cases familial; both autosomal recessive and autosomal dominant modes of inheritance described. Associated congenital anomalies seen in up to 20%

CLINICAL MANIFESTATIONS

- Typically have Hx constipation beginning in infancy. Delayed passage of meconium in first 24–48 hrs of life common
- Neonate w/ Hirschsprung disease (HD) may present w/ progressive abdominal distention and vomiting, which may be bilious
- Older child may present w/ Hx constipation
- Anal sphincter usually tight in pts w/ HD. Absence of stool in rectal ampulla, unlike pt w/ functional constipation, whose rectal ampulla typically filled w/ stool
- Enterocolitis (EC) associated w/ HD presents w/ abdominal distention, vomiting, diarrhea, which may be explosive. Pt may have fever, rectal bleeding; may appear toxic

LABORATORY AND RADIOLOGIC FEATURES

- *Abdominal x ray:* dilated bowel w/ absence of gas in rectum
- *Barium enema (BE):* dilated proximal bowel w/ contracted aganglionic distal bowel. Funnel-shaped transition zone may be seen between normal and aganglionic bowel. Pt should not have rectal exam done or be given enemas prior to BE, and enema catheter balloon should not be inflated, in order to avoid obliteration of transition zone making Dx more difficult
- *Anorectal manometry:* contraction rather than expected normal relaxation of internal anal sphincter in response to distention of rectal ampulla
- *Rectal biopsy:* absence of ganglion cells in submucosal and myenteric plexuses diagnostic. Acetylcholinesterase staining ↑. Suction biopsy can be performed safely as outpt procedure w/o general anesthesia; reliable so long as adequate specimen obtained

DIFFERENTIAL DIAGNOSIS

- Anal atresia
- Neonatal small left colon syndrome
- Meconium plug syndrome
- Meconium ileus
- Malrotation
- Hypermagnesemia
- Hypothyroidism
- Intestinal neuronal dysplasia
- Functional constipation

TREATMENT

- Definitive treatment includes performance of pull-through procedure in which aganglionic segment of bowel resected, and normally innervated bowel brought down to distal rectum

- Whether to do definitive reconstructive procedure at time of Dx, or to initially do diverting colostomy and perform pull-through procedure at later date, at discretion of surgeon
- EC managed by saline enemas, placement of rectal tube, administration of broad-spectrum antibiotics, including coverage for anaerobes. Pt may need volume support or blood transfusion as well

COMPLICATIONS

- Colonic volvulus
- Intestinal perforation, particularly perforation of appendix
- Undiagnosed HD in older child may be associated w/ chronic abdominal distention, growth failure
- EC may be presenting feature of HD, or may occur following surgical reconstruction. Delayed Dx HD beyond neonatal period ↑ risk serious morbidity or mortality from EC
- Some pts may have continued symptoms of constipation or fecal soiling following surgical reconstruction
- Pts w/ extensive small bowel involvement may have malabsorption and may require long-term total parenteral nutrition (TPN). Such pts may develop TPN-associated complications, such as cholestasis and infection, and may experience problems w/ growth

WHEN TO REFER

- Pts w/ clinical findings suggestive of HD may initially be evaluated by family physician or general pediatrician
- Pts in whom results of evaluation unclear should be referred to pediatric gastroenterologist or pediatric surgeon for definitive Dx
- Once Dx made, pt should be referred to pediatric surgeon for surgical reconstruction

DEFINITION

- Group of rare, diverse disorders characterized by localized or generalized proliferation of histiocytes

HISTIOCYTOSIS SOCIETY CLASSIFICATION OF HISTIOCYTOSIS SYNDROMES IN CHILDREN

- *Class I:* Langerhans-cell histiocytosis (LCH; replaces term *histiocytosis X, eosinophilic granuloma, Letterer-Siwe disease, Hand-Schuller-Christian syndrome,* others)
- *Class II:* histiocytoses of mononuclear phagocytes other than Langerhans cells:
    - familial hemophagocytic syndrome
    - infection-associated hemophagocytic syndrome
    - sinus histiocytosis w/ massive lymphadenopathy (Rosai-Dorfman)
    - juvenile xanthogranuloma
    - reticulohistiocytoma
    - miscellaneous/other/unclassified
- *Class III:* malignant histiocytic disorders
- *Note:* class II, III disorders extremely uncommon and not discussed further

BACKGROUND

- Generally thought to be rare disorder; ~1,200 new cases/y in US; however, accurate incidence rates not available
- Affects all ages and both sexes; incidence appears highest in pediatric, adolescent age groups
- Etiology unknown. Mounting evidence that most if not all cases of clonal nature; however, LCH not generally classified as malignant disorder

- Dx on basis of biopsy. Presumptive Dx made on basis of light microscopy; definitive Dx requires demonstration of Birbeck granules by electron microscopy or presence of CD1a antigen by special staining technique

CLINICAL MANIFESTATIONS

- Highly diverse clinical presentation depending on location and extent of involvement. Systemic manifestations may include fever, weight loss
- *Bone:* involved ~80% of cases. Often painful swelling w/ radiographic appearance of well-circumscribed lytic lesion. Common sites include skull, orbit, mandible, long bones, axial skeleton. Associated findings include proptosis, chronic otitis media, mastoid involvement mimicking mastoiditis, "floating teeth" from jaw involvement, rarely spinal cord compression from vertebral involvement
- *Skin:* involved ~60% of cases. May resemble seborrheic dermatitis; frequently involves scalp, posterior auricular areas or groin/diaper area
- *Posterior pituitary:* diabetes insipidus unusual at Dx, but frequent sign of progression (~25–50%)
- *Organ systems:* w/ or w/o organ dysfunction. Sites include lung, liver, spleen, GI tract, bone marrow, thymus, CNS
- Soft tissue mass
- Lymph node enlargement

EVALUATION OF NEWLY DIAGNOSED LCH PT

- CBC and differential
- Liver function testing
- Urine osmolality after overnight water deprivation

- PA and lateral chest radiograph
- Radiographic skeletal survey
- Other tests appropriate based on Sx, areas of known involvement

PROGNOSIS

- Many cases resolve spontaneously or after local Tx; others develop chronic relapsing course. Predictors for subsequent course not clearly defined
- Poor prognostic indicators include young age (<2 yrs), extensive disease w/ evidence of organ dysfunction

TREATMENT

- Film guidelines hampered by lack of randomized, controlled trials
- Localized disease may respond to biopsy or curettage only. Progressive or recurrent symptomatic localized disease may respond to local irradiation at low doses, intralesional corticosteroid injection, topical corticosteroids or systemic Tx
- Extensive disease or evidence of organ dysfunction often treated systematically. Numerous Tx have been employed including vinblastine w/ or w/o corticosteroid, etoposide, methotrexate, 6-mercaptopurine, others. One study suggests ↓ rate of development of diabetes insipidus w/ use of combination chemotherapy compared to historical controls

WHEN TO REFER

- Localized disease may be observed after biopsy confirmation and appropriate new Dx evaluation
- Extensive disease, young age, progressive or recurrent disease requiring systemic Tx should be referred

BACKGROUND

- Dimorphic fungus *Histoplasma capsulatum* causes granulomatous infections w/ protean manifestations (see table)
- Occurs in children worldwide; in US, most common in Mississippi and Ohio River valleys
- *Risk factors:* midwestern US, exposure to places frequented by birds or bats, eg, roosts, caves, old barns, parks, schoolyards
- Proper Dx/classification of illness critical in determining which children require antifungal chemotherapy (see table)

CLINICAL MANIFESTATIONS

- *Normal host, asymptomatic infection:* as many as 99% primary histoplasmosis infections asymptomatic; even after heavy exposure to *H. capsulatum,* up to 50% of infections asymptomatic. Calcifications of liver, spleen still may occur after subclinical infections. No Tx required
- *Normal host, self-limited symptomatic infection:* of few who become symptomatic: ≥80% have acute pulmonary histoplasmosis (influenzalike symptoms of chills, fever, headache, myalgia, nonproductive cough; chest radiographs usually showing enlarged hilar or mediastinal lymph nodes and small, patchy infiltrates, but occasionally normal); ≤10% have erythema multiforme, erythema nodosum, or pericarditis. Illness generally occurs 12–16 (range: 7–21) d after exposure, resolves 3–10 d later. Rarely requires antifungal Tx
- *Normal host, rare manifestations of histoplasmosis:* marked enlargement of mediastinal lymph nodes (mediastinal granuloma) may cause bronchial, esophageal, or superior vena cava obstruction. Most masses slowly resolve spontaneously; whether antifungal Tx speeds resolution unknown. Surgical intervention rarely required. Fibrosing mediastinitis following histoplasmosis very rare in childhood; neither surgery nor antifungal Tx useful
- *Normal host, progressive disseminated histoplasmosis of infancy:* life-threatening form of infection seen almost exclusively in children ≤12 mos of age, characterized by unexplained persistent fever, weight loss or failure to thrive, hepatosplenomegaly, pancytopenia (but pulmonary findings notably uncommon). Antifungal Tx life saving

- *Disseminated histoplasmosis in the immunocompromised child:* frequently results in progressive disseminated disease. Clinical and laboratory signs of disease nonspecific: persistent fever, weight loss, hepatosplenomegaly. Pulmonary findings may be absent in as many as 50% immunocompromised children w/ disseminated histoplasmosis. Antifungal chemotherapy life saving

DIAGNOSTIC TESTS

- *Microbiologic and histologic tests:* cultures are "gold standard" proof of *H. capsulatum* infection, but insensitive, often too slow (10–14 d) to be useful in prompt clinical decision making. Yield markedly improved in disseminated disease; centrifugation-lysis blood cultures (eg, DuPont Isolator system) 50–75% sensitive, bone marrow aspirate cultures 75% sensitive, combination of the two 90–95% sensitive in disseminated disease. Histology more rapid; lung, liver, or bone marrow biopsy may show small budding yeast on silver stain (much more likely positive in disseminated disease)
- *Serologic tests for antibodies:* in normal hosts, *H. capsulatum* antibodies demonstrable within 4–6 wks (by complement fixation or gel immunodiffusion) in 90% w/ acute self-limited pulmonary histoplasmosis and in majority of infants w/ progressive disseminated histoplasmosis of infancy. Antibody tests on immunocompromised children w/ disseminated disease less likely to be positive (50–80%). Detectable antibody titers in children w/ suggestive clinical illnesses most probably reflects true recent disease rather than coincidental persistent seropositivity
- *Detection of* H. capsulatum *antigen:* assay most valuable in prompt Dx progressive disseminated histoplasmosis of infancy or disseminated histoplasmosis of immunocompromised host in whom early Tx mandatory. Also valuable for identification of relapse in HIV-infected pts undergoing chronic suppressive Tx. Antigen testing generally not required in diagnostic approach of less severely ill patients w/ self-limited disease. Antigen assay now commercially available through Histoplasmosis Reference Laboratory (Dr. L. Joseph Wheat, Indiana University School of Medicine; 1–800-HISTO DG)

- *Histoplasmin skin test:* of epidemiologic value only; should *not* be used to diagnose histoplasmosis

DIFFERENTIAL DIAGNOSIS

- Tuberculosis
- Other endemic mycoses (blastomycosis, coccidioidomycosis)
- Lymphoma

TREATMENT

- *Indications for Tx:* see table
- *Antifungal agents:* amphotericin B drug of choice for severe disease. *Dosage:* first dose 0.25 mg/kg over 2–4 hrs, then daily dose increased by 0.25 mg/kg to target of 0.75–1.0 mg/kg/d. Multiple adverse effects may occur; consult w/ expert in pediatric infectious diseases. *Liposomal amphotericin B* recently licensed; appears less nephrotoxic, but uncertain role in pediatric histoplasmosis. *Antifungal azoles (ketoconazole, fluconazole, itraconazole)* relatively potent, much less nephrotoxic, improved pharmacokinetic parameters (eg, oral absorption) compared w/ amphotericin B; however, not w/o toxicity. Role of azoles in Tx histoplasmosis not clearly defined by appropriate large clinical trials; limited data available suggest itraconazole most useful, but amphotericin B remains best choice for initial Tx of severe histoplasmosis
- *Length of Tx:* remains undetermined, but good success obtained w/ 4 wks IV amphotericin B (ie, total dose 28 mg/kg) for progressive disseminated histoplasmosis of infancy or for immunocompromised children w/ disseminated disease. For rare older child w/ severe self-limited pulmonary disease who requires Tx, oral itraconazole (or less preferably, ketoconazole) given for 4–6 mos may suffice. For HIV-infected child w/ histoplasmosis: several weeks IV amphotericin B, followed by lifelong suppressive Tx w/ either daily itraconazole or weekly IV amphotericin B

WHEN TO REFER

- Progressive disseminated histoplasmosis of infancy
- Disseminated histoplasmosis in immunosuppressed host
- Unusual complication in normal host

Classification	Antifungal Tx Indicated
Normal host	
Asymptomatic	No
Self-limited symptomatic infection	
Pulmonary	Rarely
Arthritis/erythema nodosum	No
Pericarditis	No
Rare manifestations	
Mediastinal granuloma	Possibly
Fibrosing mediastinitis	No
Progressive disseminated histoplasmosis of infancy	Yes

Classification	Antifungal Tx Indicated
Immunocompromised host	
Disseminated histoplasmosis in children w/	
Leukemia, malignancy	Yes
Immunosuppressive therapy	Yes
HIV infection	Yes (lifelong)

BACKGROUND

- *Definition:* malignant lymphoma that usually arises in germinal centers of peripheral lymph node and spreads along lymphatics until it disseminates to lung, liver, spleen, bone, bone marrow
- Cause of Hodgkin disease unknown
- Bimodally distributed w/ one peak extending from adolescence to ~30 yrs of age and second peak in seventh and eighth decades
- Rare in infants and young children
- Some cases in siblings or in skipped generations
- *Malignant cell:* Reed-Sternberg cell
- Reed-Sternberg cells usually transformed B lymphocytes, many of which contain EBV genomes; sometimes they are T cells
- Highly responsive to radiation and/or chemotherapy
- Treatment depends on age and disease extent
- Majority of pts cured

CLINICAL MANIFESTATIONS

- Nontender swelling in cervical, supraclavicular, axillary, or rarely (5%) inguinal or femoral node
- Generalized adenopathy w/ hepatosplenomegaly
- >10% weight loss ("B" symptom)
- Fever of unknown origin (FUO) >3 wks ("B" symptom)
- Anorexia
- Night sweats
- Pruritus
- Difficulty breathing, cough, neck vein distention
- Parneoplastic nephrotic syndrome, cerebellar ataxia, or autoimmune hemolytic anemia, idiopathic thrombocytopenic purpura

LABORATORY FEATURES

- *Node biopsy:* 1/4 characteristic multicellular infiltrates (Rye histologic classification):
  - lymphocyte predominant
  - nodular sclerosing
  - mixed cellularity
  - lymphocyte depletion
- *Chest x ray:* normal or anterior mediastinal mass, peritracheal and/or hilar adenopathy, pulmonary nodules, pleural effusion
- *CBC:* normal or mild anemia, reactive left shift and thrombocytosis or rarely mild pancytopenia
- *Elevated acute-phase reactants:* ESR, ferritin, copper
- *Abdominal CT:* normal or adenopathy; hepatosplenomegaly w/ nodules
- *Bone marrow:* normal, reactive, multicellular infiltrate, or fibrotic

STAGING

- Hx, examination, laboratory studies, biopsy material lead to a stage. Stage called "clinical stage" if based on clinical and laboratory findings or "pathologic stage" if sites documented by biopsy and/or laparotomy and splenectomy
- Ann Arbor staging system:
  - stage I: single node or contiguous group of nodes
  - stage II: ≥2 node groups on same side of diaphragm
  - stage III: nodal or nodal and splenic disease on both sides of diaphragm
  - stage IV: visceral dissemination
    - "A": no symptoms
    - "B": documented FUO and >10% weight loss
    - "e": single site of extranodal disease

DIFFERENTIAL DIAGNOSIS

- Non-Hodgkin lymphoma (esp large cell NHL)
- Infectious mononucleosis
- Reactive adenopathy
- Phenytoin-induced pseudolymphoma
- Tuberculosis

TREATMENT

- Treatment plan depends on age and stage
- *Young age, low stage:* no splenectomy, 4–6 mos chemotherapy w/ or w/o moderate dose radiation to sites of disease
- *Older adolescent, young adult, low stage:* extended field higher dose (3,600–4,400 cGy) radiation or 4–6 mos chemotherapy w/ or w/o moderate dose radiation to sites of disease
- *Advanced disease:* 6–12 mos multiagent chemotherapy w/ or w/o consolidating radiation Tx
- *Chemotherapy combinations:* MOPP or COPP (mechlorethamine, or cyclophosphamide, onocvin, prednisone, procarabine), ABVD (adriamycin, bleomycin, vinblastine, dacarbazine), or combinations or variants of either/both. Used to treat pts who have had recurrence after radiation or who have had exposure to only one four-drug combination. High-dose chemotherapy and autologous marrow or stem cell rescue used in pts w/ multiple recurrences or recurrences after combined radiation and chemotherapy treatment

COMPLICATIONS

- *From tumor:* superior vena cava syndrome, anergy, inanition, paraneoplastic syndromes
- *From splenectomy:* hyperacute pneumococcal or *H. influenzae* infection; adhesions
- *From radiation:* restrictive cardiac or pulmonary disease, growth arrest in irradiated fields, sarcomas, breast cancer, hypothyroidism, infertility
- *From chemotherapy:* 2° acute myeloid leukemia, non-Hodgkin lymphoma, cardiomyopathy

WHEN TO REFER

- For biopsy if malignancy most likely Dx
- After biopsy showing Hodgkin disease

BACKGROUND

- Prevalence varies w/definition of infection/age group
- *Most significant risk factor in genital area of children/adolescents:* sexual behavior/exposure (ie, number of sexual partners); rates of perinatal transmission of HPV to genital area do occur, but rare; up to 50% of children w/external genital warts (EGW) have Hx of sexual abuse

CLINICAL MANIFESTATIONS

- Wide range clinical manifestations ranging from easily visible EGW to subclinical infections associated w/abnormal cytology/histology
- *EGW:* benign lesions, easily detected by naked eye; include condyloma acuminatum: soft, pink/whitish sessilelike tumors on mucosal surfaces, keratotic fissures/irregular on squamous epithelia; papular wart: dome-shaped, usually flesh-colored, 1–4 mm papule
- Subclinical lesions can be diagnosed w/aid of colposcopy/confirmed by histology; colposcopic descriptions of HPV-associated disease include slightly raised acetowhite (white only w/application of 3–5% acetic acid) lesions w/granular surfaces/flat acetowhite lesions w/particular vessel patterns (mosaicism, punctation)
- Routine colposcopic examination not recommended because specificity of colposcopy low in women w/normal cytology; histology remains gold standard for Dx SIL of cervical, vulvar, vaginal, anal area. Referral for colposcopy based on the Bethesda system for rating cytology (replaced older nomenclature because of low rate of agreement in Dx using older systems)
  - New nomenclature: old nomenclature:
    - ASCUS (atypical cells of unknown significance): atypia
    - LSIL (low-grade squamous intraepithelial lesions): condyloma, cervical intraepithelial neoplasia (CIN) I, mild dysplasia
    - HSIL (high-grade squamous intraepithelial lesions): CIN II-III, moderate/severe dysplasia, carcinoma in situ
- *Latency:* HPV DNA detected w/o any evidence clinical disease (normal colposcopy, cytology, histology)

LABORATORY FEATURES

- Detection depends on sensitivity/specificity of test used
- *Only currently commercially available/FDA-approved test:* HybridCapture HPV Diagnostic System (Digene Diagnostics); test uses mixture of two groups: low-risk types (6,11,42,43,44)/high-risk, cancer-related types (16,18,31,33,35,45,51,52,56)
- HPV testing not currently recommended to assist in Dx SIL/EGW

DIFFERENTIAL DIAGNOSIS OF EGWS

- *Normal anatomic variants:* pearly penile papules, vestibular papillae, sebaceous glands
- *Acquired lesions:* molluscum contagiosum, Crohn's disease, seborrheic keratosis, lichen planus, lichen nitidus, skin tags, melanocytic nevi, pseudo verrucous papules, condyloma lata, Bowenoid papulosis, SILs of vulva, Bushchke-Lowenstein tumor, psoriasis, seborrheic dermatitis, erythroplasia of Queyrat on glans penis, squamous cell carcinoma

COMPLICATIONS

- EGW benign lesions/do not have oncogenic potential
- Invasive cancer most significant complication of untreated SIL; HPV-associated cancers include cervical, vulvar, anal, vaginal

PREVENTION

- Because of ubiquitous nature of HPV infection, condoms not been shown to prevent majority HPV infections

TREATMENT

- LSIL verified by biopsy can be followed; persistent lesions (>18–24 mos)/HSIL should be referred for treatment (cryotherapy, laser etc)
- EGW that do not respond to any Tx/when Dx in question should be referred for biopsy

WHEN TO REFER

- All women w/ASCUS should have repeat cytology within 2–3 mos; second repeat ASCUS, LSIL, HSIL/invasive cancer should be referred for colposcopy/biopsy
- Children w/EGW should be referred for sexual abuse evaluation

Prevalence of Genital HPV Infections in Children and Adolescents*

Group	Condyloma	HPV DNA	Abnormal cytology
Neonates	rare reported cases	0–30%	NA
Infants (<12 mos)	<1%	0–30%	NA
Nonsexually abused children	0	0	0
Sexually abused children	1.8%	33%	33%
Nonsexually active adolescents (<20 yrs)	NA	0–3%	0
Sexually active adolescents (<20 yrs)	3%	13–38%	0.8–3%

NA = No data available in unselected populations.
*Modified from Obstet and Gynecology Clinics of NA, Vol. 23, no. 3, Sept. 1996, p. 679

Treatment for External Genital Warts

Treatment	Advantage	Disadvantage
podophyllin	relatively simple to use	contraindicated in pregnancy/on mucosal surfaces
TCA/BCA	relatively simple to use	pain, ulcerations may occur
cryotherapy (liquid nitrogen/nitrous oxide)	relatively simple to use	over-/underapplication; requires equipment and pain control
surgical removal	prompt results	results depend on provider skill; requires equipment and pain control
podofilox, imiquimod	self-applied	safety in pregnancy not known
5% fluorouracil	self-applied; use for intravaginal warts only; not useful for EGW	contraindicated in pregnancy; ulcerations may occur

*All treatment schedules subject to clinical recurrences.

BACKGROUND

- Warts, or verruca, are common viral infections of skin
- Caused by DNA virus, human papillomavirus (HPV)
- Verruca occur in 5–10% of population
- Spread through direct and indirect routes, including close physical contact and fomites (eg, locker room floors)
- Contagion depends on host/viral factors, including quantity of virus, location of verruca, skin injury, cell-mediated immunity
- Local trauma contributes to spread; ie, shaving, picking, biting involved areas may cause local spread
- >70 species of papillomavirus exist

Type of Verruca	HPV Type
Verruca vulgaris (common warts)	2, 4, 27, 29
Verruca plana (flat warts)	3, 10, 28, 49
Verruca plantaris (plantar warts)	1

CLINICAL MANIFESTATIONS

- Common warts:
  – location: exposed surfaces of hands, arms, legs, face
  – morphology: skin-colored, rough, scaly papules that may be solitary or multiple. Size from few mm to several cm. Some w/filiform, or threadlike, projections
- Flat warts:
  – location: face and legs most common, but can occur in any location
  – morphology: usually multiple skin-colored or hyperpigmented, flat-topped, slightly scaly papules 1–5 mm
- Plantar warts:
  – location: plantar surface of feet
  – morphology: hyperkeratotic papules and plaques. Often black small dots (thrombosed vessels) evident. Size from few mm to several cm. Multiple warts may fuse to form large mosaic warts

DIFFERENTIAL DIAGNOSIS

- Flat warts can be confused w/pigmented moles, epidermal nevi, tinea versicolor, molluscum contagiosum, lichen planus, lichen nitidus
- Common, plantar warts differentiated from corns, calluses by interruption of normal skin lines in the former. Paring warts w/#15 blade scalpel aids in differentiation

MANAGEMENT/EDUCATION

- *Basic Principle:* no specific antiviral Tx currently available. All current Tx act indirectly to remove infected skin, irritate skin, increase immunologic responsiveness
- *No Treatment:* most warts resolve w/o Tx. Time to resolution unpredictable w/~25% warts resolving in 3–6 mos, 65–75% resolving in 3 yrs
- *Keratolytics:* common, plantar warts: salicylic acid as 15–40% topical gel, solution, or plaster applied daily for weeks to months w/occlusion and paring between applications. Flat warts: daily topical application of tretinoin cream or gel. Advantages: relatively painless, low risk, inexpensive, home Tx. Disadvantage: slow response, irritation
- *Destructive therapy:*
  – cryotherapy: common warts: Liquid nitrogen 20–30 sec freeze-thaw w/repeat Tx q2–4 wks until warts resolved. Flat warts: 10 sec freeze-thaw. Advantages: quick office procedure. Disadvantages: pain, scarring, recurrence, pigment changes
  – surgical excision or laser ablation: surgical excision, CO_2 laser ablation, pulsed dye laser treatments. Advantages: sometimes effective in recalcitrant warts. Disadvantages: expensive, requires anesthesia, pain, scarring, recurrence
- Immunotherapy:
  – contact sensitization: topical diphencyprone (DPCP) or squaric acid to induce contact dermatitis. Local immune response leads to resolution of 60–80% of warts. Advantages: inexpensive, home Tx. Disadvantages: experimental Tx, medications must be compounded, irritation, slow response
  – interferon: topical imiquimod cream. Advantages: home Tx, little pain, approved for mucosal warts. Disadvantages: expensive, irritation, efficacy not proven for nonmucosal surfaces
  – cimetidine: oral cimetidine, 30–40 mg/kg/d × 8 wks has been reported anecdotally to be effective, but large controlled trials lacking. Advantages: inexpensive oral medication. Disadvantages: unproven efficacy, slow response

COMPLICATIONS

- Warts can embarrass child and negatively impact self-esteem
- Pain (infrequent except w/plantar warts)
- Complications of destructive Tx include scarring, dyspigmentation of skin
- Recurrence rate 5–10% w/all Tx, more for plantar and flat warts

WHEN TO REFER

- Most pts can be managed initially w/topical Tx w/o referral
- Referral to pediatric dermatologist/dermatologist for multiple recalcitrant or painful warts

BACKGROUND

- Accounts for 5% of all childhood poisonings (25% of all poisonings <5 yrs of age)
- Highest incidence 5 mos–5 yrs of age
- Volume ingested <30 mL

- >90% either asymptomatic/have minimal symptoms (cough [40%]/drowsiness [10%])
- Pulmonary/CNS most commonly involved
- Fatalities (90% occur in children <5 yrs of age) almost always due to respiratory failure following aspiration associated w/emesis (lack of emesis/presence of intact gag reflex do not exclude aspiration)
- Positive correlation between volume ingested, severity of pulmonary toxicity, extent of chest radiographic abnormalities

Common hydrocarbons		
Aliphatics	**Aromatics/Terpenes**	**Halogenated Hydrocarbons**

Low viscosity	High viscosity	Low viscosity	Low viscosity
gasoline	asphalt	benzene	carbon tetrachloride
kerosene	motor and diesel oil	toluene	methylene chloride
mineral spirits	fuel oil	turpentine	trichloroethane
mineral seal oil	grease	xylene	trichloroethylene
naphthas	lubrication oils		
furniture polish	tar		
lighter fluid	petroleum jelly		
cleaning fluid			

- Low viscosity most important chemical property determining risk of aspiration
- Low viscosity aliphatics most commonly aspirated after ingestion
- Low viscosity aliphatics poorly absorbed by GI tract; aromatic/halogenated hydrocarbons well absorbed, accounting for greater CNS toxicity
- High viscosity aliphatics: no major risk of pulmonary/CNS toxicity

CLINICAL MANIFESTATIONS

- Fever
- Respiratory distress:
  – tachypnea, cough, dyspnea, retractions, grunting, coarse/decreased breath sounds, crackles, wheezing, rhonchi (within min/hrs)
  – cyanosis, hemoptysis, respiratory failure (rare, within 24–48 hrs)
  – poor clinical correlation between symptoms, physical findings, chest radiograph
- CNS abnormalities (reported in 30%):
  – weakness, altered mental status, excitement, somnolence, tremor (rare: coma <3%, seizure <1%)
  – due to hypoxia following ingestion/aspiration of aliphatic hydrocarbons
  – due to systemic absorption after ingestion of aromatic/halogenated hydrocarbons
- GI abnormalities:
  – nausea (65%), burning/irritation of mouth and throat, abdominal pain, diarrhea, bloody stools
- Uncommon findings (usually associated w/aromatic/halogenated hydrocarbons):
  – renal (renal tubular acidosis, proteinuria, hematuria)
  – metabolic acidosis
  – cardiac (arrhythmia)
  – hematologic (hemolytic anemia, pancytopenia, disseminated intravascular coagulopathy)
  – hepatic (↑ liver function enzymes)

LABORATORY FEATURES

- Chest radiograph:
  – abnormalities in 15–40% (regardless of physical findings)
  – most common abnormality bilateral symmetric basal patchy airspace consolidation (65% of abnormal films); hyperinflation/atelectasis (rarely, pleural effusion, pneumothorax, pneumomediastinum, pneumatocele); may progress to diffuse alveolitis/bronchopneumonia
  – 60% of findings within 1st hour (90% within 3 hrs, 98% within 12 hrs)
  – resolution usually within several days/abnormalities may persist for months
  – no consistent correlation between radiologic findings/clinical course
- Hypoxemia w/o hypercapnia
- Mixed metabolic/respiratory acidosis (seen in severe hypoxemia)
- Elevated WBC count w/left shift (80% of children w/hydrocarbon ingestion)
- Uncommon findings (usually associated w/aromatic/halogenated hydrocarbons):
  – ketonuria, proteinuria, glucosuria, cellular casts, hemoglobinuria, hematuria, pancytopenia, hemolytic anemia, disseminated intravascular coagulopathy, hypoglycemia, fatty infiltration of liver

DIAGNOSIS

- Hx of exposure w/odor of hydrocarbon on child's breath
- Aspiration suggested by hx vomiting, choking, gagging shortly following ingestion

MANAGEMENT

- Identify precise hydrocarbon/volume ingested
- Contact local/regional poison control center
- Aliphatic hydrocarbons
  – observation, supportive care, hospitalization if >2 mL/kg (consider outpt management if <2 mL/kg)
  – emesis/gastric lavage contraindicated
  – catharsis, use of activated charcoal, antiemetics necessary
- Aromatic/halogenated hydrocarbons, aliphatic hydrocarbons containing toxins (eg, organophosphates, heavy metals)
  – <2 mL/kg body wt: observation, supportive care, hospitalization
  – >2 mL/kg body weight: supportive care, hospitalization
    ○ if awake, alert pt; within 30 min of ingestion:
      * ipecac-induced emesis (gastric lavage carries ↑ risk for aspiration)
      * activated charcoal, catharsis
    ○ if systemic toxicity (esp altered consciousness); within several hours of ingestion:
      * endotracheal intubation by skilled anesthesiologist to protect airway
      * gastric lavage following intubation
      * activated charcoal and catharsis
      * specific antidote
- Fever control
- Respiratory support
- Use of steroids, antibiotics unproven, not recommended; chest physical therapy not beneficial.
- Anticipatory guidance and parental education

COMPLICATIONS

- Usually full recovery in 3–8 d
- 2° bacterial pneumonia 2–4 d after aspiration
- Subclinical small airway obstruction may be detectable by spirometry years after recovery
- Pneumatocele formation (<5% of aspiration pts) 3–15 d after aspiration; treatment unnecessary; may require weeks to months for resolution
- Rarely, hepatic necrosis, disseminated intravascular coagulopathy

WHEN TO REFER

- All pts suspected of hydrocarbon ingestion should be observed ×4–6h in office setting
- Asymptomatic pts w/normal chest radiograph/normal oximetry at least 3 hrs after ingestion may be observed at home
- All symptomatic pts/pts w/abnormal chest radiographs should be admitted to hospital
- All pts at risk for systemic toxicity (aromatic/halogenated hydrocarbons/aliphatic hydrocarbons containing toxins) should be admitted to hospital
- All pts w/aspiration require formal pulmonary function testing, consultation w/pediatric pulmonologist

BACKGROUND

- Usually present at birth, but can appear at any age
- May be bilateral
- Associated w/ any condition causing ascites including presence of ventriculoperitoneal shunt

CLINICAL MANIFESTATIONS

- Usually asymptomatic scrotal swelling
- Swelling may be inguinoscrotal or inguinal, which makes differentiation from hernia more difficult
- Usually caused by a patent processus vaginalus, so may change in size
- Usually not reducible. Will not reduce w/ "squelch" of hernia
- Transilluminates

DIFFERENTIAL DIAGNOSIS

- Inguinal hernia (in which case swelling not exclusively scrotal)
- Testicular tumor (does not transilluminate)
- Testicular torsion
- Varicocele

TREATMENT

- Observation. Often resolves spontaneously. Parents warned about possible hernia
- Operative repair if hernia appears or hydrocele persists
- Hernia may appear at any time and become incarcerated

WHEN TO REFER

- If Dx secure, routine referral not necessary
- Refer if hernia appears
- Refer if hydrocele not getting smaller after the first year of life

BACKGROUND

• Pathologic CSF collection within intracranial spaces, particularly ventricles
• 3 physiologic origins:
  – ↑ CSF production
  – obstruction to normal CSF flow pattern within ventricular system
  – CSF absorption at level of arachnoid granulations
• Often seen in former premature infants w/ Hx intraventricular hemorrhage, in children w/ tumors of CNS, in children w/ congenital abnormalities of CNS (eg, acqueductal stenosis)

CLINICAL MANIFESTATIONS

• *Infant:* ↑ head circumference crossing percentile lines, along w/ bulging anterior fontanel, fussiness, crankiness, poor feeding; later, unilateral/bilateral sixth cranial nerve palsies ("sunsetting" may be seen as earlier manifestation in older children)
• *Older children:* headache, nausea, vomiting, sixth nerve palsies; later on, papilledema
• In chronic cases, frontal bossing may be present

LABORATORY FEATURES

• In infant, head circumference (crosses centile lines on head growth chart)
• *In infant, cranial ultrasonography:* ↑ ventricular size (reliable index to follow)
• In older children, cranial imaging w/ CT/MRI confirms presence ↑ ventricular size; MRI may also image obstructing structures, ↑ size of choroid plexus in cases of overproduction, excess fluid over cortical surface in instances ↓ absorption

DIFFERENTIAL DIAGNOSIS

• Megalencephaly (large brain/large head circumference w/o large ventricles):
  – familial
  – pathologic: neurofibromatosis, Alexander disease, Canavan disease, mucopolysaccharidoses
  – idiopathic
• Ventriculomegaly (enlarged ventricles after early brain injury)
• Bony overgrowth of skull (thalassemia, osteopetrosis)

TREATMENT

• *In infant post-IVH:* serial lumbar punctures (w/ or w/o diuretics) successful in many instances; if ventricular enlargement continues, surgical Tx indicated
• *In overproduction (choroid plexus papilloma):* loop diuretics (ie, furosemide) coupled w/ carbonic anhydrase inhibitors (ie, acetazolamide); if unsuccessful, resection of choroid plexus may be needed
• *In deficient absorption:* carbonic anhydrase inhibitors used; if unsuccessful, add loop diuretic
• In obstruction, alternate outflow pathway required (may begin as external ventricular drainage, but usually requires placement of shunt, ventriculoperitoneal/ventriculoatrial); if obstruction ° to small congenital stenosis, ventriculoscopy may reopen pathways/avoid need for shunt

COMPLICATIONS

• Untreated hydrocephalus can lead to serious brain injury/later psychomotor retardation
• Shunts can malfunction, leading to recurrence of hydrocephalus; shunt infection rare (can lead to ventriculitis)

WHEN TO REFER

• To neurosurgeon when overproduction/↓ absorption hydrocephalus types fail to respond to medical Tx
• In instances of obstruction

DAVID R. CHAVEZ AND LOWELL R. KING

BACKGROUND

- Prenatal ultrasound discovers possible urologic anomalies at incidence of 1/500
- Hydronephrosis more common in male fetus
- *Most common lesion: prenatal pyelocalyectasis:* ureteropelvic junction (UPJ) obstruction; UPJ obstruction confirmed by postnatal investigation in up to 39% of infants w/prenatally detected GU abnormalities
- Permanent kidneys (metanephros) begin development in 5th wk of gestation after ureteral bud grows into renal blastema
- 43% of nephrons (350,500) present by 20th wk of gestation; 767,000 nephrons present by 28th wk of gestation, nephrogenesis completed by 36th wk
- Prognosis for pregnancy good if hydronephrosis unilateral
- Prenatal intervention for severe hydronephrosis still controversial; prenatal vesicoamniotic shunt placed 20–34 wk gestation for oligohydramnios does not consistently achieve renal salvage; wide variety of GU congenital anomalies found unexpectedly postnatally (prune belly syndrome, 1° megacystis, duplex anomalies, cloacal malformations) instead of presumed antenatal Dx posterior urethral valves
- Ureteral obstruction during latter half of gestation results in hydronephrosis, whereas severe renal dysplasia occurs if obstruction begins early midtrimester

CLINICAL MANIFESTATIONS

- Oligohydramnios not always present (suggestive of significant GU anomaly if present); incidence of oligohydramnios: 0.4%–5.0%
- Oligohydramnios beginning early in gestation associated w/poorer prognosis in terms of both renal/pulmonary development than that occurring in late gestation (third trimester)
- Level of fetal obstruction dictates ultrasound findings:
  – ureteropelvic junction: hydronephrosis
  – midureter: hydroureteronephrosis
  – ureterovesical junction: hydroureteronephrosis
  – bladder neck/posterior urethra: bilateral hydroureteronephrosis, full bladder w/thickened wall; severe cases may present w/urinary ascites/oligohydramnios

LABORATORY FEATURES

- Fetal urine electrolytes sometimes predictive of fetal renal function
- Sequential sampling of fetal urine electrolytes considered if:
  – no other major congenital anomalies found
  – bilateral hydroureteronephrosis w/distended bladder
  – unilateral hydroureteronephrosis w/distended bladder/no contralateral kidney
- Favorable prognostic signs:
  – Na < 100 mEq/L
  – Cl < 90 mEg/L
  – Osm < 210 mOsm
  – urine output > 2 mL/hr
  – beta-microglobulin < 4 mg/L
  – Nl echogenicity in kidneys
  – Nl amniotic fluid volume
- Unfavorable prognostic signs:
  – Na > 100 mEq/L
  – Cl > 90 mEq/L
  – Osm > 210 mOsm
  – urine output < 2 mL/hr
  – beta-microglobulin > 4 mg/L
  – oligohydramnios
  – macroscopic cysts in kidneys
  – ↑ renal echogenicity

DIFFERENTIAL DIAGNOSIS

- Ureteropelvic junction obstruction vs. nonobstructed dilation
- Multicystic dysplastic kidney
- *Megaureters:* obstructed/nonobstructed
- Vesicoureteral reflux
- Ureterocele
- Prune belly syndrome
- Ectopic ureter
- Posterior urethral valves
- Anterior urethral valve
- Urethral atresia

TREATMENT

- Prenatal intervention rarely indicated; consider referral to specialized center for vesicoamniotic shunt if:
  – Nl chromosomes
  – favorable fetal urine parameters
  – no macroscopic renal cysts
- Complications of vesicoamniotic shunts:
  – preterm labor
  – sepsis
  – stent migration/obstruction
  – perforation of abdominal viscera
  – fetal demise ~5%
- Postnatally treatment dictated by level of obstruction, size of neonate/lung development

- Place all babies on antibacterial prophylaxis until vesicoureteral reflux excluded
- *Common scenario:* anuric baby boy w/persistent hydroureteronephrosis/distended bladder on postnatal renal ultrasound, likely Dx posterior urethral valves
- *First step:* catheter drainage; pass 5 Fr feeding tube into bladder; always document position of catheter after placement; sometimes catheter coils in dilated prostatic urethra because of hypertrophied bladder neck
- Obtain voiding cystourethrogram (VCUG) to look for urethral posterior valves/vesicoureteral reflux; urine culture/urine analysis can be collected at this time; if catheter drainage fails to improve azotemia higher diversion (vesicostomy/cutaneous ureterostomies) may be required
- Postobstructive diuresis will follow if obstruction bilateral
  – creatinine at birth will be equal to maternal creatinine
- If neonate voiding/no abdominal mass present allow first 48–72 hrs for hydration, then obtain postnatal renal ultrasound
- If postnatal hydronephrosis/hydroureteronephrosis still present, proceed w/VCUG after initiating amoxicillin prophylaxis until vesicoureteral reflux excluded
- To diagnose ureteropelvic junction obstruction (UPJ) DTPA/MAG 3 lasix renal scan w/continuous bladder catheter drainage should be arranged within first month of life; if only one kidney present/bilateral UPJ obstruction suspected, renal scan should be performed sooner

COMPLICATIONS

- *Pulmonary hypoplasia:* also be suspicious of GU anomalies if newborn has pneumothorax
- Renal dysplasia
- Urinary ascites
- Obstructive uropathy, which may lead to hypertension/chronic renal failure
- *Potter syndrome:* bilateral renal agenesis fatal; facial features molded by uterine wall
- Urosepsis

WHEN TO REFER

- Ideally pediatric urologist should be made aware of fetus w/hydronephrosis prenatally; this will allow discussion of possible future interventions neonate may require

F. BRUDER STAPLETON

BACKGROUND

- Urinary stones develop in children of all ages
- Boys, girls affected equally
- Positive family Hx urinary stones present in 50–60% of children w/urolithiasis
- Hypercalciuria most common cause of urolithiasis in children, adults
- Causes of urolithiasis in children include:
  - hypercalciuria: 42%
  - infection: 13%
  - cystinuria: 5%
  - hyperoxaluria: 5%
  - uric acid: 4%
  - idiopathic: 19%
  - others: 12%

CLINICAL MANIFESTATIONS

- Isolated microscopic/macroscopic hematuria may occur w/o evidence of urinary stones in children w/hypercalciuria
- Hematuria occurs in 60–90% of children w/stones
- Pain present in only 50% of children w/urinary stones; most common in older children, although stone-related pain may mimic infantile colic
- Infection a presenting manifestation of urolithiasis, most common in preschool children
- Crystalluria common in children w/urolithiasis

LABORATORY FEATURES

- Normal values for 24 hr urine excretion in children:
  - calcium: <4 mg/kg/d
  - uric acid: <0.57 mg/dl GFR
  - oxalate: <50 mg/1.73 m^2/d
  - cystine: <60 mg/d
  - citrate: >400 mg/g creatinine
  - urine volume: >20 mL/kg/d
- Urine calcium to creatinine ratio (mg/mg) may be useful for screening for hy-

percalciuria in younger children. In children >2 yrs, normal fasting Uca/Ucr ratios are <0.2
- Normal urine calcium to creatinine ratios <0.8 from 0–6 mos, <0.6 from 6–12 mos of age
- Serum studies should include creatinine, calcium, phosphorus, uric acid, magnesium, potassium, sodium, chloride, bicarbonate concentrations. Parathyroid hormone studied for hypercalciuria, hypercalcemia and/or hypophosphaturia
- Obtain urinary studies when pt ambulatory, ingesting routine diet, urine culture negative
- All children suspected of having urinary stones should have renal, bladder ultrasound examination, routine abdominal x-ray

DIFFERENTIAL DIAGNOSIS

- Selected causes of hypercalciuria in children include:
  - hypercalcemia
  - hypophosphatemia
  - metabolic acidosis
  - expansion of extracellular fluid volume
  - immobilization
  - hypertension
  - distal renal tubular acidosis
  - generalized renal tubular dysfunction
  - hyperalimentation
  - ACTH
  - methylxanthines
  - hypomagnesemia
  - furosemide therapy
  - juvenile rheumatoid arthritis
  - endocrine:
    - diabetes mellitus
    - hyperparathyroidism
    - hyperadrenocorticism
  - vitamin D excess
  - sarcoidosis
  - neoplasms
  - medullary sponge kidney

TREATMENT

- Medical treatment of hypercalciuria and urinary stones:
  - general: high fluid intake, low sodium diet, low oxalate diet, high potassium diet
  - thiazide diuretics: if hypercalciuria found in child w/urolithiasis, hydrochlorothiazide 1–2 mg/kg/d lowers urinary calcium excretion. Care given to assure normal serum potassium, follow serum triglycerides and cholesterol. Length of Tx unknown, but may require many years
  - potassium citrate: potassium citrate given to children w/↓ urinary citrate excretion

COMPLICATIONS

- Stones in urinary tract require urologic consultation for possible lithotripsy or surgical removal
- Hydrochlorothiazide may produce hypokalemia, may raise plasma lipids
- Long-term effects of untreated hypercalciuria on bone mineralization uncertain, but do not appear to warrant thiazide Tx in all children w/hypercalciuria

WHEN TO REFER

- All children w/urolithiasis evaluated to discern whether metabolic or urologic condition present
- When stone present in urinary tract, referral to pediatric urologist or nephrologist indicated
- Because of age-related variability of normal laboratory values, consultation for evaluation of urolithiasis often helpful

BACKGROUND

- In adults, each 1 mg/dl ↓ in total cholesterol ↓ coronary risk 2%
- *Familial hypercholesterolemia:* autosomal dominant
    - 1/500 population
    - males develop coronary artery disease in 30s–40s; females 40s–50s
- *Familial combined hypercholesterolemia (↑ cholesterol / ↑ triglycerides):* autosomal dominant
    - 1/200–300 population
- Hyperlipidemia frequently nonfamilial; 2° to diabetes mellitus, nephrotic syndrome, liver disease, hypothyroidism, Cushing syndrome

LABORATORY

- *Total cholesterol determination:* no fasting required
- *Lipid profile:* fast overnight
- Types of hyperlipidemia determined by lipid profile:
    - I: greatly ↑ triglycerides (>1,000 mg/dl); 2° to ↑ chylomicrons; rare
    - IIA: ↑ LDL-C (≥130 mg/dl); common
    - IIB: ↑ LDL-C (≥130 mg/dl); ↑ triglycerides (>125 mg/dl); common
    - III: ↑ total cholesterol (≥ 200 mg/dl); ↑ triglycerides (≥ 125 mg/dl) rare; 2° to homozygous apolipoprotein E_2, diabetes mellitus, renal disease
    - IV: ↑ triglycerides (≥ 125 mg/dl); common
    - V: markedly ↑ triglycerides (≥1,000 mg/dl); 2° to ↑ chylomicrons/VLDL; uncommon

SCREENING/PREVENTION

- *National Cholesterol Education Program (NCEP):* testing <age 2 not indicated
- *NCEP:* all children >2 yrs should be on moderately restricted diet (↓ fat, ↓ cholesterol: total fat ≤30% total calories; saturated fat <10% calories; polyunsaturated up to 10% (rest monounsaturated); cholesterol <300 mg/dl/d); carbs 55%; protein 15–20%; total calories to achieve desirable body weight
- Indications for screening during childhood:
    - parent w/total cholesterol ≥240 mg/dl
    - family Hx premature cardiovascular disease
    - family Hx dyslipidemia
    - medical condition predisposing to cardiovascular disease/dyslipidemia (diabetes mellitus, liver/renal disease, hypothyroidism, Cushing syndrome, steroid ingestion)
- Desirable lipid levels ≤21 yrs of age:

Lipid	Desirable	Borderline	Undesirable
Total cholesterol	<170 mg/dl	170–199 mg/dl	≥200 mg/dl
LDL-C	<110 mg/dl	110–129 mg/dl	≥130 mg/dl
HDL-C	>45 mg/dl	35–45 mg/dl	<35 mg/dl
Triglycerides	<125 mg/dl	—	≥125 mg/dl

- Screening follow-up:
    - if total cholesterol <170 mg/dl, retest 5 yrs
    - if total cholesterol 170–199 mg/dl, repeat in 2–4 wks w/full lipid profile: if LDL-C ≤ 110 mg/dl, no testing × 5 yrs; if LDL-C 110–130 mg/dl, step-one diet/repeat lipids in 1 yr
        ○ step-one diet: ≤30% fat; 55% carbs; protein 15–20%; total calories = 1,000 + (100 × age in years)

TREATMENT

- *Three mainstays of Tx:* diet, exercise, attention to possible 2° causes of hyperlipidemia
- *Treatment goal:* LDL-C ≤ 110 mg/dl (ideal)/110–130 mg/dl (minimally acceptable)
- *Exercise:* daily regular
- *Diet:* if step one fails, move to step two diet: ↓ saturated fats ≤ 7% total calories, total cholesterol qd ≤ 200 mg
- Exercise/diet failure if LDL-C > 160 mg/dl in 6–12 mos

- Drug Tx:
    - indications: in children at least 10 yrs of age w/type IIA or type IIB:
        ○ LDL-C = 160–189 mg/dl + family Hx cardiovascular disease
        ○ LDL-C = 160–189 mg/dl w/2 of following: smoking, hypertension, LDL-C <35 mg/dl, obesity (>30% ideal weight), diabetes mellitus, physical inactivity, male gender, renal disease
        ○ LDL ≥ 190 mg/dl
    - agents
        ○ bile acid binding agents: although often poorly tolerated, still front-line Tx for IIA (not IIB, since may ↑ triglycerides). Examples: cholysteramine 1 scoop (4 g) to start, ↑ to 2–4 scoops as tolerated; 6 scoops max.
        ○ niacin (IIA, IIB, IV, V): start 50 mg/d, ↑ q4wks, continue to 1,500–3,000 mg/m² or until LDL-C < 160 mg/dl (IIA, IIB) or triglycerides <300 mg/dl (IV); reduce dose if LDL-C <130 mg/dl/triglycerides <125 mg/dl
        ○ "statins": many available
    - example: atorvastatin (Lipitor): initial dose 10 mg hs w/↑ to 80 mg (max.) to ↓

LDL-C <160 mg/dl; if LDL-C ↓ <130 mg/dl ↓ drug dose
    - toxicities: liver/muscle (rhabdomyolysis)/kidney; serum ALT prior to Tx; 6 + 12 wks post start of Tx then q6mos
        ○ fibric acid derivatives: little indication in childhood

WHEN TO REFER

- Refer pt/family to dietician if:
    - understanding of nutrition poor after initial attempts at dietary control
    - parent compliant, but needs help w/ menu planning
    - parent compliant, but needs help specific to age of child
- Refer pt/family to lipid specialist:
    - if primary care physician uncomfortable w/medical Tx when indicated
    - if multiple risk factors present
    - if lipid profile very unusual (examples: LDL > 190 mg/dl or <50 mg/dl; fasting triglycerides >500 mg/dl; HDL <25 mg/dl)
    - if family desires additional consultation

HYPERTENSION, EVALUATION AND MANAGEMENT

BEN H. BROUHARD

BACKGROUND

- Occurs in 5% of children
- Etiology has multiple inputs (eg, genetic, ions, sympathetic nervous system)
- Normal values determined for all age groups
- Hypertensive children <10 yrs of age often have 2° cause
- Hypertensive adolescents often have essential or idiopathic hypertension

CLINICAL MANIFESTATIONS

- Rare; children usually asymptomatic
- Occasionally headache, blurred vision, usually occur w/ rapid rises to very high pressures
- Clinical manifestations reflect primary etiology

LABORATORY FEATURES

- *Essential hypertension:* no laboratory abnormalities
- *2° hypertension:* abnormalities related to primary etiology
- *Screening laboratory:* serum creatinine, UA, electrolytes, CBC, renal ultrasound
- Screening for associated cardiovascular risk factors: EKG (echo), fasting lipid profile

DIFFERENTIAL DIAGNOSIS

- Transient ↑ BP due to situation (eg, anxiety, full bladder)
- Error in measurement (eg, too small cuff size)

COMPLICATIONS

- *Untreated hypertension:* stroke, heart failure, renal failure

TREATMENT

- Nonpharmacologic Tx:
  - salt restriction: 2 g/d
  - weight reduction
  - stress reduction
  - exercise
- Pharmacologic:
  - diuretics (eg, thiazides)
  - beta blockers (eg, propranolol)
  - calcium channel blockers (eg, nifedipine)
  - peripheral alpha blockers (eg, prazosin)
  - central alpha agonists (eg, clonidine)
  - peripheral vasodilator (eg, hydralazine)
  - angiotensin-converting enzyme inhibitors (eg, captopril)
  - angiotension receptor blockers (e.g. cozaar)

WHEN TO REFER

- Children <10 yrs of age w/ persistently ↑ BP
- Hypertensive emergency
- Pt on 3 medications w uncontrolled BP

J. WILLIAMSON BALFE

BACKGROUND

- Definition:
  - *normal BP:* systolic/diastolic levels <90th percentile for age/sex
  - *high-normal BP:* systolic and/or diastolic BP 90–95th percentile for age/sex
  - *high BP/hypertension:* systolic and/or diastolic BP ≥95th percentile for age/sex on 3 occasions
- Severe hypertension (diastolic BP > 10 mmHg >95th percentile) should lead physician to consider admission for treatment/workup
- Common in adults (10–15% of population), usually 1°/essential hypertension; in children, hypertension rare, usually 2° hypertension resulting from organ dysfunction/correctable damage
- *Risk factors:* prematurity, family Hx hypertension, obesity, Hx renal disease

CLINICAL FINDINGS

- Hx: functional inquiry for renal disorders (recurrent UTIs, polyuria, nocturia), endocrine disease (hyperthyroidism/pheochromocytoma)
- *Physical examination:* be certain proper sized cuff used (two-thirds of upper-arm length); exclude coarctation of aorta by measuring arm/leg pressures; abdominal bruit suggests renal artery stenosis, fundoscopic examination for hemorrhages, exudates, papilledema; café-au-lait skin lesions suggest neurofibromatosis

LABORATORY FEATURES

- UA (protein, blood, microscopy)
- *CBC:* anemia suggests renal disease
- *Electrolytes:* hypokalemic metabolic alkalosis suggests renal artery stenosis
- Creatinine to assess glomerular filtration rate
- Heart size assessed by chest x-ray, EKG/echocardiogram
- Other tests ordered as indicated:
  - renal ultrasound to assess structural renal disease
  - renal scan (DMSA, DTPA) to assess renal structure/function
  - 24 hr urine for VMA/catecholamines
  - plasma renin activity (can be done w/captopril stimulation)
  - renal angiogram/renal vein renins to exclude renal artery stenosis

DIFFERENTIAL DIAGNOSIS

- Conditions associated w/acute transient hypertension or intermittent hypertension:
  - *renal:* acute poststreptococcal glomerulonephritis, hemolytic uremic syndrome, anaphylactoid purpura, acute renal failure

  - *metabolic:* hyperthyroidism (systolic), hypercalcemia, hypernatremia
  - *neurologic:* dysautonomia, increased intracranial pressure (any cause), Guillain-Barré syndrome
  - *drug related:* sympathomimetic agents (eg, cold preparations, nose drops), licorice (nonsynthetic), oral contraceptives
  - *miscellaneous:* burns, Stevens-Johnson syndrome, cyclic vomiting, any stress in hypertension-prone individual
- Causes of 2° hypertension in children:
  - *renal origin:* parenchymal nephropathy (glomerulonephritides), structural renal malformation (polycystic kidney disease), obstructive uropathy (ureteropelvic junction obstruction, reflux nephropathy), pyelonephritis, segmental hypoplasia, renovascular disease, Wilms tumor, trauma
  - *cardiovascular:* coarctation of the aorta, patent ductus arteriosus, polycythemia, Takayasu arteritis
  - *endocrine:* obesity, pheochromocytoma, hyperthyroidism, congenital adrenal hyperplasia, 17-hydroxylase deficiency, 1° hyperaldosteronism, Cushing syndrome
  - *neurogenic tumors:* neurofibromatosis, neuroblastoma
  - *miscellaneous:* drug exposure, sympathomimetic agents, glucocorticoids, fracture immobilization, heavy metal exposure (lead, calcium)
  - *CNS:* ↑ intracranial pressure, dysautonomia

TREATMENT

- Mild–moderate hypertension (90–95th percentile systolic/diastolic BP for age):
  - *calcium channel blockers:*
    ○ amlodipine: 5 mg tablet, dissolves in water; initial dose: 0.1–0.2 mg/kg/d po as single dose; maintenance: 0.1–0.3 mg/kg/d po as single dose
    ○ nifedipine: capsules: 5 mg/10 mg; prolonged action tablets: 10/20 mg; XL (24 hr action) tablets: 30/60 mg; dose: 0.5 mg/kg/d po div q8h, increase gradually prn to 1–1.5 mg/kg/d po; usual adult dose = 10–30 mg/dose; for rapid action, use bite/swallow capsule
  - *beta adrenergic blockers:*
    ○ nadolol: 40/80 mg tablets, suspension: 1 mg/kg/d po 1×/d; increase dose by 1 mg/kg/d q3–4d prn; max. dose = 320 mg/d
    ○ propranolol: 10/40 mg tablets; 0.5–4 mg/kg/d po div tid or qid
  - *angiotensin-converting enzyme inhibitors:*
    ○ captopril: 12.5, 25, 50 mg tablets, dissolves in water; initial dose: 0.1–0.3 mg/kg/dose po tid; maintenance dose: 0.3–4 mg/kg/d po div tid
    ○ enalapril: 2.5, 5, 10, 20 mg tablets; initial dose: 0.1 mg/kg/d po as single daily

dose or div bid; maintenance: 0.1–0.5 mg/kg/d as single daily dose or div bid; max. adult dose: 40 mg/d
  - *diuretics:*
    ○ hydrochlorothiazide: 25/50 mg tablets; dose: 2–4 mg/kg/d po div bid; combine w/spironolactone in equal mg dose to prevent hypokalemia
- Severe hypertension (>99th percentile, systolic/diastolic, for age; symptomatic):
  - first line:
    ○ nifedipine capsule: 0.2–0.5 mg/kg po bite/swallow q8h (max. = 10 mg/dose) *and/or*
    ○ hydralazine: 0.15–0.8 mg/kg/dose IV q4h (max. = 25 mg/dose; onset 10–30 min)
  - second line:
    ○ diazoxide: 1–3 mg/kg/dose, IV push q15–30min prn (max. = 4 doses; onset in minutes)
    ○ labetalol: 1–3 mg/kg/hr, continuous IV infusion
    ○ nitroprusside: 0.5–8 μg/kg/min by continuous IV infusion; requires ICU monitoring

COMPLICATIONS

- *Long-term untreated:* end-organ damage (esp cardiovascular/renal); shortened life span; major risk factor for atherosclerosis in later life
- *Severe hypertension emergent complications:* CVAs/heart failure

PREVENTION

- After age 2–3 yrs, BP measurement should be part of well-child physical examination
- Encourage healthy diet, low in sodium/fat, high in fiber
- Prevent obesity
- Correct 2° forms of hypertension if possible
- Adequately monitor long-term antihypertensive Tx (may require home BP monitoring/monthly office BP assessment; ambulatory BP monitoring useful in certain situations)

WHEN TO REFER

- Acute forms of hypertension readily manageable; if hypertension persistent/evidence of end-organ injury, refer to appropriate specialist; if pt ≤10 yrs of age/↑ BP persistent, 2° cause will usually be found (75% renal etiology)

BACKGROUND

• Hemorrhage into anterior chamber of eye (hyphema) usually results from blunt or penetrating ocular injury to children of any age. Blood originates from ciliary body and/or iris. Injury may be accompanied by iridocyclitis, lens dislocation, cataract formation, vitreous hemorrhage or retinal detachment. Hyphemas may occur at birth from traumatic forceps delivery or hemorrhage from fetal ocular blood vessels
• Child abuse must always be considered
• Nontraumatic hyphemas far less common; can be associated w/ juvenile xanthogranuloma of iris, neovascular vessels of iris (rubeosis), leukemia, retinoblastoma, medulloepithelioma of iris or ciliary body, rarely, melanoma
• Blood usually absorbs within 5–7 d

CLINICAL MANIFESTATIONS

• ↓ visual acuity (may be evident only when comparing vision of both eyes)
• Blood in anterior chamber may be seen (1) as reddish haze throughout chamber, (2) layer of blood inferiorly, or (3) completely filling chamber, thus precluding visualization of posterior segment structures
• ↑ intraocular pressure (IOP) from impaired aqueous drainage caused by presence of blood, or, soft eye due to ↓ aqueous production 2° to ciliary body trauma
• Distorted or poorly reactive pupil
• Pain from trauma or from ↑ IOP
• *Somnolence:* common in children. If deep or prolonged, consider neurologic complications
• Rupture of globe must be ruled out if any of above manifestations pronounced

LABORATORY FEATURES

• For pts of African, Hispanic, Mediterranean origin, sickle-cell preparation or Hgb electrophoresis mandatory

COMPLICATIONS

• 2° glaucoma
• Corneal blood staining and opacification
• Stimulus deprivation ambylopia can occur in infants and young children if corneal blood staining and opacification prolonged or if long delay in clearing large hyphema
• Atrophy of optic nerve
• Rebleeding ↑ incidence of aforementioned complications. Peak time for rebleeding 2–5 d after injury
• Presence of sickle-cell trait or disease makes glaucoma and optic nerve atrophy more likely and more difficult to treat

TREATMENT

• Bed rest either at home or in hospital w/ head or bed elevated. Bathroom privileges granted
• Shield placed over affected eye(s)
• Avoid aspirin, NSAIDs, quick-acting miotic or mydriatic agents. Acetaminophen w/ or w/o codeine may be used for pain
• Daily examination by ophthalmologist to determine if rebleeding has occurred, measure IOP, treat glaucoma if present, document any changes. Treatment more aggressive with sickle cell trait or disease.

WHEN TO REFER

If hyphema visible/vision impaired, place light cover/shield over eye without pressing globe; refer patient promptly to an ophthalmologist for examination, treatment.

PROGNOSIS

Visual prognosis generally good if hyphema small, no bleeding, hemoglobin normal, blood clears quickly/spontaneously.

BACKGROUND

• *Hypoglycemia*: acute, life-threatening medical emergency; consequences may include coma, seizures, permanent brain damage
• In pediatric age group, only need to consider fasting hypoglycemia
• Clinically significant reactive (postprandial) hypoglycemia rare except in association w/ gastric surgery (eg, Nissin fundoplication)
• Hypoglycemia not a disease entity; therefore, Dx underlying cause essential part of urgent Tx

CLINICAL MANIFESTATIONS, DEFINITIONS

• *Sx, two categories:* adrenergic and CNS
• *Adrenergic* signs include tachycardia, sweating, tremulousness, mydriasis, hypothermia, anxiety
• *CNS* signs include hunger, lethargy, irritability, confusion, coma, seizures
• In newborns and young infants, Sx often nonspecific
• Hypoglycemia usually defined as plasma glucose <40 mg/dL; this definition means only that severe Sx usually occur only w/ glucose <40 mg/dL
• Normoglycemia defined as plasma glucose 70–95 mg/dL (use as therapeutic target)
• Use same standards in neonates (controversy exists, but no good justification to use lower standards for hypoglycemia in newborns)

DIFFERENTIAL DIAGNOSIS

• Normal infant or child, excessively fasted
• Ingestions, medications, surreptitious insulin
• Neonatal developmental delay, peripartum stress
• Congenital metabolic and endocrine disorders

LABORATORY TESTS

• *Caution:* glucose strip tests useful for screening, but must be confirmed w/ lab measurement because accuracy never better than ±15 mg/dL
• When drawing lab glucose sample save extra 1–2 tubes for critical sample (see below) if Dx not known
• Also obtain first voided urine as part of critical sample

• *Use of Critical Blood and Urine Samples for Dx* (typical timing of hypoglycemia in parentheses)
• Obtain extra blood and urine at, or immediately after initial Tx
• general tests to order:
  – serum/plasma: glucose, bicarbonate, lactate, free fatty acids, beta-hydroxybutyrate
  – urine: ketone test (dipstick or Acetest tablets)
  – save extra blood and urine in case specific tests needed
• *Acidemia* (bicarbonate < 18 mmol/L):
  – *keto-acidosis* (BOB > 2.0 mmol/L)
    ○ normal (>20 hr)
    ○ pituitary/adrenal insufficiency (<16–20 hrs)
    ○ type 3, 6, or 9 glycogen storage disorders (3–12 hrs)
  – *lactic-acidosis* (lactate > 2–4 mmol/L):
    ○ type 1 glycogen storage disease (<3–6 hrs)
    ○ fructose-1,6-diphosphatase deficiency (8–16 hrs)
    ○ ethanol ingestion (6–12 hrs)
• *No Acidemia* (bicarbonate >18 mmol/L and urine ketones < "large"):
  – *low ketones and high free fatty acids* (BOB < 2.0, FFA > 2.0 mmol/L):
    ○ genetic defect in beta-oxidation (>12 hrs)
    ○ primary carnitine deficiency (>12 hrs)
    ○ normal newborn, day 1 (1–12 hrs)
  – *low ketones and low free fatty acids* (BOB < 2.0, FFA < 2.0 mmol/L):
    ○ exogenous insulin/oral hypoglycemic drug (varies)
    ○ congenital hyperinsulinism (1–20 hrs)
    ○ infant of diabetic mother (day 1, 1–12 hrs)
    ○ birth asphyxia/maternal toxemia (varies, resolves in weeks)
    ○ occasional neonatal hypopituitarism (1–8 hrs)
    ○ beta-blocker drugs
• Depending on suspected Dx, other uses of clinical samples include hormones (insulin, C-peptide, growth hormone, cortisol) or combination of serum carnitine and serum acyl-carnitine profile, ammonia and liver function tests, and urinary organic acid profile (for beta-oxidation disorders). Glucagon test (1 mg IV) at time of hypoglycemia useful in identifying hyperinsulinism (inappropriate glycemic response > 30 mg/dL)

TREATMENT

• *Acute, nonspecific Tx:*
  – IV dextrose, 0.25–0.5 g/kg bolus then D5 at maintenance or greater to keep blood sugar > 70–80 mg/dL (rate = 1–2× hepatic glucose production, ie, 5–10 mg/kg/min). *Caution:* some pts, esp w/ hyperinsulinism, may have increased glucose utilization and need higher glucose infusion rates
  – glucagon, 1 mg subcut, IM, or IV. *Caution:* may be used *only* for known hyperinsulinism, eg, emergency Tx for insulin-treated diabetic
• *Maintenance Tx* (depends on Dx):
  – GSD 3, 6, 9: frequent feedings, uncooked cornstarch
  – GSD 1a: frequent feedings, uncooked cornstarch, continuous intragastric dextrose infusions, restrict dietary lactose and sucrose, allopurinol for hyperuricemia
  – GSD 1b: same as GSD 1a, but G-CSF may improve associated neutropenia
  – fructose-1,6-diphosphatase deficiency: avoid fasts >10–12 hrs, limit sucrose
  – genetic defect in beta-oxidation: avoid fasts >12 hrs
  – primary carnitine deficiency: carnitine po 100 mg/kg/d (useful only in this disease)

COMPLICATIONS

• *General:* permanent brain damage, seizures may occur
• Disease specific:
  – GSD1a and 1b: late nephropathy and/or hepatic tumors
  – GSD-3: one-third cases develop myopathy and cardiomyopathy
  – genetic defect in beta-oxidation: severe forms associated w/ myopathy and cardiomyopathy

WHEN TO REFER

• Common problems can usually be managed w/o referral (eg, transient hypoglycemia in normal newborns, insulin reaction in diabetics)
• If Dx unknown and underlying endocrine/metabolic disorder suspected, obtain consult to assist in rapid Dx
• Refer pts w/ chronic forms of hypoglycemia

GENERAL NOTES

- Hypopigmented lesions less common in neonate than pigmented lesions
- Unless lesions widespread/other abnormalities present, usually little medical significance
- Clinical examination usually adequate for Dx

HYPOPIGMENTED MACULES

BACKGROUND

- ≥1 hypopigmented macules present 0.4–0.8% newborns
- Ash leaf (hypopigmented) macules present 90% pts w/ tuberous sclerosis; may be earliest sign
- Due to ↓ melanocytic activity in epidermis

CLINICAL MANIFESTATIONS

- Oval/linear white macules ranging from few mm to many cm
- Commonly located on trunk/extremities
- Wood light examination highlights lesions; particularly useful in lightly pigmented individuals

MANAGEMENT

- Evaluate for tuberous sclerosis if other Sx present (eg, seizures, developmental delay)/lesions numerous/café-au-lait macules present

NEVUS ANEMICUS

BACKGROUND

- Appear at birth/early childhood
- Due to ↓ sensitivity of involved area to endogenous vasodilators

CLINICAL MANIFESTATIONS

- Well-circumscribed, hypopigmented macule often several cm in diameter
- Border obscured by gentle pressure
- Rubbing lesion does not lead to expected red flare response seen in surrounding normal skin
- Wood light does not highlight lesion

TREATMENT

- None necessary

NEVUS DEPIGMENTOSUS

BACKGROUND

- Also known as nevus achromicus
- Rare cases of associated CNS deficits reported
- M = F
- Present at birth/stable throughout life
- Due to absence of melanocytes in affected epidermis

CLINICAL MANIFESTATIONS

- Localized, well-defined, depigmented macule of any size/often w/dermatomal/segmental distribution
- Lesions highlighted under Wood light

DIFFERENTIAL DIAGNOSIS

- Segmental vitiligo
- Piebaldism
- Waardenburg syndrome
- Hypomelanosis of Ito

MANAGEMENT

- No treatment necessary

HYPOMELANOSIS OF ITO

BACKGROUND

- Also known as incontinentia pigmenti achromians; disorder unrelated to X-linked disorder, incontinentia pigmenti (Bloch-Sulzberger disease)
- Up to 50% pts have associated neurologic, musculoskeletal, ocular abnormalities
- F:M ratio 2.5:1
- Due to ↓ melanocytic activity in epidermis

CLINICAL MANIFESTATIONS

- Hypopigmented macules forming distinctive whorled/swirled pattern over trunk, extremities
- Café-au-lait–like hyperpigmentation in similar swirled pattern may be present in other areas/instead of hypopigmentation (Linear and Whorled Hypermelanosis)

MANAGEMENT

- Hypopigmentation may improve over time
- Careful physical examination/well child follow-up to detect associated abnormalities
- Mosaicism may underlie most cases demonstrated in skin/blood samples; no specific chromosomal syndrome identified; obtain studies if lesions extensive/if other abnormalities present

WHEN TO REFER

- When diagnosis in doubt

BACKGROUND

- Anterior and posterior pituitary glands differ in origin, anatomy, function, control
- Most anterior pituitary gland hormones stimulated by hypothalamic releasing factors; prolactin inhibited by prolactin inhibitory factor (PIF)
- Vasopressin secreted from axons extending from paraventricular and supraoptic nuclei in brain to posterior pituitary gland
- Combined anterior and posterior pituitary deficiencies, if not due to congenital defect, likely indicate serious acquired pathology
- Anterior pituitary deficiency:
  – congenital anterior pituitary deficiency may be due to deficient hypothalamic releasing factor (most common), pituitary aplasia or hypoplasia (rare), or GH gene defect
  – acquired anterior pituitary deficiency due to tumor, surgery, injury, infection, or CNS irradiation after long-term survival from childhood cancer
  – most common (1/4,000) anterior pituitary deficiency: isolated growth hormone deficiency (GHD)
  – TRF/TSH, CRF/ACTH, or GnRH/LH and FSH deficiencies usually associated w/GHD
- Posterior pituitary deficiency of vasopressin; central diabetes insipidus:
  – may be congenital, in isolated or familiar patterns, and may combine w/congenital anterior pituitary deficiencies, often w/midline anatomic defect
  – may be acquired w/CNS tumors or infiltrations (eg, histiocytosis X)

CLINICAL MANIFESTATIONS

- Growth failure due to GHD: pathology more common if height far below 3rd percentile, has ↓ growth rate (crossing to lower percentile on growth chart) or has short height for family pattern
- Fasting hypoglycemia, often w/seizures, due to ↓ gluconeogenesis of GHD
- Microphallus (penis <2 cm) may occur in affected newborn males
- Late onset of growth failure ominous because it occurs w/CNS tumors or other pathology

- 2° TSH or 3° TRF deficiencies cause hypothyroidism
- Delayed or absent puberty occurs w/LH or FSH (2°) or GnRH (3° hypogonadism) deficiencies
- Kallmann syndrome combines hypothalamic GnRH deficiency and anosmia or hyposmia
- Isolated cortisol deficiency w/ACTH (2°) or CRF (3°) deficiency
- Hyperprolactinemia occurs w/absent hypothalamic PIF
- Hypoprolactinemia occurs if pituitary lactotrophs affected by pituitary disease

LABORATORY FEATURES

- GH deficiency:
  – peak GH above 10 ng/mL after arginine, L-dopa, clonidine (or dangerous insulin tolerance test) stimulation r/o classic GH deficiency
  – low serum IGF-1 or IGFBP-3 suggests GH deficiency in absence of malnutrition
- Hypothyroidism:
  – serum free T4 low; serum TSH low
- Hypogonadotropic hypogonadism:
  – serum LH and FSH low
  – anosmia or hyposmia on scent testing suggests Kallmann syndrome
- Isolated cortisol deficiency:
  – serum cortisol low in morning, evening, as is serum ACTH
- Basal serum prolactin low in pituitary disease
- Serum prolactin high in hypothalamic PIF deficiency

DIFFERENTIAL DIAGNOSIS

- Growth failure:
  – any chronic disease can cause
  – constitutional delay in growth causes short stature but growth rate normal for bone age
  – IUGR can cause short stature but growth usually at least in lower normal range
  – hypothyroidism/Cushing syndrome can cause growth failure

- 2° or 3° hypothyroidism:
  – 1° hypothyroidism (TSH↑)
- Hypogonadotropic hypogonadism:
  – constitutional delay in puberty will ultimately allow spontaneous pubertal development
  – 1° hypogonadism or Turner syndrome or Klinefelter syndrome will not
- Cortisol deficiency:
  – early or mild Addison disease may retain some mineralocorticoid function
  – adrenal hypoplasia
  – various enzymatic deficiencies of congenital adrenal hyperplasia

TREATMENT

- Growth hormone treatment for GHD
- Thyroxine replacement for hypothyroidism
- Gonadal steroids for 2° sexual development in delayed puberty
- Glucocorticoid replacement for cortisol deficiency

COMPLICATIONS

- GHD-slipped capital femoral epiphyses or pseudo-tumor cerebri w/GH treatment
- Hypothyroidism: advanced bone age/craniosynostosis w/excessive thyroxine replacement
- Delayed puberty: osteopenia if sex steroids deficient, advanced bone age if sex steroids excessive
- Cortisol deficiency: Cushing syndrome occurs if cortisol replacement excessive

WHEN TO REFER

- Severe growth failure with adequate nutrition and no systemic disease referred to pediatric endocrinologist
- Hypothyroidism: 2° or 3° hypothyroidism referred to r/o hypothalamic-pituitary tumor
- Delayed puberty: testing and treatment usually referred to pediatric endocrinologist
- Cortisol deficiency: rare threatening condition always referred to pediatric endocrinologist
- Hyperprolactinemia: in absence of drug-induced etiology, referred to eliminate pituitary tumor

HYPOSPADIAS

BACKGROUND

- *Incidence:* 8.2/1,000 male births in US. May have true geographic variance—lower in Europe and Mexico
- Etiology unknown. ↑ risk w/ ↑ maternal age, male-male twinning. May be related to failure of appropriate hCG stimulation of fetal testes and subsequent delay or ↓ testosterone production
- Multifactorial mode of inheritance, w/ incidence of second cases higher if more than one closely related family member (father, brother) affected
- Isolated defect in most children. Dx made on physical examination. Buccal smears and karyotyping unnecessary. *Exception: Boys w/ hypospadias associated w/ bilateral undescended testes—r/o girl w/ adrenogenital syndrome.* Chromosomal anomalies may be suspected in boys w/ single testicles or dysmorphic facies

CLINICAL FEATURES

- Urethral meatus located on ventral aspect of penile shaft from glans to perineum (glanular, coronal, midshaft, penoscrotal, perineal). Usually associated w/ chordee (penile curvature) of varying degrees
- Associated anomalies:
  – vesicoureteral reflux: usually low grade and unassociated w/ renal damage. Routine evaluation not recommended
  – enlarged utricle: significance unclear and does not require routine cystoscopic evaluation
  – chordee: severity related to degree of hypospadias. Present in 35% of boys w/ hypospadias. Chordee may occur independent of hypospadias

MANAGEMENT

- Surgical correction should be performed as early as possible. Penile size limiting factor
- Hormonal stimulation w/ testosterone may be used in boys w/ small phallus or w/ limited skin availability
- Repair can be performed as an outpt procedure. Staged repairs and hospitalization

may be required in some cases of proximal hypospadias or pts undergoing redo procedures following prior failed repairs
- Urethral stent may be used for few days postop; secured to glans and drains into diaper. Transparent dressing applied to penis and may be removed at time of stent removal
- Long-acting local anesthetics may be administered in form of penile block or caudal injection to provide 4–6 hrs pain relief. Pain following interval can be managed successfully w/ oral acetaminophen and codeine

COMPLICATIONS

- Persistent chordee may be prevented w/ complete penile release and demonstration of correction during surgery by artificial erection. Necessitates reexploration and possible urethral reconstruction w/ grafts
- Meatal stenosis probably result of devascularization of tip of neourethra. Usually correctable w/ meatoplasty
- Urethrocutaneous fistula most common complication. Reoperation should be delayed until tissue reaction has subsided (6 mos)

WHEN TO REFER

- At Dx, *circumcision should be avoided,* and pediatric urology consultation should be obtained as outpt
- If associated w/ bilateral undescended testes, consider female w/ congenital adrenal hyperplasia

EPISPADIAS

BACKGROUND

- Forms part of exstrophy/epispadias complex. Varies from glandular defect to penopubic variants w/ complete incontinence
- *Incidence:* 1/117,000 males, 1/484,000 females

CLINICAL FEATURES

- In penopubic (complete) forms bladder may prolapse through large urethral outlet and resemble mild form of exstrophy. Pts managed as bladder exstrophy w/ early reconstruction

- *Males:* urethral meatus located on dorsal aspect of penis. Glandular variant rarely associated w/ incontinence. Penopubic (complete) types usually associated w/ urinary incontinence
- All forms associated w/ varying degrees of dorsal curvature and divergence of pubic symphysis
- *Females:* in mild variants, urethral orifice patulous. Severest forms associated w/ open urethra and incompetent sphincter. Clitoris bifid, mons flattened, labia split
- Associated anomalies:
  – vesicoureteral reflux: noted 30–40% pts. Inherent deficiency of ureterovesical junction

MANAGEMENT

- Urethroplasty in epispadias similar to that performed in exstrophy. Reconstruction performed ~ age 1 in boys, w/ penile lengthening and repositioning of urethra below corpora. In girls, reconstruction to bring clitoral halves together, urethroplasty and monsplasty may be required
- In incontinent pts, continence dependent on bladder capacity. Bladder neck reconstruction to provide bladder outlet resistance combined w/ ureteral reimplantation, and delayed until child emotionally ready to be dry. Adequate bladder capacity essential for successful bladder neck plasty. If bladder capacity not age appropriately adequate, augmentation or continent diversion may be required

COMPLICATIONS

- *Urethral fistula:* 8–12% of boys following urethroplasty. Requires operative repair, performed as outpt. Fistula rates appear to be ↓ w/ newer surgical techniques
- *Dorsal chordee:* may recur following initial reconstruction and may require later surgical release to provide more dependent penile angle

WHEN TO REFER

- Pediatric urology consult should be obtained at time of initial Dx
- If bladder prolapse present, pt should be treated as exstrophy w/ early closure and staged reconstruction

HYPOTHERMIA

STEPHEN LUDWIG

BACKGROUND

- Hypothermia defined as core temperature of <35.5° C. Populations at risk are those whose temperature-regulating mechanism not developed or impaired
- Children at risk:
  - neonates
  - immobilizing conditions
  - brain injury
  - malnutrition
  - alcohol ingestion
  - drug ingestion (barbiturates, phenothiazines)
  - endocrinopathy (Addison disease, hypothyroidism)
  - metabolic disorders (hypoglycemia)
  - sepsis
- Children who are normal may also be prone to hypothermia from profound cold exposure (eg, being outdoors in frigid conditions) and from prolonged exposure (eg, indoor exposure in unheated conditions). Hypothermia must also be considered in conjunction w/drowning, multiple trauma. Although most hypothermia occurs in winter, during spring, fall, combination of wet, wind can lead to excessive loss of body heat

CLINICAL MANIFESTATIONS

- Clinical manifestations vary w/degree of hypothermia. Between 35 and 32° C there is shivering, vasoconstriction, teeth chattering, clumsiness. May also be amnesia and impaired judgment
- Below 32° C shivering stops; findings include apathy, disorientation. Pulse, BP fall; may be dysrythmia including atrial fibrillation, sinus bradycardia. There is hypoventilation, loss of protective airway reflexes
- Below 28° C there is coma, absent brain stem reflexes, nonreactive pupils, areflexia, loss of pulse, BP. At this degree of hypothermia, pt may be indistinguishable from dead pt, leading to maxim that no one should be pronounced dead until warm and w/o cardiovascular function

LABORATORY FEATURES

- Important to have thermometer that measures true core temperature. Many standard thermometers do not record sufficiently low enough
- Following laboratory tests should be obtained:
  - arterial blood gas corrected for temperature
  - CBC and platelet count
  - coagulation profile
  - electrolytes, BUN, creatinine, glucose, amylase
  - drug screen, alcohol level—if appropriate
  - EKG: look for Osborne J wave, a "camel hump" appearing just after the QRS
  - chest radiograph

DIFFERENTIAL DIAGNOSIS

- Conditions that may mimic hypothermia include hypoglycemia, drug intoxication, psychiatric disorders, hypothyroidism, Addison disease. Note these are same conditions that may contribute to true hypothermia. Only true test is to obtain accurate rectal or core temperature

TREATMENT

- General principles of CPR should be followed: ABCs. Handle pt as gently as possible. Correction of acidosis need only be to pH 7.25
- Specific treatment varies depending on condition of pt. Three methods: (1) passive external rewarming—blankets, warm environment, (2) active external rewarming—radiant heat, forced warm air, heating blankets, limited immersion, and (3) active core rewarming—heated O_2, warm IV fluids to 43° C, peritoneal lavage, extracorporeal rewarming
- If pt has perfusing cardiac rhythm and core temp >32° C, passive methods sufficient. If core temp <32° C, active core rewarming suggested. If child does not have perfusing cardiac rhythm, extracorporeal rewarming necessary. Aim for increasing body temperature 1° C/hr

COMPLICATIONS

- Hypothermia can lead to death. Poor prognostic factors include asystole, evidence of DIC, or hyperkalemia >10 mEq/L. Many complications can occur. Most common are cardiac dysrythmias, volume instability, coagulopathy

WHEN TO REFER

- Any pt hypothermic to level of 32° C or lower should be referred to 3° care pediatric center

BACKGROUND

	Congenital Hypothyroidism	Acquired Hypothyroidism
Age onset	At birth (begins prenatally)	Infancy through childhood; peak at adolescence
Sex	Female 2:1	Female 2:1
Incidence	1/4,000	1/500
Etiology	Thyroid dysgenesis: 85%	Chronic lymphocytic (Hashimoto) thyroiditis: 95%
	Dyshormonogenesis: 10%	Radiation injury: 3%
	Maternal antibody mediated hypothyroidism: 5%	Goitrogen ingestion: 2%
Positive Family Hx	15%	30%

CLINICAL MANIFESTATIONS

	Congenital Hypothyroidism	Acquired Hypothyroidism
Symptoms	Prolonged jaundice	Slow growth
	Constipation	Drop in school performance
	Lethargy	Sluggishness
	Feeding problems	Cold intolerance
Signs	Large fontanels	Short stature
	Macroglossia	Goiter
	Umbilical hernia	Delayed pubertal development
	Hypotonia	Slow reflexes

LABORATORY FEATURES

- Blood:
  - ↓ free T4 (normal range 0.70–1.80 ng/dL) or
  - ↓ total T4 (normal range 5.0–13.0 μg/dL) and normal or ↓ T3 resin uptake
  - remember that normal range higher in first few weeks of life
  - ↑ TSH (normal range 0.4–5.0 mU/L)
  - antithyroid antibodies: positive in autoimmune thyroid disease: antiperoxidase and antithyroglobulin antibodies
- Thyroid scan:
  - congenital hypothyroidism: not routinely necessary; can be used to delineate underlying etiology, eg, aplasia, ectopic gland, dyshormonogenesis
  - acquired hypothyroidism: may be helpful w/ nodular goiter
- Ultrasound:
  - congenital hypothyroidism: not routine, can confirm aplasia or goiter
  - acquired hypothyroidism: not routinely indicated; shows variable hypoechogenicity w/ autoimmune thyroid disease
- *Bone age radiograph:* useful for dating onset of hypothyroidism and for following skeletal maturation w/ treatment

DIFFERENTIAL DIAGNOSIS

- Congenital hypothyroidism:
  - storage diseases (eg, mucopolysaccharidoses)
  - cerebral palsy
  - Down syndrome
- Acquired hypothyroidism:
  - constitutional delay of growth and puberty
  - simple (exogenous) obesity
  - hypopituitarism

TREATMENT GUIDELINES

Age	l-thyroxine (mcg/kg/d)
Neonate	10–15
0–1 yr	5–8
1–3 yrs	3–6
3–10 yrs	3–4
>10 yrs	1.5–3

- Monitoring:
  - clinical: follow growth and development carefully
  - laboratory: follow free T4 (or total T4) and TSH at regular intervals: infants, q1–2mos; childhood: q3–6 mos
  - radiology: bone age x ray q1–2 yrs

COMPLICATIONS OF DELAYED DIAGNOSIS

- Congenital hypothyroidism:
  - mental retardation
  - incoordination, ataxia
  - speech disorders
  - short attention span
  - hearing loss
- Acquired hypothyroidism:
  - poor school performance
  - behavior problems
  - short adult height
  - empty sella syndrome

WHEN TO REFER

- *Congenital hypothyroidism:* these infants, usually detected through newborn screening programs, managed in consultation w/ pediatric endocrinologist at least through first 3 yrs of life
- *Acquired hypothyroidism:* refer when disorder severe or longstanding at Dx, initial diagnostic tests indeterminate, or response to treatment not as expected

BACKGROUND

- Diverse group of disorders characterized by scaling skin
- *Cause:* ↓ epidermal desquamation or ↑ epidermal proliferation
- Usually inheritable condition presenting at birth or in infancy: five major inheritable ichthyoses (see table) and multiple syndromes in which ichthyosis associated w/other anomalies
- Rarely presents as acquired disorder related to underlying systemic disease (Hodgkin lymphoma and other malignancies, HIV, leprosy, sarcoidosis, hypothyroidism, malnutrition, dermatomyositis, SLE) or medication (retinoids, cimetidine, allopurinol, nicotinic acid)

CLINICAL MANIFESTATIONS

- *IV:* diffuse, fine white scales; fishlike scales on extensors; spares flexures; hyperlinear, thickened palms and soles; associated w/atopy and keratosis pilaris
- *XLI:* thick, "dirty" scales more extensive on extensors
- *LI:* usually collodion baby (born within a translucent membrane that gradually peels off); after membrane shed, diffuse thick, large, dark, platelike scales; severely affects forehead, lower extremities, flexures
- *NBCIE:* usually collodion baby; after membrane shed, generalized erythroderma and fine white scales; darker, larger scales over legs; palms, soles, flexures may be affected
- *EHK:* at birth, widespread blisters, erosions, erythroderma; after neonatal period, thick, warty, spinous, brown hyperkeratosis w/marked flexural, palmoplantar involvement

LABORATORY FEATURES

- *Skin biopsy for light microscopy:* thickness of stratum corneum and granular layer, presence or absence of nuclei in stratum corneum can be helpful in establishing Dx IV, XLI, LI, NBCIE; finding of markedly thickened stratum corneum, vacuolation of suprabasal layer classic for EHK
- *Skin biopsy for electron microscopy:* "crumbly" keratohyaline granules seen in IV; numerous lipid droplets in corneocytes and abnormal lamellar bodies seen in NBCIE; subrabasal clumped tonofilaments seen in EHK
- *Serum cholesterol sulfate levels:* ↑ in XLI
- *Serum electrophoresis:* ↑ mobility of low-density lipoproteins in XLI
- *Prenatal Dx:* available for XLI, LI, NBCIE, EHK

DIFFERENTIAL DIAGNOSIS

- Ichthyoses must be distinguished from one another
- Collodion baby can be initial presentation of LI, NBCIE, or rare syndromes such as Netherton IBIDs
- In newborn period EHK must be distinguished from epidermolysis bullosa, staphylococcal scalded skin

TREATMENT

- General measures:
  – dry skin care: brief baths or wet dressings, emollients, humidified air
  – keratolytics: urea, salicylic acid (risk for systemic absorption), alpha-hydroxy acid
- Topical and systemic retinoids for EHK, LI, NBCIE
- Topical and oral antibiotics for EHK
- Humidified incubator; dry skin care; pain management; artificial tears; monitoring of hydration, temperature, calorie intake, and electrolytes for collodion baby
- Wound dressings, padding to decrease friction for newborn EHK
- Surgical correction of ectropion, eclabium

COMPLICATIONS

- *XLI:* prolonged birth labor; asymptomatic corneal opacities in most pts, in some heterozygote female carriers; cryptorchidism in 12% of pts, ↑ risk for testicular carcinoma w/or w/o cryptorchidism
- *LI:* hypohidrosis, heat intolerance; eclabium, ectropion common; may develop corneal erosions, keratitis, conjunctivitis; scarring alopecia
- *NBCIE:* hypohidrosis, heat intolerance; may have scarring alopecia, ectropion, eclabium, nail dystrophy; ↑ risk for basal, squamous cell carcinoma
- *EHK:* bacterial infection of erosions; bacterial colonization of flexural hyperkeratosis

WHEN TO REFER

- Mild disease (eg, IV) no referral
- In more extensive disease, dermatology referral indicated to establish specific Dx, guide topical Tx, prescribe systemic Tx
- Genetics referral indicated to establish specific Dx, provide genetic counseling
- Ophthalmology, plastic surgery referrals for ectropion, eclabium

	Ichthyosis vulgaris (IV)	X-linked ichthyosis (XI)	Lamellar ichthyosis (LI)	Nonbullous congenital ichthyosiform erythroderma (NBCIE)	Epidermolytic hyperkeratosis (EHK) or bullous ichthyosiform erythroderma
Inheritance	AD	X-linked recessive	AR	AR	AD (sporadic mutations)
Incidence	1/250	1/2,000–1/6,000 males	1/100,000	1/100,000	1/100,000–1/300,000
Onset	3–12 mos	birth–3 mos	birth	birth	birth
Course	usually mild; improves w/age and warm, humid climate	may worsen w/age; improves w/warm, humid climate	chronic	milder w/age	w/age, blisters and erythroderma remit; hyperkeratosis worsens

BACKGROUND

- Most frequently found 2–10 yrs of age w/peak incidence 2–4 yrs
- At <10 yrs of age M:F ratio 1:1; >10, girls predominate
- Commonly follows viral illness
- *Infectious agents associated w/immune thrombocytopenia:* cytomegalovirus, Epstein-Barr virus, HIV, rubella, measles, varicella, mumps, some hepatitis viruses
- Predictors of chronicity (disease lasting >6 mos)

	Acute	Chronic
Onset	Acute, postinfectious	Insidious
Age	<10 yrs	>10 yrs
Sex	Male or female	Female 3:1
Season	Spring	None
Platelet count	<20,000 m/L	20,000–75,000 mL
Immunoglobulin	Normal IgA	↓ IgA
Platelet antibody	High	Moderately high
Steroid response	Good	Poor

- *Recovery:* 50% by 1 mo, 90% by 6 mos
- *Mortality:* 0–1.2%

CLINICAL MANIFESTATIONS

- *Bleeding:* usually abrupt onset
- *Petechiae:* major component of bleeding manifestation
- *Common sites of bleeding:* dermal/mucosal esp nasal, buccal, GI, vaginal
- *Uncommon sites:* CNS
- Absence of lymphadenopathy, hepatosplenomegaly

LABORATORY FEATURES

- *Thrombocytopenia:* platelet count usually <20,000/mL, frequently <5,000–10,000/mL, platelets large
- *Hgb:* usually normal; if ↓, suspect ongoing blood loss/associated autoimmune hemolytic anemia (Evan syndrome)
- *RBC indices:* mean corpuscular volume (MCV) normal; ↑ MCV suggests aplastic anemia/leukemia
- *WBC count/differential:* normal
- *Peripheral blood smear:* must be reviewed by experienced individual; should be normal except for ↓ platelets
- *Bone marrow:* generally not needed unless corticosteroids become part of management, even then may not be needed; normal to ↑ megakaryocytes; no abnormal cells; occasionally mild eosinophilia; should be performed if any concern about aplastic anemia/leukemia based on Hx, physical examination, laboratory data
- *Platelet antibody:* ↑; costly study, rarely indicated
- *Other:* sedimentation rate, antinuclear antibody, anti-phospholipid antibody, various viral titers optional depending on concerns regarding underlying etiology

DIFFERENTIAL DIAGNOSIS

- Drug-induced thrombocytopenia
- Thrombotic thrombocytopenic purpura
- Hemolytic uremic syndrome
- Thrombocytopenia absent radius (TAR) syndrome (if <1 yr of age)
- Wiskott-Aldrich syndrome
- Collagen vascular disease
- Malignancy
- Aplastic anemia
- Autoimmune thyroiditis w/immune thrombocytopenia
- Subacute bacterial endocarditis w/immune thrombocytopenia
- Antiphospholipid antibody syndrome

TREATMENT

- *Principal options:* no treatment; corticosteroids; IV gamma globulin
- *No treatment:* pts w/stable Hgb, minimal bruising/bleeding; otherwise consider use of corticosteroids/IV gamma globulin
- *Corticosteroids:* ↑ platelet count quickly in most cases; may require bone marrow before starting if any concern at all about leukemia; steroids induce remission in 60% of children w/acute lymphocytic leukemia; dose: prednisone, 2–4 mg/kg/d, po × 2 wks; alternatively methylprednisolone, 30 mg/kg/d IV × 3 d; advantage: inexpensive; disadvantage: possible need for bone marrow
- *IV gamma globulin:* dose: 0.8 g/kg/IV given once as effective as other dose regimens. Advantage: produces most rapid increase in platelet count; disadvantage: very expensive; has been reported to transmit some hepatitis viruses (rare); can cause fever/severe headache, allergic-type reactions
- Corticosteroids should not be continued for >2 wks (4 wks absolute max.); IV gamma globulin may be repeated, if initially effective, as needed
- *Alternative Tx:* anti-D globulin: advantage: inexpensive; disadvantage: may have slower onset of action, will induce mild hemolytic anemia, can be used only if D⊕ antigen positive

COMPLICATIONS

- Small percentage of children require transfusion
- *CNS hemorrhage (incidence 0.2%):* most serious complication, 50% mortality

WHEN TO REFER

- Most pts managed w/o referral
- If steroids used as part of management, referral may be necessary for performance/interpretation of bone marrow findings if CBC physical findings atypical for ITP
- Referral indicated for serious complications, if Dx in doubt, if disease fails to respond readily to initial management, if disease becomes chronic

BACKGROUND

- Not rare. In aggregate, 1° immunodeficiency occurs in as many as 1/400
- 2° immunodeficiency (eg, HIV infection, anti-inflammatory, or immunosuppressive Tx) even more common
- May present at any age
- Does not always present w/severe infection

CLINICAL MANIFESTATIONS

- 1° immunodeficiency may present w/↑ susceptibility to infection, autoimmune or inflammatory manifestations, and/or as part of syndrome complex
  - ↑ susceptibility to infection:
    ○ chronic/recurrent infections w/o other explanation (eg, >1 pneumonia per decade of life, recurrent otitis media after first year of life or at frequency increasing after first year of life, infections at >1 anatomic site)
    ○ infections w/organisms of low virulence (eg, *Pneumocystis carinii,* invasive or persistent candidiasis)
    ○ infection of unusual severity (eg, empyema, chicken pox requiring hospitalization)
  - autoimmune or inflammatory manifestations:
    ○ target cells: hemolytic anemia, thrombocytopenia, thyroiditis
    ○ target tissues: inflammatory bowel disease; vasculitis; systemic lupus erythematosus; rheumatoid arthritis
  - syndrome complexes in which immunodeficiency may be presenting feature

Examples of immunodeficiency syndromes

Syndrome	Clinical presentation	Immunologic abnormality
DiGeorge syndrome	Congenital heart disease	Thymic hypoplasia
Wiskott-Aldrich syndrome	Thrombocytopenia, eczema	Variable T and B lymphocyte dysfunction
Ataxia-telangiectasia	Ataxia; telangiectasia	Lymphopenia; antibody deficiency
Ivemark syndrome	Congenital heart disease; bilateral 3-lobed lungs	Asplenia
Polyendocrinopathy syndrome	Endocrine organ dysfunction	Chronic mucocutaneous candidiasis

DIFFERENTIAL DIAGNOSIS

- Immune system considered to have 4 functional compartments:
  - antibody
  - cell-mediated immunity
  - phagocytic cells
  - complement
- Types of infections, associated illnesses seen in pt help focus workup on specific compartments

LABORATORY EVALUATION

- Although immunodeficiency can be suspected on clinical grounds, specific Dx rarely evident w/o use of laboratory
- Screening tests performed in almost all pts:
  - CBC w/differential
  - quantitation of serum immunoglobulins (IgG, IgA, IgM)
- Always consider possibility of 2° immunodeficiency:
  - HIV infection
  - Tx w/anti-inflammatory (corticosteroids), immunosuppressive (cyclosporin A) or cytotoxic (chemotherapy, radiation) drugs
  - lymphoreticular neoplasms
  - viral infections (infectious mononucleosis)
- Other tests guided by clinical features of pt

Patterns of illness associated w/1° immunodeficiency

Functional abnormality	Illnesses	
	Infection	Other
Antibody	Sinopulmonary (pyogenic bacteria); GI (enteroviruses, giardiasis)	Autoimmune disease (autoantibodies, inflammatory disease)
Cell-mediated immunity	Pneumonia (pyogenic bacteria, *Pneumocystis carinii,* viruses); GI (viruses); skin, mucous membranes (fungi)	
Complement	Sepsis and other blood borne (streptococci, pneumococci, neisseria)	Autoimmune disease (systemic lupus erythematosus, glomerulonephritis)
Phagocytosis	Skin, reticuloendothelial system (staphylococci, enteric bacteria, fungi, mycobacteria)	

Screening tests for 1° immunodeficiency

Suspected abnormality	Diagnostic tests
Antibody	Quantitative IgG, IgA, IgM[1,2]
	Antibody response to immunization
Cell-mediated immunity	CBC w/differential
	Lymphocyte enumeration (CD4, CD8)
	HIV serology
	Delayed-type hypersensitivity skin tests[3]
Complement	Total hemolytic complement (CH_{50})[4]
Phagocytosis	CBC w/differential[5]
	Nitroblue tetrazolium (NBT) dye test

[1]Clue to immunodeficiency may be low normal IgG level in individual w/recurrent infections.
[2]Measurement of IgG subclass levels rarely helpful.
[3]Unreliable in children <1 yr old.
[4]Measurements of C3 and C4 do not substitute for the CH_{50}, a functional test of all components of classical complement pathway.
[5]Presence of Howell-Jolly bodies may indicate splenic dysfunction.

WHEN TO REFER

- If screening tests abnormal, refer to specialist for confirmatory diagnostic testing, counseling, development of long-term management plan. Thereafter, much of care can be coordinated through primary care physician
- In rare cases, clinical presentation may be so suggestive of immunodeficiency (eg, severe, recurrent infections w/o other explanation) that referral indicated even if all screening tests normal

BACKGROUND

- Superficial infection localized in sub-corneal epidermis
- Most common bacterial skin infection in children. Accounts for 1–2% of visits to pediatricians; comprises 10% of skin problems, 50–60% of bacterial skin infections
- Nonbullous impetigo (impetigo contagiosa) > 70% of cases
- Most common in warm, humid climates
- *Staphylococcus aureus* in 85% lesions; sole pathogen 50–60% cases. Nonbullous impetigo due to non–phage group 2 types; bullous impetigo caused predominantly by phage group 2 *S. aureus*. *Streptococcus pyogenes* in 30% nonbullous lesions; sole pathogen in 5% cases. Serotypes of *S. pyogenes* that cause impetigo different from those that cause pharyngitis
- *Staphylococcus aureus* spreads from nose to infect skin, whereas *S. pyogenes* may colonize clinically normal skin 10 d before development of impetigo. Nasopharynx may become colonized w/*S. pyogenes* 15–20 d after appearance of impetigo
- Nonbullous impetigo develops on traumatized skin (eg, at varicella lesions, insect bites, abrasions, lacerations, burns), or develops secondarily on previously diseased skin. Lesions of bullous impetigo develop on intact skin as manifestation of localized toxin production (exfoliatin or epidermolytic toxins A or B)
- *Transmission:* direct contact w/ infected lesions. Fomites can also contribute to spread of infection
- No sex/racial predilection. *S. aureus* causes impetigo in individuals of all ages. *S. pyogenes* most common in preschool age children, unusual < 2 yrs of age except in highly endemic areas
- Resolves w/o scarring within ~ 2 wks. Occasionally lasts several weeks due to autoinoculation

CLINICAL MANIFESTATIONS

- Nonbullous impetigo begins as tiny vesicle/pustule, develops rapidly into honey-color crusted plaque few mm–few cm in diameter. Removal of crust reveals superficial, slightly oozing, red erosion
  - regional adenopathy found in up to 90%
- Bullous impetigo presents w/flaccid, transparent bullae on skin of moist, intertriginous areas, occasionally on face/extremities. Bullae rupture easily, leaving narrow rim of scale at edge of shallow, moist, erythematous erosion
  - Regional adenopathy absent
- Constitutional symptoms generally absent
- Little to no pain or surrounding erythema
- Pruritis may be present

- Infection may generalize when superimposed on previously diseased or traumatized skin (eg, atopic dermatitis, chicken pox, arthropod bites)
- Heals w/o scarring
- Postinflammatory pigmentary changes may persist weeks to months

LABORATORY FEATURES

- Organism identified by culturing blister fluid or exudate beneath lifted edge of crusted plaque
- *Histopathologic features:* vesicopustule or bulla containing neutrophils in subcorneal or granular region of epidermis. Acantholytic cells may be present at base of vesicle or bulla. Underlying stratum malpighii is spongiotic, mixed papillary dermal infiltrate of lymphocytes; neutrophils surround blood vessels of superficial dermal plexus.
- Antideoxyribonuclease B (anti-DNAase B) is test of choice for detecting preceding streptococcal impetigo

DIFFERENTIAL DIAGNOSIS

- Nummular eczema
- Contact dermatitis
- Arthropod bite w/hypersensitivity reaction
- Thermal injury
- Ecthyma
- Ecthyma gangrenosum
- Pemphigus foliaceus
- Subcorneal pustular dermatosis
- Anthrax
- Cutaneous diphtheria

TREATMENT

- Areas w/high prevalence of erythromycin-resistant strains of *S. aureus*:
  - superficial, localized, nonbullous impetigo located away from mouth: topical mupirocin 3 ×/d × 7–10 d
  - if constitutional symptoms present, lesions more widespread/complicated by extension to deeper tissues, administer an oral antibiotic active against β-lactamase:
    ○ dicloxacillin, 12.5–50 mg/kg/d div 4 daily doses.
    ○ cephalexin, 25–50 mg/kg/d div 2–4 daily doses.
- If local rate of resistance to erythromycin low among isolates of *S. aureus*, also consider:
  - erythromycin ethylsuccinate, 30–50 mg/kg/d div 3–4 daily doses.
- Erythromycin or clindamycin (15 mg/kg/d div 3–4 daily doses) suitable for penicillin-allergic pts.
- Clindamycin also useful in infections w/strains of *S. aureus* known to produce toxins, in pts w/recurrent staphylococcal infections or infections w/anaerobic organisms

- Cefadroxil, cefprozil, loracarbef, clarithromycin, amoxicillin/clavulanate are second-line agents. Cefuroxime may be useful in uncommon instance of moderately severe skin infection due to a β-lactamase–producing gram-negative organism w/proven susceptibility to cefuroxime.
- 7 d Tx generally adequate. If satisfactory clinical response not achieved, swab beneath lifted edge of crusted lesion to obtain gram stain, culture and antibiotic susceptibility profile of pathogen(s)
- Recurrent impetigo:
  - evaluate for carriage of *S. aureus* in nares, perineum, axillae.
  - nasal carriage can be eliminated temporarily by applying mupirocin formulated in white petrolatum and lanolin in nares 2–4 ×/d × 5 d.
  - rifampin in combination w/penicillinase-resistant systemic antibiotic may provide additive/synergistic activity for eradication of *S. aureus* from nares. Avoid rifampin monotherapy due to emergence of resistant strains of *S. aureus*
- Bullous impetigo in neonate best treated parenterally
- Treatment does not prevent development of glomerulonephritis in index case, but may prevent spread of nephritogenic strain to others

COMPLICATIONS

- Cellulitis
- Lymphangitis, suppurative lymphadenitis, guttate psoriasis, scarlet fever (associated w/streptococcal disease). No correlation between number of lesions and clinical involvement of lymphatics or development of cellulitis
- *Following hematogenous spread:* osteomyelitis, septic arthritis, pneumonia, septicemia
- Acute poststreptococcal glomerulonephritis. Clinical character of impetigo lesions not different between those that lead to glomerulonephritis and those that do not:
  - most commonly affected age group: school-aged children 3–7 yrs of age
  - latent period from onset of impetigo: 18–21 d.
  - strains of *S. pyogenes* associated w/endemic impetigo in US have little/no nephritogenic potential
- Acute rheumatic fever does not occur following impetigo

WHEN TO REFER

- Chronic recurrent lesions
- Unusual organism(s)

INCONTINENTIA PIGMENTI

JEROME L. GORSKI

BACKGROUND

- Inherited multisystemic developmental disease that affects tissues derived from embryonic neuroectoderm
- An X-linked dominant disease; nearly all affected pts female
- Half of affected females inherit disease from carrier female; half have new mutation
- Most common mutation maps to distal long arm of X chromosome (Xq28); rare form associated w/X autosome transloca- tions w/Xp11.21 breakpoints
- Disease typically results in male lethali- ty; affected females have excess of second trimester male miscarriages
- Rare affected males may have 47, XXY chromosomal constitution (Klinefelter syn- drome), or somatic mosaicism

CLINICAL MANIFESTATIONS

- Confirmed Dx based on presence of spe- cific dermatologic findings and positive family Hx and/or presence of additional neurologic, ophthamologic, or dental anom- alies (see Complications)
- Linear erythematous vesiculobullous le- sions specific for disease and diagnostic when additional systemic findings present
- Additional supporting dermatologic signs include linear verruciform eruptions in in- fancy, linear irregularly patterned hyper- pigmented whorls and swirls in childhood, linear epidermal and dermal atrophy, seg- mental alopecia, nail dystrophy
- ~ 80% affected pts have additional multi- systemic abnormalities (see Complications)
- Severity of clinical manifestations varies considerably among affected females

LABORATORY FEATURES

- Peripheral blood smear shows eosino- philia in infancy
- Vesicular lesion biopsy shows intraepi- dermal accumulation of eosinophils and oc- casional basophils (seldom necessary)
- Biopsies of hyperpigmented region shows melanin in the papillary dermis and vacuoli- zation of basal-cell layer (seldom necessary)

DIFFERENTIAL DIAGNOSIS

- Full clinical picture of disease unique; however, it must be distinguished from other conditions presenting w/infantile vesicular or linear cutaneous lesions including:
  - bacterial vesicular infections
  - epidermolysis bullosa
  - bullous mastocytosis
  - focal dermal hypoplasia
  - X-linked chondrodysplasia punctata
  - congenital varicella
  - Letterer-Siwe disease
  - congenital reticulohistiocytosis
  - hypomelanosis of Ito
  - linear epidermal nevus

COMPLICATIONS

- ~ 80% pts have additional multisystemic abnormalities
- Neurologic abnormalities (30%) include congenital and postnatal microcephaly, hy- potonia, seizures, hydrocephalus, mental retardation
- Ophthalmologic abnormalities (35%) in- clude progressive neovascularization, stra- bismus, cataracts, glaucoma
- Dental anomalies (65%) include delayed eruption, hypodontia or adontia, enamel hypoplasia, abnormally shaped teeth

TREATMENT

- Periodic ophthalmologic evaluations for progressive neovascularization
- Ophthalmologic surgery for ocular anom- alies
- Orthodontia for hypodontia and abnor- mally shaped teeth
- Special education referrals for learning difficulties and mental retardation
- Genetic counseling for affected females and at-risk family members
- Dermatologic anomalies rarely require cosmetic plastic surgery

COUNSELING

- Reproductive risks of affected female includes:
  - 25% chance of having affected female
  - 25% chance of having normal female
  - 25% chance of having normal male
  - 25% chance of having an affected and spontaneously miscarried male fetus
- Genetic counseling for affected females and at-risk family members

WHEN TO REFER

- Equivocal cases should be referred to medical geneticist to confirm Dx
- All affected females should be referred to pediatric ophthalmologist for detection and treatment of associated eye anomalies
- All affected and at-risk females should be referred to medical geneticist for genetic counseling
- Affected females w/dental anomalies should be referred to dentist for orthodonture

BACKGROUND

- Infectious mononucleosis most frequently occurs in adolescent and young adult years
- Epstein-Barr virus (EBV), predominant cause of infectious mononucleosis, infects most children asymptomatically during the first 6 yrs of life. Infection during adolescence and young adulthood is much more likely to produce infectious mononucleosis
- Although EBV is transmitted efficiently in general population, its clinical presentation as infectious mononucleosis does not occur commonly even among family members or other contacts living close to contact case

CLINICAL MANIFESTATIONS

- Typically, fever, sore throat, malaise, fatigue accompanied by signs of tonsillopharyngitis, lymphadenopathy, hepatosplenomegaly
- Tonsillopharyngitis often exudative (50% of time), severe
- Adenopathy most prominently involves cervical lymph nodes (anterior and posterior), usually nontender, lacks overlying skin erythema
- Organomegaly most striking in second–fourth wks of illness
- Strong correlation noted in young adults between administration of ampicillin and subsequent development of maculopapular rash not as apparent among pediatric pts

LABORATORY FEATURES

- *CBC:* absolute lymphocytosis ($\geq$ 50% lymphocytes) w/total leukocytes $\geq$ 5,000/mm^3
- *CBC:* Prominent formation of atypical lymphocytes (typically $\geq$ 10% of total leukocytes)
- *Serology:* positive test result for Paul-Bunnell heterophile antibodies (positive "differential heterophile")
- *Serology:* very young children ($\leq$ 3 yrs of age) frequently do not develop detectable heterophile antibody response
- *Serology:* for pts w/atypical manifestations, lymphoproliferative diseases, or severe illness and for those w/negative heterophile tests and prolonged or serious illness, specific laboratory testing for EBV infection (antibody testing in most cases) warranted
- *Serology:* liver transaminases often mildly ↑

- Epstein-Barr virus antigen detection in tissues or blood cells (not throat secretions) rarely indicated and usually only for pts w/presumed EBV-associated lymphoproliferative disorders

DIFFERENTIAL DIAGNOSIS

- Traditional presentation of infectious mononucleosis should not produce a diagnostic problem
- Diagnostic difficulties may arise early in clinical course, when few typical manifestations apparent; when principal typical feature absent or extremely prominent; or when organ or system uncommonly affected shows extensive involvement
- Bacterial or viral tonsillopharyngitis
- Lymphocytic leukemoid reactions (that occur w/pertussis or infectious lymphocytosis)
- Acute leukemia, lymphoproliferative disorders
- Drug-induced hypersensitivity reactions (from dilantin [phenylhydantoin] derivatives or isoniazid [INH]) or serum sickness.
- Acute brucellosis, 2° syphilis, leptospirosis
- Infectious mononucleosislike episodes due to *Toxoplasma gondii* or cytomegalovirus
- Bell palsy, acute meningoencephalitis, idiopathic thrombocytopenia purpura—when occur as early, single manifestations (ie, before full clinical picture appears)

TREATMENT

- For *routine* infectious mononucleosis, control or minimize symptomatology:
  - ibuprofen, acetaminophen to control fever and alleviate discomfort
  - gargling w/warm saline water
  - reduction of activity and bed rest, as dictated by pt tolerance
  - avoidance of contact sport, activities w/potential for trauma or stress to abdomen (vigorous exercise, heavy lifting) during period spleen palpable
  - oral penicillin V (alternative: erythromycin but *not* ampicillin) ×10 d for group A beta-hemolytic streptococcal superinfection of pharynx
  - corticosteroids not recommended
- For *complicated* infectious mononucleosis (eg, stridor from massively enlarged tonsils or paratracheal adenopathy, hematologic or neurologic complications):

  - short-term corticosteroid Tx (po or IV in doses equivalent to 40 mg/m^2/d w/tapering to complete over 1–2 wks)
  - artificial airway (preferred over emergency tonsillectomy) for complete airway obstruction
  - splenectomy, or as more recently shown nonoperative means, for traumatic or spontaneous splenic rupture

COMPLICATIONS

- Complications characteristically short lived and produce no permanent sequelae
- Complications noted ~ one-fifth of children w/infectious mononucleosis in this descending frequency:
  - respiratory (pneumonia, severe airway obstruction)
  - neurologic (seizures, meningitis/encephalitis, peripheral facial nerve paralysis, Guillain-Barré syndrome)
  - hematologic (thrombocytopenia w/hemorrhages, hemolytic anemia)
  - infectious (bacteremia, recurrent tonsillopharyngitis)
  - hepatic (jaundice)
  - renal (glomerulonephritis)
  - peritonsillar abscess
  - splenic rupture rare event in children, although rate unclear; for adults rate of splenic rupture ~ 0.2 % of cases

WHEN TO REFER

- Clinical course of most pts one of gradual, uneventful recovery after acute phase lasting several days–3/4 wks
- Referral recommended when a serious complication occurs, Dx unclear in face of serious manifestations, in-pt monitoring and management warranted, or IV Tx/fluids needed
- Referral recommended when significant clinical manifestations persist *w/o* improvement into third or fourth week after clinical onset. (Hematologic changes and hepatosplenomegaly not uncommonly detected 4–8 wks or, in some cases, even longer after clinical onset. However, signs of improvement usually present by weeks 3/4, if not earlier, of disease course)

DEBRA A. TRISTRAM

BACKGROUND

• Influenza viruses = DNA viruses. Currently three known types: A, B, C, but A, B responsible for epidemic disease. Influenza contains one of two neuraminidases (N1, N2) and one of three hemaglutinins (H1, H2, H3) to which humans make specific antibody. Changes in antigens occur frequently and can result in susceptibility to type of influenza with which persons previously infected or immunized
• *Incubation:* 1–3 d
• Highly contagious. Spread by respiratory droplets. Attack rates: healthy children 10–40%, w/1% hospitalization rates. Greater in high-risk individuals. Can be spread nosocomially through hands, respiratory equipment
• *Recovery:* usually within 7–10 d in otherwise healthy persons
• *Mortality:* can be seen among persons w/ chronic conditions and persons <6 mos of age, >65 yrs of age

CLINICAL MANIFESTATIONS

• Abrupt onset fever, chills, malaise, myalgias w/ dry cough
• *Subsequent development of respiratory symptoms:* sore throat, nasal congestion, cough
• Less common features:
  – conjunctivitis
  – GI symptoms: nausea, vomiting, abdominal pain
  – acute febrile illness w/o localizing signs in infants and young children
  – croup
  – pneumonia

LABORATORY FEATURES

• Normal or low peripheral white count
• Rapid detection methods:
  – respiratory secretion specimen for influenza type-specific fluorescent monoclonal antibody testing. Usually available within 24 hrs of laboratory receipt of sample. Not available at all laboratory facilities
• Viral culture:
  – requires respiratory sample for tissue culture. Virus identification 2–6 d
• Paired serum samples:
  – requires acute blood sample and convalescent sample 3–4 wks after illness

DIFFERENTIAL DIAGNOSIS

• Other viral diseases:
  – RSV
  – adenoviruses
  – enteroviruses
  – CMV
• Bacterial disease:
  – Legionella
  – *Mycoplasma pneumonia*
  – *Chlamydia pneumoniae*
  – early sepsis w/ *Neisseria meningiditis, Staphylococcus aureus, Streptococcus pneumoniae*

PREVENTION: INFECTION CONTROL AND PROPHYLAXIS

• *Hospitalized or institutionalized pts:* contact isolation during duration of symptoms. Strict hand washing due to spread by infectious respiratory secretions
• *Vaccine:* combination of most recently isolated virus types:
  – inactivated whole virus (whole) or purified surface antigens ("split")
  – satisfactory response in children <12 yrs of age w/ 2-dose regimen
  – efficacy in healthy subjects against homologous challenge: 70–80%. Not studied in children <6 mos
  – side effects: local, mild pain, swelling 10%; febrile reactions in children <13 yrs of age uncommon
  – indicated in high-risk groups
    ○ contraindicated in individuals w/ egg allergy, allergy to neomycin, etc
• Recommended target groups to receive yearly immunization:
  – persons w/:
    ○ cystic fibrosis, asthma, other chronic respiratory conditions
    ○ diabetes, other chronic metabolic diseases
    ○ cardiac diseases, particularly pts w/ pulmonary hypertension
    ○ immunodeficiencies
    ○ illnesses requiring chronic salicylate use (eg, JRA)
  – persons residing w/ high-risk individual
  – health care workers
  – residents of long-term care facilities housing persons of any age w/ chronic medical conditions
  – persons >65 yrs of age
• Considered groups:
  – persons providing important community services
  – women ≥6 mos pregnant or have just delivered during influenza season
  – people in schools or colleges (to prevent outbreaks)
  – international travelers to tropics or Southern Hemisphere April–September

Influenza Vaccination

Age	Vaccine Type	Dose/Route
<6 mos	not recommended	–
6 mos–3 yrs	split virus	0.25 mL/IM, 1–2 doses*
3–8 yrs	split virus	0.5 mL/IM, 1–2 doses*
9–12 yrs	split virus	0.5 mL/IM, 1 dose
>12 yrs	whole or split virus	0.5 mL/IM, 1 dose

*2 doses recommended for naive subjects; 1 may be sufficient for children w/ past Hx influenza

• *Alternatives to vaccination:* antiviral drugs amantidine and rimantidine:
  – effective only against replication of influenza A, not influenza B
  – used for pts w/ allergy to vaccine components or w/ other impediment to immunization
  – treatment or prophylaxis should begin as soon as possible after symptoms begin or after exposure to be most effective (within 48 hrs). continue for 2–7 d
  – prophylaxis may be important in preventing outbreaks in closed communities, eg, nursing homes

Amantidine and Rimantidine Dosing for Prophylaxis or Treatment of Influenza Infections

	1–9 yrs of age*	Children ≥10 yrs of age	
		weight <40 kg	weight >40 kg
Prophylaxis and treatment	5 mg/kg/d to max 150 mg in 1 dose or 2 div doses	5 mg/kg/d in 1 dose or 2 div doses	200 mg/d in 1 dose or 2 div doses

*No information in use for children <1 yr of age

• ↓ dosage in pts w/ renal insufficiency (both drugs) and hepatic dysfunction (rimantidine only): see PDR for information
• Side effects of amantidine and rimantidine:
  – CNS: can be mild and end w/ cessation of drug
  – higher incidence of seizures in pts w. epilepsy
  – side effects greater in amantidine than rimantidine recipients
  – may alter metabolism of other medications

TREATMENT

• *Most pts require symptomatic relief only:* antipyretics, antitussives, oral fluids
• Antibiotics indicated only for those w/ documented or strongly suspected bacterial superinfection
• *Medications:* amantidine or rimantidine. Treatment regimen same as that of prophylaxis:
  – suggested recipients of treatment same as for immunization plus those w/ severe disease

COMPLICATIONS

• Bacterial superinfection
  – acute otitis media
  – pneumonia
• Reye syndrome, particularly in individuals w/ Hx salicylate use
• Acute myositis, particularly following influenza, type B
• Alteration in metabolism of some medications (eg, theophylline, phenobarbital) resulting in development of toxicity due to high levels

WHEN TO REFER

• Most pts do not require referral
• Referral considered for high-risk individuals w/ severe disease, when Dx in doubt, complications develop, or pt has rapid clinical deterioration

ANTONELLA TOSTI AND BIANCA MARIA PIRACCINI

BACKGROUND

- Lateral nail ingrowing most frequently found among young adults, esp males, w/ peak incidence 14–18 yrs of age
- Condition usually affects great toes; often bilateral
- Distal embedding common complication of nail avulsion
- Idiopathic distal embedding occasionally observed in children

Predisposing Factors

- Congenital malalignment of big toenail. Condition frequently inherited as autosomal dominant trait. One or both great toenails show lateral deviation of nail plate from central axis of digit
- Congenital excessive convexity of nails
- Hypertrophic lateral nail fold
- Abnormally long toes
- Hyperhidrosis

Causes

- Trauma
- Ill-fitting footwear
- Incorrect nail cutting

Pathogenesis

- Edge of nail plate forms spicules that penetrate into lateral nail fold epithelium (lateral ingrowing) or into hyponychium, resulting in inflammatory reaction

CLINICAL MANIFESTATIONS

Lateral Ingrowing

- *Stage I:* erythema, swelling, pain of affected lateral nail fold
- *Stage II:* growth of pseudopyogenic granuloma that emerges from lateral nail fold; associated w/ pain, seropurulent exudation
- *Stage III:* epithelization of granulation tissue. Nail fold hypertrophic, partially covers nail plate

DIFFERENTIAL DIAGNOSIS

- Acute bacterial paronychia
- Herpethic whitlow
- Retinoid- or antiretroviral-induced pseudopyogenic granuloma
- Hallopeau acrodermatitis
- Acute contact dermatitis
- Digital ischemia

TREATMENT

- Excessive granulation tissue can be reduced by topical application mupirocin 2% ointment, 1×/d × 1 wk. Medium-strength topical steroid can be added to reduce inflammation and pain
- Alternatively, pseudopyogenic granuloma can be destroyed by cryotherapy or electrodesiccation
- Embedded spicula should always be removed either by cutting lateral nail or by inserting nonabsorbent cotton under nail plate to elevate lateral edge
- When condition recurrent, chemical destruction of lateral matrix, using 85% aqueous phenol solution advisable
- Selective surgical excision of lateral matrix horn appropriate, but requires great skill on part of operator

COMPLICATIONS

- Infections, common
- Onychomycosis, uncommon

PREVENTION

- Instruct pts to cut nails at right angle w/o cutting lateral corners
- Cotton can be placed along lateral nail fold to avoid further embedding
- Lateral edges of nail plate can be uplifted by fixing acrylic band to nail plate surface

WHEN TO REFER

- Podiatric or surgical referral indicated for severe or recalcitrant cases

BACKGROUND

- Most frequently used illicit substance among early adolescents following alcohol and tobacco
- 21.6% 8th grade students acknowledge lifetime use (1995 *Monitoring the Future*)
- use ↑ among early adolescents in past decade
- Substances used easily obtainable, inexpensive, legally available household products
- Inhalant abuse often considered "childish behavior" not addressed by health professionals

CATEGORIES OF INHALANTS

- *Solvents:* aromatic, halogenated hydrocarbons:
  - trichloroethane: typewriter correction fluid, vegetable cooking sprays, analgesic sprays, room fresheners
  - carbon tetrachloride: paint removers, paint thinner
  - toluene, benzene, acetone: paint thinners, furniture stripping solutions, nail polish remover, automotive additives, transmission fluid, spray paint
- *Fuels:* alkylated hydrocarbons:
  - butane: cigarette lighter fluid
  - propane: fuel for backyard grill, lanterns
  - gasoline, kerosene: fuels for household products, lawn mowers, heaters
- Anesthetics:
  - nitrous oxide: propellant in canned whipped toppings, analgesic sprays
- Means of use:
  - "huffing": cloth soaked w/ substance placed over mouth and nose for inhalation
  - "bagging": paper bag containing liquid placed over mouth and nose for inhalation
  - "whippets": cartridges or balloons containing nitrous oxide for inhalation
  - "fire breathing": igniting exhaled fuels such as propane or butane
  - "snorting": inhalation of substance from small container such as nail polish remover

CLINICAL MANIFESTATIONS

- *Intoxication:* immediate in onset following inhalation
- *Disorientation:* hydrocarbons lipophilic and accumulate rapidly in brain tissues causing neuronal membrane dysfunction. Additionally, mild hypoxia noted w/ use
- *Tachycardia, hypertension:* cardiac sensitization to catecholamine release results in rapid pulse rate, transient ↑ BP
- *Arrhythmia:* cardiac sensitization to catecholamine effects may produce acute arrhythmia leading to sudden cardiac failure
- *Nasal, oropharyngeal irritation:* chemical burns to nose and oropharynx noted w/repeated use. Examiner may also note presence of pigment in nose and oropharynx w/ paint and typewriter correction use
- *Gastric irritation:* GI distress, vomiting often noted w/ use of fuels
- *Chemical pneumonitis:* cough, tachypnea, respiratory distress may be noted immediately following use or may be delayed for up to 12 hrs following inhalation

LABORATORY MANIFESTATIONS

- *Renal:* cellular damage may result in ↑ BUN, creatinine
- *Hepatic:* cellular damage w/ resulting ↑ LFTs may be noted w/ hydrocarbon use

TREATMENT

- Acute inhalation:
  - administer oxygen for support of respiratory depression
  - chest x ray: on admission and at 6 hrs to determine chemical pneumonitis
  - baseline renal and liver function studies to monitor effects
  - EKG: if chest pain reported or arrhythmia suspected

COMPLICATIONS

- *Sudden cardiac death:* due to irreversible arrhythmia resulting in cardiac failure immediately following use
- *Chronic hepatic failure:* due to hepatic cellular damage from repeated use
- *Chronic renal failure:* due to renal cellular damage from repeated use

WHEN TO REFER

- Most pts managed w/o referral
- Education, prevention, early intervention may deter significant inhalant use
- If inhalant use one component of pattern of persistent substance use, referral to substance abuse specialist or treatment program indicated
- Referral indicated if serious complications from inhalant use identified

BACKGROUND

- Intertrigo describes superficial inflammatory process occurring in body folds or creases; folds/creases include axillae, antecubital/popliteal fossae, groin, intergluteal cleft, umbilicus, postauricular folds, inframammary creases, folds of eyelids, neck, abdomen, as well as finger/toe webs
- Moisture, heat, friction predispose to development of intertrigo
- Can occur at any age from infancy through adulthood; infants may present w/diaper dermatitis 2° to occlusion by diaper leading to maceration
- Many cutaneous disorders present w/lesions that may be confined to intertriginous areas of body
- Due to maceration that develops, 2° infection by bacteria, yeast, fungi may occur
- Factors such as obesity, occlusive clothing, incontinence, overheating due to environmental heat/humidity may lead to ↑ moisture, friction

CLINICAL MANIFESTATIONS

- Burning/itching most common complaints
- Skin becomes erythematous/macerated leading to erosions, fissures, sometimes weeping exudate
- Complete cutaneous examination necessary to elicit accurate Dx; many 1° dermatoses have lesions outside of intertriginous areas

LABORATORY FEATURES

- Laboratory examination directed at determining 1°/2° infectious etiology, such as yeast, fungus, bacteria; tests include KOH examination, fungal culture, or bacterial culture
- Wood light examination can diagnose erythrasma, revealing coral red fluorescence
- Skin biopsy may be indicated in eruptions recalcitrant to Tx

DIFFERENTIAL DIAGNOSIS

- Infectious
- Fungal
  - Candidiasis
  - Dermatophyte (Tinea corporis)
- Bacterial
  - beta hemolytic streptococcal intertrigo most commonly occurs in perianal area (also known as perianal streptococcal dermatitis), although may occur in other folds including groin, axillae, neck, postauricular areas
  - erythrasma, caused by *Corynebacterium minutissimum*. Presents w/scaly, dry, reddish brown patches, favoring axillae, genital creases, toe web spaces, esp the fourth toe web space
  - Staphylococci, pseudomonas may also present in intertriginous areas
- 1° dermatoses
  - seborrheic dermatitis
  - inverse psoriasis
  - contact dermatitis
  - irritant diaper dermatitis

TREATMENT

- Treatment of intertrigo aimed at minimizing friction/moisture. Methods include avoiding exposure to high heat/humidity, wearing loose cotton clothing, loss of weight when obesity predisposing factor
- Cool compresses soothing/can ↓ inflammation
- Steroid lotion/cream containing hydrocortisone 0.5% or 1% can briefly be used to decrease inflammation; more potent topical preparations including fluorinated preparations should be avoided in body creases where skin thinner/absorption greater
- Candidal/tinea infections should be treated w/topical antifungal; many topical antifungal preparations, such as imidazoles, effective against candida/dermaytophytes; nystatin, while effective against yeast, not effective in treating dermatophyte infections
- Erythrasma treated w/topical applications w/erythromycin, clindamycin, miconazole cream, econazole cream, Whitfield's ointment; oral erythromycin, as well as tetracycline in children ≥8 yrs also effective
- Streptococcal infections should be treated w/oral penicillin (erythromycin in penicillin-allergic pts)
- 1° dermatoses should be treated w/low-potency topical steroids

COMPLICATIONS

- 2° infection w/bacteria/yeast most common complication

WHEN TO REFER

- Pts w/recalcitrant eruptions should be referred for further evaluation/need for possible biopsy

INTERVERTEBRAL DISK INFECTIONS

GERALD W. FISCHER

BACKGROUND

- Most of data collected to date suggest diskitis infectious process
- Highest attack rates occur in young children; incidence peaks around ~1–3 yrs of age, w/ suggestion of second peak in older children 11–15 yrs of age
- Disk highly vascular in children >6 yrs of age and hematogenous spread of organisms to disk space most probable mechanism of infection
- Microtrauma to disk may provide areas more susceptible to infection
- *Staphylococcus aureus* most common isolate from biopsy and blood cultures; other bacteria including anaerobes and streptococci sporadically isolated from disk biopsies

CLINICAL MANIFESTATIONS

- Most children have low-grade fever
- *Two most common clinical presentations:* back pain and/or tenderness and hip and/or leg complaints w/ limp or refusal to walk
- Two-thirds of children w/ diskitis >8 yrs of age present w/ back symptomatology
- Most young children present w/ irritability, limp, or refusal to walk
- Physical examination generally reveals paraspinous muscle spasm

LABORATORY FEATURES

- ESR usually ↑ (30–50 mm/h)
- WBC count moderately ↑ or normal
- Blood cultures always indicated in febrile toxic pt
- Radiographs of spine may not show disk space narrowing for 3–8 wks, but may demonstrate vertebral body destruction associated w/ vertebral body osteomyelitis
- Bone scan may be useful to identify diskitis in first 1–2 wks of symptoms
- MRI can help distinguish diskitis from vertebral body osteomyelitis

DIFFERENTIAL DIAGNOSIS

- Vertebral body osteomyelitis
- Psoas muscle, paraspinus muscle abscess
- Sacroilitis
- Other serious bacterial infections such as septic arthritis, osteomyelitis, meningitis, etc (depending on clinical presentation)
- Noninfectious systemic disease (eg, malignancy, JRA, etc)
- Noninfectious musculoskeletal disease (toxic synovitis of hip, etc)

TREATMENT

- Resolution generally occurs w/ mobilization and bed rest alone in uncomplicated diskitis
- Antibiotic Tx for *S. aureus* recommended if child toxic. Nafcillin 150 mg/kg/d IV div q6h × 2–4 wks
- Antibiotic appropriate for specific pathogen if organism isolated from blood or tissue specimen

COMPLICATIONS

- Collapse of disk space common after diskitis and may reexpand over several months or years postresolution
- *Most serious complication:* not identifying more serious bacterial or systemic process

Risk Factor	Benign Diskitis*	Serious Bacterial Process**
Age	<8 yrs	≥8 yrs
Fever	<38°C	≥39°C
WBC count	Normal	Elevated, left shift
ESR	<50 mm/hr	≥50 mm/hr
Clinical appearance	Not ill	Toxic
Imaging	Disk space involvement	Bone destruction, paraspinus infection

*Benign diskitis defined as that process which responds to bed rest and immobilization; other diseases are ruled out and disk space narrowing is only abnormality detected.

**Serious bacterial processes included vertebral body osteomyelitis, brucellosis, psoas muscle abscess, etc

WHEN TO REFER

- Most pts w/ diskitis require referral for orthopedic support (immobilization, etc)
- Referral to infectious disease specialist may be indicated for evaluation for osteomyelitis or systemic infection

LESLI A. TAYLOR

BACKGROUND

- Three types of intussusception:
  - idiopathic ileo-colic intussusception w/o pathologic lead point most common form in children:
    - ○ Peyer patches usual nonpathologic lead point
    - ○ typical age group 3–12 mos of age
    - ○ 2–4 cases/1,000 live births; male predominance 3:2
    - ○ seasonal incidence w/ peaks in spring and summer and in winter
    - ○ associated w/ viral gastroenteritis and upper respiratory infections
    - ○ can progress to lethal perforation, peritonitis, septic shock in 48–60 hrs if untreated
  - pathologic lead point: Meckel diverticulum, polyp, intestinal duplication, hematoma associated w/Henoch-Schönlein purpura
  - small bowel intussusception rare cause of postop bowel obstruction

CLINICAL MANIFESTATIONS

- Well infant who becomes irritable w/severe, episodic crampy abdominal pain
- Vomiting in 80%
- Abdominal mass in 85%
- Lethargy (may be profound)
- Fever (disturbed mucosal integrity and translocation of endotoxins)
- Current jelly stool: mucus mixed w/blood from ischemic mucosa
- Small bowel obstruction
- Peritonitis, septic shock if late presentation

LABORATORY FEATURES

- WBC may be slightly ↑, but not diagnostic; usually markedly ↑ if perforation has occurred
- Abdominal plain films may be nonspecific or show intussusceptum outlined by air
- Air-fluid levels of small bowel obstruction if late presentation

DIFFERENTIAL DIAGNOSIS

- Small bowel obstruction of another cause
- Lymphoma

TREATMENT

- Barium or air enema by experienced radiologist if no peritoneal signs or evidence of perforation
- Surgery if perforated on presentation, irreducible by radiologist or perforation by enema. Appendectomy usually performed if cecum normal
- Overnight observation if enema reduction successful

COMPLICATIONS

- Perforation during enema reduction
- Inability to reduce operatively requiring resection, 1° anastomosis
- Recurrence 5–7% following enema reduction or surgical management

WHEN TO REFER

- Refer to surgeon early so determination for radiologic vs. surgical management made

BACKGROUND

- Due to lack of dietary iron, impaired absorption of iron or excessive blood losses
- Most frequently observed 6 mos–24 mos of age. Also common in adolescents esp females
- More common in low birth weight infants and children in lower socioeconomic groups

CLINICAL MANIFESTATIONS

- Pallor
- Irritability
- Listlessness
- Anorexia
- Reduced activity
- Reduced interest in environment
- Impaired cognitive performance

LABORATORY FEATURES

- *Hemoglobin (Hgb) and MCV:* reduced below age-associated normal value
- *Red cell distribution width (RDW):* elevated
- *Serum iron:* usually reduced (<30 µg/dl for young children); normal values vary w/age. Recent dietary intake of iron may transiently normalize parameter
- *Total iron binding capacity (TIBC):* elevated
- *Transferrin saturation:* reduced (<16%)
- *Serum ferritin:* reduced (<10–12 ng/mL). Acute-phase reactant, may be elevated in setting of inflammation even in presence of iron deficiency
- *Erythrocyte protoporphyrin (EP):* elevated (≥70–80 µg/dl of whole blood). Also elevated, usually to greater degree, in lead poisoning

DIFFERENTIAL DIAGNOSIS

- Thalassemia trait
- Lead poisoning
- Anemia of chronic disease (anemia of inflammation)
- Sideroblastic anemia

	Thal trait	Lead poisoning	Iron deficiency	Anemia of chronic disease
Hemoglobin	reduced	reduced	reduced	reduced
MCV	reduced	reduced	reduced	normal/slightly reduced
RDW	normal	normal	increased	normal
Serum iron	normal	normal	reduced	reduced
TIBC	normal	normal	>400 µg/dl	normal
Transferrin saturation	normal	normal	<16%	reduced
Serum ferritin	normal	normal	<10–12 ng/ml	elevated
EP	normal	elevated	>70–80 µg/dl	elevated
Serum lead	<15 µg/dl	>15 µg/dl	<15 µg/dl	<15 µg/dl

TREATMENT

- *Determine etiology of iron deficiency:* blood loss (GI, pulmonary, coagulopathy) or inadequate dietary iron
- *Oral iron replacement therapy:* ferrous sulfate in drop, elixir, syrup, tablet form
  - *Dosage:* 2–3 mg/kg/d of elemental iron div bid or tid
  - simultaneous administration of vitamin C enhances absorption
  - avoid administering w/tea, coffee, milk (reduce absorption)
  - response proportional to degree of anemia
  - with moderate to severe iron deficiency reticulocyte count increases within 2–3 d and peaks at 7–10 d treatment
  - hemoglobin rises within 2–4 wks Tx and Hgb, MCV, and EP should be corrected following 3 mos Tx
  - continue treatment 2–4 mos to replenish body iron stores
  - advantages: cost, ease of administration
  - disadvantages: possible GI irritation, diarrhea, constipation, temporary staining of teeth if not administered to back of tongue
- *Parenteral iron Tx:* iron dextran (imferon, 50 mg elemental Fe per mL)
  - dosage: in mL = weight (kg) × desired rise in Hgb (g/dl) × 0.075 administered into buttock using z track or IV
  - advantage: absorption assured
  - disadvantages: staining of skin w/IM injection, pain at injection site, potential bronchospasm or anaphylactic reactions; associated complaints of headache, nausea, vomiting, chills, fever, myalgias, arthralgias, dizziness, urticaria
- *Blood transfusion:* rarely warranted, usually in setting of severe anemia (Hgb <4–5 g/dl) and impending congestive heart failure. Best administered as partial exchange transfusion or in small aliquots w/diuretics administered midway through transfusion
  - advantage: rapid rise in hemoglobin
  - disadvantage: risk of cardiovascular compromise, transfusion-associated infection

COMPLICATIONS

- Risk of congestive heart failure in setting of profound anemia (rare)
- Potential side effects or toxicity of treatment

PREVENTION

- Oral iron supplements for preterm infants
- Iron supplementation of infant diets: iron-fortified formulas, iron-enriched dry cereals

WHEN TO REFER

- Vast majority pts managed w/o referral
- When Dx in doubt
- W/failure to respond to documented administration of oral iron
- W/chronic iron deficiency for evaluation of iron losses or lack of iron absorption

BACKGROUND

• Consists of number of syndromes that present in children as idiopathic peripheral arthritis
• Incidence rate for North America ~12/100,000, w/ prevalence 95/100,000 (95% confidence intervals 50–150)
• Age distribution varies w/ onset type w/ overall peak frequency 1.5–2 yrs of age; often suggestion in some studies of bimodal distribution w/ second peak 9–15 yrs
• No significant risk factors; 2° cases in first-degree relatives rare, although strong associations w/ certain HLA types exist, particularly in children w/ oligoarticular onset
• Pathogenesis of JRA clearly immunoinflammatory involving elements of both the B and T cell pathways, although no unequivocal etiologic factor has been identified (always been strong suspicion of viral trigger in some instances of this disease, eg, rubella)

CLINICAL MANIFESTATIONS

• JRA defined as arthritis beginning before 16 yrs of age. Arthritis defined clinically as presence of joint swelling or effusion, or presence of ≥2 of following signs: limitation of joint motion, tenderness or pain on motion, ↑ heat in ≥1 joints
• Polyarthritis defined as presentation w/ involvement ≥5 joints
• Oligoarthritis or pauciarticular onset defined as disease beginning ≤4 joints, often in only single large joint such as knee
• Systemic disease involves presence of objective arthritis plus intermittent fever of 2 wks' duration, almost always accompanied by rash of JRA evidence of internal organ involvement, such as hepatosplenomegaly

Classification of JRA

	Polyarthritis	Oligoarthritis	Systemic Disease
Frequency	30%	55%	15%
No. of joints	≥5	≤4	Variable
F:M ratio	3:1	5:1	1:1
Systemic involvement	Moderate	Not present	Prominent
Uveitis	5%	20%	Rare
RF	10% (↑ w/ age)	Rare	Rare
Antinuclear antibodies	40–50%	75–85% (in girls w/uveitis)	10%

• Onset types not only helpful diagnostically, but also in terms of prognosis and thereby selection of Tx. Defined by the manifestations of disease within first 6 mos after onset
• Course of disease equally important in terms of eventual prognosis, defined as types of manifestations of disease after first 6 mos during subsequent 2–5 y interval. Course of disease based on number of joints involved during that period of time, persistence of systemic features, development of specific complications such as chronic uveitis, devastating autoimmune inflammation of uveal tract of eye (iris, ciliary body, choroid). JRA leading cause of blindness in children after that attributed to accidents/congenital malformations

LABORATORY FEATURES

• Acute-Phase Reactants:
  – as in any inflammatory disorder, acute-phase reactants such as ESR, C-reactive protein, hypergammaglobulinemia may reflect activity of disease in youngsters w/ active arthritis. Small number of children w/ JRA (~4%) may have associated selective IgA deficiency
  – systemic onset of juvenile rheumatoid arthritis often associated w/ leukocytosis/neutrophilia, which may reach levels of 40,000–50,000 WBC/mm³, anemia of chronic illness w/ Hgbs ranging down to level of 7.5 g/dL. Thrombocytosis w/ platelet counts 500,000/cmm to occasionally in excess of 1 million accompany active systemic disease
• Autoimmune antibodies:
  – two most important associated laboratory abnormalities: positive antinuclear antibody (ANA) test/positive rheumatoid factor (RF) test
  – ANA seropositivity strongly associated w/↑ risk chronic uveitis in children w/ olioarticular onset. Titers generally moderate w/ homogeneous to speckled pattern. Antigens associated w/seropositivity have not been specifically identified
  – RF seropositivity tends to be associated w/later age of onset/poorer functional outcome. Almost entirely limited to one specific subtype, that of polyarticular RF-positive disease
• HLA antigens (MHC locus):
  – RF-positive polyarticular disease in majority of children also associated w/ HLA-DR4 subtypes (DRB1*0401 and 0404). ANA-positive oligoarthritis w/ uveitis also associated w/ specific HLA types, predominantly DRB1*1104, DPB1*0201, DQA1*0501

DIFFERENTIAL DIAGNOSIS

• Children w/ systemic onset disease, esp those who do not present w/ arthritis during initial phases of illness, easily confused w/ bacteremic entities, other connective tissue diseases such as systemic lupus erythematosus, dermatomyositis, acute leukemia, malignancies
• Children w/ oligoarthritis, particularly those w/ single joint involvement, should be distinguished from low-grade septic arthritis, intraarticular tumor (rare), or traumatic effusion, and in some cases other causes of joint swelling such as hemophilia
• Polyarticular onset often easiest type of JRA to diagnose
• Consideration should always be given in any of these presentations to the possibility of infectious diseases such as Lyme disease or parvovirus B19 infection

TREATMENT

• Basic approach to child w/ JRA to suppress inflammation w/ NSAID and begin basic program of education, coordination of care, physical Tx, occupational Tx where indicated, adequate rest, both general and joint specific w/ splinting. School issues often loom as greatest impediments to instituting quality program
• For children who do not respond to simple use of NSAID, additional Tx chosen based on therapeutic pyramid. Second-line agents often involve drugs such as hydroxychloroquine. IM gold effective/formerly much used in resistant disease. Its use has been almost totally supplanted at present time by methotrexate given 10 mg/m² 1×/wk, usually po early am on empty stomach, but occasionally SubQ and recently etanercept (soluble TNFα p75FP). Azathiaprine and cyclophosphamide should be reserved for very rare child who has not responded to any other means of Tx. Acceptable experimental Tx at present time often includes use of IV pulse steroid, IV immunoglobulin, or cyclosporin A. Systemic steroids should only be used in child w/ overwhelming systemic or articular disease in whom other forms of Tx have failed. Ophthalmic use of gluccocorticoids almost always indicated for chronic uveitis

COMPLICATIONS

• Most frequent complication of JRA joint specific w/ ↑ growth of that limb, particularly if joint involved is knee; progressive joint destruction due to unremitting disease; joint contracture; muscle atrophy. Both localized/generalized osteopenia w/ disorder bone mineralization occur in these children
• Chronic uveitis most common complication of child w/ oligoarticular onset. Tx should always be in conjunction w/ experienced ophthalmologist
• Resistant disease may be as frequent as 5% of overall pts, although as many as 45% may still have active arthritis 15–20 yrs later. However, functional disability limiting lifestyle and educational and work options in young adult who has had JRA probably <10–15%. Death from JRA or from complication of Tx <1% in North America; much higher in certain European countries related to effects of amyloidosis and, in particular, renal failure

WHEN TO REFER

• As JRA represents series of complex diseases, whose chronicity is measured in years, not months, and whose courses are highly variable w/ many confounding factors, all children should be referred at onset to pediatric rheumatologist. Probably half can thereafter be supervised predominantly by primary care physician w/ only periodic visits to specialist. Family involvement and case coordination at community level essential for success. Other half of cases represent complex therapeutic and prognostic decisions and need to be seen more frequently at tertiary care center
• All children at onset should be referred to experienced ophthalmologist for complete eye examination including slit lamp biomicroscopy for detection of early uveitis. Depending on type of onset, course of disease, children should be seen periodically thereafter (q3–4 mos for number of years for those w/ early-onset oligoarthritis, particularly if ANA seropositive)
• Although prosthetic joint replacement seldom indicated in children until general growth has ceased, most children w/ complex joint disease, limb inequality, or contractures profit from early referral to pediatric orthopedic surgeon w/ appropriate follow-up thereafter
• Children w/ cervical spine disease evidenced by pain on motion or limitation of motion may have developed apophyseal joint disease and subluxation of cervical spine, particularly at atlantoaxial level. These children demand special care and splinting, esp when riding in automobile. Intubation prior to surgery particularly hazardous in this subgroup

KAWASAKI DISEASE

BACKGROUND

- Acute systemic vasculitis primarily affecting infants/young children
- Peak age 1–2 yrs; 80% <4 yrs of age
- M:F ratio: 1.5:1
- Occurs in all ethnic groups; children of Asian ancestry at greatest risk
- Many clinical/epidemiologic features suggest infectious etiology, but cause remains unknown; superantigen toxins produced by *Staphylococcus aureus*/*Streptococcus pyogenes* may be involved in pathogenesis

CLINICAL MANIFESTATIONS (DIAGNOSTIC CRITERIA)

- Fever of at least 5 d duration
- Plus presence of at least 4 of following 5 conditions:
  - bilateral conjunctival injection
  - changes of lips/oral mucosa (dry, red fissured lips, strawberry tongue, or oropharyngeal erythema)
  - changes of peripheral extremities (erythema of palms/soles, edema of hands/feet, periungual desquamation)
  - polymorphous rash
  - cervical lymphadenopathy
- Illness not explained by other known disease processes

ASSOCIATED CLINICAL FEATURES

- Irritability
- Arthritis/arthralgia
- Aseptic meningitis
- Urethritis w/ sterile pyuria
- Hepatitis
- Hydrops of gallbladder
- Acute anterior uveitis
- Peripheral ischemia

CARDIOVASCULAR INVOLVEMENT

- *Up to 50% have cardiac manifestations:* myocarditis, pericarditis, conduction disturbances, mitral/aortic regurgitation
- *Most serious cardiac complication (occurring up to 20% of untreated pts):* aneurysmal dilatation of coronary arteries
- Coronary aneurysms may be present as early as 7 d after fever onset; peak prevalence 2–4 wks after onset of disease

LABORATORY FEATURES

- Laboratory features nonspecific/nondiagnostic
- During acute febrile phase of illness, most pts have mild anemia, leukocytosis w/ left shift, ↑ ESR
- Platelet count begins ↑ in second wk of illness; in untreated pt, may exceed 1 million/μL

DIFFERENTIAL DIAGNOSIS

- Scarlet fever
- Toxic shock syndrome
- Measles
- Infectious mononucleosis
- Stevens-Johnson syndrome

TREATMENT

- *IV immunoglobulin:* Dose: 2 g/kg as single IV infusion over 10–12 hrs; initiate Tx as soon as Dx made, preferably within 10 d of symptom onset; IVIG produces rapid resolution of fever/other clinical manifestations of acute febrile phase, reverses laboratory indices of systemic inflammation; IVIG reduces incidence of coronary artery aneurysms from ~20% to 3–4%, promotes resolution of preexisting aneurysms
- *Aspirin:* Dose: 3–5 mg/kg/d; in pts w/ no coronary artery abnormalities, continue aspirin 6–8 wks or until platelet count, ESR return to normal; in pts w/coronary aneurysms despite IVIG Tx, aspirin continued indefinitely or until 1 yr after aneurysms resolve
- *Cardiac care:* echocardiogram should be obtained at Dx, 3 wks, 8 wks after treatment

COMPLICATIONS

- US mortality rate <0.1%; most fatalities occur within 6 wks of onset of symptoms/consequence of coronary thrombosis
- Long-term prognosis unknown, but affected children may be at ↑ risk for atherosclerotic disease

WHEN TO REFER

- Care of all pts should involve pediatric cardiologist experienced in Dx/treatment of carditis associated w/ Kawasaki disease, in performance/interpretation of echocardiographic studies of coronary arteries in children
- Pts should be treated in setting w/ physicians/staff experienced w/ administration of IVIG/treatment of side effects of IVIG

OVERVIEW

- Pain about anterior aspect of knee common in adolescents
- Definite cause not always identifiable
- Exam should assess hip rotation to exclude slipped capital femoral epiphysis
- Truly "idiopathic" group may represent overuse from unresolved, submaximal stress on tissue already in baseline state of stress due to adolescent growth spurt; best treated by staged program that includes activity modification, pain control, subsequent rehabilitation of tight/weak structures

PATELLOFEMORAL DYSFUNCTION

- Common/often baffling to diagnose due to paucity of objective findings
- *Typical Hx:* poorly localized anterior knee pain aggravated by stair climbing/other activities that apply stress across bent knee
- Exam may show few, if any, objective signs; maltracking may be evident; abnormalities are often subtle; tenderness may be present over patella facets, patella compression may cause pain; much of exam entails r/o other causes of knee pain
- *Screening radiographs:* AP/lateral views of knee, tangential view of patella; CT scans w/knee extended/flexed 20°, kinematic MRI exam may be required for pts w/persistent pain
- Usually responds to nonoperative Tx based on strengthening quadriceps while avoiding/minimizing stress across patellofemoral joint; closed kinetic chain exercises, such as step downs/partial squats, keep foot in contact w/ground/diminish patellofemoral contact forces; stretching program prescribed for hamstring/iliotibial band tightness
- Recalcitrant patellofemoral dysfunction requires surgical procedures that realign quadriceps mechanism

SINDING-LARSEN-JOHANSSON SYNDROME

- Overuse syndrome w/microscopic tears/avulsion injury at junction of patella tendon and inferior pole of patella; similar to jumper's knee seen in older adolescents/adults
- Prognosis uniformly good in children; older adolescent/adult may require operative intervention
- *Typical pt:* 9–12-year-old boy complaining of activity-related pain localized to inferior pole of patella
- Exam normal except for localized tenderness
- Radiographs may show areas of heterotopic ossification at inferior pole of patella
- *Treatment:* activity modification (complete resolution of symptoms universal, but may take several months)
- Similar overuse process may occur at superior pole of patella; not as common; except for difference in location, Hx, exam, treatment, expected results similar

BIPARTITE PATELLA

- Usually incidental radiographic finding; during the adolescent years, may be source of anterior knee pain
- Presents after fall/injury w/tenderness/swelling localized to superolateral corner of patella
- *Treatment based on degree of tenderness:* 3–4 wks immobilization w/knee in extension sufficient
- In chronic cases, complaints of pain after running/jumping; activity modification may resolve symptoms, but some cases require excision of superolateral fragment w/reattachment of quadriceps tendon

PATHOLOGIC PLICA

- *Plica:* normal fold in synovium
- Medial patella plica most likely to become symptomatic
- As a result of direct blow/repetitive stress, plica becomes thickened/fibrotic causing medial anterior knee pain
- Hx of popping, snapping, pseudolocking may be elicited
- Exam reveals clicking sensation as knee flexes in 40–60° arc; w/knee flexed 60°, tender plica brought into prominent position/may be palpated medial to patella
- Nonoperative Tx often successful, includes activity modification/anti-inflammatory medications
- Arthroscopic excision appropriate for persistent symptoms

OSTEOCHONDRITIS DISSECANS

- Usually occurs in medial femoral condyle
- Most likely results from repetitive stress, ultimately causing stress fracture of subchondral bone, subsequent vascular compromise, osteonecrosis
- May progress to fissure/separation in articular cartilage
- Continued stress results in complete separation, commonly known as loose body in joint
- Onset mostly during childhood
- If presenting during adolescence, articular cartilage may have buckled, but frequently not yet separated
- Symptoms often vague/poorly localized
- Dx important because during growing years potential to heal
- Pain/stiffness after running/sports activities; occasionally swelling
- Exam may demonstrate mild effusion/quadriceps atrophy
- Dx usually by radiographs; in addition to AP/lateral view, tunnel view helpful in outlining lesions in posterolateral aspect of medial femoral condyle
- Prognosis dependent on size of lesion/age of child; lesions <1 cm in diameter do well; those >2 cm have poor prognosis for healing w/o surgery; younger children have more potential to heal; after distal femoral physis closes, lesion very unlikely to heal
- *Nonoperative management:* modify activity so symptoms do not occur; no sports for 3–12 mos; successful nonoperative management results in normal knee; long-term results after surgical Tx less predictable; indications for operative Tx include loose body, unstable lesion, persistent symptoms despite compliant nonoperative care

DENNIS P. GROGAN

BACKGROUND

- Benign, self-limited disease of tarsal navicular bone; originally described by Köhler in 1908
- Diagnosed by combination of clinical/radiographic findings
- More common in boys; may occur bilaterally
- *Peak incidence:* 4–5 yrs of age
- Ossification center of navicular appears at age 2 in girls/age 3 in boys
- Etiology thought to be related to late ossification of navicular (last bone in foot to ossify) and its position at apex of medial longitudinal arch of foot, making navicular subject to chronic repetitive compression forces, leading to vascular compression, ischemia, bone necrosis

CLINICAL MANIFESTATIONS

- Pain on medial aspect of foot
- Antalgic limp
- Pain/tenderness to palpation over navicular
- May have localized swelling over navicular; may also involve insertion of posterior tibial tendon into navicular
- Important to examine ROM of various joints of foot to exclude other sites of possible pathology

RADIOGRAPHIC FEATURES

- AP/lateral radiographs make Dx; comparison to radiographs of opposite foot often helpful
- Typical changes involve only navicular w/sclerosis, increased density, fragmentation, flattening/irregular rarefaction, leading to narrowing in AP diameter as seen on lateral view
- Significant delay in ossification evident when compared to opposite uninvolved navicular
- In young children early ossification center may seem to disappear
- Irregular ossification of navicular not uncommon
- Dx should only be made when clinical examination concurs w/ radiographic findings

DIFFERENTIAL DIAGNOSIS

- Painful accessory navicular
- Trauma (fracture)
- Medial ankle sprain
- Juvenile rheumatoid arthritis
- Other inflammatory arthritis

TREATMENT

- Depends on severity of complaints/physical findings
- Short leg cast 4–6 wks produces relief/shortens symptom duration; benefit from medial arch support if still symptomatic after period of cast immobilization
- Medial arch support/other orthotic device may be utilized for child w/ minimal complaints
- Weight-bearing activities allowed as tolerated by symptoms
- Natural Hx excellent; symptoms resolve within several months in most children; navicular reconstitutes itself within 1–3 yrs, becoming radiographically normal by skeletal maturity w/ no residual deformity/disability

COMPLICATIONS

- Minimal/limited to occasional pt w/ minor radiographic irregularity of navicular

WHEN TO REFER

- Symptomatic pt w/ radiographic findings consistent w/ Köhler disease; refer to orthopedic surgeon for treatment/follow-up

BACKGROUND

- Abnormal forward bending of spine w/ >5° of anterior vertebral wedging
- Multiple etiologies:
  - late childhood/adolescence most likely Scheuermann disease or postural round back
  - infancy and early childhood: congenital, neuromuscular (polio, spinal muscular atrophy, cerebral palsy), infectious (esp tuberculosis), "associated" (achondroplasia, mucopolysaccharidoses, spina bifida, osteogenesis imperfecta)
  - congenital:
    - type I: failure of formation of anterior portion of spine (hemivertebra)
    - type II: failure of segmentation of anterior portion of spine (unsegmented bar)
- 30% congenital curves progressive. Type I much more likely than type II to progress
  - neuromuscular: progression of deformity correlates w/ severity of underlying disorder. Polio now seen almost exclusively in children born outside US
  - infectious: Tuberculosis (Pott paraplegia) most common cause of nontraumatic paraplegia in world. Progressive kyphosis unusual in US
  - "associated": progression of deformity correlates w/ severity of underlying disorder (see individual entities)

CLINICAL MANIFESTATIONS

- Posterior spinal prominence w/ exaggerated forward bend
- When located in thoracic spine can cause pulmonary problems (performance on pulmonary function testing, exercise tolerance)
- Pain may be prominent feature
- *Progressive neurologic deterioration greatest risk:* earliest signs reflex changes, weakness/fatigability
- Congenital associated w/ urinary tract abnormalities (20%), congenital heart defects (15%), dysraphism (10%), extremity deformity (15%)

LABORATORY FEATURES

- Renal ultrasound or other urographic study *mandatory* for all congenital kyphosis
- Echocardiogram if any suspicion of cardiac involvement
- X rays of entire spine for congenital deformity. Extremity films if clinically indicated
- Sedimentation rate or c-reactive protein, CBC, blood and tissue cultures, tuberculin skin test for infectious kyphosis
- Pulmonary function tests if deformity progressive and surgery contemplated

DIFFERENTIAL DIAGNOSIS

- Tumor
- Postirradiation kyphosis
- Postlaminectomy kyphosis

TREATMENT

- *Orthosis:* ineffective for congenital deformity. May slow or prevent progression in neuromuscular or "associated" kyphosis but frequently not well tolerated. Can help limit progression in infectious kyphosis
- Spinal fusion is only treatment for progression of congenital kyphosis. Correction and instrumentation of congenital kyphosis may be associated w/ neurologic injury
- Spinal fusion w/ instrumentation is preferred treatment for progressive kyphosis in neuromuscular disorders or "associated" entities when orthoses ineffective
- Debridement, fusion of infectious kyphosis can limit deformity but not necessary for cure
- Antituberculous Tx w/ recumbency or orthotic treatment can be curative in Pott disease

COMPLICATIONS

- Paraplegia if progressive in thoracic spine (75% nonprogressive)
- Pulmonary compromise w/ thoracic involvement
- Sepsis can occur w/ infectious etiology, but may become walled off and form paravertebral abscess
- Progressive deformity prior to skeletal maturity that requires fusion may lead to excessive shortening of spine, progression of curve beyond the segments or reverse deformity (hypokyphosis, lordosis)

PREVENTION

- Early institution of preferred therapeutic measures in each category can prevent progression of deformity and its complications

WHEN TO REFER

- All children w/ kyphosis, other than postural round back, must be immediately referred to orthopedist

LACTIC ACIDOSIS

DEFINITION

- Lactic acid (LA) level >3.5 mmol/L (normal <2), usually w/ blood pH <7.35

CLINICAL MANIFESTATIONS

- *Those common to all acidoses:* initially tachycardia, then (pH <7.20) bradycardia; impaired myocardial contractility; vasodilation ("warm shock")
- Often sudden in onset; severity correlates w/ mortality
- Lactic acidosis (LAc) common in very ill patients; ↑ in LA heralds shock/circulatory collapse
- Hypoxemia (SAO_2 <75%) precipitates LAc

DIFFERENTIAL DIAGNOSIS

- LAc not single disease entity, rather a symptom
- Overloaded "normal" machinery:
  – ↑ production: main mechanism hypoxemia; may be due to ↑ tissue O_2 demand (seizures, strenuous exercise, tumor mass)
  – ↓ clearance: liver/kidney failure, diabetes mellitus, tumors (liver infiltration)
- "Poisoned" machinery: oral hypoglycemics (biguanides); salicylates, acetaminophen; alcohols (ethanol, methanol, ethylene glycol); isoniazid, streptozotocin; diabetes mellitus
- "Absent" machinery, which can occur via several pathways:
  – glycolytic pathway (glycogen storage disease GSDI, fructose 1,6-diphosphatase deficiency)
  – Pyruvic acid metabolism, so-called primary lactic acidoses (PDH, pyruvate carboxylase deficiency)
  – organic acidurias (methylmalonic, isovaleric, 3-hydroxy-methyl-glutaryl aciduria), aminoacidopathies (MSUD)
  – fatty acid oxidation defects (MCAD, LCHAD)
  – mitochondrial disorders

INDICATIONS FOR LA LEVEL

- As monitoring tool for severity, progress, prognosis where LAc expected (eg, hypoxia, major trauma, sepsis, liver failure)
- As diagnostic tool when LAc suspected because of:
  – high anion gap unexplained by diabetes, renal failure, known poisoning
  – unexplained ketosis/hypoglycemia, particularly in neonate
  – unexplained thrombocytopenia, neutropenia, hepatomegaly
  – suspected metabolic disorder (sick neonate, recurrent neurologic decompensation, seizures, protracted vomiting, suspected "sepsis")

SPECIMEN COLLECTION

- Venous or arterial (venous 5–10% higher); use tourniquet; collect in special tube (10 mg NaF, 2 mg K oxalate) or rapidly precipitate w/ perchloric acid; keep on ice/process within 15 min

LABORATORY WORKUP

- If LA used as monitoring tool, obtain screening panel: LA, chemistry profile (glucose, electrolytes, renal, liver function tests), ammonia, ketones
- If toxin suspected, obtain plasma osmolality, toxic screen, UA; calculate anion/osmolal gaps
- If genetic disorder suspected, obtain metabolic panel:
  – pyruvate/lactate ratio
  – urine organic acids
  – plasma acylcaritine profile
  – plasma amino acids/ammonia
- Save urine/plasma sample until Dx made

INTERPRETATION

- *Intermediate LA (2–3.5):* repeat (transient ↑ in dehydration, brief hypoxia, seizure)
- LA highest in mitochondrial disorders, disorders of pyruvate metabolism/glycogen storage (urea cycle disorders do not cause significant acidosis)
- High anion gap w/ high osmolal gap (>10) suggests alcohol (eg, ethylene glycol/methanol) poisoning; oxalate crystalluria suggests ethylene glycol
- ↑ LA level w/ hyperuricemia/hepatomegaly in newborn suggests GSDI; muscle biopsy may be necessary in mitochondrial disorders
- Nonspecific associated findings w/ LAc include hyperuricemia, hyperkalemia, hyperphosphatemia, abnormal WBC count

TREATMENT

- *Palliative Tx (correcting acidosis):* buys time/does not ↓ mortality; IV bicarbonate used when pH <7.20; target: serum bicarbonate 10/pH >7.20; occasionally bicarbonate-based dialysis needed. LA metabolism enhanced w/ folate/thiamine (alcohol ingestions)
- *Definitive Tx:* identify, reverse underlying disorder; improve oxygenation

WHEN TO REFER

- Consult Genetics if metabolic disorder suspected/diagnosed
- Consult Gastroenterology if glycogen storage disease suspected/diagnosed

JAY A. PERMAN AND BARBARA S. DUDLEY

BACKGROUND

- Occurs 2° to malabsorption of lactose, principal carbohydrate of mammalian milk
- Lactose hydrolyzed in small intestine by brush border enzyme lactase
- Intestinal lactase levels highest immediately after birth, ↓ w/weaning until very low levels by adulthood
- Minority of human groups maintain high levels of lactase
- Lactose intolerance *not a disease*
- Most common 2° to lactose in diet of normal child who genetically down-regulates lactase activity during postnatal development
- May occur as temporary condition in infants/lactase-persistent children postweaning, most commonly due to intestinal injury

CLINICAL MANIFESTATIONS

- Symptoms variable/may include all of the following:
  - abdominal distention
  - diarrhea
  - flatulence
  - abdominal pain
- Diarrhea not invariably present
- Symptoms influenced by amount of lactose consumed by other dietary accompaniments that influence gastric emptying

LABORATORY FEATURES

- Lactose breath hydrogen (H_2) test: Lactose malabsorption indicated by rise in H_2 concentration in expired air following administration of test dose of lactose after overnight fast; most sensitive/specific test for lactose malabsorption; commercial kits for office/home use available

- *Other screening tests:*
  - lactose tolerance test: lactose malabsorption indicated by ↑ blood glucose following oral test dose; necessitates multiple blood samples/yields unacceptable number of false-positive/false-negative results
  - stool-reducing substances/stool pH: performed on liquid portion of fresh diarrheal stool; best suited for office Dx of 2°/acquired lactase deficiency in infant w/diarrhea currently consuming lactose in diet
- *Diagnostic method most commonly used:* dietary lactose exclusion
- Pitfalls:
  - insufficient duration of dietary exclusion; may result in false-negative result
  - dietary manipulation may coincide w/resolution of symptoms, resulting in inappropriate continuation of restricted diet

DIFFERENTIAL DIAGNOSIS

- Irritable bowel syndrome
- Recurrent abdominal pain
- Chronic nonspecific diarrhea (toddler's diarrhea)
- Other causes of carbohydrate malabsorption (eg, fructose, sorbitol malabsorption)
- Peptic disease/inflammatory bowel disease

TREATMENT

- Recognize dairy products not essential in diet
- When continuation of lactose-containing foods desired by child/necessary to nutrition:
  - reduce dietary lactose content below level at which symptoms recur in individual child

  - consume whole milk rather than skim/chocolate milk/milk w/meals; all slow gastric emptying
  - prehydrolyzed milks containing lactase enzyme from microbial organisms
  - dairy products w/naturally reduced lactose content, eg, aged cheeses (cheddar, swiss, others)
  - yogurt (unpasteurized) w/lactase activity from inoculated organisms
  - lactase drops/caplets (commercially available, taken prior to ingestion of lactose-containing food; dosage must be individualized
  - deliberate daily lactose consumption in an attempt to induce adaptation of colonic microflora w/subsequent reduction of symptoms
  - unnecessary to discourage use of milk in children from population w/high rate lactose malabsorption unless intolerance evident within individual children

COMPLICATIONS

- Dehydration/electrolyte imbalance possible in infants w/diarrhea attributable to/exacerbated by 2° lactase deficiency
- Complications unlikely in children w/1° lactase deficiency in absence of inappropriate management/incorrect Dx, eg, overly vigorous/unnecessary restriction of lactose-containing foods leading to iatrogenic failure to thrive/inadequate caloric intake

WHEN TO REFER

- Most pts managed w/o referral
- Referral indicated when Dx in doubt/symptoms referable to GI tract persist

BACKGROUND

- Parainfluenza virus infections most important cause of this syndrome of lower respiratory illness (LRI); parainfluenza virus type 1 responsible for most widespread community outbreaks
- Outbreaks caused by parainfluenza viruses types 1 and 2 occur in late summer through the fall mos of year in US. Endemic parainfluenza virus type 3 (PIV3) infections occur throughout year; PIV3 outbreaks tend to occur in spring or fall mos
- Influenza A virus infections can be associated w/croup, including severe croup; influenza important antecedent of bacterial tracheitis
- Although viruses differ in propensity to cause croup, any respiratory viral infection can be associated w/croup syndrome
- Incidence of viral croup highest in healthy children 6 mos–3 yrs of age; males at ↑ risk of manifesting syndrome
- Children <4 mos of age who manifest croup should be assessed for possibility of associated anatomic abnormality of glottis, subglottis, or trachea
- Some children susceptible to recurrent bouts of croup symptoms, usually in association w/mild viral respiratory infections of varying etiologies. Children typically designated as having spasmodic croup when no underlying anatomic predisposing factor present
- Viral respiratory infection most common cause of croup syndrome, but bacterial epiglottitis, bacterial tracheitis important, life-threatening causes of airway obstruction w/clinical findings of severe croup. Typically, rate of progression of airway obstruction much more rapid in pts w/epiglottitis or bacterial tracheitis and substantially greater evidence of systemic toxicity exists. Retropharyngeal abscess also may present w/airway obstruction, features of croup

CLINICAL MANIFESTATIONS

- Laryngotracheobronchitis (croup) characterized in milder cases by Sx of laryngitis, hoarse voice or hoarse cry, usually in association w/typical "barking seal" cough
- Development of inspiratory stridor hallmark of more severe illness; children w/stridor usually demonstrate evidence of obstruction to inhalation manifest by progressively severe chest wall retractions (supraclavicular, then subcostal, then intercostal, then sternal)
- Manifestations of croup usually appear after 2–3 d antecedent period of nasal congestion, rhinorrhea. Fever (101–103°F) relatively common, but children may be afebrile
- Sx croup also prominent in bacterial epiglottitis (or supraglottitis) and in bacterial tracheitis. Substantial fever present in these conditions together w/additional signs of marked systemic toxicity
- Children w/bacterial epiglottitis usually develop life-threatening airway obstruction within first 6–18 hrs after onset of fever. Bacterial tracheitis may be manifest as severe and rapidly progressive croup syndrome in child who has had antecedent URI or viral croup symptoms w/or w/o lower grade fever

LABORATORY FEATURES

- Laboratory parameters usually unremarkable in children w/viral infection associated croup. Total WBC, differential normal; ESR, CRP normal (although these not usually measured)

- Children w/bacterial epiglottitis or bacterial tracheitis more likely to manifest ↑ WBC, w/↑ ANC, immature neutrophils; CRP frequently ↑, when assayed
- Accurate differentiation of viral croup from epiglottitis or bacterial tracheitis based primarily on assessment of clinical Hx together w/appropriate, cautious direct examination of supraglottic structures (epiglottitis) and tracheal secretions (bacterial tracheitis)
- Lateral radiographs of soft tissues of pharynx, neck should not be used routinely to help differentiate viral croup and epiglottitis. When illness severity, tempo suggest possibility of epiglottitis, direct examination of epiglottitis under controlled circumstances appropriate diagnostic approach. Likewise, direct observation of copious, thick, purulent secretions in tracheal lumen hallmark of bacterial tracheitis. Lateral soft tissue x rays helpful in Dx retropharyngeal abscess

DIFFERENTIAL DIAGNOSIS

- Bacterial epiglottitis/supraglottitis
- Bacterial tracheitis
- Retropharyngeal abscess
- Laryngeal diphtheria
- Laryngeal papillomatosis
- Congenital or acquired anatomic airway obstruction:
  – subglottic stenosis
  – subglottic hemangioma or cyst
  – laryngomalacia
- Foreign body aspiration
- Angioedema

TREATMENT

- No antiviral treatment known to modify clinical course of viral croup due to parainfluenza viruses
- Influenza A virus infections can be treated w/amantadine or rimantadine, but not known whether such treatment would prevent emergence of croup; no evidence that course of established croup due to influenza A virus infection can be modified by amantadine or rimantadine treatment
- Provision of humidified environment (typically cool mist) has been mainstay of home, outpt management for many years
- Short-term treatment w/injected or inhaled corticosteroids demonstrated to have clinical benefit in children w/viral croup, although magnitude of average benefit not great. Because the clinical course of syndrome usually benign w/o corticosteroid administration, routine use of these agents in mild to moderate croup not required or indicated. Among children whose illness severity warrants ER evaluation, corticosteroids can be used as adjunct to management (single dose 0.3–0.6 mg/kg dexamethasone IV or IM)
- Inhaled epinephrine (racemic epinephrine used typically) also reasonable for children w/more severe viral croup. Because rebound airway obstruction can follow epinephrine administration, observation in ER for 2–4 hrs post treatment required. Most children given inhaled epinephrine should probably receive corticosteroids as well
- A subset of children w/viral croup require close observation in hospital, but endotracheal intubation required in <2% of children w/uncomplicated viral croup
- Careful clinical monitoring of severity of airway obstruction, clinical condition of child mandatory. Overreliance on monitoring w/pulse oximetry must be avoided because oxygenation

can be maintained in face of impending respiratory failure. Careful clinical monitoring should allow intubation to be accomplished as planned procedure under controlled conditions in OR. Most children require intubation for <72 hrs
- In contrast, establishment of safe airway, usually by endotracheal intubation, the 1° treatment of epiglottitis, bacterial tracheitis. Likewise, surgical drainage of 1° importance in retropharyngeal abscess. Antibiotic treatment indicated for bacterial epiglottitis, tracheitis, retropharyngeal abscess. *Streptococcus pyogenes* (group A streptococci), *Streptococcus pneumoniae* probably most common causes of epiglottitis in current era of effective immunization for *Haemophilus influenzae* type b. *Staphylococcus aureus* most important cause of life-threatening bacterial tracheitis; *S. pyogenes, S. pneumoniae, H. influenzae, Moraxella catarrhalis* also implicated etiologically
- For epiglottitis, bacterial tracheitis, oxacillin or nafcillin and a third-generation cephalosporin would provide appropriate coverage pending culture and sensitivity data. Cefuroxime would be acceptable alternative
- Retropharyngeal abscess typically polymicrobial in etiology w/streptococci, anaerobic bacteria isolated in most cases. Initial antibiotic regimen active against organisms indicated. Ampicillin/sulbactam or combination of third-generation cephalosporin and clindamycin among suitable alternatives

PREVENTION

- No currently licensed vaccines for preventing parainfluenza virus croup. Inactivated influenza virus vaccines can reduce morbidity due to influenza virus infections, but routine use of influenza vaccine not currently recommended for healthy children in US
- Immunization for *Haemophilus influenzae type b* (Hib) has dramatically reduced incidence of invasive Hib infections including epiglottitis

COMPLICATIONS

- Most cases of parainfluenza virus croup resolve spontaneously over 24–72 hrs. Occasionally airway obstruction severe enough to warrant brief period of endotracheal intubation
- Children w/bacterial epiglottitis or bacterial tracheitis can develop life-threatening airway obstruction very acutely, usually during rapidly progressive clinical course. Children w/these infections must be managed in hospital. Endotracheal intubation routinely indicated in epiglottitis, together w/effective antibiotic treatment. Endotracheal intubation usually required for Dx, treatment of bacterial tracheitis. Bacterial tracheitis can be complicated by staphylococcal pneumonia, empyema, pyopneumothorax

WHEN TO REFER

- Need for referral relates to 1 to 3 features: (1) severity of airway obstruction, its rate of progression, (2) occurrence of illness in children <~4 mos of age, (3) illnesses w/prolonged clinical course. Occurrence of severe and rapidly progressive airway obstruction indicates that provision of endotracheal airway may be required for both Dx, management. Illness in very young children or protracted clinical courses suggest possibility of associated anatomic airway defect. Clinical Hx suggestive of possible foreign body aspiration may necessitate early endoscopic evaluation

LEAD TOXICITY

W. CLAYTON BORDLEY

BACKGROUND

- 2.2% of US population have blood lead levels (BLLs) ≥10 mcg/dl, including ~890,000 children aged 1–5 yrs
- ↑ risk for children who are poor, non-Hispanic black, Mexican American, live in large metropolitan areas/older housing
- Children <6, esp <2 at highest risk due to normal hand-mouth activities, ↑ susceptibility of developing CNS, ↑ GI absorption
- Lead enters body primarily through ingestion, less commonly by inhalation

Common potential sources of lead

Environmental
Lead-containing paint
Soil/dust near lead-painted homes, roadways, industries

Plumbing leachate (eg, from leaded pipes/well pumps)
Ceramicware with lead-containing glazes
Leaded gasoline
Plastic miniblinds

Occupational
Plumbers, pipe fitters
Lead-related industry (eg, miners, battery manufacturers)
Auto repairers
Glass manufacturers
Shipbuilders
Steel welders/cutters
Bridge construction workers
Firing range instructors

Hobbies
Glazed pottery making
Target shooters at firing ranges

Lead soldering
Preparing lead shot, sinkers, or toys
Stained-glass making
Home remodeling

Substance Use
Folk remedies
"Health foods"

Cosmetics
Moonshine whiskey

- Lead absorption enhanced by calcium/iron deficiencies, high-fat diet, fasting
- Lead crosses placenta/can cause fetal loss w/adverse effects on development
- Lead primarily affects CNS, heme synthesis, vitamin D metabolism, kidney; 95% of total body lead deposited in bones
- No threshold for toxic effects of lead has been identified

CLINICAL MANIFESTATIONS

- Most children w/lead toxicity asymptomatic
- Symptoms of mild toxicity, when they exist, nonspecific; include fatigue, irritability, weakness, abdominal discomfort, anorexia, headache, constipation, dizziness
- Long-standing mild toxicity strongly associated w/various neurobehavioral abnormalities including speech/hearing impairment, developmental delay, behavioral changes
- Cognitive deficits caused by lead exposure may be irreversible
- Severe toxicity (BLLS > 70–100 mcg/dl) may result in acute encephalopathy, often accompanied by seizures/coma

LABORATORY FEATURES

- BLL measurement: essential screening/diagnostic test for lead exposure
- BLLs of ≥10 mcg/dl abnormal
- Erythrocyte protoporphyrin lacks adequate sensitivity/specificity to use as screening test
- Children w/BLLs ≥ 20 mcg/dl should also have following laboratory studies: CBC, BUN, serum creatinine, U/A
- Iron deficiency anemia often coexists in pts w/lead exposure
- Abdominal radiographs only useful if acute ingestion suspected

DIFFERENTIAL DIAGNOSIS

- Nonspecific nature of symptoms when they exist make differential Dx extensive

TREATMENT

- Child w/elevated BLLs on screening test should undergo diagnostic testing according to following schedule:

If result of screening test (mcg/dl) is:	Perform diagnostic test on venous blood within:
10–19	2–3 mos
20–44	1 mo–1 wk
45–59	48 hrs
60–69	24 hrs
≥70	emergently

- Additional treatment determined by diagnostic BLL as follows:

BLL (mcg/dl)	Action
<10	• Reassess risk status or rescreen in 1 yr
10–14	• Provide family education to decrease exposure • Repeat BLL within 3 mos
15–19	• Take detailed environmental Hx • Provide family education to decrease exposure • Repeat BLL within 2 mos • If BLLs persist in this range, proceed according to actions for BLLs 20–44
20–44	• Conduct complete medical evaluation (see below) • Provide family education to decrease exposure • Referral to health department for environmental investigation and case management • If BLL > 25 mcg/dl, consider chelation (not currently recommended for BLLs <45 mcg/dl) after consultation
45–69	• Same as 20–44 mcg/dl • Begin chelation Tx
70 or higher	• Immediate hospitalization for chelation Tx • Rest of management should be noted for the management of children w/BLLs 45–69 mcg/dl

- Complete medical evaluation should include
  – careful Hx w/emphasis on symptoms, mouthing activities, pica, developmental milestones, previous BLL measurements
  – environmental Hx
  – nutritional assessment w/attention to iron, calcium, fat intake
  – supportive labs as needed (eg., CBC, iron studies, BUN, creatinine, urinalysis)

Chelation agents

Generic name	Abbreviation
Edetate disodium calcium	CaEDTA
Dimercaprol	BAL
D-penicillamine	D-penicillamine
Succimer	DMSA

- Patients w/acute encephalopathy require management in pediatric ICU

COMPLICATIONS

- Chronic lead exposure associated w/developmental delay, ↓ IQ, behavioral changes, hearing deficits
- Lead encephalopathy (ie, w/BLLs > 100 mcg/dl) often result in seizures, irreversible brain damage, coma, death

PREVENTION

- 1° prevention accomplished through anticipatory guidance focused on educating parents about
  – common/uncommon sources of lead in environment
  – optimal nutrition to ↓ lead absorption (sufficient calcium/iron, low fat, appropriate spacing of meals/snacks)
- Public health efforts to prevent lead exposure through removal of lead hazards should be supported
- 2° prevention accomplished through screening of children at ages 1 and 2 and children 36–72 mos of age who have not been previously screened. Two strategies can be considered: universal screening of all children w/BLL measurements or universal risk assessment/targeted BLL testing of those determined to be at risk
- Community-specific risk: assessment questionnaires exist in many areas/may utilize zip codes, other geographic determinations to identify high-risk populations
- All risk assessment questionnaires should include following three questions
  – does your child live in or regularly visit a house or child-care facility built before 1950?
  – does your child live in or regularly visit a house or child-care facility built before 1978 that is being or has recently been renovated or remodeled?
  – does your child have sibling or playmate who has or did have lead poisoning?

WHEN TO REFER

- Children w/BLLs ≥ 20 mcg/dl should be referred to health department to receive detailed environmental investigation/case management
- Physicians unfamiliar w/use of chelation medications should seek consultation prior to initiating these drugs; each requires careful attention to dosing, tolerance, therapeutic monitoring

LEGG-CALVÉ-PERTHES DISEASE

JOHN A. HERRING

BACKGROUND

- Avascular necrosis of femoral head
- Most often presents 5–10 yrs of age (can present as young as 3/as old as 5)
- >80% male
- *Most typical:* very active boy, small for age
- First symptoms may follow minor trauma; trauma probably not etiologic
- Prognosis related to age at onset
- Younger children (<6) usually do well w/ milder symptoms; older children (>9) have more difficult course

CLINICAL MANIFESTATIONS

- Painless limp
- Vague hip/knee pain
- Knee pain alone
- ↓ ROM of hip, abduction/internal rotation

LABORATORY FEATURES

- Initial radiograph may be negative
- After few weeks plain film of pelvis shows ↑ density of femoral head
- Technetium bone scan/MRI gives earlier Dx but usually unnecessary
- Ultrasound examination shows joint effusion early in process

DIFFERENTIAL DIAGNOSIS

- *Multiple epiphyseal dysplasia:* suspect w/ positive family Hx
- Hypothyroidism
- Sickle-cell disease w/ avascular necrosis
- Steroid-induced avascular necrosis

TREATMENT

- *Symptomatic treatment:* reduction of activities, NSAIDs, crutches for short periods
- *Containment treatment indicated for children >6 yrs at onset:* braces used/surgical procedures such as femoral osteotomy/pelvic osteotomy necessary in more severe cases
- Methods such as Snyder slings, wheelchair use, brace immobilization for multiple years outmoded/not efficacious

COMPLICATIONS

- Most recover w/o permanent disability
- Symptoms resolve over 12–18 mos; after that occasional ache/limp is complaint; older children have more protracted course; small percentage continue to have painful hip in adolescence

PREVENTION

- None known

WHEN TO REFER

- Referral to pediatric orthopedist indicated when Dx made; few weeks delay in referral do not compromise outcome

LEPTOSPIROSIS

MICHAEL GREEN

BACKGROUND

- Uncommon but important infectious syndrome
- Illness caused by spirochetes belonging to genus *Leptospira*
- Animals—major reservoir for leptospirosis
- Risk of contracting disease historically limited to individuals exposed to ill animals/ stagnant water contaminated w/ urine from infected animals
- Rats—most common animal vector
- ↑ recognition of acquisition in urban settings in children/adults exposed to dogs w/ chronic leptospiruria

CLINICAL MANIFESTATIONS

- Biphasic clinical course
- Protean manifestations
- Initial presentation w/ nonspecific, influenzalike illness w/fever, headache, myalgia, conjunctival suffusion
- Initial stage resolves spontaneously within 4–7 d
- Second, or "immune stage", begins after several afebrile days
- Immune stage (anicteric/icteric [Weil syndrome]) lasts 1–30 d

Anicteric	Icteric
aseptic meningitis	jaundice
uveitis	hemorrhage
rash	renal failure
fever	myocarditis

- Fatalities uncommon/limited to pts w/ icteric disease

LABORATORY FINDINGS

- Wide variety of nonspecific laboratory abnormalities that vary w/ phase/severity of illness

DIFFERENTIAL DIAGNOSIS

- Large number of flulike illnesses
- Other causes of aseptic meningitis
- Kawasaki disease

DIAGNOSIS

- Culture of blood, CSF in first 7–10 d; urine after 7 d illness on special media
- Serum antibody develops in second week of illness; development of titer may be weak/delayed in some pts

TREATMENT

- Majority of episodes self-limited
- In vitro data suggest penicillin/tetracycline (doxycycline) should be effective Tx in humans
- Uniform agreement on treatment if Dx considered possible/probable during first 5–7 d of illness
- Recent data support consideration of treatment in pts presenting w/ more prolonged illness
- Jarisch-Herxheimer reaction has been rarely observed in some penicillin-treated pts
- Need for careful monitoring for development of renal failure, hemorrhage, myocarditis

COMPLICATIONS

- Renal failure
- CHF (rarely in Weil syndrome)

PREVENTION

- Sanitation to reduce rodent population
- Immunization of domestic animals does not prevent infection/potential spread to humans
- Protective clothing, boots, gloves to reduce occupational exposures
- Avoidance of potentially contaminated pools
- Chemoprophylaxis w/ doxycycline effective but not usually indicated

WHEN TO REFER

- If strong consideration of diagnosis, refer to infectious disease consultant

BACKGROUND

- Also known as childhood leukemia
- 2,000 cases diagnosed/y in US
- 3–4/100,000 children affected
- Etiology largely unknown
- Peak age range 3–7 yrs
- *Remission rate:* >95%
- *Outcome:* 70% children curable
- Adverse features:
  - age <1 yr
  - WBC > 100,000
  - chromosome alterations: t(4,11), t(9,22), hypodiploidy
  - poor response to initial Tx at day 7 (marrow or blood)
  - failure to go into remission by day 28
  - any relapse

CLINICAL MANIFESTATIONS

- *Common symptoms:* malaise, bone pain, refusal to walk, fever, bleeding
- *Duration:* may be present for several weeks
- *Signs:* pallor, petechiae, shoddy lymphadenopathy, hepatosplenomegaly
- Children w/ ALL often appear more ill compared to those w/ idiopathic thrombocytopenic purpura (ITP)

LABORATORY FEATURES

- *Anemia:* mild–severe
- *Thrombocytopenia:* not isolated as in ITP
- *Leukopenia or leukocytosis:* blasts may be seen in differential
- *Neutropenia:* frequent
- *Blood smear:* RBCs may demonstrate tear drops, blasts may be seen, platelets normal–small in size
- *Chest x ray:* may demonstrate anterior mediastinal mass w/ tracheal compression
- *Chemistry profile:* may reflect various aspects of acute tumor lysis syndrome (may be seen prior to initiation of Tx): hyperkalemia, azotemia, hyperuricemia, hypocalcemia, hyperphosphatemia; liver enzymes including LDH commonly ↑
- *Bone marrow:* required for Dx; usually shows complete replacement w/ lymphoblasts w/ very few normal hematopoietic elements; studies including flow cytometric analysis/cytogenetics standard
- *CSF:* spinal tap required prior to initiating Tx; may demonstrate lymphoblasts

DIFFERENTIAL DIAGNOSIS

- Viral syndrome
- Mononucleosis
- Idiopathic thrombocytopenic purpura
- Aplastic anemia
- Rheumatoid arthritis, lupus
- Evan syndrome (ITP w/ autoimmune hemolytic anemia)
- Autoimmune pancytopenia

TREATMENT

- *1° chemotherapy:* organized into phases including induction, consolidation/CNS prophylaxis, delayed intensification, maintenance; Tx lasts 2–3 yrs; most Tx can be delivered in ambulatory setting
- *Commonly used agents:* vincristine, prednisone, L-asparaginase, doxorubicin, methotrexate, ara-C, cyclophosphamide, 6-mercaptopurine
- *CNS prophylaxis:* can be accomplished through intrathecal chemotherapy alone in many children; some high-risk children still require cranial radiation for best results
- *Intensity of Tx:* determined by risk group (see table)
- *Bone marrow/stem cell transplantation:* utilized mainly for children who suffer relapse and are in second remission/in very high-risk children in first remission, eg, t(9,22), t(4,11)

COMPLICATIONS

- *Blood component support:* commonly needed in induction but rare after that; RBC transfusion for Hgb <8 g/dL, platelet transfusion for <15,000/mm³ (use irradiated, filtered components)
- *Fever and neutropenia:* encountered commonly during induction, consolidation, delayed intensification; requires hospitalization w/urgent administration of broad-spectrum antibiotics such as piperacillin/gentamicin
- *Pneumocystis pneumonia:* due to immunosuppression; rare if sulfamethoxazole-trimethoprim prophylaxis administered
- *Chicken pox (primary varicella):* risk only in nonimmune child; exposure to varicella should be treated within 72 hrs w/ VZIG; symptomatic varicella should be treated in hospital w/ IV acyclovir
- *Neuropsychological:* rare; usually 2° to cranial irradiation; manifested by intellectual impairment/learning disabilities; more common in children <3, particularly in girls

WHEN TO REFER

- As soon as Dx acute leukemia seriously entertained
- Thrombocytopenia w/ concomitant anemia/neutropenia
- Pancytopenia
- Whenever diagnostic bone marrow examination required because it is best performed at treating institution where referring pediatric oncology specialist located/all required diagnostic studies available

Acute lymphocytic leukemia risk groups

Standard	High	Very High
age 1–10	age > 10	age < 1
WBC < 50,000	WBC > 50,000	t(4,11), t(9,22)
	poor disease response (day 7)	hypodiploidy

BEVERLY J. LANGE

BACKGROUND

- AML commonly referred to as bone marrow cancer
- French/America/British (FAB) classification:
  - M0 = acute undifferentiated leukemia (CD13+ or CD33+)
  - M1 = acute minimally differentiated granulocytic leukemia
  - M2 = acute granulocytic leukemia
  - M3 = acute promyelocytic leukemia (APL)
  - M4 = acute myelomoncytic leukemia
  - M5 = acute monoblastic leukemia
  - M6 = acute erythroleukemia
  - M7 = acute megakaryobolastic leukemia
- Incidence 4–5/10^6/y among children; minor peak in infancy; thereafter risk ↑ w/age
- In most cases cause unknown
- High-risk groups:
  - Down syndrome
  - Fanconi anemia
  - monozygotic twin of neonate/infant w/ AML
  - severe congenital neutropenia treated w/ G-CSF
  - cancer pts treated w/ alkylating agents
  - cancer pts treated w/ inhibitors of topoisomerase II
- 75–85% enter remission
- 35–50% cured
- 80% Down syndrome pts w/ AML cured

CLINICAL MANIFESTATIONS

- Pallor
- Petechiae, purpura, epistaxis, hemorrhagic diathesis (APL)
- Bone pain
- Chloroma (soft tissue mass)
- Leukemia cutis (skin nodules), esp infants
- Gingival hypertrophy
- Dyspnea (pulmonary leukostasis, WBC > 200,000/mL^3)
- Cerebrovascular accident (APL or WBC > 200,000/mL^3)

LABORATORY FEATURES

- Anemia
- Thrombocytopenia
- Leukopenia to extreme leukocytosis
- Blasts noted on peripheral smear
- Auer rods in cells
- Marrow >30% phenotypically myeloid blasts
- DIC or coagulopathy

DIFFERENTIAL DIAGNOSIS

- Acute lymphoblastic leukemia
- Disseminated alveolar rhabdomyosarcoma
- Idiopathic thrombocytopenic purpura
- Aplastic anemia
- Sepsis w/ DIC
- Megaloblastic anemia

TREATMENT

- No standard treatment, but some general principles have emerged
- *Remission induction:* cytosine arabinoside and anthracycline ± 6-thioguanine w/ or w/o etoposide
- *Remission consolidation:* repeat induction or introduce high-dose cytosine arabinoside–containing regimen
- *Postremission:* high-dose chemotherapy containing cytosine arabinoside or preferably, bone marrow transplant from matched related sibling/parent
- CNS prophylaxis w/ intrathecal cytosine arabinoside
- *Exception 1:* acute promyelocytic leukemia treated w/ all transretinoic acid and moderate-dose chemotherapy
- *Exception 2:* infants/children w/Down syndrome respond to moderate-dose chemotherapy; do not benefit from bone marrow transplantation
- Frequent red cell/platelet transfusions
- Empiric antibacterial/antifungal Tx
- *Recurrent AML:* alternative donor (cord blood; matched unrelated donor) bone marrow transplant or other high-dose chemotherapy

COMPLICATIONS

- Treatment-related mortality 10–20%
- *At Dx:* sepsis, hemorrhage, DIC, stroke
- *During treatment:* sepsis, bacterial, fungal infection, hemorrhage, stroke; veno-occlusive disease
- *After treatment:* relapse; late cardiac effects; complications of marrow transplant (chronic graft vs. host disease)

WHEN TO REFER

- When Hx, physical, CBC make leukemia most likely Dx

BACKGROUND

- *3 varieties blood-sucking lice infest humans:* Pediculus humanis var *capitis* (head louse), *P humanis* var *corporis* (body louse), *Phthirus pubis* (pubic louse)
- Body lice rare in children, associated w/ dirty infested clothing; Tx improved hygiene
- Head lice common pediatric problem, includes 10–12 million cases annually, mostly ages 3–12
- *Head lice infestation risks:* girls > boys, whites > blacks; affects all socioeconomic levels, not associated w/ poor hygiene
- *Life cycle of lice:* wingless 1–4 mm insects pierce skin/inject saliva w/ anticoagulant, then suck human blood; eggs laid in oval sacs strongly attached to hair shafts (nits). Lice hatch 7–8 d, mature 8–9 d, then repeat breeding/feeding cycle
- *Acquisition of head lice:* contact w/ infected person; also from environmental surfaces used by infected person (combs, hats, pillows, headrests)
- *Costs of head lice:* $80 million annually for head lice treatments; major infection control issue in schools
- Resistance to standard Tx recently reported/of ↑ concern

CLINICAL MANIFESTATIONS

- Scalp pruritis hallmark of disease
- Inflammatory papules form at lice feeding sites
- Amount of pruritis/irritation depends on immune response of host
- Posterior cervical adenopathy common
- Superinfection at excoriation sites common
- Dx made by observing nits/lice on scalp, best seen in postauricular/neckline areas

LABORATORY FEATURES

- No lab tests necessary/indicated

DIFFERENTIAL DIAGNOSIS

- Benign hair casts can be confused w/ nits (hair casts easily removable)
- Scalp pruritis/irritation nonspecific, w/ causes such as eczema, seborrhea, tinea, folliculitis, bug bites

TREATMENT

- Traditional treatments:
  – permethrin 1% (Nix-Burroughs Wellcome):
    ○ dose: 2 oz/adult, apply cream after shampoo, leave on 10 min, rinse
    ○ notes: OTC cream rinse, safe; single application, activity up to 10 d/thus useful against nits; initial treatment of choice; problem of ↑ resistance
  – natural pyrethrins (RID, R&C, A-200):
    ○ dose: use as directed; most are 10-min shampoos; retreat 7–10 d
    ○ notes: OTC; safe; no residual activity; retreatment needed as nits hatch; failure rates 10–30%
  – lindane 0.1% (Kwell shampoo):
    ○ dose: suds left on 4–10 min: retreatment usually recommended 7–10 d
    ○ notes: neurotoxicity potential; not for use in very young child, pregnancy
- Nonstandard Tx Tried for "Resistant" Strains:
  – Permethrin 5% (Elimite-Allergan):
    ○ dose: apply cream to dry scalp, cover w/ shower cap, leave on overnight, wash out
    ○ notes: treatment for scabies; probably safe as head surface areas, less than usual body application surface area
  – petrolatum:
    ○ dose: apply generously to entire scalp, cover w/shower cap, leave on overnight
    ○ notes: mechanism of action suffocation of lice; safe; very messy, hard to wash out of hair; dishwashing detergents helpful

  – trimethoprim-sulfamethoxazole:
    ○ dose: 8/40 mg/kg/d in 2 div doses × 7 d
    ○ notes: not approved usage; theoretically may work by killing bacteria in louse's gut
  – Ivermectin (Merck):
    ○ dose: single oral dose of antihelminth Tx
    ○ note: not FDA-approved usage; may be useful in extremely resistant cases
- Addendum treatment issues:
  – "nit picking" time consuming/difficult; removal of visible nits useful in controlling epidemics in schools. Process helped by presoaking hair w/ 1:1 solution of vinegar/commercial products of weak acids (eg, Step 2, Genderm; R&C Lice Treatment Kit, Reed & Carnick; Clear Total Lice Elimination System, Care Technologies), use of special fine-toothed combs
  – treatment of contacts individualized, usually only needed if symptomatic, may treat prophylactically persons who share beds
  – reasonable environment measures indicated: combs/brushes washed 10 min in hot soapy water, bedclothes washed using hot dryer cycle, vacuuming carpets/chairs/car seats; noncleanable objects such as hats/stuffed animals stored in plastic 14 d. Sprays rarely indicated
  – eyelash infestation treated w/ thick petrolatum
  – after successful treatment, irritation of scalp may persist. Topical steroid creams some help in selected cases
- Useful informational resources:
  – National Pediculosis Association (www.headlice.org); Care Technologies Inc. (www.clearcare.com)

WHEN TO REFER

- Most pts managed w/o referral

BACKGROUND

- Most pediatric cases occur in neonates/ among immunocompromised children including children receiving corticosteroids, cyclosporin A, prostaglandins
- Neonatal infection early-onset (<7 d of age) late-onset infection (after 7 d)
- *Listeria monocytogenes* serovariants 1/2a, 4a, 4b most common
- Incidence in US 13/100,000 live births
- Epidemics of food-borne listeriosis have disproportionately high numbers of early-onset perinatal cases
- Mortality 30–50%, early-onset infection; 5–15% late-onset neonatal infection
- Pts w/ AIDS have 1,000-fold ↑ risk invasive listeriosis

CLINICAL MANIFESTATIONS

- *During pregnancy:* maternal influenza-like illness w/ fever, chills, fatigue, headache, muscle pains, often precedes premature delivery
- *Early-onset neonatal:* in severe infection granulomatous skin rash over trunk can be found (granulomatous infantisepticum)
- *Late-onset neonatal:* clinical manifestations may be mild, fever prominent
- Although listeria gram-positive organism, may have clinical features of endotoxic shock

Characteristic	Early Onset	Late Onset	Immunocompromised Host
Usual age at onset	<1 d	12–30 d	Variable
Sex	Males 2:1	Males 2:1	Male or female
Preterm infants	Common	Uncommon	Uncommon
Features in infants:			
Meconium stain	Common	Rare	NA
Pneumonia	Common	Uncommon	NA
Meningitis	20%	90%	50%

LABORATORY FEATURES

- ↑ neutrophils; thrombocytopenia, anemia in severe early-onset sepsis
- *CSF:* in meningitis cell count usually >2,000
- *Infected body fluids including CSF/bronchial secretions:* short, gram-positive intracellular organisms w/variable length, rounded ends; because organism irregularly decolorized, sometimes misidentified as gram-positive cocci
- Organism in blood, CSF/other normally sterile body fluids identified using standard isolation techniques. Use of enrichment media not indicated except as tool to identify food-borne source

DIFFERENTIAL DIAGNOSIS

- Clinical features similar to early/late-onset group B streptococcal infection
- Meningitis may resemble viral meningoencephalitis/mycobacterial infection because of relatively mild/delayed onset of clinical symptoms
- In immunocompromised host other opportunistic infections (cytomegalovirus/systemic fungal infection)

TREATMENT

- Ampicillin plus aminoglycoside

DOSAGE

Early-onset neonatal listeriosis

- Ampicillin:
  - first week of life w/ body weight <2,000 g: 100 mg/kg/d (div 2 equal doses)
  - first week of life w/ body weight >2,000 g: 150 mg/kg/d (div 3×/d)
  - second week of life: 150 mg/kg/d/200 mg/kg/d for infants under/over 2,000 g body weight, respectively
- Aminoglycoside:
  - doses vary w/ agent chosen: for gentamicin 5 mg/kg/d (div 2 equal doses) for first week of life/7.5 mg/kg/d (div 3 equal doses) for second week of life
    - treatment × 14 d recommended

Late-onset neonatal listeriosis and meningitis

- Ampicillin (200–400 mg/kg/d div 4–6 equal doses) in combination w/ an aminoglycoside
- Lumbar puncture repeated daily until organism cleared
- *Corticosteroids:* no information suggests dexamethasone of value
- Treatment for 14–21 d recommended
- *Alternative Tx:* trimethoprim-sulfamethoxazole; advantage: penetration of antibiotic into intracellular environment where organism may survive; disadvantage: may ↑ risk of bilirubin toxicity

COMPLICATIONS

- High mortality rate for early-onset neonatal sepsis. High morbidity associated w/ other complications of prematurity
- Complications from neonatal meningitis infrequent; in older children/adults, high incidence of prolonged ataxia, hydrocephalus, rhombdoencephalitis

WHEN TO REFER

- *Early-onset neonatal listeriosis:* requires intensive neonatal management w/ consultation to neonatologist/pediatric infectious disease specialist
- *Late-onset neonatal listeriosis:* referral indicated if organism persists in CSF on Gram stain/culture after 48 hrs, if clinical condition fails to show clear improvement within 48 hrs
- Onset beyond neonatal period raises concerns about immunodeficient status including HIV infection
- Report cases to public health authorities; food-borne outbreaks identified by unusual ↑ incidence of perinatal listeriosis

BACKGROUND

- Usually seen in skeletally immature athlete
- Overuse injury due to excessive throwing
- May present w/ acute/chronic symptoms
- Most often seen in baseball pitchers; may occur in any throwing athlete
- Similar syndrome seen in gymnasts

PATHOGENESIS

- Rapid acceleration of arm produces extreme valgus force on elbow, producing tension on medial side/compression of lateral side of joint
- Tension across medial side of joint:
  - flexor, pronator muscle group places stress on medial epicondyle
  - hypertrophy, fragmentation of medial epicondyle in child
  - avulsion of medial epicondyle in adolescent
  - medial collateral ligament strain may occur
  - ulnar nerve may become inflamed w/ chronic stretching
- Compression across lateral joint (capitellum, radial head):
  - less common than medial side problems
  - lateral changes more common in older adolescents
  - osteochondritis dissecans of radial head/capitellum
  - loose body formation

CLINICAL MANIFESTATIONS

- Ache/soreness in elbow
- Loss of full extension
- Sudden painful injury to medial side of elbow (avulsion of flexor pronator mass/medial epicondyle)
- Pain, numbness in ulnar nerve distribution
- Mechanical symptoms due to loose body

EXAMINATION

- Loss of full extension of elbow
- Tenderness over medial epicondyle
- Tender over lateral elbow
- Joint swelling
- Exquisite pain, tenderness, swelling in medial epicondyle avulsion

RADIOGRAPHY

- AP, lateral view of elbow
- Changes may occur in medial/lateral side of joint
- Acute changes:
  - avulsion of medial epicondyle
  - acute osteochondral fracture of capitellum/radial head
- Chronic changes:
  - hypertrophy/fragmentation of medial epicondyle
  - hypertrophy of capitellum/radial head
  - osteochondritis dissecans of radial head/capitellum
  - loose bodies

DIFFERENTIAL DIAGNOSIS

- Panner disease:
  - usually in 8–11 yr old age group
  - irregular ossification of capitellum
  - not due to overuse or trauma
  - minimal symptoms

TREATMENT

- Conservative:
  - usually successful if no radiographic changes present
    - rest
    - ↓ frequency/force of throwing
    - change mechanics of throwing
    - occasional immobilization
    - NSAIDs
- Operative:
  - may be required if radiographic changes present
    - osteochondritis dissecans, loose bodies
    - arthroscopy/arthrotomy
    - possible open reduction, internal fixation of displaced medial epicondylar avulsion
- Rehabilitation:
  - preventable problem
  - education of parents, coaches, players
  - restrict throwing: number/types of pitches in games, practice
  - changes in technique: vertical release better than sidearm release
  - restore mobility/strength of involved extremity
  - change in position often necessary

WHEN TO REFER

- Severe symptoms
- Significant radiographic changes
- No response to regimen of restricted throwing

BACKGROUND

• Uncommon in infants and children, w/ incidence ↓ due to improved medical and surgical Tx; est <1/100,000 pediatric admissions
• Among children, median age now ~8–9 yrs, w/ fewer children < age 5
• Boys may be at slightly greater risk than girls; in adults, males 2× risk
• Significant risk factors include aspiration, hematogenous spread of bacteria from other sites, underlying immune compromise

CLINICAL MANIFESTATIONS

• Fever in 80–100%
• Cough in 53–67%; usually nonproductive at first, but can become purulent if rupture into bronchus
• Tachypnea, dyspnea, chest pain common
• Hemoptysis present ~10% pts
• Chest auscultation frequently unrevealing, but may be diminished lung sounds in presence of large abscess

LABORATORY FEATURES

• ESR ↑ nonspecifically, as is WBC count w/ left shift
• Blood culture positive up to 10% pts
• Chest x ray usually all that is needed for Dx: thickened cavity w/ air-fluid level
• CT can better define extent of abscess and aid in differential Dx
• Needle aspiration of abscess yields positive culture in >90% pts not previously treated w/ antibiotics. Pretreatment lowers yield to ~70%
• Bronchoscopy may be useful, esp if foreign body suspected

• Microbiology:
  – infections w/ multiple organisms found frequently
  – anaerobic infections very common, so take care to handle and culture abscess fluid appropriately
  – after anaerobes, common bacteria are *Staphylococcus aureus, Pseudomonas aeruginosa, Streptococcus pneumoniae,* nontypable *Haemophilus influenzae,* alpha-hemolytic *Streptococcus,* other gram-negative rods (*Klebsiella, Escherichia coli, Serratia*)
  – fungal infections (*Candida, Aspergillus, Mucor*) more likely seen in immunocompromised pts
  – tuberculosis was one of most common causes of lung abscesses; incidence ↓ w/ improved screening measures

DIFFERENTIAL DIAGNOSIS

• Pneumonia
• Loculated empyema
• Bronchopleural fistula w/ purulent pleural effusion
• *Cystic lesions:* congenital cyst, hydatid cyst, pseudocyst
• Pneumatoceole
• Saccular bronchiectasis
• Metastatic disease from Ewing sarcoma or osteosarcoma

TREATMENT

• Medical:
  – normal host: clindamycin, ampicillin/sulbactam, or ticarcillin/clavulanate for initial empiric Tx

  – immunocompromised host: add gram-negative coverage (aminoglycoside, cephalosporin)
  – pts w/ cystic fibrosis: be sure antibiotic choice covers *Pseudomonas*
  – Tx continued for min. 2–3 wks for uncomplicated course that responds rapidly to antibiotics; 4–6 wks or longer for complicated course
• *Surgical:* when medical management fails (defined as no response to parenteral antibiotics after 1–3 wk trial), or if abscess close to mediastinum, surgery may be indicated. Possible procedures include drainage of the abscess, wedge resection, or lobectomy

COMPLICATIONS

• Rupture into bronchus, mediastinum, or pleural space. Rupture into bronchus dangerous if pt unable to handle volume of abscess cavity. Rupture into mediastinum can be life threatening, esp if cardiac involvement. Rupture into pleural space may cause long-lasting pleuritic pain
• Mortality rate 5–10% and higher in those w/ underlying host resistance

WHEN TO REFER

• All pts should be hospitalized for parenteral antibiotics
• Referral may be needed for aspiration of abscess fluids for diagnostic and therapeutic purposes
• Pts should be referred if they fail to respond to medical management

LYME DISEASE

EUGENE D. SHAPIRO

BACKGROUND

- Most common vector-borne disease in US
- Caused by spirochete, *Borrelia burgdorferi;* transmitted by *Ixodes scapularis* (deer tick)
- Most cases occur in southern New England/Middle Atlantic states; some occur in Upper Midwest (rarely in Pacific states)
- Incidence highest during peak activity of ticks (spring–fall)
- Risk of disease from recognized deer tick bites low (1–2% overall); infected ticks (15–50% in endemic areas) must feed for ≥48 hrs before transmission risk substantial (most attached ticks recognized/removed sooner); analysis of ticks for infection/antimicrobial prophylaxis for persons bitten not indicated
- Prognosis for children treated for Lyme disease excellent; most common reason for treatment failure: misdiagnosis

CLINICAL MANIFESTATIONS

- See table
- Pts may present w/ any stage (w/o Hx or Sx of earlier stages)
- Single erythema migrans rash (flat, expanding erythematous circular rash at site of bite, may have central clearing, may reach >12 in in diameter, lasts for weeks if untreated)
- Multiple erythema migrans (multiple smaller circular lesions) indicative of bacteremic spread of spirochete

- Carditis very rare manifestation in children
- Arthritis affects knee (>90% of time), may also affect other joints, may recur if untreated; presentation often subacute, although may present like acute septic arthritis; Hx preceding erythema migrans now rare (because antimicrobial treatment of early disease prevents late disease); arthritis may recur

LABORATORY FEATURES

- Laboratory findings nonspecific; WBC/ESR may be normal; mild CSF pleocytosis common, even w/ no neurologic symptoms; in arthritis, WBC count in joint fluid varies 10,000–>100,000/cc
- Antibody tests not indicated if symptoms nonspecific (eg, chronic fatigue/arthralgia)/in pts w/ erythema migrans (rash pathognomonic, antibody titers often negative early in disease); antibody tests (enzyme-linked immunosorbent assay, confirmed w/ Western immunoblot) necessary to diagnose later stages of disease

DIFFERENTIAL DIAGNOSIS

- Ringworm, nummular eczema, insect/spider bites, granuloma annulare, erythema multiforme for erythema migrans
- Bell palsy, septic arthritis, juvenile rheumatoid arthritis, serum sickness, Henoch-Schöenlein purpura, viral meningitis/cardi-

tis, collagen vascular disease, rheumatic fever for early disseminated/late disease

TREATMENT

- Doxycycline (not for children <8 yrs of age) or amoxicillin × 2–3 wks for erythema migrans, seventh nerve palsy, × 4 wks for arthritis; erythromycin, cefuroxime alternatives
- Ceftriaxone or aqueous penicillin G parenterally × 2–3 wks for meningitis
- NSAIDs (eg, ibuprofen) may help alleviate symptoms
- Dermatitis in sun-exposed areas may occur in pts who take doxycycline

COMPLICATIONS

- Jarisch-Herxheimer reaction (↑ fever/myalgia) during first 24–48 hrs of treatment caused by organism lysis. Do not discontinue antibiotics

PREVENTION

- In endemic areas minimize exposure to ticks/check for, remove ticks daily

WHEN TO REFER

- If pt has meningitis, carditis, recurrent arthritis

Manifestations of Lyme disease			
Stage of Disease	**Time After Initial Infection**	**Sx**	
Early localized (~two-thirds of cases)	1–3 wks	Single erythema migrans rash (may be accompanied by fever, arthralgia, myalgia, fatigue, headache)	
Early disseminated (~one-quarter of cases)	3–7 wks	Multiple erythema migrans	
		Seventh/other cranial nerve palsy	(often accompanied by fever,
		Aseptic meningitis	arthralgia, myalgia, fatigue, headache)
		Carditis (heart block)	
Late (~one-tenth of cases)	2–6 mos/longer	Arthritis	

DAN VON ALLMEN

BACKGROUND

- Lymphangiomas: broad category of malformations that range from simple small, well-circumscribed, SubQ lesions to large poorly defined masses occupying chest, abdomen, or extremities
- Pure lymphangiomas originate from developing lymphatic system that begins in wk 6 of gestation as paired sacs in neck/iliac regions
- By wk 8 of gestation paired thoracic ducts connect retroperitoneal lymph sac w/sacs in neck; subsequently cephalad portion of right thoracic duct/caudal portion of left thoracic duct regress, leaving single thoracic lymphatic duct that enters venous system on left; abnormal development can lead to lymphangioma formation
- Benign lymphatic tumors may occur anywhere on body
- Two-thirds of lymphangiomas diagnosed at birth

CLINICAL MANIFESTATIONS

- Typically present as soft asymptomatic masses that can occur anywhere on body
- Usually nontender/transilluminate
- Commonly septa are visible within lesion
- Most common manifestation occurs in neck; frequently referred to as cystic hygroma
- Groin axilla and mediastinum also common sites

- Most common complication of lymphangiomas infection; when infections occur, lesions become tender/erythematous; child may develop systemic symptoms including fever/lethargy; CBC reveals ↑ WBC count/ shift to left; causative organism usually streptococcal/staphylococcal species

DIFFERENTIAL DIAGNOSIS

- Most lymphangiomas very characteristic in appearance/texture, making differential Dx limited
- In some cases difficult to distinguish between lymphangioma and teratoma
- Small SubQ lesions on extremities may be confused w/lipomas/dermoid cysts

TREATMENT

- Treatment for lymphangiomas surgical
- Acute infections treated w/appropriate antibiotics to cover gram-positive organisms but ultimately lesion must be removed surgically
- Lymphangiomas may be well circumscribed, making total excision very straightforward, or may be poorly defined, making excision much more difficult
- Although tumor not malignant (does not invade normal structures), can surround normal structures such as nerves/vessels that must be preserved

- Because tumor not malignant, normal structures should not be sacrificed during removal; mass should be simply debulked in cases where surrounding structures prevent complete resection

COMPLICATIONS

- Infection/recurrence most common complications; infection caused by gram-positive organisms/responds rapidly to antibiotics
- Risk of recurrence following surgical removal determined by extent of original resection; lesion completely excised, recurrence very unlikely; if lesion merely debulked, lymphatic fluid may reaccumulate
- Extent of surgical scarring obviously related to size/location of lesion

WHEN TO REFER

- Infants should be referred to pediatric surgeon when lesions diagnosed; timing of surgical removal may vary depending on size/location of lesion, but ultimately surgical resection necessary

BACKGROUND

- Febrile illness known to occur in human beings since antiquity
- Caused by 1/4 species of intraerythrocytic protozoan parasites: *P. vivax, P. ovale, P. falciparum, P. malariae*
- Parasite life cycle requires two hosts, mosquitoes/human beings
- Female anopheline mosquitoes serve as vectors/hosts for sexual reproduction of parasites
- After transmission to human beings, parasites undergo one asexual reproductive cycle in liver parenchymal cells (exoerythrocytic schizogony); subsequent asexual reproductive cycles occur in erythrocytes (erythrocytic schizogony)
- Disease widely distributed in tropical/subtropical countries; threat to ~40% of world's population
- Disease caused by *P. falciparum* life threatening in nonimmune hosts
- Most deaths occur in children 1–5 yrs of age

CLINICAL MANIFESTATIONS

- Exoerythrocytic schizogony produces no symptoms
- Erythrocytic schizogony produces paroxysms of chills/fever
- Any fever pattern possible but *P. vivax, P. ovale, P. falciparum* may cause fever w/ periodicity of 48 hrs (tertian); *P. malariae* causes fever w/ characteristic periodicity of 72 hrs (quartan)
- Other manifestations include headache, nausea, vomiting, tachycardia, frequent micturition
- Pt also may have postural hypotension, herpes labialis, anemia, hepatosplenomegaly, jaundice, hypoglycemia

- *P. falciparum* infections may cause pernicious forms of malaria w/ mortality rates as high as 50%
- *P. vivax, P. ovale* infections cause self-limited disease lasting several days–3 mos; may relapse due to persistence of exoerythrocytic parasites in liver
- *P. malariae* infections usually mild but may persist for many years, may cause nephrotic syndrome

LABORATORY FEATURES

- Blood films stained w/ Wright/Geimsa (preferred) stains show intraerythrocytic parasites w/ sufficient detail to allow identification of different species
- The ParaSite-F (dipstick) test positive in 90% pts w/ *P. falciparum* infections
- During paroxysm, leukocytosis may occur; between paroxysms, leukopenia the rule/thrombocytopenia common
- Liver function tests may be abnormal

DIFFERENTIAL DIAGNOSIS

- Any febrile illness, particularly influenza

TREATMENT

- Chemotherapeutic agents may be useful; include quinoline derivatives (quinine, chloroquine, amodiaquine, mefloquine, primaquine), dihydrofolate reductase inhibitors (pyrimethamine, proguanil), sulfonamides, artemisinin derivatives, antibiotics (erythromycin, tetracycline derivatives, lincomycin derivatives, fluoroquinolines)
- Chloroquine drug of choice for *P. vivax, P. ovale, P. malariae* infections in 4 doses spread over 3 d to achieve total dose 25 mg/kg, not to exceed 1.5 g. To eliminate possibility of relapse, pt should also receive primaquine (0.3 mg of base/kg × 14 d); pts receiving primaquine must be observed for evidence of G-6-PD-associated hemolytic anemia
- Pts infected w/ *P. falciparum* (frequently resistant to chloroquine) may be treated w/ quinine (30 mg quinine sulfate/kg div 3 doses/d × 10–14 d, up to max dose 650 mg 3 ×/d × 10–14 d) or mefloquine (15 mg/kg as single dose, up to max dose 1,250 mg); primaquine not necessary because exoerythrocytic stage of *P. falciparum* does not persist in liver
- Chemoprophylaxis should be used by people traveling to endemic areas; recommendations change frequently/up-to-date advice should be sought from public health department/travel clinic

COMPLICATIONS

- Cerebral malaria (severe delirium, coma, convulsions, severe hyperpyrexia)
- Blackwater fever (hemoglobinuric acute renal failure)
- Extensive vascular involvement of GI tract accompanied by nausea, vomiting, acute diarrhea
- Algid malaria (extreme prostration)
- Acute respiratory distress syndrome

WHEN TO REFER

- When one of pernicious complications of malaria present
- When treatment not promptly successful (within 1–2 d)
- When pt relapses

MAPLE SYRUP URINE DISEASE

JULIE E. HOOVER AND NANCY BRAVERMAN

BACKGROUND

- Maple syrup urine disease (MSUD) caused by deficiency of enzyme branched-chain alpha-ketoacid dehydrogenase (BCKD) required to metabolize branched chain amino acids (BCAAs, ie., leucine, isoleucine, valine)
- BCAAs found in all dietary protein sources; also component of body's endogenous protein stores
- Symptoms caused by buildup of toxic form (alpha-ketoacids) of BCAAs/leucine itself; leucine particularly toxic to CNS
- Marked ↑ alpha-ketoacids/leucine occurs when MSUD pt consumes excess BCAAs/catabolizes protein stores in times of stress (ie, fever, infection, surgery)
- MSUD named for urine odor produced by ↑ 2-oxo-3-methylvaleric acid
- Incidence of 1/200,000; incidence in North American Mennonites 1/176; M = F
- Autosomal recessive
- Five forms of MSUD characterized by age of onset, severity, response to thiamine, cofactor of BCKD; each form runs true within family

Type	Onset	Severity
Classical*	week 1 of life	life threatening
Intermediate	infancy to adulthood	milder than classical
Intermittent	infancy to adulthood; episodic w/illness	mild; episodic
Thiamine responsive	infancy to adulthood	thiamine supplement ameliorates metabolic complications
Lipoamide dehydrogenase (E3) deficiency**	infancy	milder than classical

*Most common form; described in Mennonite population.
**Rarest form.

- MSUD included in newborn screen of only 21 states; screening measures leucine in dried blood
- Pts w/classical MSUD often symptomatic before abnormal newborn screen found

CLINICAL MANIFESTATIONS

- *Classical:* irritability, poor feeding, lethargy, hypotonia alternating w/hypertonia, seizures, progress to cerebral edema, coma, death if untreated; survivors often have severe psychomotor retardation; chance of normal outcome depends on early Dx, treatment; unfortunately, early Dx usually 2° to anticipatory treatment of newborn w/affected sibling
- *Intermediate:* failure to thrive, ataxia, vomiting, psychomotor retardation; laboratory abnormalities usually milder than classical form
- *Intermittent:* episodic lethargy/ataxia associated w/intercurrent illness/excessive protein intake; laboratory abnormalities usually only w/acute exacerbations
- *Thiamine responsive:* mildest form; responds to thiamine
- *Lipoamide dehydrogenase (E3) deficiency:* similar to intermediate form w/lactic acidosis

LABORATORY FEATURES

- Abnormal newborn screen; may be false negative if first screen collected before 24 hrs of feeds
- *Spot urine test:* 2,4-dinitrophenylhydrazine (DNPH) combines w/alpha-keto acids of BCAAs to make white precipitate
- *Plasma amino acid analysis:* ↑ BCAAs and unique amino acid, alloisoleucine
- *Urine organic acid analysis:* ↑ 2-oxoisocaproic, 2-oxo-3-methylvaleric, 2-oxoisovaleric, 2-hydroxyisovaleric, 2-hydroxyisocaproic, 2-hydroxy-3-methylvaleric acid, all by-products of unmetabolized BCAAs
- Hypoglycemia, metabolic acidosis, ketosis, hyperammonemia

DIFFERENTIAL DIAGNOSIS

- MSUD presentation quite similar to that of many serious illnesses including sepsis, toxic ingestion, stroke, other inborn errors of metabolism; prudent to consider entire category of metabolic disease as potential Dx for severely compromised infant/child
- Consider metabolic disease in any child:
  – ill enough to treat presumptively for sepsis
  – w/unexplained recurrent episodes of severe illness, esp if responsive to IV fluids/glucose
  – who avoids high-protein food/has unexplained behavioral changes after high-protein meals
  – diagnosed w/developmental delay

TREATMENT

- Acute management:
  – stop all protein sources (Subacutely, patients respond well to BCAA-free formula with supplemental isoleucine and valine.)
  – supply adequate calories (glucose) to prevent catabolism at around 70% RDA; use insulin if hyperglycemia occurs rather than decrease calories
  – consider hemodialysis to remove toxic BCAA/ketoacids
  – consult geneticist w/metabolic expertise/have nephrologist/intensivist readily available; if pt deteriorates (inc. lethargy or ammonia), condition may be critical, require intensive care management
- Chronic management:
  – restrict intake of BCAAs to that required only for growth; consult w/dietitian
  – supply adequate amount of other amino acids, calories for growth/to prevent catabolism based on RDA w/light activity (infant, 100–120 kcal/kg; toddler, 90–100 kcal/kg; child, 70–90 kcal/kg; teen, 40–55 kcal/kg; adult, 30–40 kcal/kg)
  – education of pt's caregivers regarding potential life-threatening exacerbations of MSUD w/otherwise minor illnesses

COMPLICATIONS

- Severe psychomotor retardation, pancreatitis, seizures, coma, death in untreated classical form
- Outcome based on time interval to Dx; some w/classical form have normal IQ if diagnosed in first 10 d of life

PREVENTION

- Know your state's procedure for notification/follow-up of abnormal newborn screens
- Any abnormal results necessitate immediate direct patient follow-up for feeding status, activity, weight; immediate referral to genetic center if any abnormalities noted; repeat newborn screen
- Prenatal Dx available via enzyme assays on chorionic villi samples/cultured amniocytes; offered primarily to parents w/prior affected child

WHEN TO REFER

- After notification of abnormal newborn screen in face of clinically compromised infant
- W/acute/chronic poor feeding, vomiting, tachypnea, lethargy, abnormal scent of urine, ketoacidosis, hyperammonemia; also symptoms episodic in nature associated w/metabolic stress/large protein loads
- Where? To center w/metabolic geneticist, nutritionist w/metabolic disease expertise, facilities to evaluate plasma amino acids/urine organic acids, nephrologist, intensive care resources including hemodialysis

BACKGROUND

- Defective fibrillin (component of microfibrils)
- Autosomal dominant trait w/variable expression
- New mutation rate ~15% w/tendency toward more severe phenotype
- Prevalence 1/10,000, occurring in all races/ethnic groups

- Dx usually made during adolescence/adulthood
- Median cumulative probability of survival 72 yrs
- Infantile Marfan syndrome more severe; mean age at Dx 3.2 mos; mean age at death 16.3 mos, usually due to CHF; only 30% family Hx Marfan syndrome

CLINICAL MANIFESTATIONS

- Index case:
  - if no family Hx mutation known to cause, requires major criteria in at least two organ systems/involvement of third organ system
  - if family Hx mutation known to cause, requires one major criterion/involvement of second organ system
- Family Hx of Marfan syndrome:
  - requires one major criterion/involvement of second organ system

System	Major Criteria	Minor Criteria
Skeletal (To be involved, at least 2 major criteria components *or* 1 major criteria component and 2 minor criteria must be present)	At least 4 of the following: Pectus carinatum Pectus excavatum requiring surgery Reduced upper to lower body segment ratio *or* arm span to height ratio >1.05 Wrist and thumb signs Scoliosis >20° *or* spondylolisthesis Reduced extension of elbows (<170°) Medial displacement of medial malleolus causing pes planus (flatfeet) Protrusio acetabulae (deep hip sockets)	Pectus excavatum of moderate severity Joint hypermobility Highly arched palate w/dental crowding Facial appearance: dolichocephaly (narrow head), malar hypoplasia, enophthalmos, retrognathia, down-slanting palpebral fissures
Ocular (To be involved, ectopia lentis *or* at least 2 minor criteria must be present)	Ectopia lentis (dislocated lenses)	Abnormally flat cornea Increased axial length of globe Hypoplastic iris or ciliary muscle causing ↓ miosis
Cardiovascular (To be involved, a single major or minor criterion must be present)	Dilation of ascending aorta involving sinuses of Valsalva Dissection of ascending aorta	Mitral valve prolapse Dilation of main pulmonary artery in absence of valvar PS, peripheral pulmonary artery stenosis, or other obvious cause before age 40 Calcification of mitral annulus before age 40 Dilation or dissection of descending thoracic aorta before age 50
Pulmonary (To be involved, one minor criterion must be present)	None	Spontaneous pneumothorax Apical blebs
Skin and Integument (To be involved, one minor criterion must be present)	None	Striae atrophicae (stretch marks) not associated w/marked weight changes, pregnancy, or repetitive stress Recurrent or incisional herniae
Dura	Lumbosacral dural ectasia (by CT or MRI)	None
Family/Genetic History (To be involved, one major criterion must be present)	Parent, child, or sibling who meets these criteria independently Fibrillin-1 (FBN1) mutation known to cause Marfan syndrome Haplotype around FBN1, inherited by descent, known to be associated w/unequivocally diagnosed Marfan syndrome in the family	None

LABORATORY FEATURES

- *Echocardiography (required):* assess aortic root size in suspected pts (compare w/normal values for age/body surface area); at least annual echocardiogram to assess aortic root size in known pts
- *Chest x ray (required):* examine lung parenchyma for evidence of bullous disease; heart size/contour affected by pectus deformities; chest x ray cannot be used to exclude aortic root dilation
- *Pulmonary function tests (required):* pectus deformity/scoliosis may cause restrictive ventilation defect
- Dilated eye examination w/slit lamp to screen for ectopia lentis (required)

DIFFERENTIAL DIAGNOSIS

- Congenital contractural arachnodactyly
- Familial aortic dissection
- Familial ectopia lentis
- Familial Marfan-like habitus
- Familial mitral valve prolapse syndrome
- Familial thoracic aortic aneurysm
- Homocystinuria
- MASS phenotype (*m*yopia, *m*itral valve, *a*orta, *s*kin, *s*keleton)
- Shprintzen-Goldberg syndrome
- Stickler syndrome

TREATMENT

- Long-term beta blockade slows rate of aortic root dilation/↓ risk of death, aortic dissection/rupture, development of audible aortic regurgitation, need for cardiac surgery, CHF
- Regardless of aortic root size, pts w/Marfan syndrome should be treated w/beta blocker at youngest age possible
- Adjust beta-blocker dose as tolerated to significantly blunt heart rate response to exercise
- Infective endocarditis prophylaxis for individuals w/aortic/mitral regurgitation

COMPLICATIONS

- Aortic dilation begins during infancy/childhood
- Aortic dissection/rupture most common during fourth decade
- Heart failure/infective endocarditis 2° to aortic or mitral valve disease
- Visual impairment 2° to dislocated lenses
- Spontaneous pneumothorax
- Skeletal injuries

PREVENTION

- Beta-adrenergic blockade/composite aortic root replacement ↓ risk of aortic complications
- Endocarditis prophylaxis

- Competitive athletics:
  - if no family Hx premature sudden death, no aortic root dilation, no mitral regurgitation may compete in low static/low dynamic sports (eg, bowling, golf, riflery)/moderate static/low dynamic sports (eg, archery); measure aortic root dimension q6mos
  - may compete only in low static/low dynamic sports if aorta dilated
  - no contact sports due to risk of lens dislocation, retinal detachment, skeletal injury, pneumothorax, aortic dissection
  - avoid weight lifting, other isometric exercise, maximal exercise, which raise BP/↑ aortic wall stress
  - additional recommendations exist for athlete w/aortic/mitral regurgitation

WHEN TO REFER

- Annual follow-up by multidisciplinary team including cardiologist, orthopedic surgeon, ophthalmologist recommended for stable pt
- Pt w/significant aortic root dilation, increasing aortic root size, significant valve disease, pregnancy must be seen more frequently
- Replacement of aortic valve/ascending aorta w/composite graft indicated for:
  - aortic dissection
  - aortic root diameter >55 mm
  - progressive aortic dilation, aortic regurgitation

BACKGROUND

- Most frequently used illegal drug in US
- After constant declines in use by adolescents 1979–1992, trend toward ↑ use documented in 8th, 10th, 12th graders

Percentage students reporting marijuana use in past year

	1991	1998
8th graders	6.2	16.9
10th graders	16.5	31.1
12th graders	23.9	37.5

THE DRUG

- *Source/active ingredient:* derived from dried/shredded flowers, leaves of *Cannabis sativa,* the hemp plant
- Delta-9-tetrahydrocannabinol (THC) active ingredient in all forms of marijuana, including hashish (sticky resin from female plant leaves/flowers); sensimilla (buds/flowering tops of female plants cultivated to obtain high THC levels); hash oil (tarlike liquid distilled from hashish)
- Potency of all forms of marijuana has risen since 1960s (hashish, sensimilla, hash oil are most potent forms)
- *Methods of use:* rolled into cigarette (joint), smoked in pipe/water pipe (bong), filled into sliced cigar (blunt), baked into foods, brewed into tea
- Effects of use:
  - used mostly for sense of relaxation/well-being; effects may be unpredictable depending on user's expectations, potency of drug, dose/method of administration
- physical reactions: ↑ heart rate, conjunctival injection, dry mouth/throat, dilated pupils, sleepiness, loss of coordination/balance, ↓ reaction time
  - effects of intoxication: time, auditory/visual distortions; impaired learning, cognitive functions; ↑ appetite; euphoria; mood fluctuations; depersonalization; hallucinations
  - withdrawal symptoms: usually mild, may last up to a month, include sleep disturbances, anxiety, sweating, irritability, nausea, vomiting, anorexia
  - potential toxic reactions: anxiety, panic, organic brain syndrome, delusions, hallucinations, paranoia, precipitation of seizures in epileptics, precipitation of psychotic episodes in schizophrenics
- Adverse effects:
  - pulmonary: greater burden of carbon monoxide/tar than tobacco; chronic use leads to bronchoconstriction, bronchitis, ↓ pulmonary function; postulated link between chronic marijuana smoke exposure/lung cancer w/ metaplastic cell changes seen in human/animal studies
  - endocrine/immune functions: ↑ anovulatory cycles, antagonistic effects on insulin, ↓ sperm count/motility, ↑ abnormal morphology of sperm, gynecomastia, possible suppression of immune function
  - neurobehavioral: impaired memory, learning ability, perception w/ long-term use; "amotivational syndrome"/passive withdrawal from usual work, recreational activities (controversial whether marijuana causes or if behaviors preexistent); high correlation w/ heavy use/truancy/poor school performance; correlation of dependence/depression, suicidal ideation, family disruption, injuries, risky sexual behaviors
  - drug interactions: can potentiate sedation when used w/ alcohol, diazepam, antihistamines, phenothiazines, barbiturates, narcotics; potentiates stimulation when used w/cocaine/amphetamines; antagonistic w/effects of phenytoin, propranolol, insulin

TREATMENT

- Acute intoxication:
  - effects generally abate 2–3 hrs after smoking/up to 24 hrs after ingestion
  - no specific detoxification treatment
  - THC may be detected by urine drug screens
  - screens may be positive in long-term users for up to 1–2 mos because of metabolite storage in fat tissue
- Abuse/dependence:
  - all treatment options aim to interrupt use, institute sobriety, assist in developing drug-free lifestyle
  - outpt/inpt treatment may be required, with outpt treatment w/ individual/group Tx used most often

PREVENTION

- Inclusion of alcohol/other drug abuse screening, topic discussion as part of anticipatory guidance/at visits for issues such as poorly explained trauma important
- Screening may be done by interview/written screening instruments
- *Specific screening strategy:* "Have you used marijuana 5 or more times in your life?" If the answer positive, then ask, "Have you used in the past 6 months?" If the answer positive, consider further evaluation for possible treatment
- Patient-physician discussion, peer counseling, computer-assisted instruction effective ways to educate about health risks associated w/ drug use; pediatricians can provide assistance to teens in coping w/ peer pressure/aid parents w/ strategies on how to anticipate, avoid/cope w/ behavior issues; pediatricians can strengthen protective factors among adolescents by encouraging their participation in organized activities at school, w/ religious groups, in maintenance of family rituals

MASTOCYTOSIS: URTICARIA PIGMENTOSA

SONALI G. HANSON AND MOISE L. LEVY

BACKGROUND

- Group of clinical disorders characterized by accumulation of mast cells; urticaria pigmentosa (UP) most common form of cutaneous mastocytosis
- Most commonly results in cutaneous manifestations during childhood but may develop at any age/involve any organ system
- In general, children w onset < age 10 have better prognosis than adults (almost always purely cutaneous disease that resolves spontaneously)
- Accumulations of mast cells in skin most often appear during first 2 yrs of life; may be congenital
- In adults, skin lesions seldom disappear; 30–55% pts have evidence of systemic involvement
- Equal in both sexes
- All races affected
- Clinical features subdivided into systemic/cutaneous mastocytosis
- Generally isolated occurrence; rare familial cases have been reported
- Etiology unknown

CLINICAL MANIFESTATIONS

- Lesions of UP typically pigmented; may urticate spontaneously/after trauma
- Pts may have few–thousands of lesions
- Lesions found on any body surface; most commonly oval/round, red-brown macules, papules; plaques/nodules may occur, as well as vesicles/bullae
- Most lesions found on trunk, followed by extremities; face and scalp usually spared; lesions rare on palms/soles
- Individual lesions in very young children tend to be larger than those of adults; may blister
- Frequently clustering of papules to form plaques w/cobblestone appearance in which normal skin markings exaggerated. In older children/adults, individual lesions tend to be smaller, macular, relatively stable, although large, red-brown plaques may form
- Underlying color ranges from that of surrounding skin to varying hues of yellow, tan, brown hyperpigmentation (becomes more pronounced after repeated cycles of urtication)
- Pruritus, most common symptom, tends to be paroxysmal, frequently remains localized to sites of mast cell infiltration
- Dermatographism almost constant feature but not diagnostic; most pronounced over sites infiltrated by ↑ number mast cells
- *Darier sign:* exaggerated tendency for area of skin infiltrated by larger than normal number of mast cells to become erythematous/urticate upon stroking; extremely useful/fairly sensitive diagnostic sign
- Flushing, telangectasia, petechiae, ecchymoses may occur in lesions or in clinically normal skin

LABORATORY FEATURES

- Skin biopsy from area of apparent cutaneous involvement frequently reveals mast cells in dermal papillae/around superficial blood vessels, sometimes extending into deeper portion of dermis; ↑ melanin is epidermal/tends to be distributed in basal/lower Malphigian layers
- Injection of anesthetic directly into site to be biopsied can result in mast cell degranulation; should be avoided because would make histopathologic identification of mast cells difficult
- In great majority of pts, laboratory evaluation beyond confirmatory skin biopsy not indicated; treatment generally based on clinical symptoms

DIFFERENTIAL DIAGNOSIS

- 2° syphilis
- Café-au-lait macules
- Insect bites
- Juvenile xanthogranuloma

TREATMENT

- Symptomatic/must be tailored to individual pt
- Avoidance of potential mast cell degranulators such as aspirin, codeine, opiates, procaine, spicy foods, cheese, excessive ingestion of alcohol, polymyxin B, as well as hot baths/vigorous rubbing after bathing
- Traditional antihistamines (H_1 blockers) in usual doses for flushing/pruritus (ie, hydroxyzine 2–4 mg/kg/d in div doses, diphenhydramine 5 mg/kg/d in div doses)
- Oral cromolyn sodium (20–40 mg/kg/d in 4 div doses up to 2 yrs of age; 100 mg qid, children 2–12 yrs old) for diarrhea/abdominal pain
- H_2 blockers such as ranitidine/cimetidine as adjunct to H_1 blockers, and for gastric/duodenal manifestations
- Local corticosteroid treatment may have limited use; systemic corticosteroids may be helpful
- Oral calcium channel blockers such as nifedipene/ketotifen have been used because mast cell degranulation is a calcium-dependent process
- Psoralin and UVA irradiation (PUVA)

COMPLICATIONS

- Be aware of possibility of multisystem involvement (symptoms include nausea, vomiting, diarrhea, abdominal pain, weight loss, headache, fatigue, episodic flushing, tachycardia, hypotension, dizziness, syncope)
- Baseline radiologic survey recommended for pts w/ extensive cutaneous involvement regardless of presence of systemic symptoms, to identify asymptomatic bony lesions early/thereby prevent unnecessarily extensive evaluation if bony changes discovered incidentally later in life (ie, for diagnoses such as osteoporosis, metastatic carcinoma, multiple myeloma, Paget disease of bone)
- Circulatory collapse/airway compromise in pts w/ systemic disease
- Development of leukemia/related malignant condition affecting tissues of reticuloendothelial system in adult pts w/ mastocytosis

WHEN TO REFER

- If clinical Dx in doubt, may need to refer for cutaneous biopsy

MASTOIDITIS

CHARLES M. MYER III

BACKGROUND

- Incidence ↓ markedly since development of numerous broad-spectrum antimicrobial agents/relatively common use of tympanostomy tubes
- All cases of acute otitis media associated w/ inflammation of mastoid air cell system; this is not clinical mastoiditis
- Progression of acute inflammatory process may produce periostitis, possibly, subperiosteal abscess; this represents mastoiditis in clinical setting

CLINICAL MANIFESTATIONS

- Pts usually present w/ Sx of acute otitis media, tenderness/erythema (cellulitis) overlying mastoid, loss of postauricular crease
- Worsening noted by displacement of pinna outward/forward; edema/sagging of posterior/superior external auditory canal wall; fluctuance of skin behind auricle indicative of subperiosteal abscess
- Be suspicious of masked mastoiditis in pts who present w/ persistent/recurrent pain 2 wks after initiating appropriate antimicrobial Tx for acute otitis media

IMAGING/LABORATORY FEATURES

- In pts who do not improve w/ IV antimicrobial Tx/those who develop subperiosteal abscess, CT scan obtained to delineate intratemporal anatomy, evaluate for potential intracranial complications; scan done w/ and w/o contrast, w/soft tissue/bone windows
- In acute mastoiditis, will be breakdown of mastoid septa due to coalescence

DIFFERENTIAL DIAGNOSIS

- Acute external otitis w/ periauricular cellulitis
- Temporal bone trauma
- Langerhan cell histiocytosis
- Temporal bone rhabdomyosarcoma
- First branchial cleft anomaly

TREATMENT

- Once identified, child should undergo urgent tympanocentesis for culture/susceptibility studies in addition to ventilating tube placement
- IV antimicrobial Tx should cover *Haemophilus influenzae, Staphylococcus aureus, Streptococcus pneumoniae;* appropriate agents w/broad-spectrum coverage: ampicillin w/sulbactam, ceftriaxone
- Improvement noted usually within 24–36 hrs; marked by ↓ postauricular swelling/tenderness, ↓ middle ear pain/drainage
- May be switched to oral antimicrobial Tx in 5 d w/ continued improvement; antimicrobial agent choice based on culture/susceptibility studies, continued for another 10 d
- When child fails to improve or if subperiosteal abscess develops, CT scan obtained prior to surgical intervention (see Imaging/Laboratory Features)

COMPLICATIONS

- Once coalescent mastoiditis has developed (destruction of bony trabeculae of mastoid air cell system) potential for spread; may see collection of pus in postauricular region (subperiosteal abscess), in neck deep to sternocleidomastoid muscle (Bezold abscess), or extending medial to petrous portion of temporal bone (petrositis); may be associated labyrinthitis/facial nerve paralysis 2° to inflammatory products; intracranial spread of infection may occur w/ development of meningitis, epidural abscess, brain abscess, subdural abscess

WHEN TO REFER

- Any child w/ suspicion of acute mastoiditis should be evaluated by otolaryngologist

BACKGROUND

- Most common tumors of infants/children
- ~1–2% of all pigmented lesions of newborn are congenital nevi, composed of cells derived from neural crest/thought by some to be derived from epidermal melanocytes
- Predisposition to development of malignant melanoma (incidence: 3–17%); lifetime risk for melanoma ↑ in congenital nevi, esp giant congenital nevus, thought to be at least fivefold
- Congenital nevi classified according to size:
  – giant congenital nevi: >120 cm/those that cover area such as scalp, trunk, extremity; synonyms: "coat sleeve," "bathing trunk," "caplike," "giant hairy"
  – large congenital nevi: >1.5 cm, <120 cm
  – small congenital nevi: <1.5 cm in surface area

CLINICAL MANIFESTATIONS

Giant congenital nevi

- Variegate pigmentation from blue black to dark brown to areas of hypopigmentation; surface verrucous, usually covered w/coarse black hair
- As child gets older, nevi become darker, more hairy, more verrucous
- Nevi that overlie spinal column frequently associated w/neurologic abnormalities/spina bifida
- Verrucous blue-back nodules often develop in nevi/can grow at alarming rates; in infants <6 mos usually benign course even though histology quite atypical/can be interpreted as malignant; infants >6 mos in age may have different prognosis

Large congenital nevi

- Also show variation in color but less blue black than giant congenital nevus; surface becomes verrucous w/increasing age; hair also develops
- Melanoma can develop; incidence varies but thought to be less than in giant variety

Small congenital nevi

- Present as *macules* w/sharply defined borders; color varies from tan to brown/may be freckling
- Resemble café-au-lait spots
- Hair will develop
- Nodulation uncommon; melanoma reported/incidence < giant congenital nevi

HISTOLOGY

- Melanocytic cells seen in all congenital nevi; found within epidermis/dermis as single as well as nests of cells
- Nevic cells found streaming between collagen bundles found in hair, blood vessels of erector muscle, sweat glands; can be found in deep muscle, fascia
- One pattern of nevic cell infiltration is dermal sparing of epidermal-dermal interface; pattern does not affect course of nevi
- Lower dermal cells almost always smaller in size than those at surface
- Nodules that develop may show significant pigmentation/cytologically atypical, equate to melanoma

DIFFERENTIAL DIAGNOSIS

- Café-au-lait spots
- Nevus of Ota/Ito
- Mongolian spot
- Epithelial nevus
- Vascular nevus
- Lentigo
- Pigmented neurofibroma

TREATMENT

- No accepted universal treatment standard; some advocate total excision of all nevi (impossibility in many cases); some recommend conservative approach of selective excision of clinically atypical areas, new growth, nodule formation
- Suggested management:
  – careful monitoring of nevus w/photos/measurements on defined schedule
  – remove altered/growing areas by surgical excision; electrodesiccation, laser, curettage should never be performed
  – counseling for all pts/parents esp those w/disfiguring nevi
  – small congenital nevi can be excised in toto, eliminating any risk of malignancy
  – systematic follow-up, good lines of communication between parent/physician essential

COMPLICATIONS

- Major complication development of malignant melanoma
- Other complications associated w/neurological defects including spina bifida

WHEN TO REFER

- Nodule development in nevus at any age
- Neurologic manifestations
- Crusting/bleeding from any site

MENINGITIS, BACTERIAL

ELAINE I. TUOMANEN

BACKGROUND

- Pediatric emergency
- Most frequently occurs <5 yrs of age
- Etiology changes w/ age

Age	Etiology	Antibiotic Tx
<2 mos	Escherichia coli	ampicillin and aminoglycoside or cefotaxime/ ceftazidime
	Listeria monocytogenes	
	Group B streptococcus	
>2 mos–5 y	Streptococcus pneumoniae	cefotaxime/ ceftriaxone
	Neisseria meningitidis	
teenage	Neisseria meningitidis	cefotaxime/ ceftriaxone
>50 y	Streptococcus pneumoniae	cefotaxime/ ceftriaxone

- Mortality rate 10–30%
- Recovery complicated by neurologic sequelae in 30%; most commonly, high-frequency hearing loss
- ↑ S. pneumoniae beta lactam antibiotic resistance requires addition of vancomycin to initial Tx in some geographic locations

CLINICAL MANIFESTATIONS

- *Early:* fever, irritability, poor feeding
- *Late:* stiff neck, bulging fontanelle, seizures, petechiae
- *Young adult:* headache, rapid ↓ in mentation, petechiae suggest meningococcemia

LABORATORY FEATURES

- CSF analysis mandatory:
  - tube 1: *cell count abnormal if:*
    - <1 mo of age: >30 cells/mm^3 (90% mononuclear)
    - all others: >5 cells/mm^3
  - tube 2: *chemistry abnormal if:*
    - ↓ glucose: <50% simultaneous blood level
    - ↑ protein: >40 mg/dL
  - tube 3: *culture abnormal if:*
    - any bacterial growth
    - request assay of sensitivity of isolate to penicillin
- Blood culture usually positive

DIFFERENTIAL DIAGNOSIS

- Viral meningitis
- Sepsis w/o meningitis

TREATMENT

- Immediate referral to ER
- IV antibiotics in ER

Antibiotic	Dose	Duration
cefotaxime	75 mg/kg q8h	7–10 d
ceftriaxone	100 mg/kg q24h	7–10 d

As alternative to beta lactam in cases of anaphylactoid allergy:

chloramphenicol	25 mg/kg q6h	7–10 d

Suspected beta lactam–resistant strain:

vancomycin	15 mg/kg q6h	7–10 d

- IV dexamethasone recommended in children >2 mos of age; administer just *before* first antibiotic dose: 0.15 mg/kg q6h × 2–4 d

- Immediate admission; respiratory isolation; ICU necessary hemodynamically/neurologically unstable
- *Chemoprophylaxis:* pt, household, childcare contacts: within 24 h administer rifampin, 10 mg/kg/dose (max 600 mg) q12h × 2 d

COMPLICATIONS

- Seizures
- Shock/DIC
- Cerebral edema

SUSPECT TREATMENT FAILURE

- Fever >48 h w/o 2° infection site
- Clinical deterioration on antibiotics
- Antibiotic-resistant strains in CSF not adequately treated by high-dose beta lactams; requires vancomycin
- *Action:* repeat CSF analysis/add vancomycin until sensitivities of bacterial isolate confirmed

PREVENTION

- *Haemophilus influenzae* vaccine has nearly eradicated type B as cause of meningitis
- Vaccination available for memingococcus types a/c; most disease type B
- Vaccination available for pneumococcus 23-valent; not effective <2 yrs of age

WHEN TO REFER

- If management of disease/complications not possible

MENINGOCOCCEMIA

MARSHA S. ANDERSON

BACKGROUND

- Usually severe, rapidly progressing, sometimes fatal infection of blood, w/ apparent sepsis associated w/ fever/petechiae/purpura
- Meningitis, arthritis, pericarditis, pneumonitis, pharyngitis, conjunctivitis may occur
- Causative organism *Neisseria meningitidis*, gram-negative diplococcus, sometimes described as kidney bean shaped. Bacteria grow best on chocolate or blood agar
- Young children–young adults most commonly affected (50% <2 yrs of age); persons w/o protective antibody at risk
- Young healthy adults w/asymptomatic nasal colonization most common reservoir of infection
- Serogroups B/C most common serogroups in US and are increasing
- Consider screening for complement deficiency, especially if unusual serotype
- Functionally/anatomically asplenic persons at ↑ risk

CLINICAL MANIFESTATIONS

- Fever, petechiae, purpura (some present w/o rash)
- Headache, vomiting, myalgias, lethargy, malaise also common
- Stick neck, seizures, photophobia in pts w/ meningitis
- *Neonates:* irritability, lethargy, poor feeding
- Circulatory collapse on presentation/ shortly after antibiotic Tx common

LABORATORY FEATURES

- Isolation of organism from blood culture definitive; susceptibility testing required because of penicillin-resistant isolates
- Petechiae lesion Gram stain often shows gram-negative diplococci
- ↑ WBC counts w/ left shift/occasionally neutropenia; often thrombocytopenia/abnormal coagulation studies (DIC)
- W/ meningitis typically CSF pleocytosis. Occasionally normal-appearing spinal fluid, but positive CSF cultures

DIFFERENTIAL DIAGNOSIS

- Acute rheumatic fever
- Subacute bacterial endocarditis
- Henoch-Schönlein purpura
- Rocky Mountain spotted fever
- Miliary tuberculosis
- Collagen vascular/neoplastic
- Gonococcemia
- 2° syphilis
- Rat bite fever
- Malaria
- Typhoid fever
- Other bacterial sepsis

TREATMENT

- Treat shock w/ fluid/pressors (central line if indicated)
- Lumbar puncture unless contraindicated by severe thrombocytopenia, cardiovascular instability, ↑ intracranial pressure
- *Empiric Tx:* ceftriaxone IV, 100 mg/kg/d div q12h or cefotaxime IV, 200 mg/kg/d div q6h. If meningitis present consider adding vancomycin, 60 mg/kg/d div q6h for possible cephalosporin-resistant pneumococcus (until cultures definitive)
- Penicillin alone should not be initially used
- Repeat blood culture to document sterilization
- For susceptible meningococcal strains, 7 d IV Tx adequate (even if meningitis present); dosing maintained at meningitic levels if meningitis present; for meningococcemia alone, ceftriaxone IV, 50 mg/kg/d qd, cefotaxime, 150 mg/kg/d div q8h, or penicillin G, 250,000 U/kg/d div q4h
- Neonates need dosing adjustment depending on postnatal age, weight, prematurity
- Chemoprophylaxis to prevent meningococcal disease recommended:
  – household contacts of index case
  – day-care center contacts
  – health care workers w/ intimate exposure to secretions (ie, intubation, mouth-to-mouth resuscitation)
  – index pt (unless treated w/cephalosporins) to eradicate nasal colonization (generally given during last 2 Tx d)

CHEMOPROPHYLACTIC OPTION REGIMENS

- *Rifampin:* po 10 mg/kg/dose (not to exceed 600 mg/dose) q12h × 4 doses; contraindicated in pregnancy; stains body secretions orange; may stain contact lenses orange; may cause birth control pills to be ineffective; multiple drug interactions
- *Ceftriaxone:* <15 yrs 125 mg IM; >15 yrs 250 mg IM as single dose
- *Ciprofloxacin:* 500 mg po as single dose *(adults only);* contraindicated in pregnancy
- Evaluate ill contacts for meningococcal disease

COMPLICATIONS

- Arthritis, 2–4%; infectious/immune complex mediated
- Pericarditis/myocarditis, 2–5%
- Pneumonia
- Neurologic:
  – vascular thrombosis/cerebral infarction
  – hydrocephalus
  – cerebral edema/herniation
  – hearing loss or other cranial nerve abnormalities
  – subdural effusions/empyema
  – seizures
  – spasticity or hemiplegia
- Loss of digits, limbs, or skin necrosis
- Waterhouse-Fredrichson syndrome

WHEN TO REFER

- Most/all, w/ suspected meningococcemia admitted to ICU for monitoring
- Report to county health department immediately
- Vaccine effective for pts >2 yrs of age (only protective against serogroups A, C, W–135, and Y).

BACKGROUND

- CNS viral infection referred to as meningitis, encephalitis, meningoencephalitis, encephalomyelitis, depending on clinical involvement area
- Meningoencephalitis most often uncommon complication of many very common viral infections, including enteroviruses (echoviruses, Coxsackie A/B, enterovirus 71, polio), herpes simplex, human herpes virus 6, varicella zoster, Epstein-Barr, adenoviruses, influenza A/B, measles, mumps
  - arboviruses, spread during summer months by mosquitoes, also cause meningoencephalitis; arboviruses reported in US include Eastern equine, St. Louis, Western equine, Venezuelan equine, California, Powassan, Colorado tick fever encephalitis, West Nile
  - rabies, herpes virus simiae (herpes B), lymphocytic choriomeningitis viruses, unusual causes of meningoencephalitis in US, spread to humans from mammals
- Infection to CNS through lymphatics/ bloodstream (eg, enteroviruses/arboviruses), through retrograde invasion along peripheral nerves (eg, herpes simplex/rabies), may occur as postinfectious/parainfectious process immunologically mediated (eg, varicella)
- Prognosis generally favorable except in meningoencephalitis caused by herpes simplex, some arboviruses, esp Eastern equine encephalitis, rabies, herpes B

CLINICAL MANIFESTATIONS

- Fever, headache, seizures, alteration in awareness, agitation, other signs of cerebral/cerebellar dysfunction
- Meningismus (meningitis)/peripheral weakness (myelitis) may also occur
- Varicella postinfectious encephalitis most often affects cerebellum/results in ataxia
- Herpes simplex encephalitis most often affects temporal lobes

LABORATORY FEATURES

- CSF pleocytosis usually present (mononuclear cells predominate)
- Localized CNS hemorrhage may result in CSF RBCs
- MRI usually demonstrates temporal lobe involvement in herpes simplex disease
- EEG may demonstrate localized/diffuse pathology
- Serology/viral cultures of stool, throat, CSF should be done to determine etiology

DIFFERENTIAL DIAGNOSIS

- Bacterial infection of the CNS, eg, tuberculosis, syphilis, borrelia, cat scratch disease, *H. influenzae, S. pneumoniae, N. meningitidis,* mycoplasma, chlamydia, rickettsiae
- CNS fungal infection, including cryptococcus
- CNS protozoal/helminthic infection, including naegleria, acanthamoeba, toxoplasma, plasmodium, trypanosoma, trichinosis, schistosomiasis, strongyloides
- Metabolic derangements, including hypoglycemia, uremia, hepatic encephalopathy
- Toxic ingestion
- Reye syndrome, toxic shock syndrome
- Tumor, abscess, hemorrhage

TREATMENT

- Need for treatment depends on cause/ complications
- No specific Tx available for encephalitis due to arboviruses, enteroviruses, adenovirus, Epstein-Barr virus, influenza B, measles, mumps, lymphocytic choriomeningitis virus, rabies
- Antiviral Tx unnecessary for immunologically mediated postviral encephalitis
- Herpes simplex: acyclovir, 1,500 mg/m^2/d div q8h
- Influenza A: amantadine, 5–8 mg/kg/d (max. 200 mg/d) div q12h

COMPLICATIONS

- Seizures, ↑ intracranial pressure, inappropriate secretion of antidiuretic hormone, respiratory decompensation

WHEN TO REFER

- Except postviral cerebellar ataxia, usually following varicella, pts w/viral encephalitis should be hospitalized often in consultation w/neurologist/pediatric infectious disease specialist because of need for specific Dx/management of complications

BACKGROUND

- Occurs in 1.5–2% of children
- Any process that affects brain development/function, constitutional/acquired, can produce mental retardation
- Aberration detected in early years if serious; etiology more likely to be identified in that setting
- 6 mechanisms considered for causation:
  - hereditary disorders
  - embryodysgenesis/chromosomal abnormality
  - serious preterm birth, placental difficulties
  - head injury, CNS infection
  - psychosocial deprivation
  - unknown
- If recognized later in life, w/ mild expression, origin may not be clear

CLINICAL MANIFESTATIONS

- Refers to person having (per AAMR definition) significantly subaverage intellectual functioning, existing concurrently w/ related limitations in 2/more of following adaptive skill areas: communication, self-care, home living, social skills, community use, self-direction, health/safety, functional academics, leisure, work
- ≥85% involved persons have "mild" retardation (IQ 50–70), 10% moderately affected; only 5% have severe/profound retardation
- Ultimately necessary to obtain appropriate/accurate evaluation of child w/ delays in development causing concern; planning of lifelong supports at stake

LABORATORY FEATURES

- Various laboratory studies helpful in understanding child's Dx/courses
- Include study of chromosomes in setting of unusual phenotype/CNS imaging if obscure brain disorder
- Urine screening for mucopolysaccharide/amino acid abnormalities
- Blood studies for thyroid, amino acids, lactate, variety of enzyme levels
- EEG, EMG, spinal fluid study, biopsies of skin, muscle, nerve, can have value in special situation

DIFFERENTIAL DIAGNOSIS

- Mental retardation can be simulated by situations that confound psychological testing, language development, personal social progress:
  - serious behavior disorders (w/ atypical responses or interaction)
  - early-onset hearing impairment
  - developmental aphasia, apraxia
  - serious chronic illness that hinders developmental experiences

TREATMENT

- Educational planning based on thoughtful assessment of child
- Support services as needed (habilitative Tx)
- Assistive technology, to enhance function/communication
- Health care that seeks preventive intervention/avoidance of 2° conditions
- Assistance to child/family for optimal personal growth
- Specialized Tx in particular situations, such as cardiovascular surgery in Down syndrome, bone marrow transplant in inborn errors of metabolism

COMPLICATIONS

- *Most common concern:* difficulty w/ adaptation/personal adjustment, leading to behavioral disorder
- Variety of "2° conditions" can occur as complications/contingencies of involved syndromes (skin, neuromuscular, skeletal, pulmonary, renal, etc)
- Serious "comorbidities" can add to difficulties for some persons, such as seizures, cerebral palsy, visual impairment

PREVENTION

- *Most central:* soundly implemented prenatal/newborn care
- Appropriate experiences (+ early education) for small child
- Reinforcement of family/its resources
- Thoughtful continuing health care for children (the "medical home"), including immunization, good nutrition, bicycle helmets, developmental review
- Preparation of youth for eventual responsibilities of parenthood
- Public health supports including folic acid supplement, pregnancy/newborn screening, lead control, alcohol education
- Genetic counseling when special risk involved

WHEN TO REFER

- If child's developmental course seriously altered, developmental pediatrician/neurologist can given useful insight
- If function/development lags, consultation w/ developmentally oriented physical therapist, occupational therapist/speech therapist can provide family/school w/ guidance/Tx for long-term care
- Clinical child psychologist needed in many situations, for measurement/counseling
- Often most/all these professionals can be found together in child development center/program

METATARSUS ADDUCTUS (METATARSUS VARUS)

GEORGE H. THOMPSON

BACKGROUND

- Most common foot deformity in infants/toddlers (1–3 yrs of age)
- Deformity usually due to in utero positioning
- *More common in first-born infants:* increased molding effect from primigranda uterus, abdominal wall
- ~5% incidence metatarsus adductus in subsequent siblings
- Occurs equally in males/females; 50% have bilateral involvement
- Questionable association w/ hip dysplasia/muscular torticollis; hips/neck require careful evaluation
- *Natural Hx:* 85% resolve spontaneously by 3 yrs of age

CLINICAL MANIFESTATIONS

- Adducted forefoot; convex lateral border; prominent base fifth metatarsal; concave medial border; neutral/slight valgus hindfoot
- Occasional mild separation between great/second toes
- *Variable forefoot flexibility:* passive flexibility assessed by stabilizing hindfoot in neutral position/applying gentle pressure over head of first metatarsal (not great toe); active flexibility elicited by stroking medial border of foot, producing withdrawal response
  - type I: forefoot actively/passively corrects past neutral (forefoot abduction)
  - type II: active forefoot correction to neutral position; passive correction past neutral
  - type III: rigid, uncorrectable deformity
- Vertical, medial midfoot skin crease: usually seen in rigid deformities

LABORATORY FEATURES

- No laboratory studies necessary

RADIOGRAPHIC FEATURES

- Radiographs not necessary for most deformities: does not demonstrate forefoot flexibility
- Indicated for rigid deformities, in those not improving w/ conservative management, in older children
- *AP/lateral weight-bearing/simulated weight-bearing radiographic views:* requires careful positioning, in infants; non-weight-bearing radiographs of *no* value

DIFFERENTIAL DIAGNOSIS

- *Metatarsus adductus:* forefoot adduction only
- *Metatarsus varus:* metatarsus adductus but w/mild forefoot supination; usually more severe deformity
- *Skewfoot:* complex deformity w/ forefoot adduction/supination, neutral midfoot/valgus hindfoot; rigid deformity that requires radiographs
- *Cavus foot:* elevated medial longitudinal arch w/mild forefoot adduction; usually associated w/underlying neuromuscular disorder, such as spinal dysraphism in young children; requires careful spinal/neurologic evaluation

TREATMENT

- *Metatarsus adductus/metatarsus varus:* recognize feet that need treatment—usually based on forefoot flexibility:
  - type I: observation; passive stretching into overcorrected/abducted position (usually not beneficial)
  - type II: observation/corrective orthosis: outflared shoe/commercial orthoses; usually worn 20–22 hrs/d × 6–8 wks; highly successful; passive stretching exercises of no value
  - type III: birth–4 yrs: serial short leg casts for 6–8 wks; perhaps longer in older children; cast change q1–2wks; best results when initiated <8 mos of age; Denis-Browne bar not recommended following operation
  - 4–5 yrs: surgery: soft tissue releases: abductor hallucis recession, medial release, tarsometatarsal/intermetatarsal release
  - 6+ yrs: surgery: metatarsal osteotomies/midfoot osteotomies

RESULTS

- Minimal, if any, disability even if complete correction not achieved spontaneously/w/ treatment. No pain, normal shoe wear

COMPLICATIONS

- *Nonoperative treatment:* mild recurrence; occasionally "searching" great toe seen for 1–2 yrs but this resolves w/ growth/development
- *Operative complications:* wound infection, incomplete correction

WHEN TO REFER

- Rigid forefoot deformity
- Infants w/ hindfoot valgus/cavus deformity
- Older child not improving w/ growth

BACKGROUND

1° Milia

- Represent miniature epidermal inclusion cysts that arise spontaneously from infundibulum of vellus hairs at level of sebaceous duct
- Caused by retention of keratin in superficial dermis
- 40–50% newborns during first few months of life

2° Milia

- May develop from any epithelial structure including hair, sweat duct, sebaceous duct/epidermis
- Usually follow trauma that results in full thickness epidermal injury/subepidermal blister
- Represent retention cysts caused by proliferative tendencies of skin after injury

CLINICAL MANIFESTATIONS

1° Milia

- Multiple/solitary 1–2 mm globoid firm papules
- May involve any cutaneous site
- Most common on face of newborns during first few months of life
- Solitary lesions (2–4 mm) on foreskin, nipple, scrotum, labia majora
- Resolve spontaneously w/normal desquamation of skin

2° Milia

- Look similar to 1° milia but appear in areas of trauma such as abrasions, lacerations, surgical scars, blistering disorders
- May be first clue to Dx scarring blistering disorders including epidermolysis bullosa, porphyria, immunobullous diseases (chronic bullous dermatosis of childhood, bullous pernphigoid, dermatitis herpetiformis)

LABORATORY FEATURES

1° and 2° Milia

- Skin biopsies show small epidermal cysts lined by stratified epithelium few cell layers thick
- Cysts contain lamellae of keratin
- Usually skin connected to vellus hair follicle

WHEN TO REFER

- Widespread 1° milia
- Progressive 2° milia
- Pt desires removal

JOSEPH G. MORELLI

BACKGROUND

- Caused by obstruction of eccrine sweat duct
- Neonates esp prone
- Incidence highest in hot humid climates where up to 30% may be affected
- May also occur in desert climates
- Individual susceptibility quite variable
- Easily reproducible by occlusion of skin under polyethylene 3–4 d
- No sex preference

CLINICAL MANIFESTATIONS

- Miliaria crystallina:
  - clear thin-walled 1–2 mm vesicles
  - no inflammation
  - develop in crops
  - usually on trunk
  - vesicles resolve within 24 h followed by superficial desquamation
- Miliaria rubra:
  - erythematous 1–4 mm papules
  - sometimes large wheallike lesions occur
  - may become pustular
  - may be present in large numbers
  - seen in areas of friction w/ clothing and in flexural areas
  - in infants lesions most commonly seen on neck, groin, axilla
  - discomfort often described as prickly sensation, thus term *prickly heat*

HISTOLOGY

- Miliaria crystallina:
  - obstruction of eccrine sweat duct within stratum corneum
- Miliaria rubra:
  - obstruction of eccrine sweat duct within epidermis and upper dermis

DIFFERENTIAL DIAGNOSIS

- Miliaria crystallina:
  - none
- Miliaria rubra:
  - erythema toxicum
  - viral exanthems
  - folliculitis
  - irritant reactions

TREATMENT

- No treatment usually necessary
- Powders/shake solution may be beneficial
- Avoid overheating

COMPLICATIONS

- 2° bacterial infection
- Disturbance of heat regulation

WHEN TO REFER

- Referral usually not necessary

MILK PROTEIN SENSITIVITY

LARRY W. WILLIAMS

BACKGROUND

- Dx describes infants who may have spectrum of adverse reactions to protein in formula
- *Other names:* "formula protein–induced enterocolitis," "allergic proctocolitis," "allergic colitis"
- Infants fed cow's milk formula, soy formula, or, uncommonly, breast milk (reactive to traces of immunogenic cow's milk protein from nursing mother's diet) may be affected
- Almost all affected infants rapidly recover if offending protein identified/excluded from diet for 6 mos; most then tolerate implicated protein
- Pathophysiology unclear; proof of antibody-mediated/cell-mediated immune causation lacking, but most assume immune mechanism; IgE probably not involved

CLINICAL MANIFESTATIONS

- Typically infants <4 mos of age
- Presentation variable w/ features of diarrhea, vomiting, malabsorption, failure to thrive
- Occult blood in stool common/gross blood may be seen
- Affected infants often mistakenly thought to have relapsing viral gastroenteritis/lactase deficiency
- Symptoms typically resolve within 48 hrs of stopping offending formula

- Large minority of cow's milk–sensitive infants also sensitive to soy protein; cross-reactivity differs from IgE-mediated food sensitivity, where simultaneous milk/soy allergy much less common

DIFFERENTIAL DIAGNOSIS

- *Infectious enteritis:* viral, bacterial, protozoal
- *2° malabsorption:* may follow an infectious process
- Severe combined immunodeficiency (may present at 3–6 mos w/ bloody diarrhea/failure to thrive)

DIAGNOSTIC MANEUVERS

- No diagnostic laboratory test
- Change of formula to hydration solution/casein hydrolysate (Nutramigen/Alimentum) should rapidly reduce diarrhea
- Return of symptoms when conventional formula started can occur in 2° disaccharidase deficiency/in milk protein sensitivity
- Endoscopy/biopsy not diagnostic/may reveal colitis w/ or w/o enteritis w/ mucosal/submucosal eosinophilic infiltration
- Dx depends on recurrence of symptoms when infant challenged w/ milk protein, 0.6 g/kg po (diarrhea, vomiting, increase in WBC, stool leukocytosis may occur w/ challenge)
- Impressive diarrhea/shock possible on

challenge; if performed, challenge should be limited to adequate medical facility

TREATMENT

- Implicated formula avoided for 4–6 mos
- Nutramigen/Alimentum; if not tolerated elemental (amino acid) formulas such as Vivonex required
- Reintroduction of unmodified cow's milk protein should be under medical observation; risk of severe reaction w/ milk protein; omission of initial diagnostic challenge does not avoid need for feeding under observation several months later

COMPLICATIONS

- If undiagnosed, condition may lead to failure to thrive, repeated/prolonged hospitalizations

WHEN TO REFER

- Many managed w/o referral if other significant illnesses eliminated on testing
- Referral warranted for significant weight loss before Dx suspected
- Infants w/ severe enteritis should be referred
- Infants w/ milder disease who do not tolerate trial of conventional formula within 6 mos should be referred for further evaluation

CHARLES A. BULLABOY

BACKGROUND

- *Pathology:* myxomatous proliferation of leaflet spongy layer disrupting fibrous core
- Phonocardiographic association of nonejection click(s)/mid–late systolic murmur w/ mitral valve prolapse (MVP) in 1961
- 2–5% prevalence in pediatric population; F:M ratio 2:1; autosomal dominant trait w/ varying penetrance
- Associated w/ at least 62 conditions: connective tissue (Marfan, Ehler-Danlos), cardiac (atrial septal defect), endocrine (thyroid), hematologic (Von Willebrand), genetic (Down, muscular dystrophy), skeletal

CLINICAL MANIFESTATIONS

- Asymptomatic overwhelming majority
- Consequence of hyperadrenergic tone/autonomic dysfunction: fatigue, exercise intolerance, palpitations, dizziness, near-syncope, rarely syncope, chest pain—nonanginal, nonexertional, ill defined, left precordial, sharp, fleeting/prolonged
- Transient ischemic attacks from purported microthromboembolism
- Thin gracile body habitus often w/ straight back, scoliosis, pectus, ligamentous laxity
- *Key to clinical Dx:* nonejection apical click/mid–late systolic murmur; principal cardiac feature related to ventriculovalvar disproportion; dynamic auscultation: ↓ LV volume, ↑ contractility, ↓ resistance to ejection augment click-murmur, move toward first heart sound

LABORATORY FEATURES

- *Electrocardiogram:* T-wave flattening-inversion in II, III, AVF, V5–6; ↑ QTc
- *Chest roentgenogram:* normal cardiopulmonary findings, generally not indicated unless evaluating mitral insufficiency/suspected coexisting cardiovascular malformations
- *Echocardiogram:* superior displacement of mitral valve leaflet/coaptation point above annular plane into left atrium sine qua non

DIFFERENTIAL DIAGNOSIS

- *Auscultatory mimics:* tricuspid valve prolapse, mitral regurgitation of hypertrophic cardiomyopathy/rheumatic heart disease, aortic valve click, ventricular septal defect w/ aneurysm of membranous septum
- Panic disorder w/ hyperventilation

TREATMENT

- *Prudent lifestyle:* regular exercise, avoidance of catecholamine stimulants—caffeine, nicotine, alcohol, certain OTC/"recreational" drugs
- Liberalizing fluid/salt intake for orthostatic symptoms
- *Beta blockers:* atenolol, 1–2 mg/kg/d po max 50–100 mg; for incapacitating fatigue, anxiety, palpitations w/ sinus tachycardia; wean after 3–6 mos symptom-free interval
- *Antiplatelet drugs for focal neurologic events:* ASA, 3–5 mg/kg/d po, max 325 mg; or dipyridamole, 3–5 mg/kg/d po, adult dosage 25 mg tid
- Infective endocarditis prophylaxis per American Heart Association recommendations

COMPLICATIONS

- Benign prognosis for most pts
- *Risk factors:* family Hx sudden cardiac death, syncope/neurologic incidents, mitral regurgitation, ↑ QTc, complex atrial/ventricular dysrhythmias

WHEN TO REFER

- *High-risk pts:* may require 24-hr ambulatory monitoring, exercise treadmill test, head-up tilt, cardiac catheterization/electrophysiologic study for complete evaluation
- Pts desiring to participate in competitive athletics
- Problematic chest pain/palpitations

MOLLUSCUM CONTAGIOSUM

PETER J. SUNENSHINE AND CAMILA K. JANNIGER

BACKGROUND

- Common viral infection of skin/mucous membranes in children of school age, sexually active adults, immunocompromised individuals
- Boys more often affected than girls
- Caused by pox virus of double-stranded DNA
- Two different viral strains have been reported (MCV I and II); no clinical differentiation noted between two strains
- Transmitted by fomites, close physical contact, autoinoculation
- Prevalence higher in tropical climates
- Sexually transmitted disease; however, infection commonly involves genital area of children who have not been abused
- Signs of AIDS; however, overwhelming majority of children w/molluscum contagiosum normal/healthy
- Risk factors for HIV may be discussed w/parents/HIV test offered on behalf of child
- Systemic histoplasmosis/systemic cryptococcus in AIDS pts may first be evident as cutaneous nodules virtually indistinguishable from molluscum contagiosum

CLINICAL MANIFESTATIONS

- *Papules:* 1–2 mm, smooth, discrete, dome shaped, pearly white/skin colored, sometimes reaching diameters 1–2 cm in immunocompromised; white core of papule may be expressed
- *Central umbilication:* apparent as papules enlarge
- *Erythema:* may be associated eczematous/inflammatory reaction surrounding papules
- *Distribution:* in children, lesions generally found on face (particularly eyes/mouth), trunk, extremities
- *Grouping:* usually multiple, occurring groups in one–two areas/widely disseminated; may coalesce to form plaques

- *Symptoms:* usually asymptomatic, but rarely pruritus, tenderness, pain may be present
- May involve eyelid to cause unilateral refractory conjunctivitis/rarely conjunctive nodule
- Presumptive Dx may be obtained from clinical observation/should be confirmed w/biopsy/histologic examination

LABORATORY FEATURES

- Material expressed from lesions can be placed on slide/stained by Wright, Giemsa, Gram, Papanicolaou method
- Microscopic evaluation shows characteristic pattern of numerous discrete ovoid homogeneous intracytoplasmic Feulgen-positive inclusion bodies, called molluscum bodies, which contain viral particles
- Papule well circumscribed, w/characteristic collection of virally infected keratinocytes
- Enlarged epidermal cells located above normal-appearing basal layer
- Molluscum bodies ↑ in size as infected cell moves toward surface
- Hematoxylin-eosin staining initially demonstrates enlarged cells as eosinophilic, but become basophilic as molluscum bodies enlarge/cells reach granular layer

DIFFERENTIAL DIAGNOSIS

- *Cryptococcus / histoplasmosis:* in immunocompromised, deep fungal infection may mimic this disorder
- Warts
- Intradermal nevus
- Syringoma
- Jessner lymphocytic infiltration
- Keratoacanthoma
- Trichoepithelioma
- Condyloma acuminatum
- Chalazion

TREATMENT

- Background:
  – gentle destruction: treatment modality used most; care should be taken not to be overly aggressive, esp in small children, as spontaneous resolution generally occurs in immunologically competent persons within 2–12 mos
  – lesions heal w/o scarring in absence of 2° bacterial infection; Tx warranted to prevent autoinoculation/transmission of virus to close contacts
  – >1 treatment often necessary because of recurrence/development of new lesions
  – molluscum contagiosum typically recalcitrant to Tx in HIV-infected individuals
- *Cryosurgery:* treatment of choice because cost effective, practical/gives good cosmetic results; freeze each lesion w/cotton-tipped applicator × 6–10 sec/repeat at 3 wk intervals as needed; in children, procedure can be facilitated w/eutectic mixture of local anesthetic (EMLA) such as lidocaine/prilocaine to relieve local discomfort; EMLA should be given 1 hr before treatment
- *Curettage:* this method supplies tissue specimen to confirm Dx, particularly important in immunocompromised child; EMLA may also be used; light electrodesiccation may also be employed after curettage
- *Chemical destruction:* application of retinoic acid, phenol, salicylic acid, lactic acid, cantharidin sometimes of value

COMPLICATIONS

- Recurrence
- 2° impetigo

WHEN TO REFER

- Some pts may be managed w/o referral
- Referral indicated if management fails/Dx in doubt
- Referral may be considered if associated w/immunosuppressed states such as AIDS

BACKGROUND

- Caused by rubulavirus, RNA virus in paramyxovirus family
- Spread person to person via infected droplets entering upper respiratory tract
- Most common in children 5–9 yrs of age
- Uncommon since use of mumps vaccine, although outbreaks attributed to 1° vaccine failure occur in vaccinated populations such as those in colleges/workplace

CLINICAL MANIFESTATIONS

- Incubation period ~18 d (range 14–25 d)
- Febrile URI alone in 30–70%
- Prodromal flulike illness followed by enlargement of one/more salivary glands, most commonly parotids, less often submandibular/sublingual glands
- Tenderness/swelling *covers* angle of jaw, bisected by line down through long axis of ear, ↑ 1–3 d, persists 1–3 d, subsides over next week
- Pain w/ chewing, sour/spicy foods/liquids
- Submandibulitis can be associated w/ bull-neck appearance, laryngeal/presternal edema; sublingual gland infection w/swelling of tongue/dysphagia

LABORATORY FEATURES

- *Viral isolation:* saliva, urine, CSF, fluid, blood, breast milk, infected tissues
- *Serologic testing:* enzyme immunosorbent assay (EIA), hemagglutination inhibition (HAI)/complement-fixation (CF) antibodies. Titers measured by neutralization assay, HI assay, and ELISA do not correlate well. Assessment of immunity to mumps virus remains problematical.
- Single positive mumps EIA IgM/CF against S (soluble) viral antigen indicates recent infection
- Positive EIA IgG indicates immunity
- Amylase ↑ 90% of parotitis, up to 3 wks; low levels in subclinical parotid infections
- Asymptomatic pleocytosis (up to 50% cases)

DIFFERENTIAL DIAGNOSIS

- Viral sialadenitis due to parainfluenza virus 1, 3; influenza A, Coxsackie virus A, echovirus, HIV, cytomegalovirus, lymphocytic choriomeningitis, mumps vaccine (Urabe) virus, adenovirus
- Bacterial (acute suppurative) sialadenitis due to *Staphylococcus aureus,* streptococcal species *(S. pyogenes, S. pneumoniae, S. viridans),* anaerobic bacteria (including Actinomyces sp.), gram-negative enteric bacilli, Salmonella sp., *H. influenzae, Pseudomonas pseudomallei, Bartonella henselae,* typical/atypical mycobacteria
- *Miscellaneous:* histoplasmosis, trichinosis
- *Ductal obstruction:* stone, tumor, chronic sialectasis
- Salivary gland tumor/cyst, leukemia, lymphoma
- Drugs that reduce salivary flow (anticholinergics, phenothiazines), iodides ("pyelography mumps"), isoproterenol phenylbutazone, oxyphenylbutazone, alpha-methyl DOPA, bromides, heavy metal (mercury, lead, copper) poisoning, thioruacil, thiocyanate, phenothiazines, nifedipine, cimetidine
- *Metabolic:* dehydration, malnutrition (including bulimia), obesity, diabetes mellitus, gout, uremia, hypothyroidism
- *Miscellaneous:* sarcoid (uveoparotid fever), cystic fibrosis, Kawasaki syndrome, Sjögren syndrome, benign lymphoepithelial lesion, Waldenström macroglobulinemia, systemic lupus erythematosis, pneumoparotitis, excessive starch ingestion, fibrous parotitis

TREATMENT

- *Symptomatic:* analgesics (acetaminophen, ibuprofen, naproxen), hot/cool compresses; avoid opioids if pancreatitis suspected
- *Avoid increased salivary flow:* no chewy, sour/highly seasoned foods/mucous membrane irritants such as peppermint
- *Epididymoorchitis:* cold packs, scrotal bridge for support, analgesics (opioids if necessary; see above)

COMPLICATIONS

- Symptomatic meningitis (10%), rarely, encephalomyelitis, neuritis, Guillain-Barré syndrome, cerebellar ataxia
- Orchitis (20% postpubertal males), epididymitis (85% of cases of orchitis), oophoritis (5% postpubertal females), pancreatitis (5%), rarely, thyroiditis, mastitis, arthritis, thrombocytopenic purpura, myocarditis/pericarditis, nephritis, deafness (labyrinthitis), fetal wastage
- *Prognosis:* serious dysfunction/fatalities due to encephalitis, myocarditis, nephritis exceedingly rare; testicular atrophy may occur/sterility rare

PREVENTION

- Mumps vaccine (combined w/ measles, rubella: MMR) at 12–15 mos/4–6 yrs of age; two doses ≥1 mo apart for older children lacking documented immunization/serologic immunity
- Postexposure mumps immunization of no proven effectiveness in preventing infection, but poses no risk/may prevent later infection
- Isolation w/ standard/droplet precautions for 9 d afer onset of swelling

WHEN TO REFER

- Complications requiring specialized care, eg, encephalomyelitis w/ severe CNS dysfunction, severe pancreatitis, myocarditis w/ heart failure, nephritis w/ renal failure, deafness

BACKGROUND

- Genetically determined diseases w/ quite different clinical manifestations
- *Clinical:* most show proximal ≥ distal muscle weakness/wasting; examination of family often helpful
- *Laboratory:* most have ↑ "muscle" enzymes (creatine kinase, transaminases, lactic dehydrogenase, aldolase); EMG abnormalities common but often not diagnostically required; muscle biopsy generally helpful, biochemically specific in some
- *Treatment:* generally nonspecific; should include physical/occupational Tx, genetic counseling for all, orthopedic/orthotic/prosthetic intervention where appropriate
- *When to refer:* due to their rarity, specialist nature of treatment/rapid molecular biologic developments in field, all children w/suspected dystrophy should have initial referral to neuromuscular specialist for Dx/treatment plan/family genetic counseling; specialist follow-up depends on rate of progression: 6/mo for Duchenne, yearly/less w/more benign types

Major Types	Heredity	First Manifestations
Duchenne	X-linked recessive	1–5 yrs
Becker	X-linked recessive	1st/2nd decade
Facioscapulohumeral	Autosomal dominant, some recessive	1st decade–adult
Myotonic	Autosomal dominant	Birth–adult
Limb girdle	Most autosomal recessive	1st–2nd decade

DUCHENNE MD

- *Clinical:* early milestones mildly delayed; then difficulty running; waddling gait, lordosis; frequent falls; use hands to "climb" up legs to rise from floor/chair (Gower sign), pseudohypertrophy of calves; frequent nonprogressive intellectual impairment (30% IQ <70)
- *Laboratory Dx:* ↑ "muscle" enzymes; creatine kinase several thousand IU/L; ~70% families have diagnostically specific DNA abnormalities of peripheral blood w/ deletion on Xp21 chromosome; muscle biopsy "dystrophic" changes w/ severely reduced/absent dystrophin levels
- *Progression:* wheelchair 7–10 yrs; 90% scoliosis after wheelchair confined; respiratory/cardiac muscle weakness second decade; death in second/early third decade
- *Treatment:* early regular physical Tx from parents; resting night splints to retard ankle contractures; spinal fixation when scoliosis progresses beyond 30%
- *Disputed Tx:* chronic high-dose corticosteroids delay progression; tendon releases/long leg braces delay progression to wheelchair

BECKER MD

- As for Duchenne, but onset late first decade or later, progression less severe
- Same laboratory abnormalities, muscle dystrophin mildly/moderately reduced/structurally abnormal
- Blood DNA and muscle dystrophin analyses commercially available

FACIOSCAPULOHUMERAL MD

- *Clinical:* characteristic facial weakness, inability to bury eyelashes, puff out cheeks, show teeth. Poor smile may result in social ostracization. Often winged scapula. Lower limbs less and later. Some families have intellectual, hearing impairment. Progression slow over decades
- *Laboratory:* muscle enzymes, EMG/biopsy may show only very mild abnormalities

SCAPULOHUMERAL AND SCAPULOPERONEAL MD

- Similar w/o facial involvement

MYOTONIC MD

- *Clinical:*
  - marked variability of onset and progression
  - weakness, including intrinsic hand, face/proximal muscles; nonprogressive intellectual impairment/mental retardation; cataract; characteristic facies w/ wasting of temporalis, masseter muscles, later male pattern frontal balding; cardiac conduction defects; hypersomnolence; of endocrine abnormalities
  - grip myotonia (inability to relax fingers after gripping examiner's hand
  - percussion myotonia (contraction of muscle w/ delayed relaxation after percussion of belly w/ tendon hammer)
- *Laboratory Dx:* muscle enzymes normal; muscle biopsy nonspecific; EMG, diagnostic "dive bomber" myotonic potentials; specific DNA analysis for trinucleotide repeats on chromosome 19 commercially available
- *Infantile form:* limited to children of affected mothers; severe weakness, hypotonia, mental retardation at birth; may not show myotonia/EMG changes in first year of life
- *Treatment:* myotonia may be relieved by phenytoin/procainamide; some require cardiac pacemakers; infantile form requires intensive early childhood intervention
- *Progression:* childhood form, slow over decades; infantile form, most learn to walk/show slow improvement in motor milestones over first decade; then progress like childhood

LIMB GIRDLE MD

- Clinically/genetically heterogenous group w/proximal limb muscle weakness/atrophy
- Onset first/second decade
- Laboratory abnormalities often mild
- Generally slow progression over decades

RARE DYSTROPHIES (ANALYSIS FOR SOME CAN BE PERFORMED AT RESEARCH CENTERS)

- *Severe childhood autosomal recessive MD:* males/females; phenotype similar to Duchenne. Reduced/absent adhalin in muscle
- *Congenital MD:* heterogeneous group, severe symptoms at birth/first few months of life; reduction/absence of merosin in muscle
- *Emery Deryfus MD:* autosomal dominant; slowly progressive from first decade; early contractures, cardiac involvement; reduction/absence of emerin in muscle
- *Fukuyama MD:* autosomal dominant; Japanese lineage; similar to Duchenne plus severe mental retardation

DIFFERENTIAL DIAGNOSIS

- Spinal muscular atrophy—infantile (Werdnig Hoffman)/juvenile (Kugelberg Weilander)
- Poly/dermatomyositis
- Parasitic myopathies
- Endocrine myopathies
- Acid maltase deficiency (Pompe disease)
- Congenital myopathies
- Mitochondrial myopathies
- Central core disease
- Myasthenia gravis
- Myotonia congenita

BACKGROUND

- Myasthenia gravis (MG) rare in childhood
- Three forms of MG in infants/children:
  - acquired autoimmune myasthenia gravis (juvenile myasthenia gravis, JMG):
    - accounts for 10–12% of cases of autoimmune MG in US
  - congenital myasthenia gravis (CMG):
    - heterogeneous group of syndromes
    - each due to specific architectural abnormality of neuromuscular junction/acetylcholine receptor complex
    - several distinct forms
  - transient neonatal myasthenia gravis (TNMG)
    - self-limited
    - occurs in 10–15% of infants born to mothers w/autoimmune MG
    - results from transplacental transfer of maternal anti-acetylcholine receptor (anti-AChR) antibody
    - occurs in seropositive/seronegative mothers
    - no correlation between severity of disease in mom/child
    - may be cause for arthrogryposis
- Association w/other autoimmune disorders, eg, thyroid disease, juvenile rheumatoid arthritis, juvenile diabetes mellitus
- Thymoma rare in children

CLINICAL MANIFESTIATIONS

- Fluctuating, variable fatigable weakness characteristic feature:
  - worse w/activity, improved w/rest only to recur w/resumption of activity
- Symptoms predominate in eyelids, muscles of eye movement:
  - complaints of ptosis, blurred/double vision
- Majority have "bulbar" weakness involving voice, chew, swallow
- Limb weakness common but unless severe may be difficult to ascertain

LABORATORY FEATURES

- Tensilon (edrophonium) testing improves strength in majority but not all pts
- Presence anti-AChR antibody diagnostic of autoimmune form of disease:
  - 10% of adolescents/40–50% of prepubertal pts are seronegative (may be confused for congenital form of disease)
- Decremental response to repetitive nerve stimulation signifies abnormality of neuromuscular transmission/does not specify which form of disease
- ↑ neuromuscular jitter (and blocking) on single fiber EMG most sensitive finding

DIFFERENTIAL DIAGNOSIS

- Important to distinguish autoimmune form of MG (JMG) from numerous forms of congenital MG (CMG):
  - may require therapeutic trial of IVIG/plasma exchange if pt seronegative
- Miller-Fisher variant of Landry-Guillain-Barré syndrome (oculomotor palsy, weakness)
- Brain tumor (oculomotor palsy)
- Mitochondrial myopathy (oculomotor palsy, ptosis, weakness)
- Botulism (weakness, ptosis)
- Tick paralysis (weakness)

TREATMENT

- Dependent on form of MG
- Autoimmune myasthenia gravis—similar to that used in adults:
  - cholinesterase inhibitors
    - often initial form of treatment
  - thymectomy:
    - most effective if done within 12 mos of symptom onset
  - immunosuppression (corticosteroids, cyclosporine, azathioprine):
    - must balance potential medication risk w/clinical benefit
  - transient immunomodulation (IVIG, plasma exchange):
    - short-term benefit
    - few adverse events
    - expensive
    - 1° role to reduce perioperative morbidity, to produce rapid improvement in critical situations, while waiting for immunotherapy to work, as chronic treatment in selected pts
- Congenital myasthenia gravis:
  - cholinesterase inhibitors 1° form of Tx
  - variable response in different genetic forms
  - aminopyridines (3,4-DAP) of benefit in some pts
  - immunotherapy/thymectomy not of benefit
- Transient neonatal myasthenia gravis:
  - primarily supportive care
  - occasionally requires cholinesterase inhibitors to improve strength (eg, suck, cry, respiration)
  - rarely require IVIG/exchange transfusion
  - therapeutic apheresis of mother prior to delivery may reduce severity of illness in child
  - no indication for thymectomy

COMPLICATIONS

- Severe generalized weakness may result in respiratory failure
- Numerous drugs may exacerbate myasthenic weakness, eg, aminoglycoside antibiotics, erythromycin, zithromax, beta blockers, calcium channel blockers
- *Steroid side effects:* Cushingism, growth limitation, bone demineralization, acne, weight gain
- *Immunosuppressive medication side effects:* drug specific but include bone marrow suppression, teratogenicity

WHEN TO REFER

- All pts should be referred to neurologist, preferably one w/neuromuscular expertise, to ascertain Dx/specific form of MG
- Complexities of treatment often require expertise of others such as neurologist, blood bank physician (for apheresis)

BACKGROUND

• Although >15 strains of nontuberculous mycobacterium (NTM) pathogenic for humans, infections in normal children rare/most often involve *Mycobacterium avium-intracellulare* complex (MAI)/*Mycobacterium marinum*
• *MAI:* common cause of persistent bacteremia in severely immunocompromised pts w/ AIDS
• *M. marinum* infections follow exposure to fresh/saltwater sources (home aquariums/abrasions while handling fish)/typically in older children
• MAI ubiquitous in environment, particularly around barnyards/swamps of southeastern US; age of usual infection in normal children: 1–5 yrs
• NTM infections not spread person to person

CLINICAL MANIFESTATIONS

• Subacute lymphadenitis of anterior cervical/submandibular lymph nodes usual illness following infection w/ MAI in normal children
• Lymph node swelling of >1.5 cm develops over 1–2 wks/initially nontender, nonfluctuant, not associated w/ fever/other systemic signs of illness
• *M. marinum* infections develop as nodules at site of minor trauma several weeks after exposure; in 3–5 wks, lesions enlarge to ulcerated/wartlike sores
• MAI bacteremia in AIDS pts presents w/ fever, night sweats, chills, anorexia, weight loss, weakness, generalized lymphadenopathy, hepatosplenomegaly

LABORATORY FEATURES

• W/ subacute lymphadenitis in normal children, intermediate strength tuberculin skin test may show 5–15 mm induration at 48 hrs; differentiation from tuberculosis includes lack of known exposure to active tuberculosis, negative chest x ray, absent/small tuberculin skin test reaction
• *Definitive Dx requires isolation of NTM:* biopsy of involved lymph node/skin lesion; blood culture if MAI bacteremia suspected

DIFFERENTIAL DIAGNOSIS

• *Lymphadenitis:* bacterial (*Staphylococcus aureus, Streptococcus pyogenes*), tuberculosis, cat scratch disease, mononucleosis, toxoplasmosis, histoplasmosis, brucellosis, tularemia, malignancy (esp lymphomas)
• *Skin lesions:* impetigo, sporotrichosis

TREATMENT

• For NTM lymphadenitis, complete surgical removal of all infected lymph nodes curative; surgery should be performed early in the course while lymph nodes encapsulated to avoid complications
• Medical management of NTM lymphadenitis not recommended due to resistance of MAI to most antituberculous medications
• *M. marinum* often self-limited/usually susceptible to rifampin, amikacin, ethambutol, trimethoprim-sulfamethoxazole, tetracyclines; Tx w/ two drugs × 3–4 mos usually therapeutic
• MAI bacteremia in AIDS pts treated w/ combinations of clarithromycin/azithromycin, rifabutin, ethambutol

COMPLICATIONS

• If not surgically removed, most lymph nodes infected w/ NTM eventually develop caseation w/ central erythema/fluctuance; nodes spontaneously rupture to form chronically draining fistula
• Partial biopsy may also result in chronic drainage
• If lymph node excision delayed until extensive caseation, removal of all infected material very difficult leading to high risk of recurrence; risk of surgical damage to facial nerve ↑

PREVENTION

• No methods to prevent NTM lymphadenitis
• Avoiding exposure to contaminated water sources only way to prevent *M. marinum* skin infection
• Risk of MAI bacteremia ↓ by initiating clarithromycin/azithromycin prophylaxis in AIDS pts w/ very low CD4 peripheral blood counts

WHEN TO REFER

• Pts w/ subacute lymphadenitis unresponsive to antibiotics effective for *S. aureus/S. pyogenes,* no other obvious etiology should be referred to surgeon for complete lymph node excision for culture and histology
• Infectious diseases specialist should be consulted for management of recurrent NTM lymphadenitis, *M. marinum* infections, children w/ AIDS

BACKGROUND

- Neural tube defect involving outpouching of meningeal sac containing nerve roots
- *Incidence:* 0.4–1/1,000 live births
- Multifactorial etiology w/both genetic/environmental influences (folic acid deficiency, valproic acid use early in pregnancy, diabetes mellitus, hyperthermia, alcohol use)
- Prenatal Dx available w/maternal serum alpha-fetoprotein

CLINICAL MANIFESTATIONS

- Sac-like lesion ranging from cervical to sacral levels, w/variable degrees of epithelialization
- Hydrocephalus present in at least 90% (Arnold-Chiari type II malformation)
- Neurogenic bladder/bowel in most

TREATMENT: NEONATAL

Neurosurgical
- Evaluate for hydrocephalus (serial head circumferences, head ultrasound/CT scans)
- Monitor for Arnold-Chiari problems (stridor, O_2 desaturation, dysphagia w/feeding difficulties, apnea)
- Shunt infections in 2–4%, generally within first 2 mos after shunt placement

Urologic
- Renal ultrasound/voiding cystourethrogram (VCUG) in newborns to evaluate for renal anomalies/vesicoureteral reflux
- Postvoid residuals to determine need for clean intermittent catheterization (CIC)
- May require prophylactic antibiotics if vesicoureteral reflux (VUR) present

Orthopedic
- Assess lower extremity function/position; deformities often present, may benefit from stretching/serial casting in neonatal period
- Assess for kyphosis/scoliosis; rarely kyphectomy may be required at time of back closure

TREATMENT: LONGITUDINAL

Neurosurgical
- Monitor for shunt malfunction (headache, vomiting, lethargy, changes in school performance/personality)
- Assess motor/sensory function, strength including upper extremity function, changes in bladder/bowel status, reflexes, to evaluate for complications such as tethered cord, syringomyelia, hydromyelia

Urologic
- Urologic function rarely static/requires ultrasounds, VCUGs at 6–12 mo intervals; urodynamics required to determine most appropriate management
- Usually require combination of CIC/medication (oxybutynin; ephedrine)
- Many have bacteriuria; pain, fever, foul-smelling urine, fatigue may require antibiotics; if asymptomatic, treatment involves increasing fluid intake/frequency of CIC; routine monitoring w/nitrite sticks may lead to overtreatment

Orthopedic
- Many require surgery to optimize function/allow for bracing
- *Mobility variable:* L_3/lower generally ambulatory w/moderate bracing, crutches; levels > L_3 usually rely on wheelchairs for greatest mobility

Bowel dysfunction
- Prone to constipation (may lead to encopresis)
- Management requires adequate fluids, high fiber diet, timed toileting; may require stool softeners, suppositories

Skin integrity
- Lack of sensation/decreased movement lead to decubiti
- Prevention of decubiti best management (daily skin checks, properly fitting braces/shoes, appropriate seating, sunscreens)

Obesity
- Early dietary counseling/intervention to reduce incidence of obesity
- Identify opportunities for exercise/activity, esp for those in wheelchairs

Endocrine issues
- May develop precocious puberty, usually central
- Often short stature due to ↓ growth in leg bones from paralysis (but may be due to growth hormone deficiency)

Latex allergy
- Reported incidence as high as 40% (contact *and* airborne)
- Symptoms range from local skin reactions to anaphylaxis; RAST testing available/not always reliable
- Latex gloves worst, but not only, offenders
- Reduce latex exposure in *all*/latex-free environment for those w/proven sensitivity

Seizures
- In ~15%; exclude shunt malfunction

Strabismus
- ~20% incidence; most require surgery

Learning
- ~70% normal intelligence
- Learning disabilities/ADHD in >50%
- Management requires appropriate classroom placement, behavioral strategies counseling; medications beneficial as adjunct

COMPLICATIONS

- ~5% of VP shunts malfunction per year
- Symptomatic A-C malformation occur in 10–20%
- Fractures of legs due to immobility

WHEN TO REFER

- Myelomeningocele clinic visits q3–6 mos in first year, q6–12 mos thereafter
- Shunt malfunction, symptomatic Arnold-Chiari malformation, tethered cord
- Increasing leg/back deformity, decubiti, worsening mobility, fractures
- Frequent urinary tract infections, hematuria

BACKGROUND

- Occurs in <1% of enteroviral infections; incidence may ↑ to ~4% of Coxsackie B virus infections
- Incidence reported as high as 16–20% of children dying suddenly
- Represents ~10% adult pts w/ recent-onset CHF/left ventricular dysfunction
- *Infectious etiology of myocarditis:* viral most common
  - *viral:* Coxsackie B1-5, A16; echovirus 9,11,22; adenovirus; parvovirus; influenza; respiratory syncytial virus; herpes simplex; mumps; HIV
  - *bacterial:* diphtheria, tuberculosis, typhoid fever, streptococcal, staphylococcal, pneumococcal; tetanus; pertussis, brucellosis
  - *protozoal:* trypansoma cruzi (Chagas disease); malaria; toxoplasmosis
  - *fungal:* candida; cryptococcosis, actinomycosis, coccidiomycosis; aspergillosis; histoplasmosis
  - *rickettsial:* Q fever, Rocky Mountain spotted fever
  - *metazoal:* trichinosis, schistosomiasis, echinococcosis; cysticercosis, ascariasis, filariasis, strongyloidiasis

CLINICAL MANIFESTATIONS

- Hx antecedent flulike illness/gastroenteritis
- Sx CHF including tachypnea, tachycardia, shortness of breath, diminished exercise tolerance, fatigue, malaise
- *Physical examination:* S_3 or S_4 gallop, soft apical blowing systolic murmur, rales, hepatomegaly
- *Fulminant presentation:* hypotension, shock, weak peripheral pulses, poor perfusion

LABORATORY FEATURES

- *Chest radiograph:* cardiomegaly common/heart size may be normal. ↑ pulmonary venous markings, pulmonary edema also present
- *Electrocardiogram:* usually sinus tachycardia/atrial/ventricular arrhythmias may be present; generalized low voltage; ST/T wave changes
- *Echocardiogram:* dilated, poorly contracting left ventricle; left atrial dilatation; color Doppler may reveal mitral regurgitation
- *Cardiac catheterization:* ↑ pulmonary capillary wedge/left ventricular end-diastolic pressures
- *Endomyocardial biopsy:* "gold standard" for definitive Dx/may be negative due to focal nature of inflammation; *characteristic findings:* inflammation in association w/ myocellular necrosis/degeneration

DIFFERENTIAL DIAGNOSIS

- Idiopathic dilated cardiomyopathy
- Anomalous origin of left coronary artery from pulmonary artery
- *Disorders of fatty acid metabolism:* carnitine deficiency, long (or medium) chain acyl CoA dehydrogenase deficiency
- Glycogen storage disease type IIa (Pompe)
- Familial/X-linked cardiomyopathy

TREATMENT

- Supportive Tx for mild–moderate heart failure:
  - digoxin: 10 mcg/kg/d IV/po qd/q12h
  - furosemide: 1 mg/kg/dose IV/po q6–q12h
  - captopril (may have selective advantage over other ACE inhibitors)
  - infants: initial 0.1–0.25 mg/kg/dose po q8h; titrate dose over several weeks to max 1.5–2 mg/kg/dose q8h
  - children: initial 0.3–0.5 mg/kg/dose po q8h; titrate dose to max 2 mg/kg/dose q8h
- Severe CHF:
  - dobutamine: 5–10 mcg/kg/min IV
  - dopamine: 2.5–10 mcg/kg/min IV
  - milrinone: 0.25–1 mcg/kg/min IV (dosing adjusted downward in renal insufficiency)
  - nitroprusside: 0.5–4 mcg/kg/min IV
- IV gamma globulin: 2 mg/kg IV as single dose; administer slowly to avoid volume overload
- *Corticosteroids:* efficacy controversial; consider using in pts who fail to respond to other supportive Tx
  - methylprednisolone: 10–15 mg/kg/d IV × 3 d
  - prednisone: 2 mg/kg/d po div bid

COMPLICATIONS

- Arrhythmias including atrial flutter/fibrillation, supraventricular tachycardia, ventricular ectopy, ventricular tachycardia, heart block
- Progressive heart failure
- Renal failure/multiorgan system failure

CLINICAL COURSE

- Recovery to normal/near normal ventricular function (60–70% pts)
- Recovery from acute phase but w/ persistent chronic dilated cardiomyopathy (20–30% pts)
- Death/require urgent heart transplant (10% pts)

WHEN TO REFER

- All pts should be referred to pediatric cardiologist at first sign of heart failure/cardiorespiratory symptoms suggestive of myocardial dysfunction

BACKGROUND

- *Two common presentations:* "floppy baby"/toddler w/ proximal weakness who moves slowly/clumsily
- Congenital myopathies tend to improve w/ time
- Muscular dystrophies generally display progressive weakness (exception: congenital muscular dystrophy)
- Most genetic diseases/can be treated but not cured at this time
- X-linked muscular dystrophinopathies (Duchenne/Becker) have incidence ~1/6,000 births (1/3,000 males); Becker milder/generally later onset than Duchenne
- Other childhood muscle diseases together have similar incidence
- Diagnostic testing by DNA rapidly advancing for both direct gene testing/testing of muscle proteins on biopsy specimens

CLINICAL MANIFESTATIONS

- Proximal weakness, often including Gowers sign
- Low muscle tone prominent in infantile myopathies
- Depressed deep tendon reflexes
- Enlarged calves in dystrophinopathies (Duchenne/Becker dystrophy)
- Cramps may occur due to excessive exercise in weak child (eg, walking 3 blocks)/cramps may be part of metabolic myopathy (eg, phosphofructokinase deficiency/McArdle disease)
- Neonatal/infantile presentations of myopathies typically include generalized hypotonia, "myopathic facies" (tented upper lip, ptosis), feeding difficulty, respiratory insufficiency (often w/o appearance of respiratory distress signs like retractions/w/ "paradoxical respirations")

LABORATORY FEATURES

- No single lab feature defines all muscle diseases
- ↑ CPK
- *Blood DNA tests:* a dystrophin gene deletion/duplication identifies 70% children w/ dystrophinopathies; excessive triplicate repeats of DNA base pairs identifies myotonic dystrophy
- New disease-specific markers may become available
- Electromyogram/nerve conduction velocity
- *Muscle biopsy:* in dystrophies shows muscle cell loss, pyknosis, ballooned cells, fiber/fat replacement of muscle plus absent/altered dystrophin in dystophinopathies
- Sural nerve biopsy to look for specific neuropathies (eg, inflammatory)
- Occasional presentation as unexplained ↑ "liver enzymes" (which are really also muscle enzymes, eg, LDH, SGOT, SGPT
- EKG, echocardiogram may identify associated cardiomyopathy

DIFFERENTIAL DIAGNOSIS

- Neuropathy
- Anterior horn cell disease esp spinal muscular atrophy
- Myasthenia (various forms)
- Myopathy:
  - congenital myopathies
  - congenital muscular dystrophy
  - metabolic myopathies
  - toxic myopathy (eg, steroids)
- Muscular dystrophy:
  - Duchenne-Becker dystrophy (dystrophinopathies)
  - autosomal recessive similar conditions
  - myotonic dystrophy
- Poly/Dermatomyositis
- Acute diseases (eg, flu-related myositis, Guillain-Barré syndrome)

TREATMENT

- *Medications:* prednisone, 0.75 mg/kg/d for Duchenne (optional, noncurative, slows progression of weakness, may prolong ambulation 2 yrs, typical steroid; 2 mg/kg/d for polymyositis Tx
- *Orthopedic:* tendon-lengthening procedures may be performed to return feet to plantigrade posture/then apply orthoses
- *Orthotics*
- *Adaptive:* power/standard wheelchairs, standing devices, Texas catheters, reachers/grabbers, mobile arm supports
- *Genetic counseling*

COMPLICATIONS

- *Related to weakness:* fractures, scoliosis, constipation, skin sores from orthoses/seating, joint contractures, swallowing difficulties, respiratory symptoms, obesity, sleep disorders, psychosocial difficulties
- *Related to other body systems:* cardiomyopathy, learning disabilities/mental retardation

WHEN TO REFER

- Chronic weakness
- Persistent floppy baby
- Acute weakness w/o obvious explanation
- Persistent ↑ CPK
- Recurrent muscle cramps
- Muscle biopsy should be done at specialized center (for proper selection of biopsy site plus handling/proper selection of pathologic/muscle protein stains)

BACKGROUND

- Dermatomyositis most common acquired myopathy in children; polymyositis/myositis associated w/ collagen vascular disease rare causes of myopathy in children
- Peak incidence 5–10 yrs of age
- Systemic vasculopathy affecting skin, muscle, connective tissue, GI tract, small nerves
- Not associated w/ malignancy like adult-onset disease
- Full recovery 80% w/adequate treatment
- Mortality 5%

CLINICAL MANIFESTATIONS

- Usually insidious, but rarely fulminating, onset of fever, malaise, fatigue over weeks–months prior to skin/muscle signs
- Rash beginning w/ eyelid erythema, edema (heliotrope) progressing to involve periorbital/malar regions of face and extensor surfaces of extremities
- Progressive proximal muscle weakness, stiffness/pain
- Rash/weakness variable in severity from case to case
- Early development of joint contractures
- Late development of SubQ calcifications

- Infarction of GI tract/rarely other organs leading cause of death

LABORATORY FEATURES

- Serum creatine kinase usually/not always ↑ early in course
- ESR/other tests of chronic inflammation usually normal
- Electromyography always abnormal w/ neuropathic/myopathic features
- Muscle biopsy diagnostic showing perifascicular muscle fiber atrophy/necrosis w/ inflammation

DIFFERENTIAL DIAGNOSIS

- Polymyositis
- Viral myositis
- Systemic juvenile rheumatoid arthritis
- Systemic lupus erythematosis
- Eosinophilic fasciitis
- Trichinosis
- Sarcoidosis
- Cysticercosis

TREATMENT

- *Corticosteroids:* prednisone, 2 mg/kg/d until strength improves, then qOd; slowly taper 5–10 mg q mo until strength/creatine kinase normal; maintenance Tx 10–20 mg qOd × total course 2 yrs: may cause significant side effects of steroid excess w/ Cushing syndrome, glucose intolerance, hypertension, osteoporosis w/ spinal compression fractures
- *Methotrexate:* 20 mg/m^2/wk for prednisone treatment failures/for steroid sparing; monitor liver function carefully
- IV gamma globulin: 2 g/kg/IV over 2–4 days for treatment failures/acute relapses; anecdotal evidence for efficacy
- Physical Tx to prevent contractures

COMPLICATIONS

- Calcinosis of SubQ tissues in 50%—*calcinosis universalis* severe complication
- GI infarction; rarely cardiac/renal involvement
- Late progression/relapse

WHEN TO REFER

- Most pts should be referred for electromyography/muscle biopsy
- Referral indicated for serious complications, treatment failure to initial management/complications of Tx

Clinical Feature	Dermatomyositis	Polymyositis	Myositis w/ Collagen Vascular Disease
Peak age incidence	5–10 yrs of age	>12 yrs of age	>12 yrs of age
Onset	Insidious, rarely fulminant	Insidious	Variable
Systemic Sx	Fever, malaise, fatigue	Rare	Variable CNS, renal and hemopoetic disease
Rash	Periorbital, malar, extensor surfaces	None	Variable
Weakness	Moderate–severe	Mild–moderate	Mild
Contractures	Early, severe	Late, moderate	Late, mild
Response to Tx	Good	Variable	Variable

BACKGROUND

• Commonly associated w/ acute URIs (most commonly influenza)
• Pathogenic organism traditionally been taught as *Mycoplasm pneumonia;* however, new evidence supports viral etiology
• *P. aeruginosa* may also be isolated from ruptured bullae
• In some children, same organisms isolated in acute otitis media may be isolated from bullous myringitis
• Recovery nearly 100%, although some may have residual hearing loss

CLINICAL MANIFESTATIONS

• Serous/hemorrhagic blebs can be seen around inner bony surface of external auditory canal/sometimes on tympanic membrane

• Rupture of blebs leads to serosanguinous discharge from ear
• Other symptoms of acute URI may be present (fever, malaise, ear pain)
• Hearing loss present in some pts
• Severe ear pain often present

LABORATORY FEATURES

• Cultures not necessary

DIFFERENTIAL DIAGNOSIS

• Herpes zoster oticus (Ramsay Hunt syndrome)
• Otitis externa
• Acute otitis media

TREATMENT

• Same topical ear drops used for otitis externa may be used

• If otitis media present, appropriate systemic antibiotics indicated
• Pain management w/ analgesics may be necessary

COMPLICATIONS

• Sensorineural hearing loss may be present in ~ one-third of affected ears/mixed hearing loss in another one-third[1]

WHEN TO REFER

• If hearing loss is suspected, baseline audiogram indicated

---

[1]Hoffman RA, Shepsman D: Bullous myringitis and sensorineural hearing loss. Laryngoscope 93:1544, 1983.

DENNIS P. GROGAN

BACKGROUND

• Accessory navicular one of several supernumerary bones that may normally occur in foot
• May be present 4–14% of population; most remain asymptomatic
• Usually becomes symptomatic in adolescent age group (averaging 10–12 yrs old)
• More often symptomatic in girls

CLINICAL MANIFESTATIONS

• Pain over medial aspect of foot
• Tenderness localized to bony prominence on medial aspect of foot
• May be soft tissue swelling/erythema over prominence medially
• Symptoms aggravated by activity/relieved w/ rest, immobilization
• Pain elicited by passive eversion/pronation of foot, which puts tension on insertion of posterior tibial tendon, w/ active inversion of foot against resistance
• Foot may be pronated, w/ loss of longitudinal arch

ANATOMY

• Posterior tibial tendon attaches to medial/plantar aspect of navicular. Accessory navicular medial/plantar to main body of navicular; receives significant part of insertion of posterior tibial tendon; size of accessory bone varies few millimeters–>1 cm

PATHOLOGY

• Accessory navicular connected to main portion of navicular via cartilaginous synchondrosis
• Acute trauma/more commonly, chronic stress across this synchondrosis may lead to "stress fracture" through area w/ resultant inflammation; this fracture through cartilaginous tissue has poor healing potential; area of injury is cause of symptoms

RADIOGRAPHIC FEATURES

• Separate ossification center medial/plantar to navicular
• *Radiographic views to diagnose:* AP, lateral, external oblique views of foot
• External oblique view most helpful; most clearly profiles accessory navicular
• Classification:
  – type I: small ossicle within posterior tibial tendon
  – type II: large triangular bone attached via cartilaginous synchondrosis (most commonly symptomatic)
  – type III: cornuate navicular, probably resulting from fusion of accessory navicular to main navicular

DIFFERENTIAL DIAGNOSIS

• Posterior tibial tendonitis
• Fracture of the navicular
• Chronic ankle sprain
• Köhler disease (ischemic necrosis of the tarsal navicular)
• Tarsal coalition

TREATMENT

• *Acute:* immobilization in short leg cast may be effective to ↓ inflammation/relieve pain
• *Chronic:* recommendation to ↓ activity level, cast for immobilization/orthosis to provide arch support/control of pronation may relieve symptoms
• If conservative measures not effective in providing relief, surgical resection of accessory bone should provide relief; insertion of posterior tibial tendon needs to be partially released to allow excision of accessory bone along w/ synchondrosis/prominent portion of main navicular; tendon then reattached to main navicular/will require period of cast immobilization postop to allow tendon to heal; advancement of posterior tibial tendon not necessary

COMPLICATIONS

• Delay in Dx most common complication; failure to suspect Dx/obtain correct radiographic views to make Dx are usual reasons for delay

WHEN TO REFER

• Most often accessory navicular may be found incidentally on radiographs of foot taken for another reason; no treatment indicated
• When symptomatic accessory navicular diagnosed/suspected, referral to orthopedic surgeon recommended

ACNE NEONATORUM

BACKGROUND

- *Incidence:* 20% newborns
- *Onset:* typically after 1–2 wks of life
- *Resolution:* spontaneous, usually within first year
- Etiology:
  – maternal androgen stimulation of sebaceous glands
  – Malassezia furfur

CLINICAL MANIFESTATIONS

- Comedones, inflammatory papules, pustules
- *Distribution:* cheeks, forehead, chin

LABORATORY FEATURES

- Direct microscopy of pustular lesion may show the yeast Malassezia furfur

DIFFERENTIAL DIAGNOSIS

- Miliaria rubra
- Atopic dermatitis
- Seborrheic dermatitis
- Staphylococcal pyoderma
- Milia

TREATMENT

- Daily cleansing w/soap and water
- Ketoconazole cream 2×/d if direct microscopy (+) for yeast

COMPLICATIONS

- Nodulocystic acne, esp if steroids applied
- Chronicity of lesions

WHEN TO REFER

- Referral indicated for complications, when Dx in doubt or if lesions do not spontaneously remit

ERYTHEMA TOXICUM

BACKGROUND

- *Incidence:* 50% term infants (decreased incidence in premature infants)
- *Onset:* first 24–48 hrs (range: birth–10 d)
- *Resolution:* clears in 4–5 d
- *Etiology:* unknown; hypothetical etiologies include absorption of intestinal toxins, neonatal allergy, chemical/mechanical irritation

CLINICAL

- Red, evanescent, blotchy macules, papules, and pustules
- Resembles flea bites
- *Distribution:* face, trunk, proximal extremities
- Usually spares palms and soles

LABORATORY FEATURES

- Tzanck prep of pustule reveals eosinophils
- Blood eosinophilia 7–15%
- Biopsy not indicated unless suspecting other Dx

DIFFERENTIAL DIAGNOSIS

- Neonatal pustular melanosis
- Congenital candidiasis
- Miliaria rubra
- Incontinentia pigmenti
- Eosinophilic pustular folliculitis
- Herpes simplex
- Impetigo
- Milia

TREATMENT

- None indicated
- Need to r/o infectious causes of neonatal pustules w/gram stain, bacterial and viral cultures, KOH smear and fungal culture

COMPLICATIONS

- None

WHEN TO REFER

- Atypical onset or when Dx in doubt

MILIA

BACKGROUND

- *Incidence:* 40–50% infants
- *Onset:* birth–several yrs
- *Resolution:* 1–3 mos
- *Etiology:* retention of keratin and sebaceous material within pilosebaceous apparatus

CLINICAL

- 1–2 mm tiny, white cyst
- Distribution: face, esp around eyes

LABORATORY FEATURES

- None

DIFFERENTIAL DIAGNOSIS

- Acne neonatorum
- Erythema toxicum
- Neonatal pustular melanosis

TREATMENT

- Usually none required
- For persistent lesions, gentle extrusion may be indicated

COMPLICATIONS

- None

WHEN TO REFER

- If lesions very numerous (may be associated w/congenital syndromes)
- Lesions persistent and need extrusion

BACKGROUND

- Most frequently found in preschool children (80% <6 yrs of age at onset)
- Male predominance (3:2)
- Rarely leads to renal failure
- *Characterized by relapses:* 76–97% relapse, 50% frequent (>3/y), 25% spontaneously remit
- Idiopathic nephrotic syndrome can have several histologic characteristics:
  - minimal lesion (MLNS): 80%
  - focal segmental glomerular sclerosis (FSGS): 10%
  - membranoproliferative glomerulonephritis (MPGN): 5%
  - diffuse mesangial proliferative: 3%
  - membranous nephropathy: 2%
- Nephrotic syndrome can also be 2° to 1° disease process (eg, lupus, hepatitis)

CLINICAL MANIFESTATIONS

- Edema, usually periorbital, pretibial
- Oliguria

LABORATORY FEATURES

- Proteinuria ($\geq$40 mg/m^2/hr)
- Hypoalbuminemia (<2.5 g/dL)
- Normal creatinine
- Normal serum complement (except in MPGN)
- Normal CBC
- Hypercholesterolemia

DIFFERENTIAL DIAGNOSIS

- Malnutrition
- Heart failure
- Liver failure
- Protein-losing enteropathy
- Allergy

TREATMENT

- Symptomatic treatment includes:
  - salt restriction during relapse
  - albumin infusion for (1) massive edema and (2) rehydration
  - diuretics (furosemide [Lasix] 2 mg/kg/d)
- Initial episode:
  - prednisone: 60 mg/m^2/d $\times$ 4 wks, then 40 mg/m^2 qOam $\times$ 4 wks then stop
- Relapse:
  - prednisone: 60 mg/m^2/d until proteinuria clears for 2–3 d then 40 mg/m^2 qOd $\times$ 4 wks

COMPLICATIONS

- *Thrombosis:* renal vein, peripheral veins, pulmonary embolus
- *Spontaneous bacterial peritonitis:* usually due to *S. pneumoniae* or *E. coli*; *S. pneumoniae* vaccine should be given at appropriate time

WHEN TO REFER

- Growth failure due to frequent use of daily steroids
- Failure to obtain remission after 4 wks of daily steroid Tx
- Nephrotic syndrome in child <1 yr of age
- $\uparrow$ serum creatinine for age

ANDREW J. GRIFFITH

BACKGROUND

- Highly variable degrees of severity, symmetry, progression of hearing loss
- ~1/1,000 children born w/hearing impairment in US
- 50% of cases thought to be genetic; may be associated w/any one of hundreds of genes
- One-third genetic cases thought to be inherited as part of syndrome
- Two-thirds genetic cases thought to be nonsyndromic (ie, isolated hearing loss)
- In some ethnic populations, large proportion of nonsyndromic recessive deafness may be caused by mutations in *GJB2* (Connexin 26) gene
- Nongenetic etiologies include maternal/systemic infections, untoward events during first trimester, birth, perinatal complications (eg, kernicterus), head trauma, ototoxic medications, meningitis
- X-linked/autosomal recessive cases as well as new dominant mutations may appear sporadic

CLINICAL MANIFESTATIONS

- ↓/absent responses to auditory stimuli
- Delayed development of expressive/receptive language skills
- Occasional balance difficulties, including delays in motor milestones such as walking/sitting
- Severe vertiginous episodes rare; can be manifested by head tilting, vomiting; suggest perilymph fistula from malformed inner ear to middle ear
- Meningitis can be caused by ascending infection from perilymph fistula
- Numerous different nonauditory features can be associated w/syndromic hearing loss

LABORATORY FEATURES

- UA/blood urea nitrogen, creatinine, glucose (can detect Alport syndrome, diabetes, etc)
- Thyroid function tests (hypothyroidism may indicate Pendred syndrome/cretinism)
- CBC (may indicate anemia/infection)
- Renal ultrasound (obtain if branchial/ear malformations suggest branchio-oto-renal syndrome)
- EKG (QT interval may be prolonged as part of Jervell and Lange-Neilsen syndrome)
- ESR, ANA, rheumatoid factor (↑ values may indicate autoimmune etiology)
- Viral immunologic tests (obtain if maternal CMV, rubella, HSV, syphilis, toxoplasma infection suspected)
- Audiometry/tympanometry (indicates type, severity, symmetry of hearing loss)
- Thin-section CT scan of temporal bones (may detect middle/inner ear anomalies)
- *GJB2* mutation testing (currently performed on research basis)

DIFFERENTIAL DIAGNOSIS

- Conductive hearing loss
- Central auditory processing disorders

TREATMENT

- Specific Tx directed toward causative/associated conditions (eg, infection, diabetes, etc)
- Speech/language evaluation and rehabilitation
- Conventional hearing amplification/assistive devices
- Cochlear implantation as indicated/desired

COMPLICATIONS

- Meningitis due to ascending infection from perilymph fistula
- Morbidities due to associated disorders

PREVENTION

- Newborn hearing screening for early detection, treatment, rehabilitation
- Avoid acoustic trauma/ototoxic medications
- Avoid head trauma if vestibular aqueduct(s) enlarged on CT scan
- Aggressively treat conditions such as chronic otitis media that may cause further hearing loss

WHEN TO REFER

- *Otolaryngologist:* always
- *Audiologist:* always
- *Speech therapist:* as indicated
- *Medical geneticist:* in all sporadic/familial cases where etiology could potentially be genetic
- *Ophthalmologist:* r/o Usher syndrome if etiology could be genetic/if nongenetic etiology can be associated w/ocular pathology (eg, CMV)
- *Other specialists:* as indicated by presence of associated pathology

BACKGROUND

- One of group of neuroblastic tumors (neuroblastoma, ganglioneuroblastoma, ganglioneuroma)
- Most common extracranial solid tumor in childhood (8–10% of all childhood cancers); prevalence: 1/7,000 births; 550 cases/yr in US; M:F:1.2:1
- Mean age at Dx: 22 mos; 36% <1 yr, 79% <4 yrs, 97% <10 yrs
- Some believe as many as one-half of all tumors may regress w/o Tx prior to detection
- MYCN (N-myc) oncogene amplification in 25%: associated w/advanced disease, rapid progression, poor prognosis; deletions short arm chromosome 1 (1p) common in tumor

CLINICAL MANIFESTATIONS

- Can arise anywhere along sympathetic nervous system chain or adrenal gland; 65% in abdomen, mostly adrenal
- If in abdomen: fullness, discomfort; occasionally bladder/bowel symptoms; may obstruct lymphatics, causing scrotal/leg edema
- Chest tumors: often coincidentally found on x-ray; may cause Horner syndrome (unilateral ptosis, myosis, anhidrosis), superior vena cava syndrome
- Paraspinal tumors may cause nerve root/spinal cord compression resulting in paraplegia
- Proptosis/periorbital ecchymosis frequent; 2° to retrobulbar/orbital infiltration
- Skin involvement common in stage IV-S disease
- Paraneoplastic syndrome presentation: opsomyoclonus
- Secretory diarrhea 2° to vasoactive intestinal peptide (VIP) secretion (mostly ganglioneuroblastoma/ganglioneuroma)

DIFFERENTIAL DIAGNOSIS

- Pathologic finding: "small blue round cell" also seen w/Ewing sarcoma, non-Hodgkin lymphoma, primitive neuroectodermal tumors, undifferentiated soft tissue sarcomas (eg, rhabdomyosarcoma)
- Neuroblastoma, particularly if catecholamine negative (5%), can be mimicked by other conditions, particularly disseminated bone disease (osteomyelitis, rheumatoid arthritis)
- VIP presentation can be confused w/inflammatory bowel disease
- Opsoclonus-myoclonus/atoxic syndrome presentation can resemble 1° neurologic disease

DIAGNOSIS

- To confirm Dx, biopsy of tumor needed; on occasion, bone marrow may be sufficient if marrow involved w/typical cells; some feel compatible radio/sinographs plus positive urine catecholamines sufficient for Dx
- 90–95% of tumors have ↑ urine catecholamines; at least 2 catecholamines/metabolites (eg, urine HVA/VMA) must be measured; values ≥3 SD mean for age = ↑
- Appropriate CT/MRI/bone scan used as needed
- Meta-iodobenzylguanidine (MIBG) scintigraphy highly specific for detection of tumor/metastasis; not available in all institutions
- In addition to histopathology, tumor tissue preferably studied for immunophenotype, MYCN gene copy number, tumor cell DI, expression of TRK-A

STAGING

- 3 major staging systems were used in past depending on pediatric oncology group preference; table illustrates current International Neuroblastoma Staging System (INSS)

Stage 1	Stage 2A	Stage 2B	Stage 3	Stage 4	Stage 4S
Localized tumor confined to the area of origin; complete gross excision, w/or w/o microscopic residual disease; identifiable ipsilateral/contralateral lymph nodes negative microscopically	Unilateral tumor w/incomplete gross excision; identifiable ipsilateral/contralateral lymph nodes negative microscopically	Unilateral tumor w/complete/incomplete gross excision; w/positive ipsilateral regional lymph nodes; identifiable contralateral lymph nodes negative microscopically	Tumor infiltrating across midline w/or w/o regional lymph node involvement; or unilateral tumor w/contralateral regional lymph node involvement; or midline tumor w/bilateral lymph node involvement	Dissemination of tumor to distant lymph nodes, bone, bone marrow, liver, other organs (except as defined in stage 4S)	Localized primary tumor as defined for stage 1 or 2 w/dissemination limited to liver, skin, or bone marrow

TREATMENT

- Surgery: should be undertaken only at center w/full range of pediatric surgical specialties; makes Dx, establishes staging (w/other studies), removes tumor if possible; importance of gross surgical resection remains controversial
- Chemotherapy: predominant management modality; cyclophosphamide, cisplatin, doxorubicin, epipodophyllotoxins (tenoside/VM-26, etoposide/VP-16), vincristine: most commonly employed in one/more combinations
- Radiation Tx: largely used in multimodality management of residual tumor, bulky unresectable tumor, disseminated disease

PROGNOSIS

- Low risk: infants and children w/INSS stages 1 and 2A; infants w/INSS stages 2B, 3, 4S
  – stage 1, regardless of age 90% disease-free survival w/surgery alone
  – stage 2A (all ages), 2B/3 (infants): 2 yr survival = 85%, 87%, 89%, respectively; Tx w/surgery + minimal chemotherapy
  – stage 4S: survival 57–90% regardless of type of treatment
- Intermediate risk
  – stage 2B/3 (children), 4 (infants): 40–60% survival w/aggressive multimodality Tx
- High risk
  – stage 4 (children): overall survival <15% even w/multimodality Tx

WHEN TO REFER

- All pts suspected/confirmed w/neuroblastoma should be referred to pediatric cancer treatment center w/comprehensive diagnostic treatment facilities

NEUROCUTANEOUS MELANOSIS

SONALI G. HANSON AND MOISE L. LEVY

BACKGROUND

- Rare congenital syndrome characterized by presence of large/multiple congenital melanocytic nevi, benign/malignant pigment cell tumors of leptomeninges
- Thought to represent error in morphogenesis of embryonal neuroectoderm
- Occurs sporadically/equally in males, females
- Usually presents in neonates; may not become apparent until second decade of life
- When neurologic symptoms present, clinical course characterized by progressive deterioration/early death

CLINICAL MANIFESTATIONS

- Congenital nevi in neonates/infants ~9 cm in diameter on head/6 cm on body/20 cm in adult/that are ≥3 in number
- Two-thirds have giant congenital melanocytic nevi, most commonly in lumbosacral distribution; one-third have numerous lesions w/o single giant lesion
- Almost all have nevi on posterior midline areas/on head/neck
- No malignant melanoma transformation of involved skin area
- Small proportion have neurologic Sx/2°

melanosis of nervous system; most frequently manifest by age 2 yrs; Sx ↑ intracranial pressure (irritability, lethargy, headache, recurrent vomiting, generalized seizures, ↑ head circumference, bulging anterior fontanelle, photophobia, papilledema, neck stiffness, occasionally cranial nerve palsies)
- Presence of intracranial masses may manifest as focal seizures
- ~ two-thirds develop hydrocephalus
- May experience expressive aphasia, ataxia, hemiparesis/paraparesis, paralysis, sensory loss, sciatica, bowel/bladder dysfunction
- Developmental delay may be present
- Pts presenting near puberty may have Sx intracranial mass lesions/spinal cord compression (psychiatric symptoms, expressive aphasia/dysarthria, focal seizures, localizing sensorimotor changes)
- Definitive Dx NCM requires histologic confirmation of CNS lesions

LABORATORY FEATURES

- CSF pressure may be ↑; typically ↑ protein level, normal glucose level, sterile leukocytosis
- EEG may demonstrate either focal/generalized abnormalities

- Hydrocephalus/mass lesions may be identified w/imaging
- MRI may show signal suggesting melanocytosis

DIFFERENTIAL DIAGNOSIS

- Neurofibromatosis

TREATMENT

- No specific treatment
- Palliative surgical measures, such as shunt placement to reduce intracranial pressure, may result in transient improvement

COMPLICATIONS

- Leptomeningeal melanoma may develop, w/ possibility of metastases
- Progressive neurologic deterioration even in face of histologically benign CNS lesions, due to structural damage

WHEN TO REFER

- When neurologic symptoms occur
- For ophthalmologic exam
- For evidence of developmental delay

BACKGROUND

• *Neurofibromatosis 1 (NF1/von Reckling-hausen/neurofibromatosis 2 (NF2):* autosomal dominant, genetic disorders primarily affecting cell growth/development; 50% NF1 cases spontaneous mutations (no family Hx)
• NF1/NF2 clinically/genetically different diseases

	NF1	NF2
Population incidence	1/4,000	1/40,000
Chromosome locus	17q11.2	22q11.2

CLINICAL MANIFESTATIONS

• *NF1/NF2:* wide range of manifestations
• *NF1/NF2:* manifestations often age dependent (definite Dx in prepubertal child can be ambiguous)
• Clinical Dx based on NIH Consensus criteria[1]:
• *Dx NF1:* At least two of following:
  – 6/> café-au-lait macules (>5 mm, prepubertal; >15 mm, postpubertal)
  – 2/> neurofibromas of any type/one plexiform neurofibroma
  – freckling in axillary/inguinal region
  – optic glioma
  – 2/> Lisch nodules (iris hamartomas)
  – distinctive osseous lesions—sphenoid dysplasia/thinning of long bone cortex w/ or w/o pseudarthrosis
  – first-degree relative w/ NF1 by above criteria
• *Dx NF2:* At least one of following:
  – bilateral acoustic neuromas
  – first-degree relative w/ NF2 and either unilateral acoustic neuroma/two of the following: meningioma, schwannoma, neurofibroma, presenile lens opacity

[1]Neurofibromatosis Conference statement. National Institutes of Health Consensus Development Conference. Arch Neurol 45:575–578, 1988.

LABORATORY FEATURES

• No routine tests necessary to establish Dx NF1/NF2; DNA analysis/Protein Truncation Test commercially available but rarely indicated; children w/ NF1 should be monitored for school problems/psychological testing if problems occur
• Imaging may be used to confirm Dx/detect complications of NF1/NF2:
  – bone radiographs—pseudarthrosis, kyphoscoliosis/sphenoid wing aplasia in NF1
  – neuroimaging:
    ○ NF1: CT/MRI of brain to exclude optic gliomas/other intracranial neoplasms; T2-weighted cranial MRI often reveals high-signal-intensity foci
    ○ NF2: CT scan of temporal bone/cranial MRI may detect acoustic neuroma

DIFFERENTIAL DIAGNOSIS

• Multiple café-au-lait spots
• McCune-Albright syndrome
• Tuberous sclerosis
• Noonan syndrome
• Proteus syndrome (the "elephant man")
• Multiple lipomatosis

TREATMENT

• Early detection of complications:
  – NF1: yearly physical examination including measurement of BP, ophthalmologic examination, developmental assessment
  – NF2: yearly audiogram, CT/MRI
• Treat complications in same manner as when occurring in general population

COMPLICATIONS OF NF1

• Neurofibroma:
  – cutaneous/SubQ neurofibroma: disfiguring in adolescents/compressive neuropathies
  – plexiform neurofibroma: pain, disfigurement, serious dysfunction, malignancy
• Learning disabilities 40% NF1
• *Pain:* headaches/pain associated w/neurofibroma
• *Tumors:* optic glioma the most common (15%)/brain stem glioma
• Rarely strokes/seizures
• *Disturbances of growth/sexual development:* macrocephaly, short stature, precocious puberty
• *Orthopedic:* pseudarthrosis (tibial bowing), kyphoscoliosis, bone overgrowth
• *Hypertension:* essential, renal artery stenosis/pheochromocytoma
• *Other non-CNS malignancies:* leukemia more frequent, neurofibrosarcomas (most common malignant tumor, unusual in children)
• *Miscellaneous:* pruritus (proportionate to neurofibroma burden), constipation (10%)

PREVENTION

• Genetic counseling of affected individuals/other family members

WHEN TO REFER

• Suspected NF1/NF2
• Known NF1/NF2: pts w/ Sx major complications (academic problems, persistent pain, persistent headache, seizures, hypertension, rapidly growing neurofibroma, visual/hearing disturbances, disfiguring neurofibromas, neurologic deficits, unexplained visceral complaints)

BACKGROUND

- *Definition:* absolute neutrophil count (ANC) <1,000 cells/UL
- *Ethnic variation:* ANC 200–600 cells/UL less in blacks
- Occurs at any age
- Characterized as intrinsic defects of marrow/extrinsic factors on marrow
- Can be classified as simple neutropenia/neutropenia in association w/ other immune deficits

CLINICAL MANIFESTATIONS

- Mouth, skin, ear infections; apthous stomatitis common in cyclic neutropenia
- Frequent deep infection esp pneumonia
- Always risk of septicemia (less in pt w/ cyclic neutropenia/pts w/ otherwise intact immune system)
- In absence of neutrophils, character of infection changes; physical/radiologic exam of infection dependent on white cell killing/pus formation

TREATMENT

- Neutropenia w/ no signs of fever/illness:
  – maximum immune system (check immunoglobulins, verify T-cell function w/ skin testing)
  – maximize nutrition
  – antibiotic prophylaxis often used in Kostmann syndrome/neutropenic pts who demonstrate recurrent infection; should in general be avoided
  – pneumocystis prophylaxis for neutropenia/immune compromise (trimethoprim-sulfa; 3 d/wk)
  – high risk for esophagitis; if significant epigastric pain, consider endoscopy/candida esophagitis
- Neutropenia w/ fever/obvious site of infection:
  – aggressively culture/treat w/broad-spectrum antibiotics until cultures available
  – culture leading edge of cellulitis
  – sinusitis possible sign serious opportunistic infection
  – chest disease requires admission/treatment w/broad-spectrum antibiotics/trimethoprim-sulfa if pneumocystis suspected; bronchoscopy entertained if no improvement after 48–72 hrs, rapid deterioration of lung function, unusual radiologic patterns (eg, reticulonodular/pattern suggestive of nonbacterial infection)
  – in absence of white cells, evaluation of abdomen rendered difficult; if severe abdominal pain, antibiotic anaerobic coverage used; serial examination w/ careful attention to bowel sounds, distention, tenderness in right lower quadrant (coecum commonly affected); serial KUBs performed if concern about perforation/pneumatosis intestinales
- Neutropenia w/ fever/no source of infection:
  – pt w/immune neutropenia/acute postviral neutropenia less prone to bacteremia, opportunistic infection/rapid spread of localized infection; nonetheless, should have cultures taken of blood/other sites/receive 48–72 hrs parenteral antibiotics
  – pts w/ neutropenia/immune system dysfunction treated w/ broad-spectrum antibiotics (eg, ceftriaxone) plus agents designed to treat *Pseudomonas aeriginosa*. If white cells expected to return broad-spectrum antibiotics should be continued in hospital until ANC >500 even if specific organism identified; if no expectation of return of ANC, may treat as above for 10–14 afebrile d w/ negative cultures
- Reappearance of fever after becoming afebrile cause for concern/constant vigilance; possibility of superinfection w/resistant organisms/emergence of opportunistic infection (esp Candida/other fungi)
- Failure to become afebrile suggests:
  – viral infection
  – closed space infection/infection on foreign object (eg, implanted catheter)
  – gut/mucosal barrier breached, endotoxemia
  – bacterial infection not sensitive to current antibiotic regimen
  – opportunistic infection
  – decision to move to more complex antibiotic regimens/add new medications (eg, antifungal agents) should follow observation for at least 48 hrs (unless level of toxicity increasing); continued serial physical examination/radiologic investigation warranted

Cause of Neutropenia	Potential Modalities to Raise ANC
Cyclic neutropenia	G-CSF for acute episodes
Kostmann syndrome	G-CSF for acute episodes
Schwachman syndrome	Optimize nutrition; G-CSF for acute episodes
Chronic neutropenia	Although less reliable, G-CSF for acute episodes
Viral-induced neutropenia	ANC returns spontaneously
Sepsis (bacterial overwhelming)	Aggressive antibiotic Tx
	Value of G-CSF unclear; bone marrow may be necessary to assess value
Neonatal	Fresh whole blood exchange transfusion; G-CSF under study
Immune neutropenia	Steroid treatment, IV gamma globulin
Bone marrow failure	G-CSF, GMCSF
Drug induced:	
Immunosuppressives	G-CSF, GMCSF
Anticonvulsants/sulfonamides, etc	Discontinue drug
Systemic illness	Treat illness

COMPLICATIONS

- Life-threatening sepsis
- Chronic abscess formation
- Toxicity from frequent antibiotic use including emergence of resistant organisms, ototoxicity, renal/GI toxicity

WHEN TO REFER

- Viral-induced neutropenia/immune neutropenia, usually managed w/ referral; refer if bacterial sepsis/if localized infection requires treatment to raise ANC
- Neutropenia associated w/immune deficit best managed in tertiary setting

BACKGROUND

• Common autosomal dominant multiple congenital anomaly syndrome; likely genetic heterogeneity w/ one causative gene mapped to 12q
• Offspring of affected individuals have 50% risk to inherit syndrome
• Marked variability of expression of clinical manifestations w/ age-related evolution of facial phenotype
• Incidence 1/1,000–1/2,500 live births/high proportion due to new mutation
• *Pathogenesis may be associated w/ jugular lymphatic obstruction:* webbed neck/pterygium colli may follow in utero cystic hygroma; disruption of normal tissue migration/organ placement by lymphedema may explain cryptorchidism, wide-spaced nipples, low-set posteriorly rotated ears, abnormal dermatoglyphics; abnormal lymphatics at base of developing heart may contribute to high risk of structural defect by reduction in right-sided cardiac blood flow

CLINICAL MANIFESTATIONS

• *Growth:* average length/weight at birth; failure to thrive in infancy; prepubertal growth usually parallels third centile; pubertal growth spurt often reduced/absent; delayed bone age in up to 20%; detailed growth curves available
• *Craniofacial:* age-related evolution of facial features; *newborn:* tall forehead, hypertelorism, downslanting palpebral fissures, broad depressed nasal root, small upturned nasal tip, well-grooved philtrum w/ "cupid's bow" lips, micrognathia, excess nuchal skin, low posterior hairline; *infant:* tall forehead, prominent eyes w/ level fissures, hypertelorism, hooded lids, depressed nasal root; *childhood:* often coarse, almost myopathic expression, increasingly triangular face shape w/ broad forehead tapering to small chin, longer neck w/ webbing or prominent trapezius; *adult:* subtle phenotype, triangular face, prominent nasolabial folds; at all ages, low-set, posteriorly rotated ears w/ thickened helix; eyes often striking blue or blue-green; hair may be wispy, curly/wooly
• *Cardiac:* abnormal structure in two-thirds: valvular pulmonary stenosis (50%), ASD (10%), asymmetric septal hypertrophy (10–20%); left axis deviation may be present even in structurally normal heart
• *Genitourinary:* cryptorchidism (70%) may lead to delayed puberty/deficient spermatogenesis in males; female pubertal timing/fertility generally normal
• *Skeletal:* characteristic pectus w/carinatum superiorly, excavatum inferiorly; broad thorax w/wide-spaced nipples; rounded shoulders; cubitus valgus; clinobrachydactyly
• *Lymphatic:* dysplasia, hypoplasia, aplasia of lymphatic channels, pulmonary/intestinal lymphangiectasia, in utero hydrops/cystic hygroma, excess of whorls on fingertip dermatoglyphics 2° to SubQ fluid accumulation in utero
• *Behavior/development:* motor delays: may be 2° to hypotonia/relative macrocephaly; language delay 2° to perceptual motor disabilities, mild hearing loss, or articulation abnormalities; IQ < unaffected family members, mild mental retardation in up to third of cases

LABORATORY FEATURES

• Coagulopathy 20%: factor XI deficiency, von Willebrand disease, platelet dysfunction; screen w/ PT, PTT, bleeding time

DIFFERENTIAL DIAGNOSIS

• Williams syndrome
• Intrauterine exposure to alcohol, primidone
• Aarskog syndrome
• Cardiofaciocutaneous syndrome
• Costello syndrome

TREATMENT

• Surgical correction of some cardiac defects/cryptorchidism
• Tx/correction of specific bleeding diathesis where possible
• Growth hormone Tx where growth hormone deficiency substantiated

WHEN TO REFER

• Many pts managed w/o referral
• Specialty referral may be indicated for evaluation of cardiac status, short stature/delayed puberty; investigation of excessive bruisability/workup of potential coagulopathy prior to elective surgery; orchidopexy

BACKGROUND

- ↑ among US children/adolescents; affects ~1/5 children
- Among girls, non-Hispanic blacks predominate; among boys, Mexican Americans predominate
- Occurs when energy consumed exceeds metabolic expenditure in genetically predisposed individual
- Not all obese children become obese adults; risk of adult obesity greatest for the most obese children and those obese later in adolescence
- No universally accepted definition of obesity; definition most accepted: body mass index (BMI) calculated as weight (in kilograms) divided by height (in m²); national norms exist for each age/gender
- BMI at 85th percentile conservative, may overdiagnose; BMI at 95th percentile clearly obese

CLINICAL MANIFESTATIONS

- Meets BMI criteria for obesity *or* >20% expected for height
- Look for underlying medical cause; <1% cases
- Look for complications due to overweight (e.g. hypertension)/affecting ability to follow diet/exercise recommendations (e.g. asthma)
- Look at family support, social, psychological stresses

LABORATORY FEATURES

- Generally, lab work not required
- Studies to look for medical cause should *not* be done unless suggested by historical/physical findings
- Best use of lab to evaluate complications identified in Hx/physical examination
- Screening for dyslipidemias at discretion of physician

DIFFERENTIAL DIAGNOSIS

- *Endocrine disorders:* hypothyroidism, Cushing disease, primary hyperinsulinism, pseudohypoparathyroidism
- *Genetic syndromes:* Prader-Willi, Alstrom, Laurence-Moon-Biedl, Carpenter, Cohen
- *Acquired hypothalamic lesions:* infection, trauma, neoplasms, vascular malformations
- Key points to consider:
  – obesity due to nutritional excess: pts usually tall for age, mentally normal, no other physical stigmata, often other family members obese
  – obesity due to endocrine, genetic/other hypothalamic disorder: pts usually short for age, often mentally retarded, associated physical stigmata, other family members seldom affected
- *Rule of thumb:* if pt's height has been consistently above 50th percentile, pt has obesity due to nutritional excess

TREATMENT

- Aimed primarily at modifying eating/exercise behavior
- *Very low calorie diets (<1000 Kcals/d):* considered experimental in children
- *Medications:* experience in children limited; may be important in future
- *Surgical interventions:* virtually never used in children
- Eating/exercise recommendations should be specific, tailored to child's developmental level; should involve entire family; need to increase skills/modify environment; school/other community support extremely helpful
- Enlist aid of local nutritionist/dietitian
- May need to address other psychological/social stresses
- 1–2 lbs weight loss/mo reasonable goal in most cases; ideal body weight frequently unrealistic
- Weigh weekly in office/school; monitor for complications

COMPLICATIONS

- *Obstructive sleep apnea:* becoming more common, can be life threatening, can occur even after tonsillectomy/adenoidectomy
- *Cardiovascular risk factors:* hypertension, NIDDM, dyslipidemias
- *Orthopedic problems:* Blount disease, slipped capital femoral epiphysis
- *Gallbladder disease:* uncommon
- *Skin problems:* intertrigo, benign acanthosis nigricans
- *Menstrual irregularities:* polycystic ovarian syndrome

PREVENTION

- *Critical periods for development of obesity:* ages 5–7 yrs and adolescence
- Ask about eating/exercise during routine office visits
- Discuss importance of limiting television to 1–2 hrs/d
- Suggest regularly scheduled meals/snacks, avoid eating from emotional upset/boredom
- Limit fast foods, eating out to 1–2 occasions/wk
- Remind parents that they are role models for eating/exercise patterns of their children

WHEN TO REFER

- Referral indicated for serious complications of obesity, such as obstructive sleep apnea
- Refer to mental health professional any pt w/ depression, binge eating pattern, serious emotional problem
- Many pts benefit from referral to dietitian

BACKGROUND

- *Snoring:* common indication for evaluation
- 7–9% children snore nightly
- Clinical significance of habitual snoring underappreciated
- 1–2% have clinically significant airway obstruction
- *Peak occurrence:* 3–6 yrs; uncommon <1 yr
- Role of inheritance unclear

CLINICAL MANIFESTATIONS

- Spectrum of illness ranges from benign (1°) snoring to severe partial airway obstruction w/ or w/o complete airway obstruction (apnea)
- *1° snoring (PS):* vibratory inspiratory noise created in upper airway; not associated w/ gas exchange abnormalities/clinical problems other than embarrassment
- *Upper airway resistance syndrome (UARS):* similar noise to PS except sleep disruption/daytime symptoms occur
- Obstructive sleep apnea syndrome (OSAS):
  - asleep: loud snoring w/ retractions, rib cage paradox, periods of complete airway obstruction (obstructive apnea: silent periods interrupted w/ snoring), unusual sleep positions, gas exchange abnormalities (hypoxemia/hypercapnia)
  - awake:
    - behavioral personality changes ranging from grogginess, dull, flat affect, depression, to irritability/aggressiveness
    - cognitive difficulties
    - hyponasal speech, chronic nasal obstruction, chronic mouth breathing
    - failure to thrive
    - excessive daytime sleepiness (uncommon)
    - cor pulmonale (uncommon)

LABORATORY DATA

- *Screening:* no effective screening tool other than perhaps home videotaping
- Diagnostic:
  - polysomnography
  - abnormality defined by presence of obstructive apnea, hypoventilation, hypoxemia, ↑ work of breathing/abnormal sleep parameters (frequent arousals, abnormal sleep patterns)
- Assess severity:
  - Hgb: polycythemia
  - electrolytes: evidence of CO_2 retention
  - EKG/echo: evidence of right ventricular hypertrophy

DIFFERENTIAL DIAGNOSIS

- Includes differential Dx snoring (ie, PS, UARS, OSAS); noisy breathing during sleep (laryngomalacia, nocturnal asthma); excessive daytime sleepiness (narcolepsy, poor sleep habits)

DIAGNOSIS

- Hx snoring not sufficient to separate 1° snoring for which treatment not indicated from UARS/OSAS for which Tx warranted; if primary care physician documents by clinical observation, obstructive breathing in child w/ other clinical manifestations of OSAS, reasonable to defer other diagnostic studies/proceed w/ treatment

LABORATORY EVALUATION

- Tests:
  - overnight oximetry:
    - may be difficult to maintain w/o problems w/ false alarms/artifacts
    - may miss children w/ UARS w/o significant desaturation
  - videotaping:
    - potential screening tool
  - polysomnography:
    - records EEG, sleep oximetry, respiration, end-tidal CO_2, EKG
    - "gold standard" for Dx OSAS/UARS

TREATMENT

- Hx snoring alone not sufficient indication to refer child for treatment, esp surgery; Dx OSAS/UARS must be made before surgery
- *1° snoring:* no treatment needed; counseling for parents/child
- *UARS/OSAS:* for most children, tonsillectomy/adenoidectomy treatment of choice
  - CPAP/BiPAP (nasal ventilation) for those who don't respond to T&A
  - role of nasal steroids/decongestants unclear

COMPLICATIONS

- Delayed Dx
- Intellectual impairment
- Cor pulmonale
- Failure to thrive

WHEN TO REFER

- Children w/ suspected severe OSAS, ie, pts w/ associated cor pulmonale/failure to thrive
- children <2 yrs w/ snoring
- Children w/ predisposing conditions (ie, craniofacial syndromes, CNS injury)
- Persistent symptoms following Tx for OSAS
- Initiate/titrate nocturnal noninvasive ventilation

OBSTRUCTIVE UROPATHY

DAVID R. CHAVEZ, JEFFREY E. TABER, AND LOWELL R. KING

BACKGROUND

- *Cause:* congenital most common in children (in adults generally acquired)
- Obstruction/reflux combined w/infection damages growing kidney rapidly; infected urine combined w/vesicoureteral reflux causes significant renal scarring, esp in polar regions
- Chronic obstruction causes progressive tubular dilation/cellular atrophy; by 28th day of obstruction 50% of medulla lost, marked atrophy of proximal tubules has occurred, cortex thinned; glomeruli last to be damaged/show histologic evidence by day 28
- 69 days longest reported time in humans that completely obstructed kidney has recovered some function after relief of obstruction
- Acute unilateral ureteral obstruction changes renal blood flow (RBF)/ureteral pressure in three phases:
  – RBF/ureteral pressure ↑ in phase I (1.5 hrs)
  – RBF ↓/ureteral pressure ↑ in phase II (1.5–5 hrs)
  – RBF/ureteral pressure ↓ in parrallel in phase III (>5 hrs)
- Vesicoureteral reflux can occur w/obstruction of the lower urinary tract/leads to ↑ voiding, storage pressures; persistently ↑ bladder pressures (>40 cm H_2O) have been shown to cause upper urinary tract damage; poorly compliant bladders found in pts w/urethral valves, spina bifida, non-neurogenic neurogenic bladders (Hinman-Allen syndrome)
- ~50% of nephrons must be damaged before serum creatinine increases
- Congenital ureteropelvic junction obstruction more common on left side

CLINICAL MANIFESTATIONS

- In absence of infection/acute obstruction may be no clinical signs; progressively worsening urinary tract obstruction may be clinically silent
- First indication may be UTI, palpable abdominal mass, gross hematuria, vague abdominal pain, failure to thrive, persistent enuresis
- Level of obstruction can be anywhere from intrarenal collection system to urethral meatus; very distal obstruction in male child can present as spraying, narrowing of stream, slow voiding, dribbling, ballooning of foreskin

- UPJ/UVJ (ureterovesical junction) obstruction may present as gross hematuria after minor abdominal/flank trauma/flank pain after drinking

LABORATORY FEATURES

- Variable depending on stage of obstruction; renal function may be normal/significantly ↓; hyperkalemic distal renal tubular acidosis (RTA type IV) w/obstructive uropathy
- Screening urine dipstick/spun microscopic urine analysis can often exclude intrinsic renal disease/systemic diseases (juvenile onset diabetes, group A hemolytic poststreptococcal nephritis, Henoch-Schönlein nephritis, nephritis of subacute bacterial endocarditis, hemolytic-uremic syndrome, systemic lupus erythematosus)/also screen for proteinuria, glucosuria, microscopic hematuria, renal tubular cells, red cell and granular casts/signs of infection
- Urine concentrating function, sodium reabsorption, hydrogen excretion, GFR and renal blood flow impaired in chronic obstruction

DIFFERENTIAL DIAGNOSIS

- Ureteropelvic junction obstruction
- Multicystic dysplastic kidney
- Childhood polycystic kidney disease (autosomal recessive)
- Calyceal diverticulum
- *Megaureters:* obstructing/nonobstructing
- Vesicoureteral reflux (2°)
- Ureterocele
- Prune belly syndrome
- Ectopic ureter
- Non-neurogenic neurogenic bladder (Hinman-Allen syndrome)
- Myelodysplasia w/neurogenic bladder
- Rhabdomyosarcoma of the bladder/prostate
- Posterior urethral valves
- Anterior urethral valve
- Meatal stenosis

TREATMENT

- Dictated by level of obstruction, renal function, presence or absence of infection
- Once level of obstruction has been determined (ultrasound, cystogram, IVP, CT scan, retrograde pyelogram) quantitate renal function w/functional study (radionucleotide renal scan); this does not apply to pts in acute renal failure/clinically urosep-

tic (in these prompt relief of obstruction paramount)
- Most accurate means of assessing renal function/possible recovery: percutaneous nephrostomy; if after 2–3 mos kidney not contributing ≥15% total renal function/child older than 4 yrs of age, elective nephrectomy should be considered
- In neonates, if postnatal hydronephrosis/hydroureteronephrosis present obtain VCUG after initiating amoxicillin prophylaxis (10 mg/kg/d)/will diagnose vesicoureteral reflux. If in males VCUG also examines for urethral valves
- To diagnose ureteropelvic junction obstruction (UPJ)/possibly more distal obstruction/quantitate renal function, obtain DTPA/MAG 3 lasix renal scan (w/continuous bladder catheter drainage in infants); in neonate, if only one kidney present/bilateral UPJ obstruction suspected, renal scan should be performed during first wk of life
- Postobstructive diuresis occurs after bilateral obstruction relieved but rarely becomes life threatening if child alert/able to drink fluid ad lib
- Earlier surgical repair of neonatal UPJ obstruction yields maximal improvement in renal function; other series have suggested that observation in neonates w/UPJ obstruction/good renal function safe option; "observationists" assume they can intervene in future if renal function deteriorates while still obtaining results that earlier surgery produces; this assumption not been proven in controlled randomized studies
- Priorities in children w/spina bifida:
  – preserve nephrons
  – urinary continence: in overzealous attempt to make child dry upper urinary tract may be permanently damaged

COMPLICATIONS

- Urosepsis
- Hypertension
- Renal failure
- Stone formation
- Bladder decompensation
- Stunted growth

WHEN TO REFER

- Involve pediatric urologist early if any question regarding obstruction of GU system; w/proper timing of correct intervention renal function can be stabilized/often improved

OSGOOD-SCHLATTER DISEASE AND SINDING-LARSON-JOHANSSON DISEASE

WENDI JOHNSON AND GREGORY L. LANDRY

BACKGROUND

- *Apophysis:* outgrowth of bone, including 2° ossification center
- *Traction apophysitis:* inflammation in these areas from repetitive microtrauma at bone-tendon junction during periods of rapid growth/high activity
- OSD affects tibial apophysis
- SLJD affects patellar apophysis

CLINICAL MANIFESTATIONS

- Usually athletic pts, but similar lesions occur in children w/ spastic cerebral palsy
- Ages 10–15; girls 10–11 yrs, boys 13–14 yrs
- M:F ratio = 3:2
- *Location:* OSD L > R, 25% bilateral, SLJD usually unilateral
- Dull, achy pain (rarely sharp) w/insidious onset; OSD/SLJD symptoms exacerbated by impact loading (running, jumping, stairs)
- Examination maneuvers that provoke pain:
  - OSD: palpation of tibial tubercle, resisted knee extension, passive hyperflexion, occasionally w/ passive patellar subluxation
  - SLJD: palpation of inferior pole of patella, quadriceps contraction, patellar compression
- Other examination findings:
  - full active ROM
  - tight hamstrings, quadriceps, heel cords
- Findings sometimes associated w/ OSD:
  - genu valgum
  - excessively pronated feet
  - "miserable malalignment": femoral anteversion, external tibial torsion
  - heel pain due to Sever disease (calcaneal apophysitis)

RADIOGRAPHIC FEATURES

- Indications for x ray:
  - persistent pain not responding to treatment
  - acute exacerbation of injury
- *OSD:* normal/soft tissue swelling anterior to tibial tuberosity, heterotopic bone may form anterior/superior to tubercle (ossicles)
- *SLJD:* fragmentation of inferior pole of patella
- 4 radiologic stages (OSD/SLJD):
  - I: normal
  - II: fragmentation
  - III: coalescence of fragments
  - IVa: incorporation into tibia (OSD) or patella (SLJD): b: separate calcified mass (ossicle)

DIFFERENTIAL DIAGNOSIS

- Patellar contusion
- Prepatellar bursitis
- Patellar tendonitis
- Osteomyelitis
- Patellar chondromalacia
- Tibial spine avulsion fracture
- Meniscal tear
- Fat pad impingement syndrome
- Stress fracture
- Patellofemoral pain syndrome
- Enthesopathy
- Tumor
- Pes anserine bursitis
- Bipartite patella
- Patellar subluxation

TREATMENT

- Relative rest, reduce impact loading (eg, biking, swimming), ↓ activity if limping
- Quadriceps, heel cord/hamstring stretching
- Ice 15–20 min as needed
- NSAIDs/acetaminophen for analgesia
- Arch supports/better shoes for hyperpronation
- Knee pads if kneeling
- Subjective symptomatic improvement *may* be noted w/ patellar stabilizing brace/neoprene sleeve
- If severe pain (ie, consistent limp w/ walking), crutches 2–3 wks

COMPLICATIONS

- Avulsion fracture of tibial apophysis
- Patella alta
- Genu recurvatum
- Enlarged tibial tuberosity
- Ossicles/persistent pain

WHEN TO REFER

- Immediate referral if tibial spine avulsion fracture suspected on x ray
- If not improving in 3–6 mos (most cases totally resolved in 1–2 yrs/definitely by skeletal maturity)
- If pain interferes w/ activities of daily life/unresponsive to treatment
- If pain/ossicle on x ray after skeletal maturity
- If unsure of Dx

BACKGROUND

- *Definition:* osteocartilaginous lesion affecting articular surface and subchondral bone
- *Etiology:* osteochondritis dissecans of knee and elbow:
  - micro-trauma causing subchondral fracture (osteochondral fracture: severe)
  - avascular bone from microtrauma
  - anatomic variation, predisposition
  - relation to 2° ossification centers
  - steroids (adults)

CLINICAL MANIFESTATIONS: KNEE

- Most often on lateral aspect of medial femoral condyle (medial femoral condyle affected in 69%)
- Predominantly affects males
- Poorly localized knee pain
- Mild effusion
- Mechanical symptoms (catching, clicking, popping) if articular cartilage disrupted or loose body present
- Pain to palpation of area
- Pt holds leg (tibia) in external rotation (to avoid pressure on lesion)
- Pain w/extension and internal rotation (Wilson test)
- Natural Hx:
  - developing: 10–15 yrs
  - late (loose body): 15–18 yrs
  - osteoarthritis: adult (if untreated)

CLINICAL MANIFESTATIONS: ELBOW

- Part of spectrum known as "Little League elbow" including:
  - traction apophysitis of medial epicondyle
  - avulsion of medial epicondyle
  - osteochondrosis of capitellum
  - osteochondritis dissecans of capitellum
- Clinical signs nonspecific
- Osteochondrosis vs. osteochondritis dissecans of capitellum:
  - peak age 10 yrs
  - mild flexion contracture (10–15°)
  - can be bilateral
  - 2° changes in radial head seen late
  - focal area of capitellum
  - residual deformity

LABORATORY MANIFESTATIONS

- Usually normal
- Radiographic features:
  - plain radiographs best; AP and lateral (tunnel and "sunrise" views also for knee)
  - MRI: note whether cartilage intact/note size, location, amount of fragmentation of bone lesion
  - monitor progress of treatment w/plain x rays (MRI or CT scans may confuse issue)

DIFFERENTIAL DIAGNOSIS

- Anomalous 2° ossification centers
- Chondroblastoma
- Epiphyseal osteomyelitis
- Acute osteochondral fracture
- Multiple epiphyseal dysplasia
- Spondyloepiphyseal dysplasia
- Avascular necrosis

TREATMENT: OSTEOCHONDRITITIS DISSECANS OF KNEE

- General:
  - physes open:
    ○ closed treatment 3–6 mos: intermittent immobilization; restrict sports activity
    ○ surgery if not compliant or still symptomatic at 3–6 mos
  - physes closed:
    ○ operative treatment: arthroscopic
    ○ classification dictates specific procedure
- Specific treatment based on age (3 categories):
  - category I: up to skeletal age 11 yrs (females) and 13 yrs (males):
    ○ good general prognosis
    ○ intact cartilage (most). Conservative treatment: limit activity, occasional immobilization; if failure of conservative treatment, arthroscopic drilling and 3 mos non–weight bearing; 90% heal w/drilling
    ○ if articular cartilage disrupted (rarely seen in this age group), surgery to take down lesion, debride, reduce, and rigid fixation (screw or pins); 80–90% heal
    ○ dislodged fragment w/loose body seldom seen in age group
  - category II:
    ○ skeletal age 11–15 yrs (females), 13–17 yrs (males): up to skeletal maturity
    ○ intact cartilage: prognosis good; conservative treatment rarely successful; arthroscopic drilling; 3 mos non–weight bearing; 90% heal
    ○ if articular cartilage disrupted (common): arthroscopy to assess; take down lesion, debride, bone graft (if needed), reduce fragment, rigid fixation
    ○ dislodged fragment w/loose body: arthroscopic loose body removal and treatment of defect by either: (1) abrasion, drilling (induces fibrocartilage repair), or (2) osteochondral autograft, allograft transfer, or cultured chondrocyte transfer (if defect involves a large weight-bearing area)
  - category III: skeletal age >18 yrs (after physeal closure):
    ○ prognosis: guarded
    ○ treatment: surgery
    ○ intact cartilage (rarely seen): arthroscopy to confirm intact cartilage; take down lesion, bone graft and rigid fixation (Herbert screw)
    ○ if articular cartilage disrupted (common), surgical treatment: arthroscopy to assess; take down lesion, debride, bone graft (if needed), reduce fragment, rigid fixation
    ○ dislodged fragment w/loose body: arthroscopic loose body removal and treatment of defect by either: (1) abrasion, drilling-fibrocartilage response, or (2) osteochondral autograft vs. allograft transfer vs. cultured chondrocyte transfer (if defect involves large weight-bearing area of either tibia or femur

TREATMENT: OSTEOCHONDRITITIS DISSECANS OF ELBOW

- Conservative measures for intact fragment: rest, stretching
- Moderation of activity; advise sport other than throwing (at least temporarily)
- Arthroscopic drilling intact fragment not responsive to conservative measures
- Arthroscopic removal of loose body when present: rare

COMPLICATIONS

- Osteoarthritis

WHEN TO REFER

- At Dx

OSTEOMYELITIS

SHELDON L. KAPLAN

BACKGROUND

- *Three types of pathogenesis:* acute hematogenous most common, usually involving the metaphysis of long bones/trauma often preceding event; bone inoculated via penetration; contiguous site of infection
- Clinically presents as acute, subacute/chronic osteomyelitis involving one bone most frequently
- Acute hematogenous most common *S. aureus*/group A streptococcus most common organisms in infants/children; group B streptococcus common in neonates; *P. aeruginosa* most common pathogen following penetrating inoculation of foot; Salmonella most frequent isolate in children w/ hemoglobinopathies

CLINICAL MANIFESTATIONS

- Fever, pain at site of infection, reluctance to use affected extremity, refusal to bear weight
- Nonspecific symptoms may include anorexia/vomiting
- Swelling, warmth, erythema of affected area
- Point tenderness key finding
- Unusual sites such as pelvic osteomyelitis may be difficult to detect; abdominal pain/urinary tract symptoms may be presenting complaints
- In children w/ hemoglobinopathies, Sx may be difficult to differentiate from sickle-cell crisis/bone infarction
- Vertebral osteomyelitis/disk space infection (diskitis) form spectrum of infections

LABORATORY FEATURES

- WBC count normal–↑
- ESR/C-reactive protein usually ↑
- Blood cultures positive 30–50% children w/ acute hematogenous osteomyelitis
- Bone aspiration, drainage/biopsy may yield pathogen when blood cultures sterile
- *Plain radiograph:* soft tissue swelling initially; bony erosion/lytic lesion appears 7–14 d later; periosteal new bone formation
- Technetium bone scan sensitivity ~80% except in neonate; specificity ↓ in pts w/ hemoglobinopathy
- MRI may be most sensitive radiographic technique; esp useful when plain film/bone scan nondiagnostic/surgical drainage may be required

DIFFERENTIAL DIAGNOSIS

- Cellulitis/septic arthritis
- Fracture/trauma/child abuse
- Malignancy
- Infarction w/ hemoglobinopathy
- Thrombophlebitis

TREATMENT

Organism	Antibiotic	Duration (minimum)
S. aureus*	Nafcillin, oxacillin Alternatives: clindamycin/cefazolin	3 wks and ESR < 20–30 mm/h Neonate–4 wks
Group A streptococcus	Penicillin	as above
P. aeruginosa	Ticarcillin or piperacillin plus aminoglycoside	7–10 d if adequate debridement
Salmonella	Ampicillin, if susceptible; cefotaxime, ceftriaxone trimethoprim-sulfamethoxazole	3–4 wks

*Tx can be completed w/ oral antibiotics in older infant/child if organism recovered/susceptible to appropriate agent, pt afebrile × 3 d, improving on IV antibiotic, child can tolerate oral drug, parents are reliable. Try to achieve trough SBC ≥ 1:2 (for chronic osteomyelitis oral Tx continued 6–12 mos).

INDICATIONS FOR SURGERY

- Drain purulent material from subperiosteal space/other tissue planes
- Remove sequestra/infected foreign material
- Debride/drain puncture associated infection
- In neonate early drainage of bone w/ or w/o joint critical
- Chronic osteomyelitis

COMPLICATIONS

- *Complications:* concomitant septic arthritis in infants <18–24 mos of age, chronic osteomyelitis, sequestrum, pathologic fracture, altered bone growth if growth plate injured, soft tissue infection/abscess if ruptured through bony cortex, malignancy of bone

WHEN TO REFER

- Usually orthopedic surgeon w/ pediatric experience consulted
- Unusual site, organism/subacute to chronic presentation
- Underlying illness such as hemoglobinopathy
- Pt has allergy to beta-lactam antibiotics

BACKGROUND

- Commonly known as "swimmer's ear"
- Most common >5 yrs of age
- Most prevalent in warmer climates/summer months; associated w/ some form of trauma (scratching/cleaning ear) to external ear canal that breaks protective barrier of canal skin/protective cerumen layer
- Most common organisms include *P. aeruginosa, S. aureus, S. epidermidis,* Proteus, Enterobacter, *E. coli,* diptheroids
- *Recovery:* nearly 100% in 1–2 wks provided proper treatment/care
- *Mortality:* none for routine otitis externa; higher for malignant otitis externa (necrotizing OE)
- *Always* question for Hx of immune deficiency/diabetic status

CLINICAL MANIFESTATIONS

- Itchy/painful ear accompanied by "creamy"/serous drainage; often ↓ hearing in involved ear
- Erythema involving pinna in advanced cases
- Lymphadenopathy may involve pre-/post-auricular lymph nodes
- Pain within temporomandibular joint on involved side w/ mastication

LABORATORY FEATURES

- Culture only necessary in cases not responding to routine Tx
- When culturing, send for routine bacteria/fungal cultures
- If pts diabetic/immunocompromised, evaluate glucose/check CBC

DIFFERENTIAL DIAGNOSIS

- Otitis media w/ perforation
- Chronic otitis media w/cholesteatoma/perforation
- Bullous myringitis
- Keratitis obliterans
- Malignant OE/necrotizing OE (usually adult, usually diabetic/immunocompromised, always w/ draining ear, granulation tissue at bony-cartilagenous junction, *P. aeruginosa* infection)
- Chronic/eczematoid OE often related to neomycin allergy/other eczematoid dermatologic disease
- Carcinoma of external auditory canal (EAC) skin (rare in children)

TREATMENT

- Thorough cleaning of EAC w/ suctioning/swabbing; may need to be repeated several times during treatment period
- If tympanic membrane cannot be seen, place wick in EAC to help topical medication treat entire canal; remove within 72 hrs of application/replace if EAC not responding to Tx
- Topical application of otic drops containing steroid preparation to ↓ inflammation/antibiotic to cover infecting organisms; these solutions usually prepared in acidic solution that also inhibits bacterial growth; commonly used preparations in table; drops should be used 7–10 d w/ follow-up during treatment to assure proper Tx
- Oral ciprofloxacin would add good antibacterial coverage, however not yet approved for children
- Pts should avoid water activities during treatment period, refrain from wearing hearing aids, avoid cleaning canal w/ cotton swabs
- Persistent inflammation/draining despite adequate treatment may represent allergy to topical preparation (usually neomycin); cultures may prove beneficial/change of Tx to topical anti-inflammatory steroid cream/drops alone often helps clear process
- Pain may require oral analgesic control

COMPLICATIONS

- Chronic OE may lead to stenosis of EAC
- Malignant/necrotizing OE if untreated may lead to osteomyelitis of temporal bone/skull base leading to possible death
- Spread of OE to surrounding ear structures may lead to cellulitis/chondritis; require hospital admission for aggressive IV antibiotics/local wound care

PREVENTION

- If prone to OE, lowering acidity of EAC/keeping moisture low may ↓ incidence of infection; 50:50 mixture of white vinegar/rubbing alcohol when used after swimming/bathing in several drop quantities helps lower pH/evaporate any moisture
- Avoid excessive cleansing/scratching of EAC

WHEN TO REFER

- If granulation tissue identified in EAC
- If tympanic membrane not visible/uncomfortable placing a wick
- If debris excessive/do not have equipment to clean canal properly

Ototopic Drops	Antimicrobial	Steroid Component
VoSol HC	2% acetic acid	1% Hydrocortisone
Cortisporin Otic	Polymyxin B, neomycin sulfate	Hydrocortisone
Coly-Mycin S Otic	Colistin sulfate, neomycin sulfate, thonzonium bromide	Hydrocortisone
Gentamycin	Gentamycin	
Ophthalmic drops: Tobrex	Tobramycin	Dexamethasone

BACKGROUND

- Acute otitis media w/effusion (AOME) occurs in 90% children; recurrent AOME in ~30%
- Children average 2 AOME/year in first 3 yrs of life
- Risk factors: short, straight, floppy immature eustachian tube/dysfunction of mature eustachian tube, age <5 yrs, male gender, viral upper respiratory infections (URIs), pacifier after 2 yrs of age, day care w/>6 attendees, passive smoke exposure, and/or propping the bottle
- Otitis-prone children include Native Americans, Down syndrome, cleft palate pts, first AOME <6 mos of age/3 AOME in previous 4 mos
- Pathogens in AOME:
  – *Streptococcus pneumoniae* (S. pneumo ~35% AOME cases)
  – *Haemophilus influenzae* nontypable (H. flu nt ~30%)
  – *Moraxella catarrhalis* (M. cat ~12%)
  – group A streptococcus (GAS ~5%)
  – questionable pathogens: *Mycoplasma pneumoniae/Chlamydia pneumoniae* (<5%)

CLINICAL MANIFESTATIONS

- Fever (~50%), rhinorrhea (~80%), ↓ appetite (~65%), disturbed sleep (~85%), otalgia (~35%); in infants, drainage from external ear canal may be liquefied cerumen/purulent exudate from middle ear
- Dx:
  – visualize entire tympanic membrane (TM) w/pneumatic otoscopy; nonpneumatic otoscopy leads to overdiagnosis/has <60% specificity
  – key diagnostic features of TM: red to yellow color, full to bulging position, mobility ↓ on both positive/negative insufflation

LABORATORY FEATURES

- Optional, for follow-up, not initial Dx
- *Tympanometry:* useful >6 mos of age; confirms abnormal TM mobility
- *Audiometry:* useful >3 yrs old; confirms hearing deficit

DIFFERENTIAL DIAGNOSIS

- *Ear pain/fever:* myringitis (inflammation of TM w/o middle ear involvement (ie, normal TM mobility)
- *Ear pain/external canal swelling:* external otitis difficult to distinguish from AOME w/perfora-

tion; mucopurulent secretions in external canal confirm AOME; cheesy drainage confirms external otitis; painful tragus uncommon w/AOME/common w/external otitis
- *Ear pain/normal TM:* myofacial pain syndrome/post-tonsillectomy referred pain
- *Red TM/normal TM mobility:* usually from crying; child's whole head also red
- *Abnormal mobility only on positive insufflation:* effusion but no infection

ANTIBIOTIC RESISTANCE

- Highly variable geographically
- ~50% of H.flu produce beta-lactamase that inactivates amoxicillin, cefaclor/cefprozil
- ~40% of children <2 yrs in day care have penicillin-resistant S. pneumo, also ~50% resistant to trimethoprim/sulfamethoxazole, ↑ resistance to macrolides (near 40%)/cephalosporins
- Clinicians should ask about resistance in respiratory isolates from their local laboratory

TREATMENT

- 10 d standard/5 d course option in intermittent AOME
- *Fever/pain reduction:* acetaminophen/ibuprofen; lidocaine-containing drops not better than vehicle alone
- *Respiratory symptoms:* decongestant/antihistamines do not affect middle ear effusions/infections but may help nasal congestion/allergy symptoms
- Antibiotic choices (see table) based on Hx AOME frequency:
  – intermittent AOME (>3 mos since last AOME): no treatment an option if >3 yrs of age/no fever/no otalgia (>80% spontaneous resolution); otherwise, first-tier drug
  – recurrent AOME (<3 mos since last AOME): second tier, beta-lactamase stable
  – recalcitrant AOME (failure on/within 7 d of stopping antibiotic): third-tier drug/tympanocentesis (drain abscess, culture/susceptibilities for antibiotic choice)
  – expectations of tympanocentesis: ~one-third, negative cultures; ~one-third, organisms susceptible to first-line antibiotics
- Tympanocentesis also if severe otalgia

COMPLICATIONS

- *Hearing deficit:* common/nearly always conductive/temporary; effusion damps TM vibration, amplification via ossicles; clears as effusion resolves
- *TM perforation:* common/usually heals spontaneously when infection clears; refer if drains >5d
- *Behavioral/speech problems:* not uncommon w/prolonged hearing losses
- *Adhesive otitis media:* not uncommon w/frequent AOME/usually >5 yrs old; TM atrophic/drapes across the ossicles
- *Mastoiditis:* uncommon/fever, pain behind ear, pinna of ear rotated forward/out
- *Chronic draining otitis:* rare/persisting perforation w/drainage
- *Bacteremia:* rare/predominantly <2 yrs old w/S. pneumo AOME, high fever
- *Meningitis:* very rare/at <3 yrs old, only w/S. pneumo AOME
- *Cholesteatoma:* very rare/severe TM retraction, frequent perforations result in retained squamous epithelium in a pouch in middle ear; potentially fatal condition

PREVENTION

- *General:* substitute home care for day care/avoid cigarette smoke/breast feeding
- *Vaccine:* pneumococcal 23-valent vaccine in otitis-prone children (limited efficacy but any efficacy of benefit; influenza vaccine in autumn reduces AOME by nearly one-quarter in otitis-prone children
- *Antibiotic prophylaxis:* controversial since onset of ↑ drug-resistant pneumococcus; consider in child w/>3 AOME episodes in 3 mos (up to 80% fewer AOME w/sulfisoxazole, 50–75 mg/kg hs × 6 wks); stop prophylaxis after 6 wks to reduce selection of drug-resistant organisms; sulfisoxazole preferred over amoxicillin (20 mg/kg hs) (leads to less drug-resistant pneumococcus)

WHEN TO REFER

- For PE tubes (>3 AOME in 4 mos despite short-term prophylaxis); pressure-equalizing (PE) tubes prevent ~80% of recurrent AOME
- For perforation >1 wk, retraction pocket on TM/suspicion of cholesteatoma

Antibiotic Candidates for AOME

Tier	Generic Name (trade names below)	Cost	Dosing mg/kg/d	Dose Div	S. pneumo PS/DR, 5 = best	H. flu, β-lact (–)/(+)	M. cat	GAS	Side Effects GI, 0 = least	Rash, 0 = least	Taste, 0 = least
1st	Amoxicillin	1	40–60	bid	5/2	5/0	3	5	1	1	1–3
1st	Amoxicillin	2	80–100	bid	5/4	5/0	3	5	1	1	1–3
1st	Erythromycin/sulfisoxazole	2	40 of erythromycin	tid	5/2	3/3	5	4	4	2	4
1st	Trimethoprim/sulfamethoxazole	1	10 of trimethoprim	bid	3/1	4/4	2	0	1	4	2
2nd	Cefpodoxime* proxetil, 5 or 10 d	4	10	qd or bid	5/3	5/5	5	5	2	1	4
2nd	Loracarbef†	4	30	bid	5/1	5/4	5	5	0	1	0
2nd	Azithromycin‡	3	10 on day 1, 5 on days 2–5	bid d1, qd d2–5	5/2	2/2	5	4	1	1	1
2nd	Cefixime§	4	8	qd or bid	4/0	5/5	5	5	1	1	0
2nd	Amoxicillin + clavulanate	4	45	bid	5/2	5/5	5	5	1	1	1
3rd	Amoxicillin + clavulanate§§	4.5	80–100 div bid	bid	5/4	5/5	5	5	1.5	1	1
3rd	Ceftriaxone§§§	3	50	one IM	5/1	5	5	5	2	1	N/A

Abbreviations: S. pneumo = *Streptococcus pneumoniae,* PS = penicillin susceptible, DR = drug resistant, H. flu = *Haemophilus influenzae,* beta-lact (+/-) = beta-lactamase positive/beta-lactamase negative, M.cat = *Moraxella catarrhalis,* GAS = group A streptococcus

Trade names of generic drugs: Amoxicillin = Amoxil; Erythromycin/sulfisoxazole = Pediazole; Trimethoprim/sulfamethoxazole = Bactrim, Septra, Co-trim; Cefpodoxime proxetil = Vantin, Loracarbef = Lorabid; Azithromycin = Zithromax; Cefixime = Suprax; Amoxicillin/Clavulanate = Augmentin

*Cefuroxime axetil (Ceftin) 40 mg/kg/d div bid has similar profile/possibly somewhat less efficacy vs. DR pneumococcus.

†Cefprozil (Cefzil) 30 mg/kg/d div bid alternate w/better efficacy vs. pneumococcus but w/somewhat less stability to *H. influenzae* beta-lactamase. Cefaclor (Ceclor) no longer sufficiently potent to be used as 2nd/3rd tier drug; cefdinir 2nd tier drug resistant pneumo and beta-lactamase *H. flu*

‡Clarithromycin (Biaxin) 15 mg/kg/d div bid alternate/has worse taste, higher cost, less efficacy vs. *H. influenzae.*

§Ceftibuten (Cedax) 9 mg/kg/d 1×/d alternate w/somewhat better stability to extended-spectrum beta-lactamases.

§§45 mg/kg/day div bid, plus separate prescription for amoxicillin 40–50 mg/kg/day

§§§Ceftriaxone given on 3 consecutive days level 4 activity against resistant pneumo (not yet FDA approved)

OVERUSE INJURIES OF THE LOWER LEG: STRESS FRACTURES, SHIN SPLINTS, AND TENDINITIS

ANGELA D. SMITH

BACKGROUND AND ETIOLOGY

- Occur in active children/adolescents, mainly those who participate in single sport >3×/wk; rare <8 yrs of age
- Usually gradual onset; pts typically present when pain begins to interfere w/activities
- Often related to intrinsic biomechanical problems (ie, excessive foot pronation, rigid high-arched feet, angular or rotational malalignment of lower extremities [eg, femoral torsion, tibial torsion, genu valgum, genu varum], inflexible or weak muscles)
- Extrinsic factors include inappropriate shoes; training errors such as too rapid change in training program time, speed, intensity

DIFFERENTIAL DIAGNOSIS AND CLINICAL MANIFESTATIONS

- *Stress fracture:* aching pain continues long after activity stops, often still present following morning; pain, tenderness localized to narrow area; pain usually reproduced by 3 point bending; may have been preceded by period of diffuse tenderness
- *Shin splints:* Dx of exclusion; to most sports medicine practitioners, shin splints synonymous w/posteromedial tibial stress syndrome
- *Exertional compartment syndrome:* most frequently in anterior or deep posterior compartment of lower leg; may have localized swelling and severe cramplike or aching pain; generally resolves very quickly after cessation of activity
- *Achilles tendinitis:* often related to tight gastrocnemius; in older adolescent, may have mucinous degeneration of tendon, may rupture if attempt to train through severe pain
- *Peroneal tendinitis:* from boot-top pressure (skating, skiing); overuse in sports that prominently use peroneals (skating; ballet and Irish dancing); same forces may cause fibular stress fracture
- *Flexor hallucis longus tendinitis:* primarily among dancers; pain w/resisted great toe plantarflexion; may feel nodule "catch" w/active toe flexion
- *Anterior tibial, extensor digitorum and extensor hallucis longus tendinitis:* usually from pressure from sports equipment; may develop huge overlying bursas
- *Posterior tibial tendinitis:* during growth spurt, may be related to tight gastrocnemius, esp in athletes w/flat feet and accessory naviculars (w/tight gastrocnemius, must pronate more to be plantigrade); same forces may cause distal tibial stress fracture
- *Other diagnoses in differential:* neoplasm, infection, metabolic bone disease

RADIOGRAPHIC STUDIES

- Plain x-ray rarely shows evidence of stress fracture before at least 2 wks of symptoms; may see periosteal new bone formation, localized thickening of cortex, or fracture line
- Technetium[99] bone scan may show diffusely increased uptake consistent w/posteromedial tibial stress syndrome or stress reaction, or marked focal increase of radionuclide indicative of stress fracture
- MRI very sensitive, generally not useful for these problems in childhood, adolescence

OTHER STUDIES

- Exertional compartment syndrome diagnosed by direct measurement of compartment pressure; if surgery contemplated, pressure of all lower leg compartments should be checked immediately after exercise

TREATMENT

Stress fracture (and stress reaction)
- Active rest (do only activities that cause no pain)
- Correct biomechanics (muscle flexibility, muscle strength, shoes, alignment, etc)
- Correct training errors
- Ice
- NSAIDs, only if stop activities that cause pain (do not want to mask symptoms)
- Crutches, cast, removable immobilization device, or surgery if indicated; must do one or more of these if "black line" fracture, or have pain at rest even after stopping activities that caused injury
- Ascertain (and treat if abnormal) nutritional, menstrual status; stress fracture more common in undernourished, in female athlete triad (disordered eating, amenorrhea, osteoporosis)

Shin splints/posterior tibial tendinitis
- Active rest
- Stretch gastrocnemius muscle, strengthen posterior tibial muscle

- Correct other biomechanical or training causes
- Ice, ultrasound, other physical Tx modalities; NSAIDs
- Consider compressive wrap, tape
- Orthotic shoe inserts if indicated

Other lower leg tendinitis
- Determine cause, if possible, and correct/remove it
- Active rest
- Ice, ultrasound, other modalities; NSAIDs
- Consider compressive wrap, tape
- Stretch tight calf muscles; heel cup/lift for Achilles tendinitis until stretched sufficiently
- Strengthen injured musculo-tendinous unit
- Correct any other biomechanical or training causes
- Orthotic shoe inserts if indicated
- If refractory, consider corticosteroid injection into *sheath* of tendon, not into its substance; may increase risk of rupture; injection rarely indicated
- Surgical exploration for reconstruction (Achilles) or release of sheath (FHL) rarely needed; for bursas, can almost always solve problem by operating on equipment rather than on foot

Exertional compartment syndrome
- Stretch gastrocnemius; but usually ineffective
- Quit causative sport activity
- Surgically release *all* affected compartments

COMPLICATIONS

- Completion of unicortical stress fracture into displaced fracture
- Tendon rupture
- Acute compartment syndrome (rare as complication of exertional compartment syndrome)

WHEN TO REFER

- When symptoms not responding to level of treatment you feel comfortable providing, given particular situation

BACKGROUND

- Relatively uncommon disease in pediatrics; can be mild/severe
- Etiology unknown in 25% of cases; common causes include:
  – trauma: probably most important immediate concern because of risk of serious (other) injuries; evaluate for other injuries esp if Hx blow to abdomen/any physical signs of trauma, abuse); be extra alert for Hx suggesting accident w/trauma to abdomen esp one involving bicycles, sticks/fists; *consider child abuse*
  – infections: mumps, Epstein-Barr virus, HIV
  – cystic fibrosis: even if no other signs (esp if symptoms recurrent)
  – complication of other chronic (or acute) disease: biliary tract disorders, congenital anomalies, multisystem diseases including vasculitides, metabolic diseases
  – drugs (large number of medications associated w/pancreatitis): sulfonamides, diuretics, steroids

CLINICAL MANIFESTATIONS

- Dx may require high index of suspicion
- Mild cases most notable for lack of toxicity/can even be "subclinical"
- Abdominal pain usually epigastric/can be relatively sudden in onset, often constant/prolonged
- Minimal abdominal tenderness w/no peritoneal signs reassuring
- Vomiting may/may not be present
- Food may aggravate symptoms
- Moderate to severe cases have worsening pain, may have continuing vomiting, toxic appearance, abdominal distension w/significant abdominal tenderness, peritoneal signs

BASIS OF DIAGNOSIS

- Laboratory tests:
  – ↑ serum (or urine)amylase/lipase very helpful; degree of ↑ not necessarily indicative of degree of inflammation; severe pancreatitis may be present w/normal, minimal, significantly ↑ pancreatic enzymes
  – ↑ WBC count, ↑ ESR, C-reactive protein, other nonspecific measures of inflammation
  – mild, uncomplicated cases do not have concomitant abnormalities in other blood studies; moderate to severe cases may have ↓ albumin/calcium
- Imaging studies:
  – plain abdominal film may show nonspecific ileus pattern/generally not very helpful
  – ultrasound currently most readily acceptable "standard" for Dx
  – CT scan perhaps better than ultrasound
  – endoscopic retrograde choangiopancreatography (ERCP) of potential use in evaluating recurrent disease/when anatomic abnormalities suspected; *will induce pancreatitis in significant number of pts*

DIFFERENTIAL DIAGNOSIS

- Includes virtually all causes of abdominal pain from most benign to surgical emergencies

TREATMENT

- Supportive for both mild/severe cases:
  – mild cases w/↑ amylase may be managed locally/at home under careful observation
  – ↓ oral intake (NPO for 24 hrs), followed by low-fat diet traditional, but of unproved effectiveness
- Discontinue medications associated w/pancreatitis
- Moderate–severe cases have significant morbidity/mortality; hospitalization for IV hydration, careful attention to fluid/electrolyte balance/management of pain

COMPLICATIONS

- Worsening symptoms leading to moderate/severe pancreatitis
- *Pancreatic pseudocyst:* recurrent abdominal pain as early as 2–3 wks after acute event (esp if Hx trauma)
- Recurrent attacks
- Exocrine/endocrine pancreatic insufficiency may occur w/recurrent attacks/may be sign of hereditary pancreatitis, pseudocyst formation, congenital abnormality

WHEN TO REFER

- *Refer all but most mild/incidental cases*
- Evidence of complications
- Evidence of toxicity
- Narcotics required for pain control
- GI bleeding
- Uncertainty regarding Dx
- Recurrence of Sx
- Failure to respond to supportive Tx within few days
- Concern regarding child abuse (referral to appropriate authority)

PAPULAR ACRODERMATITIS OF CHILDHOOD (Gianotti-Crosti Syndrome)   SHARON S. RAIMER

BACKGROUND

- May occur infancy–early teens; children 1–4 yrs of age most commonly affected
- Equal incidence in boys/girls
- Originally thought to be associated exclusively w/hepatitis B antigen, generally subtype ayw
- Now recognized as exanthem associated w/several infectious agents, principally viruses
- Commonly associated w/hepatitis B infection in southern Europe/Japan; association w/hepatitis B in US uncommon
- Viral infections reported in children w/Gianotti-Crosti syndrome include Epstein-Barr virus, cytomegalovirus, Coxsackie virus A16, Coxsackie virus B, parainfluenza virus, respiratory syncytial virus, hepatitis viruses A, B, C, poliovaccine enterovirus, parovirus B19, possibly HIV
- Streptococcal pharyngitis has been reported in association w/syndrome
- Cases have been reported in which no associated infectious agent could be demonstrated
- Duration of eruption generally 3–8 wks, although reported duration 15 d–11 wks
- Extent/severity of eruption does not influence duration
- Skin lesions resolve w/o sequelae

CLINICAL MANIFESTATIONS

- Appears abruptly in well child/occasionally w/symptoms of viral infection
- Skin lesions erupt 2–4 mm lichenoid papules/vesiculopapules
- Papules flesh colored to red; may appear slightly umbilicated
- Lesion symmetrically distributed on extremities, buttocks, face, occasionally ears; upper trunk/abdomen relatively spared
- Extensor surfaces more frequently affected than flexor surfaces
- Frequently demonstrate isomorphic response (Koebner phenomenon)
- Eruption develops in crops w/new papules appearing while older ones resolving
- May be pruritic; scratching may result in impetiginization
- Adenopathy variable
- Hepatomegaly uncommon

LABORATORY FEATURES

- No laboratory features specific for this syndrome
- Children generally appear clinically well; laboratory evaluations usually not indicated; clinical evaluation should direct laboratory evaluation in symptomatic children
- *Liver function tests:* consider in children living in areas endemic for hepatitis B who have not been vaccinated/when hepatomegaly, other findings/symptoms indicate

- *Viral studies:* usually not warranted for this self-limited disease
- *Histology:* skin biopsy generally not indicated; histologic features not specific but have sufficient characteristic features to support clinical Dx

DIFFERENTIAL DIAGNOSIS

- Scabies
- Molluscum contagiosum
- Lichen planus
- Lichen nitidis
- Papular erythema multiforme

TREATMENT

- No specific treatment available
- For pruritic lesions mild topical steroids/antihistamines may provide symptomatic relief
- For impetiginized lesions, antibiotics as indicated

COMPLICATIONS

- None associated w/syndrome
- Complications from associated infections rare

WHEN TO REFER

- Most pts managed w/o referral
- Referral indicated when Dx in doubt

BACKGROUND

- Most frequently occurs in young children with peak incidence in 2–3 yr olds
- More common in underdeveloped countries, areas where children have ↑ exposure to arthropods
- Incidence peaks in late spring, summer in temperate climates
- Most often associated w/flea and mosquito bites; other ectoparasite associations include lice, mites (human, cat, dog, bird, rodent, bat forms), ants, ticks, gnats, caterpillars, bedbugs
- Probably represents hypersensitivity reaction to foreign proteins inoculated into skin during bug bite; serum antibodies to insect salivary proteins and foregut endothelium have been found in affected individuals
- Both immediate and delayed hypersensitivity reactions thought important
- Repeated exposures lead to "tolerance" and resolution of symptoms
- Resolution in wks to yrs
- No mortality in uncomplicated cases

CLINICAL MANIFESTATIONS

- Significant pruritus at affected sites
- Lesions appear in crops; often symmetrical involvement
- Distribution: depends on etiology
  - *fleas:* legs, arms, areas of tight clothing (waistband); often appear in clusters of three ("breakfast, lunch, dinner" for flea)
  - *lice:* head and neck lesions predominate
  - *mosquitoes, gnats, ants:* exposed areas
  - *cat and dog mites:* arms and chest
  - *scabies:* wrists, web spaces of digits, axillae, groin, elbows

- Morphology:
  - discrete erythematous and sometimes urticarial papules
  - excoriations and superimposed crusts common
  - central puncta occasionally seen within papules
  - papulovesicles, blisters, even large bullae occasionally present
- New bites may cause old sites to "light up," become acutely inflamed
- Lichenified papules, nodules, plaques may result from chronic involvement, scratching
- Generalized "id" or autoeczematization eruption may subsequently develop; consists of small pruritic eczematoid papules

LABORATORY STUDIES

- Not usually required
- Scabies preparation and bacterial culture occasionally helpful
- IgE may be ↑
- Skin biopsy may be helpful in atypical or very persistent cases. Acanthosis, spongiosis, superficial and deep mixed perivascular infiltrate and interstitial eosinophils common findings

DIFFERENTIAL DIAGNOSIS

- Classic urticaria
- Scabies
- Early varicella
- Papular atopic dermatitis
- *Uncommon:* pityriasis lichenoides et varioliformis acuta or chronic form
- *Uncommon:* neurotic excoriations
- *Rare:* lymphomatoid papulosis, papulonecrotic tuberculid

TREATMENT

- Symptomatic:
  - oral antihistamines: cetirizine, diphenhydramine, hydroyzine, doxepin for severe cases
  - topical antipruritics: menthol, camphor, pramoxine
  - oatmeal baths
  - troublesome cases: high-potency topical steroids sparingly
  - oral thiamine: efficacy not proven
- Environmental control
  - *survey pt's environment for ectoparasites:* home, pets, yards, day-care setting
  - *flea infestation requires aggressive intervention:* vacuum all cloth furniture, floors and rugs, consider fogging house
  - insect repellent and protective clothing in appropriate cases involving mosquitoes or ticks

COMPLICATIONS

- *Common:* 2° bacterial infection
- Rare cases of typhus from flea bites
- Adverse reactions from overaggressive and inappropriate topical agents applied by parents (eg, topical benadryl creams leading to contact hypersensitivity; multiple lindane or permethrin treatments leading to irritated dry skin)

WHEN TO REFER

- Most pts managed in 1° care setting
- Evaluation by dermatologist may prove helpful in persistent cases; biopsy may reassure families that nothing serious causing eruption
- Veterinarian may be useful to r/o animal mites when family pets exist
- Professional exterminators should be involved in difficult cases to evaluate house or day-care setting for evidence of bird, rat, bat mites

PATTERNS

- Congenital
- Habitual
- Central
- Lateral

CONGENITAL DISLOCATION OF THE PATELLA

- Very uncommon
- Patella dislocates laterally
- Associated w/nail-patella syndrome
- *Additional findings:* fixed knee flexion contracture of 20–30° w/further flexion of 100–130°, mild ↑ genu valgum, external tibial torsion
- Radiographs nondiagnostic in young children (patella does not ossify until 3–5 yrs of age). Ultrasound/MRI may be necessary to confirm Dx
- *Untreated:* inefficient knee mechanics/progressive bony deformity
- Treatment requires quadricepsplasty w/release of the contracted lateral soft tissue structures, shortening of stretched-out medial structures, centralization of quadriceps mechanism

HABITUAL DISLOCATION OF THE PATELLA

- Uncommon
- Presents during first decade
- Patella dislocates laterally every time knee flexed
- Associated w/:
  - repeated IM injections w/subsequent fibrosis/contracture of vastus lateralis
  - conditions such as Down syndrome that have marked ligamentous laxity
- *Treatment:* surgical. Realignment procedure similar to that used for congenital dislocation, but in pts w/fibrosis, extensive proximal release of vastus lateralis origin may be required; in cases associated w/ligamentous laxity, some advocate transfer of semitendinosus tendon/other soft tissue

structures to act as "check rein" that prevents recurrence
- *Results:* good if patella remains located but recurrence may occur w/subsequent growth; particularly true in Down syndrome/repeat surgery usually not attempted

CENTRAL DISLOCATION OF THE PATELLA

- Very uncommon
- Direct trauma to superior pole of patella, which strips quadriceps attachment, jams superior portion of patella in joint
- *Treatment:* closed or open reduction under general anesthesia, short-term immobilization

LATERAL DISLOCATION/SUBLUXATION OF THE PATELLA

- Common, represent spectrum of similar pathomechanics
- *Age group:* primarily second/third decade
- *Predisposing factors:* female gender, ligamentous laxity, genu valgum, patella alta
  - genu valgum positions patella laterally
  - w/patella alta, patella in relatively superior position; ie, out of confines of intercondylar notch for greater degree of flexion-extension
- Mechanism of injury:
  - dislocation/subluxation: rotational stress to knee
    - athletic events/dancing: 55%
    - minor trauma: 45%; knee gave way while walking or during trivial fall; this group has greater degree of ligamentous laxity, patella alta, etc
- *Dx:* very easy–difficult; the problem obvious in child who comes to ER w/patella sitting on lateral aspect of knee; many pts, however, have patella dislocations that either spontaneously reduce/are reduced by pts themselves. The former group can only describe their injury in terms of knee "giving out" or "slipping"

- Exam:
  - acute dislocation/subluxation: (1) tenderness along superior medial border of patella, (2) hemarthrosis, (3) positive apprehension sign elicited by stretching the torn vastus medialis; w/knee extended, quadriceps muscle relaxed, examiner uses thumb to push patella laterally/knee is then flexed; positive apprehension sign noted by ↑ in pt's anxiety, pain as patella starts to subluxate. Exam should r/o other injuries that cause hemarthrosis of knee
- Radiographs:
  - in acute dislocation/subluxation: AP, lateral, tangential view of patella obtained to r/o osteochondral fractures, associated injury that occurs ~10–15% of the time, and to assess patella alta, other predisposing factors
- Treatment:
  - acute dislocation: when required, relocation of patella easily done by flexing hip, extending knee, and pushing patella medially
  - nonoperative Tx of acute dislocation starts w/aspiration of hemarthrosis, immobilization of knee in extension. Immobilization continued 2–6 wks
  - physical Tx continued until knee motion, quadriceps strength regained
  - only absolute indication for 1° surgical procedure is osteochondral fracture within joint
- Results:
  - recurrent instability following patella dislocation more likely in younger teenagers, in pts w/ligamentous laxity, in pts w/predisposing anatomic factors
  - in one study redislocation rate 60% in 11- to 14-yr-old age group, but only 33% and 28%, respectively, in 15- to 18- and 19- to 27-yr-old age group and was not observed when first dislocation occurred after age 28
  - symptomatic recurrent instability requires realignment of quadriceps mechanism

PATENT DUCTUS ARTERIOSUS

KAREN S. RHEUBAN

BACKGROUND

- Anatomy:
  - vascular structure that develops during fetal life connecting main pulmonary artery and descending aorta
  - histologically, ductal tissue demonstrates greater amounts of medial smooth muscle and thicker intima than adjacent aorta or pulmonary artery
- Physiology:
  - in fetal life only 6–8% of combined ventricular output perfuses lungs; 55–60% shunts right to left through ductus arteriosus to aorta
  - postnatal closure effected via immediate contraction of ductal smooth muscle followed over period of weeks by subintimal proliferation and eventual fibrosis to form ligamentum arteriosus. Factors contributing to ductal closure include increasing PaO_2, release of vasoactive substances, reduction in circulating prostaglandin levels attributable to removal of placental sources and breakdown in lungs. In normal-term infants, shunting rarely detected echocardiographically by 72 hrs after birth
  - clinical manifestations of patent ductus arteriosus relate to following factors: ductal size, pulmonary/systemic vascular pressure and resistance, myocardial performance in response to volume overload, altered myocardial perfusion
  - persistent patency of ductus arteriosus following birth generally results in left-to-right shunt (from aorta to pulmonary artery) when pulmonary vascular resistance less than systemic. Presence of pulmonary hypertension may, however, lead to bidirectional or right-to-left shunting at ductal level

CLINICAL FEATURES

- Neonatal patent ductus arteriosus:
  - in postnatal period, any condition that lowers arterial PaO_2 or alters prostaglandin levels may delay ductal closure
  - left-to-right shunting may produce pulmonary edema in preterm infants, worsening respiratory distress, left atrial enlargement w/stretched patent foramen ovale and left-to-right atrial level shunt. Myocardial dysfunction and subendocardial ischemia 2° to volume overload, impaired coronary perfusion, papillary muscle dysfunction w/either mitral or tricuspid insufficiency may ensue. Cardiac murmur may be audible w/↑ precordial activity and bounding pulses, although significant ductus may be present in absence of murmur. Aggressive treatment w/IV inhibitors of prostaglandin synthetase (indomethacin) or ductal ligation may greatly improve symptomatic preterm neonates w/respiratory distress. Indomethacin may be given prophylactically in selected preterm infants
  - right-to-left shunting at ductal level and at foramen ovale may occur in persistent pulmonary hypertension of newborn. No murmur attributable to ductus audible in this condition
  - left-to-right shunting through ductus arteriosus in specific congenital heart defects associated w/reduced diminished pulmonary blood flow may improve O_2 saturation until further palliative or corrective measures may be taken (as in pulmonary or tricuspid atresia). Administration of IV prostaglandin E1 to dilate ductus and relieve hypoxemia may be life saving
  - dilation of ductus arteriosus in pts w/congenital heart defects w/impaired systemic blood flow (as in hypoplastic left heart syndrome, coarctation of aorta, or critical aortic stensosis) may improve systemic perfusion and relieve acidosis. Administration of IV prostaglandin E1 may be life saving in these neonates
- Persistent patent ductus arteriosus in older infants/children
  - incidence: 5–10% of all congenital heart defects, 1/2,000 live births, possibly related to anatomic/physiologic abnormality of ductal tissue
  - small PDA generally causes no symptoms. Physical examination may demonstrate normal heart sounds w/continuous or typical "machinery" murmur. BP pulses normal, and no evidence for CHF exists. Laboratory studies may show normal or mildly abnormal EKG (top normal LV forces); chest radiograph normal or may show mild ↑ in heart size, pulmonary vascularity. Echocardiogram confirmatory; may be otherwise entirely normal or may show very mild left atrial enlargement
  - moderate-sized PDA often associated w/mild CHF, slow weight gain, mild tachypnea, easy fatigability. Physical examination shows ↑ precordial activity, thrill at base of heart, loud continuous murmur that may obscure heart sounds, mitral diastolic flow rumble, bounding pulses, hepatomegaly. Laboratory studies show left atrial enlargement, left ventricular hypertrophy on EKG, cardiomegaly, ↑ vascularity on chest radiograph. Echocardiogram confirmatory; also demonstrates left atrial, ventricular enlargement
  - large PDA associated w/Sx CHF, manifest by poor feeding, easy fatigability, tachypnea, failure to thrive. Physical findings include bounding pulses, ↑ precordial activity, loud second heart sound, either continuous murmur or systolic murmur if coexisting pulmonary hypertension present. Mitral diastolic rumble usually present. In cases w/evolving pulmonary vascular obstructive disease, may be reversal of shunt. EKG shows biventricular hypertrophy; chest radiograph may show cardiomegaly, enlarged central pulmonary arteries, varying degrees of shunt vascularity related to severity of pulmonary vascular disease

LABORATORY STUDIES

- *EKG:* LVH, LAE, in addition to RVH in cases w/pulmonary hypertension
- *Chest radiograph:* cardiomegaly, shunt vascularity, left atrial enlargement generally seen in all but those pts w/small left-to-right shunt. Pulmonary edema may be present in premature infants. Oligemic lungfields may be seen in neonates w/persistent pulmonary hypertension
- *Echocardiogram:* PDA may readily be imaged by two-dimensional echocardiography, confirmed by color-flow Doppler echocardiography. Left atrial and left ventricular enlargement, stretched patent foramen ovale w/left-to-right atrial level shunts commonly seen in cases w/moderate to large ductal shunts. Right ventricular enlargement may be seen, in presence of coexisting atrial level shunts and/or pulmonary hypertension
- *Cardiac catheterization:* cardiac catheterization rarely performed prior to surgery unless associated congenital heart disease or pulmonary hypertension exists; coil occlusion possible via cardiac catheterization

DIFFERENTIAL DIAGNOSIS

- Arteriovenous fistula (coronary, pulmonary, systemic)
- Anomalous origin of left coronary artery from pulmonary artery
- Venous hum
- Surgically created systemic-pulmonary shunt
- Aorticopulmonary window
- Coarctation of aorta
- Extreme peripheral pulmonary artery stenoses
- Pulmonary atresia w/bronchial collaterals
- Truncus arteriosus
- Total anomalous pulmonary venous return
- Ruptured sinus of Valsalva

COMPLICATIONS

- Bacterial endocarditis/endarteritis
- Aneurysm of ductus arteriosus
- Calcification of ductus arteriosus

TREATMENT

- *Preterm infants:* IV indomethacin (initial dose: 0.2 mg/kg IV followed by 2 additional age-dependent doses given 12 hrs apart; <24 hrs of age: 0.1 mg/kg IV; 1–7 d of age: 0.2 mg/kg IV; >7 d: 0.25 mg/kg). Should not be given to neonates w/serum creatinine >1.6 mg/dL, clinical bleeding, necrotizing enterocolitis because complications may include platelet dysfunction, bleeding, ↓ renal, mesenteric blood flow
- *Term infants:* IV indomethacin only in presence of CHF
- *Older infants/children:* surgical ligation and division, transcatheter occlusion (experimental)
- *All pts:* SBE precautions until ductal closure confirmed
- Anticongestive measures (digitalis, diuretics)
- Intentional dilation of ductus in neonates w/specific congenital heart defects may be accomplished via IV infusion of prostaglandin E1 (0.05–0.1 mcg/kg/min). Complications include apnea, hyperthermia, irritability

BACKGROUND

- *Definition:* pectus excavatum: abnormality of chest wall w/posterior angulation of sternum/lower costal cartilages toward spine; pectus carinatum: anterior angulation of sternum (often lower one-third)
- *Etiology:* unknown; genetic factors probably exist/one-third pts have family Hx chest wall deformity
- Pectus excavatum 10× more common than carinatum
- Incidence in males 3× > females
- Common in Marfan syndrome; evaluate particularly in males w/scoliosis; eye exam for subluxation of lens/echocardiogram for dilatation of aortic root, aortic/mitral valve regurgitation

CLINICAL MANIFESTATIONS

- Characteristic chest wall defect
- Defect noted by 1 yr of age in two-thirds
- *Symptoms:* chest wall discomfort/limited exercise tolerance for strenuous activities; some school-age children/adolescents do not interact w/peers (particularly in sports activities) due to appearance of defect
- Usually asymptomatic in infancy/childhood w/symptoms appearing in late childhood/school-age children; some pts remain asymptomatic
- Scoliosis noted in 15% of pts

LABORATORY FEATURES

- *Chest radiographs:* displacement of heart to left on posterior-anterior view; posterior angulation of sternum toward spine on lateral view
- *CT scan:* used by some to rate severity of pectus

- *Pulmonary function tests:* perform w/maximal exercise if possible
- *Echocardiography:* if heart murmur/physical features consistent w/Marfan syndrome
- Cardiopulmonary function pre/postop subject of numerous reports
- Most studies identify mild ↓ in total lung capacity/inspiratory vital capacity, which correlate w/severity of chest wall defect (measured as degree of sternal depression)
- Degree of impairment difficult to determine/probably related to severity of pectus excavatum
- Effect of repair of petus excavatum on pulmonary function controversial; several studies fail to demonstrate significant improvement
- Response to upright exercise below normal in some pts/in some has improved w/surgical repair
- ↑ in stroke volume in some w/surgical repair may be reason why exercise tolerance improves after surgery

DIFFERENTIAL DIAGNOSIS

- Evaluate for Marfan syndrome, particularly tall boys w/joint hyperextension

TREATMENT

- Indications for and timing of surgery:
  - symptomatic pectus excavatum
  - severe defect w/psychological factors, ie, child not interacting w/peers due to appearance
  - progression of defect documented by radiographic ↓ sternal-vertebral distance
  - demonstrable defect in pulmonary function w/exercise

  - most surgeons defer surgery until at least 4 yrs of age/some prefer to wait until 8–12 yrs of age
- *Surgical technique:* two methods exist for repair of excavatum:
  - cartilage resection/sternal osteotomy:
    - elevation of muscle flaps
    - excision of deformed cartilage w/preservation perichondral sheath; sternal osteotomy/elevation w/or w/o internal bar fixation; bar left in place 6 mos; some use "tripod fixation" technique involving second and third costal cartilages to maintain sternal elevation
    - in Marfan syndrome recurrence rate high if internal support bar not utilized
  - Nuss procedure (recent/1997)
    - involves elevation of sternum/cartilage w/o sternal osteotomy or cartilage resection
    - large bar maintains elevation/left in place 2 yrs
    - probably best for 6–12 yr olds w/symmetric defects
- *Pectus carinatum:* cartilage resection/sternal osteotomy

COMPLICATIONS

- Operative/early postop:
  - pneumothorax
  - pulmonary injury, bleeding, infection: rare
- Late postop:
  - recurrence: major recurrence, 3–5%

WHEN TO REFER

- *Moderate to severe defect:* allows family counseling of risks/benefits of surgery
- Symptomatic defects

BACKGROUND

- 3 million STD cases/y in adolescents
- Microbial etiology mainly chlamydia, gonorrhea; other microbes include aerobes, anaerobes of normal vaginal flora
- ~10–20% gonorrheal and chlamydial cervical infections ascend and result in development of PID, inflammation of endometrium, fallopian tubes
- Complications of PID include tubo-ovarian abscess, perihepatitis
- Long-term sequelae occur in 25%, including ectopic pregnancy, infertility, chronic pelvic pain
- Risk factors:
  - behavioral: <19 yrs old, early sexual debut, multiple partners, unprotected sex
  - contraception: oral contraception ↑ risk chlamydial cervical infection, ↓ symptomatic chlamydial PID, has no effect on fertility; IUDs ↑ PID in initial months *after* insertion
  - biologic: ↑ ectopy (↑ columnar epithelial cells → ↑ attachment for chlamydia and types of gonococci at endocervix); relative ↓ immunologic competence due to inexperience w/prior STDs or PID
- "Silent" PID (no symptoms) make up small proportion of PID cases resulting in infertility later

CLINICAL MANIFESTATIONS (SYSTEMIC AND PELVIC EXAMS)

- Minimum diagnostic criteria: empirical treatment of PID encouraged when 3 minimum criteria present:
  - lower abdominal tenderness
  - adnexal tenderness
  - cervical motion tenderness
- Additional criteria (↑ specificity of Dx):
  - oral temperature >38.3°C
  - abnormal cervical/vaginal discharge
  - ↑ ESR
  - ↑ C-reactive protein
  - laboratory documentation of cervical gonorrhea or chlamydia infection
- Elaborate criteria (specific diagnostic tools, helpful when indicated/available):
  - tubo-ovarian abscess on sonography or other radiographic tests
  - histopathologic evidence of endometritis on endometrial biopsy (rarely indicated)
  - laparoscopic abnormalities consistent w/PID (rarely indicated)

DIFFERENTIAL DIAGNOSIS

- Reproductive tract:
  - pregnancy: ectopic or intrauterine pregnancy; spontaneous abortion
  - dysmenorrhea
  - endometriosis
  - ruptured corpus luteum cyst
  - torsion of ovary
- Urinary tract:
  - urethritis, cystitis, pyelonephritis
  - ureteral calculi
- GI tract:
  - appendicitis
  - diverticulitis
  - cholecystitis
  - gastroenteritis
  - hepatitis
  - inflammatory bowel disease
- Other:
  - pneumonia
  - pleuritis
  - sickle-cell crisis
  - trauma

TREATMENT

- Hospitalization recommended:
  - possibly all adolescents to ensure compliance
  - uncertain Dx when surgical emergencies such as appendicitis and ectopic pregnancy cannot be ruled out
  - pelvic abscess suspected
  - pregnancy
  - HIV positive pt
  - illness severe or nausea/vomiting do not permit compliance w/oral medication
  - pt unable to follow or tolerate outpt regimen
  - pt has failed to respond on outpt Tx (usually within 72 hrs)
  - clinical follow-up within 72 hrs of starting antibiotic treatment cannot be arranged
- Inpt treatment:
  - cefoxitin, 2 g IV q6h or cefotetan, 2 g IV q12h *plus* doxycycline, 100 mg po or IV q12h
  - clindamycin, 900 mg IV q8h *plus* gentamicin, 2 mg/kg loading dose IM or IV; then 1.5 mg/kg IV q8h
- Outpt treatment:
  - cefoxitin, 2 g IM plus probenecid, 1 g po in single dose (or ceftriaxone, 250 mg IM, or other parenteral third-generation cephalosporin (eg, ceftizoxime or cefotaxime) *plus* doxycycline, 100 mg po 2×/d × 14 d
  - ofloxacin, 400 mg po 2 ×/d × 14 d *plus* either clindamycin, 450 mg po 4 ×/d or metronidazole, 500 mg 2 ×/d × 14 d

COMPLICATIONS

- Tubo-ovarian abscess
- PID w/pregnancy
- Incorrect Dx, esp when surgical emergency (eg, ectopic pregnancy, acute appendicitis)
- Long-term sequelae (eg, infertility, pelvic pain, ectopic pregnancy)

WHEN TO REFER

- If pregnant, refer to Ob-Gyn
- If surgically acute abdomen, refer to Ob-Gyn/surgery
- If no improvement within 72 hrs and Dx still uncertain (reevaluate/? refer)
- If PID associated w/tubo-ovarian abscess, refer to Ob-Gyn

SUMMARY

- Dx PID largely based on subjective criteria
- Imperative to overdiagnose, overtreat, reevaluate within 48–72 hrs
- Main cause of tubal infertility and preventable by encouraging delay in onset of sexual activity, encouraging use of condoms when active, screening and treating asymptomatic gonorrhea, chlamydia as part of well adolescent care—important role for pediatricians

PENILE DISORDERS, MISCELLANEOUS: BALANITIS, PHIMOSIS, PARAPHIMOSIS, AND MEATAL STENOSIS

JOHN W. BROCK III AND SAM CHANG

BACKGROUND

- *Definition:* inflammatory processes involving preputial foreskin and glans region of phallus
- May affect any age group (newborn–adults), but commonly seen in younger uncircumcised children

BALANITIS

DEFINITION

- Technically, local cellulitic inflammation only of glans penis, but often used to describe inflammation of prepuce and distal phallus
- Often associated w/ and due to phimotic opening of distal foreskin

CLINICAL MANIFESTATIONS

- Erythema, swelling, inflammation, tenderness, difficulty retracting foreskin
- Increased incidence seen in diabetics; and inflammatory process may be first manifestation of previously unrecognized diabetes

TREATMENT

- *Mild cases:* local antibiotic cream/antifungal creams effective; oral antibiotics, eg, cephalosporin or sulfa medication useful adjuncts
- *Definitive treatment:* after local inflammation has subsided, circumcision best means for solution and prevention of recurrence

PHIMOSIS

DEFINITION

- Fibrotic narrowing, contraction of preputial opening to degree that retraction very difficult or impossible. Evolution of potential space between glans and preputial foreskin is a developmental process. W/ newborns, one normally cannot retract foreskin; by 1 yr of age ~50% retractable, and by 5 yrs, >90% retractable

CLINICAL MANIFESTATIONS

- Tight contracted opening, may even impede urinary stream, often associated w/ localized cellulitic inflammatory process (balanitis)

TREATMENT

- Most effective solutions are dorsal slit, which can be performed at bedside and/or circumcision, which is most definitive

PARAPHIMOSIS

DEFINITION

- Entrapment of phimotic prepuce proximal to (behind) the coronal margin. Initially after retracting phimotic foreskin, usually can bring foreskin back over glans—at times, however, difficult, and greater the length of time that phimotic foreskin retracted, greater chance for entrapment and paraphimosis

CLINICAL MANIFESTATIONS

- Once ring of tissue kept retracted, lymphatic congestion occurs, quickly leading to swelling, pain, tenderness, edema. Process quickly progresses to venous congestion and even arterial compromise

TREATMENT

- *Initial treatment:* manual reduction of paraphimosis. Place thumbs on glans to give countertraction as second and third digits envelope phimotic ring and pull tight foreskin back over glans. May be necessary to perform emergent dorsal slit to relieve constriction
- Definitive treatment: circumcision

MEATAL STENOSIS

DEFINITION

- Meatal stenosis occurs at the urethral opening in the distal portion of glans. The meatus may become irritated and inflamed, which can then progress to meatal stenosis. Normal caliber of urethral meatus for 18 mo old child should be ≥10 Fr.

TREATMENT

- Requires dilatation of meatus

BACKGROUND

- Bimodal distribution—infants (<12 mos), teenagers
- Incidence greater in boys
- Perianal abscess:
  - may be from infected diaper rash
- Perirectal abscess:
  - infection of crypt of Morgagni at dentate line, which tracts along intersphincteric plane
  - straight tract from crypt abscess to skin
  - in older children, perirectal abscess associated w/inflammatory bowel disease, immunodeficiency states, leukopenia
  - fistula in ano is recurrence of perirectal abscess after spontaneous or surgical drainage (abscess acute phase; fistula chronic phase)
  - 50% incidence of occurrence of fistula in ano after perirectal abscess
  - fistula in ano indicates tract lined w/granulation tissue exists between skin of anal region and crypt from which abscess arose
    - spontaneous healing of fistula in ano rare

CLINICAL MANIFESTATIONS

- Perirectal or perianal abscess:
  - tender, red mass in perianal area; rarely bilateral
  - perirectal abscess may require rectal exam for Dx
  - pain
  - fever
  - may spontaneously drain pus
  - internal opening radially opposite external opening
- Fistula in ano:
  - chronic punctum w/intermittent discharge of pus and/or blood

LABORATORY FEATURES

- WBC usually normal

DIFFERENTIAL DIAGNOSIS

- Periurethral abscess: urethral obstructive disease, urinary symptoms
- Anal fissure: painful lesion in posterior midline
- Furuncle
- Pilonidal disease (rare in infants)
- Buttock rhabdomyosarcoma (very rare)

TREATMENT

- Perirectal or perianal abscess:
  - sitz baths or warm compresses if not fluctuant
  - surgical incision, drainage w/sedation, local anesthesia in infant
  - surgical incision, drainage w/general anesthesia in older child
  - spontaneously draining abscess needs surgical exploration to effect complete drainage
  - perioperative antibiotics, esp endocarditis prophylaxis
  - antibiotics alone inadequate treatment
- Fistula in ano:
  - fistulotomy or fistulectomy under general anesthesia

COMPLICATIONS

- ~50% perirectal abscesses persist as fistula in ano; require excision of fistulous tract under general anesthesia. Wound left open to granulate
- Recurrence of fistula in ano rare if treated appropriately w/fistulotomy/fistulectomy

WHEN TO REFER

- Fluctuant or spontaneously draining perianal or perirectal abscess or fistula in ano

PERICARDITIS, ACUTE

CHARLES A. BULLABOY

BACKGROUND

- *Infrequent:* reported ~1/850 hospital admissions
- *Varied and sundry etiologies:* idiopathic; infections: bacterial *(Staphylococcus aureus, H. influenzae);* viral (Coxsackie virus B5, echovirus 6, HIV); mycobacterial (tuberculosis); autoimmune (JRA, SLE); drugs (procainamide, minoxidil); traumatic; neoplastic; radiation
- Presumed immune/inflammatory response in one-third of cases w/o discernable cause; self-limited course usually lasting 2–6 wks
- Purulent pericarditis predominance in children <2 yrs of age
- Sequelae of inflammation, effusion, tamponade, fibrosis w/constriction

CLINICAL MANIFESTATIONS

- *Nonspecific as related to inciting etiology:* fever, malaise, anorexia, myalgia, tachycardia, tachypnea w/shallow respirations
- *Chest pain:* typically exacerbated by inspiration or lying flat and ameliorated by sitting upright and leaning forward
- *Pericardial friction rub:* superficial, scratchy, grating, similar to squeak of new leather at left sternal border and/or apex
- *Effusion:* distant, muffled heart tones
- Tamponade w/hemodynamic embarrassment manifest by inspiratory ↓ in systolic BP >10 torr (ie, "pulsus paradoxus"); inspiratory distention of neck veins (Kussmaul sign); compressed left lower lobe producing bronchial breath sounds below the left scapula (Ewart sign)

LABORATORY FEATURES

- *Electrocardiography:* inflammatory evolution of widespread ST-segment elevation w/reciprocal depression in aVR, V1, V2; return to baseline followed by T-wave flattening/inversion, resolution; low voltage and electrical alternans w/effusion
- *Chest roentgenogram:* "water-bottle" configuration w/large effusions
- *Echocardiography:* sensitive and specific in Dx, hemodynamic evaluation, follow-up of pericardial effusion; diastolic collapse of RA, RV, or LA signs of cardiac tamponade
- *Echocardiographically guided pericardiocentesis w/percutaneous catheter drainage or percutaneous balloon pericardiotomy:* not indicated unless doubtful Dx, tamponade, suspected bacterial or malignant pericarditis, or w/prolonged, complicated cases
- *Other:* as indicated in determining underlying disease process

DIFFERENTIAL DIAGNOSIS

- *Chest pain:* Tietze syndrome, precordial catch syndrome, trauma
- Spontaneous pneumothorax
- Pneumonia w/pleuritis
- Congenital absence of pericardium
- *Angina:* anomalous left coronary artery, Kawasaki disease
- *1° myocardial disease:* myocarditis, cardiomyopathies
- Aortic dissection

TREATMENT

- *General supportive measures:* bed rest and restricted physical endeavors until resolution of pain and fever
- NSAIDs for quieting immune/inflammatory response and pain control; continue ~2 wks
  - ASA, 80–100 mg/kg/d po div q4–6h; max 3.6 g/d
  - ibuprofen, 30–40 mg/kg/d po div q6–8h; max 2.4 g/d
  - indomethacin, 1–2.5 mg/kg/d po div q6–12 h; max 200 mg/d
- *Corticosteroids:* only w/refractory cases that fail NSAID agents; frequent rebound phenomenon when tapered; mask other illnesses
  - prednisone, 1–2 mg/kg/d po div q6–8 h; max 60 mg

COMPLICATIONS

- Tamponade
- Relapse of pericarditis or chronic effusion in up to 15% of cases upon cessation of Tx
- *Constrictive pericarditis:* rare postviral involvement; may acutely follow purulent pericarditis; leading cause worldwide is tuberculous pericarditis; difficult to distinguish from restrictive cardiomyopathy

WHEN TO REFER

- *Hemodynamically unstable pts:* require urgent pericardiocentesis
- *Bacterial pericarditis:* life-threatening illness necessitating appropriate antimicrobial Tx, pericardial drainage, intensive supportive care
- *Recurrent pericarditis:* may require prolonged immunosuppression or surgical pericardiectomy
- *Suspected constriction or restrictive cardiomyopathy:* difficult, challenging Dx, often requiring CT, MRI, cardiac catheterization w/endomyocardial biopsy or exploratory thoracotomy to ferret out

BACKGROUND

- *Periorbital cellulitis:* superficial to periorbital septum:
  - Hx trauma, insect sting, or bite in 25–33% of cases not predictive of etiology unless local wound infection
  - sinusitis, URI, or otitis present in 50% of cases but not predictive of etiology
  - unilateral >95% of cases
  - eyelid discoloration present in most cases but not helpful in predicting etiology
  - Hx immunization w/*Hemophilus influenzae* type B conjugate vaccine important. Pt who has received 2 doses w/last dose given at least 1 wk prior to onset of periorbital cellulitis very unlikely to have Hib disease
  - etiology w/o purulent wound: *Streptococcus pneumoniae* or Hib
  - etiology w/purulent wound: *Staphylococcus aureus, Streptococcus pyogenes* (necrotizing lesions of eyelid also reported)
- *Orbital cellulitis:* deep to periorbital septum, involving orbital structures:
  - sinusitis present >75% of cases
  - almost always unilateral
  - may be surgical emergency
  - etiology not identified in 75%; *S. aureus, S. pyogenes, S. pneumoniae,* anaerobes most frequent isolates

CLINICAL MANIFESTATIONS

- Obtain Hx trauma, insect bite or sting, allergy, Hib conjugate vaccine
- Complete physical examination of involved eye *must* be done
- Clinical findings:

	% pts
Swelling	100
Unilateral	98
Temperature >38.5°C	68
Chemosis	13

- Distinguishing features:

	Periorbital	Orbital
Age (mean)	<5 yrs (2.75)	>5 yrs (7.4)
Hx trauma	negative >95%	positive 25–33%
Proptosis	–	+ or —
Ophthalmoplegia	–	+ or –
Eye pain	–	+ or –
Change in vision	–	+ or –
Chemosis	+ or –	+ or –

LABORATORY FEATURES

- CT scan of orbit if signs of orbital involvement
- Laboratory evaluation unlikely to yield information useful in making early management decisions
- Lumbar puncture should be performed on children <1 yr of age unless vaccinated against Hib and w/o CNS Sx
- Specimens of blood, purulent material from wounds near involved eye, or material obtained at surgery or by aspiration of paranasal sinuses should be cultured for bacterial pathogens

DIFFERENTIAL DIAGNOSIS

- Conjunctivitis, blepharitis, allergy, trauma, insect bite or sting, sinusitis, tumor, dacryocystitis, dacryoadenitis, sty, chalazion, Chagas disease (Ramoña sign)

TREATMENT

- Pts w/orbital cellulitis should be hospitalized and receive parenteral ceftriaxone (50 mg/kg/d 1×/d) to cover pathogens associated w/acute sinusitis *plus* clindamycin (10 mg/kg per dose q8h) to cover *S. aureus* and anaerobes. Narrow coverage when etiology is known
- Selected pts w/periorbital cellulitis can be treated as outpts if no signs of orbital involvement, child does not appear toxic. Obtain blood culture, give ceftriaxone (50 mg/kg IM or IV 1×/d). If culture negative at 48 hrs, change to oral agent like ampicillin-clavulanate or trimethoprim/sulfamethoxazole to complete 7–10 d
- Pts w/purulent wound near involved eyelid should be treated w/semisynthetic penicillin like oxacillin or nafcillin, or first-generation cephalosporin like cefazolin or cephalothin, or macrolide like clindamycin to cover *S. aureus* and *S. pyogenes*

COMPLICATIONS

- *CNS:* including meningitis, brain abscess, subdural empyema, blindness or visual loss, optic nerve atrophy, cavernous sinus thrombosis
- Eyelid abscess, orbital abscess, periosteal abscess

PREVENTION

- *H. influenzae* type B conjugate vaccine

WHEN TO REFER

- If complete eye exam cannot be performed or if signs of orbital involvement, ophthalmologist should be consulted

BACKGROUND

- Peritonitis indicates inflammation of parietal, visceral peritoneal membranes. Etiology may be chemical (eg, spillage of bile, pancreatic enzymes or lymph) or infectious
- Infectious peritonitis 1° or 2°
- 1° peritonitis (spontaneous peritonitis or spontaneous bacterial peritonitis) originates outside peritoneal cavity and contaminates normally sterile peritoneal cavity by hematogenous or lymphatic spread
- 2° peritonitis results from 1° intraabdominal catastrophe, such as rupture of hollow viscus (eg, appendix) or abscess/infected cyst in solid organ
- Peritonitis may result from trauma or infected foreign body (eg, ventriculoperitoneal shunt)
- 1° peritonitis occurs almost solely in pts w/ascites (eg, cirrhotics and nephrotics)
- Bacterial agents identified in children w/1° peritonitis include *Streptococcus pneumoniae,* group A beta-hemolytic streptococci, gram-negative enteric bacilli. Multiple organisms, aerobic and anaerobic, identified in peritoneal fluid of child w/2° peritonitis
- Bacteria of genital tract, including *N. gonorrhoeae* and *Chlamydia trachomatis,* cultured from peritoneal cavity of sexually active teenage females
- Early antibiotic Tx almost always effective; prognosis relates to underlying disease(s)

CLINICAL MANIFESTATIONS

- Severe abdominal pain
- Fever (often to 40°C)
- Nausea/vomiting; diarrhea rarely
- Toxic appearance w/tachycardia, shallow respirations, altered mental acuity
- Abdominal distention w/diffuse tenderness initially; localization to lower abdomen may be seen as infection/inflammation progresses

LABORATORY FEATURES

- ↑ WBC w/predominance immature forms
- Hemoconcentration
- Metabolic acidosis
- Abdominal sonogram reveals free intraperitoneal fluid, no abscess and normal appendix
- Pneumoperitoneum if 2° peritonitis
- Paracentesis:
  - ↑ WBC (>300/mm^3); granulocyte predominance
  - fluid pH <7.35; lactate >25 mg/dL
  - gram stain positive (>40%)
  - 2° peritonitis: multiple bacterial forms on Gram stain, and ↑ amylase and bilirubin levels (vs. serum)
  - positive culture (90%)

DIFFERENTIAL DIAGNOSIS

- Acute pancreatitis
- Acute intermittent porphyria
- Acute chylous ascites (eg, postop)
- Familial Mediterranean fever
- Idiopathic panniculitis

TREATMENT

- 1° peritonitis:
  - cefotaxime, 200 mg/kg/24 h div q6–8 h IV until culture/sensitivities available
    - alternative Tx: classic: ampicillin, 100 mg/kg/24 h div q6h plus gentamicin, 7.5 mg/kg/24 h div q8h
    - preliminary data suggest that oral oflaxacin 20 mg/kg/24 h div q12h may be as effective as IV cefotaxime
- 2° peritonitis:
  - ampicillin, gentamicin (as above) plus clindamycin, 40 mg/kg/24 h div q6–8h IV
    - alternative Tx: ticarcillin/clavulanate, 300 mg/kg/24 h div q4–6 IV *or* imipenem-cilastatin, 100 mg/kg/24 h div q6–8 h IV *plus* tobramycin, 7.5 mg/kg/24 h div q8h
  - Paracentesis repeated in 48 hrs. Significant reduction in WBC and negative culture support efficacy

COMPLICATIONS

- *Fluid loculation/abscess formation:* require surgical drainage

WHEN TO REFER

- Surgical consultation when 2° peritonitis diagnosed
- 1° peritonitis in cirrhotic pt may be considered indication for hepatic replacement
- Consultation w/pediatric gastroenterologist or pediatric nephrologist for assistance in overall management of pts w/cirrhosis and nephrosis

SARAH S. LONG

BACKGROUND

- *Bordella pertussis* usual cause of pertussis and sole cause of epidemic pertussis; *B. parapertussis* responsible ~5% of cases, and respiratory viruses and *Mycoplasma pneumoniae* for occasional pertussis-like illnesses
- Most frequent in infants <1 yr of age and in adolescents
- Symptoms more severe in underimmunized individuals
- Adult w/protracted coughing illness usual (but unrecognized) index case in family
- Clinical course ~6 wks in older children and adolescents; more protracted in infants
- Mortality (0.5%) limited to infants

CLINICAL MANIFESTATIONS

- Progressively worsening cough following insignificant URI
- Afebrile
- Normal physical examination
- Well between paroxysms
- Abrupt onset of machine gun–like paroxysms of cough, sometimes followed by loud inspiratory whoop (older infant, toddler) and/or vomiting (children, adults)
- Apnea, post-tussive cyanosis, prostration, or fugue-like state esp in young infants
- Subconjunctional hemorrhages, upper body petechiae, torn frenulum sometimes from forceful coughing

LABORATORY FEATURES

- Lymphocytosis (10,000–100,000/μL) w/normal small lymphocytes
- Thrombocytosis (500,000–1,000,000/μL)
- Lymphocytosis and thrombocytosis most profound in unimmunized individuals and parallels severity of illness
- Neutrophilia or left shift not present unless 2° bacterial pneumonia
- Chest radiograph abnormal in majority of hospitalized cases w/perihilar densities (butterfly appearance); atelectasis common; extraparenchymal air not uncommon

	Pertussis	Lower respiratory tract infection
Onset prodrome	Mild URI	Abrupt, w/fever, constitutional symptoms
Onset cough	Predominant symptom	Commensurate w/other symptoms
Character cough	Paroxysmal, machine gun–like bursts on single expiration	Intermittent, nondescript, staccato
Behavior during paroxysm	Anxious, inattentive; eyes watery, bulging; w/or w/o apnea, cyanosis, loss of stature	Alert, attentive
Behavior at end paroxysm	Exhausted; altered state; w/or w/o inspiratory whoop; w/or w/o vomiting	Alert, active
Behavior between paroxysms	Normal	Not well (depends on cause and severity of infection)
Physical examination	Normal	Tachypnea, retractions, wheezes, rhonchi, rales; w/or w/o rhinorrhea, conjunctivitis, enanthem, exanthem

DIFFERENTIAL DIAGNOSIS

- Upper respiratory tract viral infections
- Lower respiratory tract viral, mycoplasmal, chlamydial infections
- Allergic syndrome (eg, cough: equivalent asthma)
- Chronic bronchitis (eg, cystic fibrosis, immune deficiency)
- Airway or cardiac anomalies

DIAGNOSIS

- Culture of nasopharyngeal secretions in Regan-Lowe or other specialized medium (special transport media required)
- Direct florescent antibody staining of nasopharyngeal secretions
- Polymerase chain reaction of gene products in nasopharyngeal secretions available at some sites

TREATMENT

- *Erythromycin:* 40–50 mg/kg d po in 4 div doses (max 2 g/d), × 14 d
- *Albuterol, corticosteroids, immunoglobulin:* use not warranted
- *Mist:* may be helpful
- *Environment:* quiet, low lighted, smoke free
- Household and other close contacts should be given erythromycin (as above) promptly, regardless of Hx immunization or age

COMPLICATIONS

- Apnea, bradycardia, seizures, encephalopathy (limited to infants, and during escalating phase of disease)
- 2° bacterial pneumonia
- Malnutrition, apathy

DECISION ON DISPOSITION

- *Infants <3 mos:* hospitalized to determine degree of distress, evolution of symptoms, ability for self-rescue
- *Infants ≥3 mos:* paroxysm must be witnessed to determine disposition

BACKGROUND

- *Pharyngitis/tonsillitis:* vague clinical term used to describe infection of upper respiratory tract w/emphasis on involvement of pharynx and tonsils
- Can be caused by viruses and bacteria (see table)
- More common in older children; unusual in infants
- Incubation period 1–5 d, usually 2–3 d
- Usually spread to contacts by close contact
- In clinical practice only need to separate streptococcal infections from all the rest
- Virus infections do not require antimicrobial treatment
- Among infections due to bacteria, those due to group A streptococcus require antimicrobial treatment

CLINICAL MANIFESTATIONS

- Classic features of streptococcal pharyngitis:
  - sudden onset
  - sore throat (pain on swallowing)
  - fever
  - headache
  - nausea, vomiting, abdominal pain (esp in children)
  - marked inflammation of throat, tonsils
  - patchy discrete exudate
  - tender, enlarged anterior cervical nodes
  - scarlet fever
- *Rare:* suggestive of other etiologies:
  - conjunctivitis
  - cough
  - laryngitis (stridor, croup)
  - diarrhea
  - nasal discharge (except in young children)
  - muscle aches/malaise
- Occurs most frequently in winter, early spring in school-age children who have close contact w/infected person
- One-third to one-half pts w/streptococcal pharyngitis do not have classic features
- *Some pts w/nonstreptococcal infections have characteristic clinical features:* pharyngoconjunctival fever (adenoviruses); herpangina, lymphonodular pharyngitis, hand, foot, mouth disease (enteroviruses)
- Etiologic Dx not clear in most cases, requiring laboratory Dx

LABORATORY FEATURES

- Very useful tests:
  - throat culture on sheep blood agar "gold standard," 90+% sensitive; less specific
  - rapid strep test on throat swab; almost 100% specific for group A streptococcal infections but less sensitive than throat culture. Does not recognize groups C and G infections
  - standard practice: do rapid test first. If positive, no need for throat culture. If negative, do throat culture
- Tests of limited usefulness:
  - WBC count. May be ↑ in streptococcal pharyngitis. Not helpful in most cases
  - determination of streptococcal antibody (usually ASO) in acute and convalescent blood samples. Rise makes retrospective Dx
- Tests of no usefulness:
  - rapid tests for Dx of some viral infections rarely helpful in pts w/pharyngitis/tonsillitis
  - viral cultures no help

Bacterial Causes
Common:
- Group A streptococcus
- Less Common
  - *Arcanobacterium hemolyticum*
  - *Chlamydia pneumoniae*
  - *Groups C & G streptococci*
  - *Mycoplasma pneumoniae*
- Unusual:
  - *Neisseria gonorrhoeae*
  - *Neisseria meningitidis*
- Not causative
  - *Chlamydia trachomatous*
  - *Haemophilus influenzae*
  - *Moraxella catarrhalis*
  - *Staphylococcus aureus*
  - *Streptococcus pneumoniae*

- Intrepretation of a positive rapid strep test or throat culture:
  - streptococci remain for wks to mos in throats of untreated or inadequately treated pts
  - "carried" streptococci not harmful to host or to contacts
  - obtain rapid strep tests and throat cultures only from pts w/sufficient clinical and epidemiologic evidence of streptococcal infection

MANAGEMENT OF NON–GROUP A STREPTOCOCCAL INFECTIONS

- Groups C, G streptococcal infections:
  - will have negative rapid strep test and positive throat culture
  - do not cause rheumatic fever
  - treatment same as for group A infections
- *A. hemolyticum, C. pneumoniae,* M. pneumoniae infections:
  - cannot be differentiated clinically from group A infections
  - no readily available laboratory tests to aid Dx
  - usual treatment supportive only

TREATMENT OF STREPTOCOCCAL INFECTIONS

- Penicillin:
  - drug of choice except in pts w/penicillin allergy; no resistant organisms
  - adequate treatment of streptococcal pharyngitis prevents spread to contacts and acute rheumatic fever
  - oral penicillins
    - penicillin V: 250 mg 2–3 ×/d in most children. Adolescents, 500 mg 2–3 ×/d
      - treat 10 full d
    - ampicillin/amoxicillin; satisfactory treatment but offers no microbiologic advantage
  - IM benzathine penicillin G. Preferred in pts unlikely to complete 10 d course of oral Tx; 600,000 units IM for pts weighing ≤27 kg, 1,200,000 units for heavier children. Combination of 900,000 units of benthazine G, 300,000 units of procaine penicillin G satisfactory for most children, less painful
- Other antimicrobial agents:
  - macrolides:
    - oral erthyromycin × 10 d acceptable for pts allergic to penicillin
    - erythromycin estolate, 20–40 mg/kg/d in 2–4 doses; or erythromycin ethyl succinate, 40 mg/kg/d in 2–4 doses. Max. dose of erythromycin is 1 g/d

Viral Causes
Common:
- Adenoviruses, types 1, 2, 3, 5
- Less common:
  - Enteroviruses
  - Epstein-Barr virus
  - Herpes simplex virus
  - Influenza viruses
  - Parainfluenza viruses
  - Respiratory syncytial virus

- Infrequent:
  - Coronaviruses
  - Rhinoviruses

  - oral cephalosporins:
    - 10 d course of oral, narrow-spectrum cephalosporin acceptable alternative
  - clindamycin:
    - 10 d course of oral clindamycin also acceptable alternative
- Unacceptable antimicrobial drugs for treatment:
  - tetracyclines, sulfonamides, trimethoprim/sulfamethoxazole

COMPLICATIONS

- Suppurative complications such as otitis media, sinusitis, cervical adenitis can accompany cases of pharyngitis due to viruses and bacteria
- Recurrence of streptococcal infections; retreat only symptomatic relapses
- Development of streptococcal toxic shock syndrome (STSS)
- Acute rheumatic fever and acute glomerulonephritis

PREVENTION

- Early treatment w/eradication of streptococcus prevents spread. Pts considered noninfectious 24 hrs after treatment started
- Sulfomamides or penicillin effective prophylactic measures for streptococcal infections but infrequently used except in pts who have had rheumatic fever or in unusual circumstances such as in military populations

WHEN TO REFER

- Almost all pts managed w/o referral
- Pts w/streptococcal toxic shock syndrome should be hospitalized immediately and referred if adequate acute care cannot be assured
- Pts w/severe complications such as cellulitis or necrotizing fasciitis should be hospitalized immediately, referred if adequate acute care and surgical consultation not available

BACKGROUND

- *Etiology:* deficiency of phenylalanine hydroxylase enzyme, which normally converts phenylalanine (PHE) to tyrosine. Degree of enzyme deficiency varies
- Autosomal recessive inheritance; gene location 12q24.1. Over 300 gene mutations identified thus far. Prenatal Dx possible if both mutations have been identified in proband child
- *Incidence:* 1/10,000–15,000 births in US

CLINICAL MANIFESTATIONS

- Progressive mental/motor retardation
- Hypopigmentation w/fair skin, blue eyes, light hair, failure to tan
- Musty odor to urine, perspiration
- Some have seizures and/or eczema

LABORATORY FEATURES

- Newborn screening (24 hrs–3 d of age). Guthrie bacterial inhibition or tandem mass spectrometry assay done in all 50 states and most industrialized countries. Detects ↑ of blood PHE of 4 mg/dl (twice upper limit of normal)
- *Confirmation:* amino acid quantitation confirms ↑ blood PHE level; tyrosine level normal or low

Classification of Hyperphenylalaninemias

	Blood Phenylalanine Level (mg/dl)	Mental Retardation	Need for Treatment
Classic PKU	>20	Virtually all	All*
Atypical (variant) PKU	6–20	Mild to moderate	Most*
Benign persistent hyperphenylalaninemia	2–6	None	None*
Biopterin defects	4–40	Normal to severe	All

*Women in these categories require careful treatment during pregnancy whenever blood phenylalanine >6 mg/dl.

DIFFERENTIAL DIAGNOSIS

- Biopterin defects can also result in hyperphenylalaninemia because they interfere w/availability of BH_4, necessary cofactor for phenylalanine hydroxylase enzyme
- Deficiency of any one of three enzymes may cause biopterin defects; two of these enzymes responsible for BH_4 synthesis and one for regenerating biologically active BH_4 from its dihydro form
- These disorders must be r/o in all newborns presenting w/hyperphenylalaninemia; treatment far more complex than for PKU, must be initiated as early as possible

TREATMENT

- Required for any pt w/blood PHE level >6 mg/dl
- If Tx begun prior to 2–3 wks of age, normal IQ achieved
- *Treatment principles:* lower PHE intake, supplement tyrosine as needed
- Major source of protein (80–90%) "medical food," powder from which infant formula and later "milk substitute" made. Contains amino acids (w/o PHE) plus fat, carbohydrate, vitamins, minerals
- Source of PHE provided in limited amounts, geared to maintain blood PHE level in therapeutic 2–6 mg/dl range. Provided by infant formula or breast milk initially. Later, source of PHE low-protein foods such as fruits and vegetables. All foods containing any protein must be weighed/measured carefully. Extensive listings available detailing PHE content of foods. Special foods modified to be low in protein useful as supplements to natural foods; these include pastas, flour for baking, rice, cookies, etc
- Both "medical food" and PHE sources distributed throughout day, so steady source of various nutrients available
- Blood tyrosine levels followed along w/PHE levels; additional tyrosine powder added to formula as needed to keep blood tyrosine level 1–2 mg/dl
- Growth, mental development, psychological adjustment carefully monitored
- Diet diaries analyzed regularly for sufficiency of all major nutrients, such as essential fatty acids, minerals, etc.
- Family, patient education should be ongoing
- During illnesses, prescribed amount of PHE cut to half or less, to minimize ↑ of PHE that occurs due to catabolic effect of illness. Intake of full amount of medical food maintained, to minimize catabolism
- Treatment must be lifelong
- Any adult PKU woman w/blood PHE level >6 mg/dl must achieve very rigid control of blood PHE level (<6 mg/dl) *before* attempting to conceive. Stringent degree of control must be maintained throughout pregnancy. Higher maternal blood levels carry serious risk of babies being born w/microcephaly, mental retardation, various birth defects including congenital heart disease. In general, incidence, severity of fetal damage directly proportional to degree of maternal blood PHE elevation

RESULTS OF TREATMENT

- *If adequate:* normal IQ
- May have minor specific deficits including visual-motor, visuospatial, executive functions, often only detected by sophisticated testing
- Higher incidence of ADHD and of ADD; virtually all affected pts benefit from methylphenidate treatment

COMPLICATIONS

- Inadequate control of PHE levels, if chronic, can result in declining IQ. In addition, behavioral and personality deterioration, including irritability, depression, anxiety, agoraphobia or even frank psychosis may occur
- Possible neurologic deterioration over time described
- Overlimitation of PHE and/or insufficient intake of "medical food" results in suboptimal protein synthesis. If deficiencies severe, slowing of growth, dermatitis, brain damage, even death can occur

WHEN TO REFER

- PKU should always be treated in center experienced in managing all aspects of disorder

PIEBALDISM, WAARDENBURG SYNDROME, AND TUBEROUS SCLEROSIS

SANDY S. TSAO AND KENNETH A. ARNDT

PIEBALDISM

BACKGROUND

- Autosomal dominant developmental disorder of neural crest-derived melanoblasts; involves defective cell proliferation/migration during embryogenesis; all races affected
- Mutation in c-*kit* proto-oncogene, which encodes for cell-surface receptor expressed on melanocytes; KIT function required for normal development of dermal melanocytes prior to melanoblast migration from neural crest and postnatally

CLINICAL MANIFESTATIONS

- Tuft of white hair over midfrontal scalp (white forelock) in 80–90% pts w/underlying hypopigmentation of scalp
- Congenital, well-demarcated, chalky-white (depigmented) nonscaly macules principally involving forehead, ventral chest and abdomen, upper arms, lower legs; roughly symmetrical about midline; islands of hyperpigmentation observed within hypopigmented macules
- Noninvolvement of central back, shoulders, hips, hands, feet
- Involved areas remain stable in shape/size over time
- Café-au-lait macules frequently observed
- No visual tract/hearing defects noted; normal retinal pigmentation

LABORATORY FEATURES

- Wood lamp examination: bright white macules w/focal areas of hyperpigmentation
- Histopathology: markedly reduced to absent melanocytes within hypopigmented macules w/paradoxical increase in melanocytes at margins of macules; normal melanocyte numbers within hyperpigmented macules

DIFFERENTIAL DIAGNOSIS

- Waardenburg syndrome
- Albinism
- Vitiligo
- Nevus depigmentosus

TREATMENT

- *No treatment:* generally stable distribution and size
- *Topical corticosteroids:* ineffective for repigmentation
- *Photochemotherapy:* ineffective for repigmentation
- *Minigrafting/autologous melanocyte transplantation:* may be successful for repigmentation of localized areas; requires experienced dermatologist for procedure
- *Depigmentation:* recommended only for pts w/extensive disease/extreme distress regarding cosmetic appearance; treatment applied to normally pigmented skin; effect permanent/irreversible; side effects include sunburns, irreversibility; requires experienced dermatologist for procedure

COMPLICATIONS

- None

PREVENTION

- Auditory testing to r/o sensorineural deafness (Waardenburg syndrome)

WHEN TO REFER

- Referral to dermatologist to confirm Dx

WAARDENBURG SYNDROME

BACKGROUND

- Autosomal dominant/autosomal recessive developmental disorder of neural crest-derived melanoblasts; type I: chromosome 2q; type II: chromosome 3p; type IV: chromosome 13q
- Frequency of 1–2/100,000
- Accounts for 0.5% cases of congenital deafness
- Type I: defect in *PAX*-3 gene, which encodes transcription factor critical for activating melanoblasts/other cellular elements to proliferate/to begin migration from neural crest; type II: defect in *MITF* (microphthalmia) gene, which encodes dimeric transcription factor critical for melanocyte development/regulation of many melanocyte-specific genes; type IV: defect in *endothelin*-3 gene

CLINICAL MANIFESTATIONS

- Congenital, well-demarcated, chalky-white (depigmented) macules similar to those observed in piebaldism
- Tuft of white hair over midfrontal scalp (white forelock) in at least 17% pts
- Pigmentary abnormalities of iris (heterochromia irides)
- Lateral displacement of inner canthi of the eyes/normal interpupillary distance (dystopia canthorum)
- Congenital sensorineural deafness of one/both ears
- Broad nasal root
- Hypertrichosis/fusion of medial eyebrows
- Four variants: type I: piebaldism-like depigmentation, heterochromia irides, dystopia canthorum, deafness; type II: same findings as type I w/o dystopia canthorum; type III (Klein-Waardenburg): piebaldism-like depigmentation, heterochromia irides, dystopia canthorum, deafness, congenital upper limb deformities; type IV: same findings as type II with Hirschsprung disease

LABORATORY FEATURES

- Wood lamp examination: bright white macules
- Histopathology: absent melanocytes

DIFFERENTIAL DIAGNOSIS

- Piebaldism
- Albinism
- Vitiligo
- Nevus depigmentosus

TREATMENT

- *No treatment:* self-limited in distribution
- *Topical corticosteroids:* ineffective for repigmentation
- *Photochemotherapy:* ineffective for repigmentation
- *Minigrafting/autologous melanocyte transplantation:* may be successful for repigmentation of localized areas; requires experienced dermatologist for procedure
- *Depigmentation:* recommended only for pts w/extensive disease/extreme distress regarding cosmetic appearance; treatment applied to normally pigmented skin; effect permanent/irreversible; side effects include sunburns, irreversibility; requires experienced dermatologist for procedure

COMPLICATIONS

- None

PREVENTION

- None

WHEN TO REFER

- Referral to dermatologist for confirmation of Dx
- Referral to ophthalmologist for optic evaluation
- Referral to ENT for auditory testing

TUBEROUS SCLEROSIS

BACKGROUND

- M:F ratio 1:1; incidence of 1/20,000 to 1/100,000; all races affected
- Autosomal dominant w/variable penetrance/spontaneous mutations; two loci identified; one on chromosome 9q34 (TSC-1)/one on chromosome 16p13.3 (TSC-2); TSC-2 encodes protein, tuberin, which functions as tumor suppressor gene

CLINICAL MANIFESTATIONS

- Congenital well-circumscribed 2 mm–12 cm macules/patches w/partial pigmentary loss/perifollicular pigmentation; earliest sign of tuberous sclerosis, present at birth (80%) or by age 2 yrs (100%); remain stable in size/shape; lance-ovate (ash-leaf), polygonal (thumbprint), confetti-like configurations most commonly on back, oriented in transverse direction, extremities, oriented in cephalocaudad direction
- Connective tissue nevi (shagreen patches; 40%) appearing between ages 2–5 yrs, presenting as flesh-toned plaques w/gooseflesh appearance
- Skin-colored papules/nodules of central face (angiofibromas; adenoma sebaceum; 70%), mouth, neck, axillae, scalp; appear after infancy
- Periungual/subungual fibromas (Koenen tumor; 22%) appearing after puberty
- Slightly red plaque (fibrous plaque; large angiofibroma) on forehead/scalp
- Patchy white hairs within scalp, eyebrows/eyelashes
- Circumscribed hypopigmentation of iris/fundus; retinal hamartomas
- Neurologic manifestations include seizures (infantile spasms; 80–90%), mental retardation (45%); cerebral calcifications (56–88%), intracranial subependymal hamartomas (cortical tubers) detected early in childhood
- Cardiac rhabdomyosarcomas (58%), renal angiomyolipomas, pulmonary lymphangiomyomatosis; liver, testicular hamartomas

LABORATORY FEATURES

- Wood lamp examination: dull white to off-white macules
- Histopathology: ash-leaf spot: normal to reduced number of melanocytes, ↓ number of melanosomes; angiofibromas: fibroblast proliferation w/associated angiogenesis and increased collagen; cortical tubers: gliomas

DIFFERENTIAL DIAGNOSIS

- Vitiligo
- Nevus depigmentosus
- Piebaldism
- Hypomelanosis of Ito

TREATMENT

- *No treatment:* hypopigmented macules stable in size/number
- *Sunscreen:* Protection of involved skin from sunburn/limitation of tanning of normally pigmented skin; UVA, UVB, titanium dioxide spf > 30 recommended
- *Topical corticosteroids:* ineffective
- *Photochemotherapy:* ineffective
- *Carbon dioxide laser surgery:* resurfacing of angiofibromas to flatten lesions

COMPLICATIONS

- Dependent on organ systems involved

PREVENTION

- Screening echocardiogram (ECHO) to r/o rhabdomyosarcoma
- Head CT to r/o intracranial calcifications, MRI to r/o cranial subependymal tubers, abdominal/chest CT to r/o organ hamartomas
- Ophthalmologic examination to r/o fundal hamartomas
- Genetic counseling of affected patients and family members
- Cutaneous screening of first-degree relatives

WHEN TO REFER

- Referral to dermatologist for confirmation of Dx/long-term follow-up

GENERAL NOTE

- Pigmented lesions common findings in newborns
- Range from self-resolving lesions of no medical significance (eg, transient neonatal pustular melanosis, mongolian spots) to lesions w/significant medical risk/serious cosmetic deformities (eg, giant congenital nevi)
- Dx usually reached by clinical examination

TRANSIENT NEONATAL PUSTULAR MELANOSIS

BACKGROUND

- Benign disorder in 0.2–4% of all term newborns
- More common in African Americans
- Pigmentation postinflammatory

CLINICAL MANIFESTATIONS

- Presents at birth w/pustules, vesicles/pigmented macules
- Usually lesions cluster over chin, forehead, neck, lower back, shins/may be anywhere

DIAGNOSIS

- If vesiculopustules present, smear will demonstrate neutrophils, cellular debris, w/o organisms
- Look for collarette of scale around pigmented macules as evidence of prior vesicopustules

TREATMENT

- None necessary; pigmented macules resolve within 3 mos

CAFÉ-AU-LAIT MACULES (CALM)

BACKGROUND

- Onset birth/early infancy
- 1.9% of newborns have single CALM (more common in African Americans); 12% have single CALM, 1.8% have 3
- 10–28% of school-age children have ≥1 CALM
- Represent increased activity of melanocytes w/o melanocytic hyperplasia

CLINICAL MANIFESTATIONS

- Uniform, well-demarcated, light brown macules of any size
- Often truncal but any body site can be involved
- Growth proportionate to body size

ASSOCIATED DISORDERS

- Neurofibromatosis type 1
- McCune-Albright syndrome
- Watson syndrome
- Many other disorders have CALM as occasional finding

MANAGEMENT

- Usually none necessary
- Consider evaluation for associated disorders if >5 CALM ≥0.5 cm/if abnormalities in other organ systems present
- If occurring in swirled/segmental pattern consider hypomelanosis of Ito (Linear and Whorled Hypermelanosis)

NEVUS SPILUS

BACKGROUND

- Present in 0.2% of newborns
- M = F
- Represent ↑ activity of melanocytes (café-au-lait–like regions) in association w/melanocytic hyperplasia (speckled regions)

CLINICAL MANIFESTATIONS

- Well-demarcated tan to brown café-au-lait–like macule w/superimposed more darkly pigmented macules/papules giving speckled appearance
- Most common on trunk/extremities
- Size: 1 cm–> 20 cm

MANAGEMENT

- Melanoma arising in nevus spilus rare but has been reported in adults
- Clinical follow-up w/biopsy if suspicious change noted

CONGENITAL MELANOCYTIC NEVI (CMN)

BACKGROUND

- Usually separated into three groups based on size: small (<1.5 cm); giant (>20 cm est adult size); intermediate (between small/giant)
- Small nevi occur in ~1% of births/giant congenital nevi rare

CLINICAL MANIFESTATIONS

- Small CMN light brown to black, usually evenly pigmented, well-demarcated macules, papules/plaques
- Intermediate/giant CMN light brown to black, well-demarcated macules/plaques often w/verrucous/multinodular surface/irregular pigmentation
- Multiple other "satellite" pigmented nevi up to several cm in diameter common w/giant CMN; may be present at birth/develop during infancy
- W/time, CMN can become thicker, darker/lighter, develop coarse hairs
- Growth of all CMN proportionate to body size

COMPLICATIONS

- Risk of melanoma in small/intermediate lesions generally considered low
- Lifetime risk of melanoma/other neural crest malignancy in giant CMN est 6–8%; risk higher in first decade
- CNS melanosis may be present in giant CMN overlying head/spine. Symptomatic CNS involvement is uncommon but carries a very poor prognosis. Asymptomatic involvement detected by MRI is common; significance unknown
- Spinal dysraphism should be excluded if lesions overlies lumbosacral spine

MANAGEMENT

- Must be individualized to each child
- CMN can be prophylactically excised/followed clinically w/aid of photographs; should be watched for suspicious change, esp new papules, nodules, focal change in pigmentation, shape; consider excising very dark/nodular areas in giant CMN in which detection of melanoma would be difficult
- Brain MRI (w/gadolinium contrast after infancy) if giant CMN overlies cranium/spine
- Evaluate for spinal dysraphism if CMN overlies lumbosacral spine

MONGOLIAN SPOTS

BACKGROUND

- Extremely common, esp in more pigmented races
- Present at birth/soon after
- May darken/enlarge during first 2 yrs of life; thereafter fade/usually become inapparent
- 3–4% of lesions persist, esp extrasacral lesions
- Pigmentation due to arrested migration of melanocytes deep in dermis

CLINICAL MANIFESTATIONS

- Indistinct, gray to blue-gray macules of any size
- Usually single, may be multiple
- Mongolian spots occur anywhere; 75% in sacrococcygeal area

TREATMENT

- None usually necessary
- Persistent/cosmetically disfiguring lesions can be treated w/Q-switched ruby laser

NEVUS OF OTA AND NEVUS OF ITO

BACKGROUND

- 75% occur in Asian pts; may be seen in all racial groups
- F:M ratio: 5:1
- 50–60% present at birth
- Pigmentation due to nevocellular melanocytes deep in dermis

CLINICAL MANIFESTATIONS

- Typically indistinct brown-gray, blue-gray/purple macule, often w/mottled appearance
- Nevus of Ota involves facial skin, conjunctiva, sclera in distribution of V1/V2
- Nevus of Ito involves truncal skin in distribution of posterior supraclavicular, lateral cutaneous brachial nerves

COMPLICATIONS

- Risk of malignancy in nevus of Ota ~ up to 25% for whites, 1% for blacks, 0.5% in Asians
- Malignancies have occurred in choroid plexus, brain, meninges, iris, ciliary body, optic chiasm
- Pts w/ocular pigmentation also at risk for glaucoma

TREATMENT

- Refer pts w/ocular pigmentation to ophthalmologist
- Cosmetic improvement achieved w/Q-switched ruby laser treatment

WHEN TO REFER

- When diagnosis in doubt

BACKGROUND

• Causative agent, *Enterobius vermicularis,* lives freely in lumen of colon, rectum
• After copulation, female worm migrates out of rectum onto perianal skin, where she experiences uterine prolapse, deposits some 10,000 fertilized eggs, dies
• Eggs, picked up by scratching fingers that later find their way to mouth of child, or—because they are very light—those that float in air and are inhaled and then swallowed, initiate infection. This leads to series of developmental stages that take 2–3 wks, culminate in adult worms living in colon and rectum, ready to reinitiate cycle
• No reservoirs of this infection; it is ubiquitous, limited to humans, primarily young children, but occasionally adults, esp members of households w/infected children
• Affects both sexes, all socioeconomic classes. No evidence of racial predilection
• In girls and women, adult female worm has been known to migrate into vagina and deposit eggs there; can cause vaginal itching. Moreover, because worm can carry on her integument enteric bacterial flora, vaginal infection w/those organisms can also develop

CLINICAL MANIFESTATIONS

• *Salient presenting symptom:* perianal itching. Not all infected individuals symptomatic; indeed most not aware of infection
• In girls and women, may be associated vulvovaginitis

LABORATORY FEATURES

• Presence of characteristic eggs detected by low-power microscopic examination of transparent—not merely translucent [!]—adhesive tape whose sticky side has been applied to perianal skin and then pasted onto glass slide
• Collection of specimen best carried out early am as child awakens because worms tend to deposit eggs at night

DIFFERENTIAL DIAGNOSIS

• *Other causes of perianal itching:* impetigo, hemorrhoids
• In cases of vulvovaginitis, r/o bacterial, yeast infections

TREATMENT

• Either pyrantel pamoate, 11 mgm/kg, or mebendazole, 100 mgm, regardless of pt's weight, administered once, equally effective
• Whichever drug used, administer again 2–3 wks in order to destroy worms that have developed after initial treatment, because it kills only adult worms, not eggs
• Recurrence of enterobiasis common, but usually results from reinfection, not failure of treatment

COMPLICATIONS

• Exceptionally rare; mostly reported anecdotally
• If female worm gets stuck in appendix or diverticulum, she may lay eggs there and these eggs continue infection, in spite of otherwise effective treatment. In such rare cases surgical removal of appendage of gut may be necessary
• Other complications have been attributed to infection, including grinding of teeth at night, enuresis; must be considered part of folklore because good epidemiologic evidence exists that any such attributed relationship spurious

PREVENTION

• None

WHEN TO REFER

• In extremely rare cases when ordinary treatment failed for one of reasons cited above

PITYRIASIS ROSEA

LEONARD KRISTAL

BACKGROUND

- Most cases occur 10–35 yrs of age. Condition occurs in childhood; unusual in infancy
- Slight female preponderance, w/3:2 F:M ratio
- Cause unknown, although presumed viral
- Most frequent during late fall, winter months
- Eruption self-limited, lasting 6–12 wks

CLINICAL MANIFESTATIONS

- Most cases begin w/development of single lesion, so-called herald patch, well-demarcated, red, round or oval, scaling lesion, 2–5 cm in diameter. Herald patch most commonly located on trunk, upper arms, neck, thighs
- Generalized eruption follows herald patch after 5–15 d, involving trunk, neck, proximal extremities; 2° eruption characterized by discrete, small, oval, pink macules w/collarette of scale following skin cleavage lines on trunk in Christmas-tree pattern
- Skin lesions, esp in children, may be papular, vesiculobullous, pustular, urticarial, even purpuric. Children may also have involvement of head, face, hands, feet
- Oral lesions uncommon
- Itching may be severe in up to 25% cases

LABORATORY FINDINGS

- Hx, physical examination sufficient for Dx because no specific laboratory abnormalities

DIFFERENTIAL DIAGNOSIS

- Tinea corporis
- 2° syphilis
- Drug eruption
- Guttate psoriasis
- Nummular eczema
- Seborrheic dermatitis
- Lichen planus

TREATMENT

- Since pityriasis is usually asymptomatic and self-limited, most pts require only reassurance about the self-limited nature of eruption
- Treatment of pruritus:
    - topical antipruritic agents such as calamine lotion, Sarna lotion, or pramoxine-containing preparations
    - oral antihistamines
    - low-potency topical corticosteroids
    - ultraviolet light for severe cases

COMPLICATIONS

- There are no complications associated w/pityriasis rosea

WHEN TO REFER

- Most pts managed w/o referral
- Referral necessary for evaluation of atypical presentations/control of severe pruritus. Eruptions lasting longer than 8–12 wks should be referred for confirmation of Dx

BACKGROUND

- Also known as "atypical pneumonias"
- *Typical age:* 2–4 mos
- Most commonly due to *Chlamydia trachomatis.* Probably also caused by *Ureaplasma urealyticum* and cytomegalovirus (CMV). Transmitted from genitally colonized mother to infant. CMV can also be acquired from breast milk
- Conjunctivitis, 15–50%, pneumonia, 5–13% of untreated infants colonized w/*C. trachomatis* at birth
- May persist several weeks–months if undiagnosed
- In very ill infant w/afebrile pneumonia of infancy, consider possible underlying immunodeficiency including HIV infection
- *Mortality rate:* 3–4%

CLINICAL MANIFESTATIONS

- *Cough:* may be paroxysmal; w/chlamydia, typical "staccato" nature
- Tachypnea, rales, indrawing of intercostal muscles
- Absence of fever
- Conjunctivitis or Hx preceding conjunctivitis esp suggestive of infection w/*C. trachomatis* (present in ~half of pts w/chlamydial pneumonia)
- Discharge may be unilateral and purulent

LABORATORY FEATURES

- Mild eosinophilia
- ↑ immunoglobulins

- Chest radiograph:
  - air trapping, bronchial wall thickening, interstitial infiltrates, atelectasis
  - rarely: reticulonodular infiltrate or miliary pattern
- Specific Dx (need referral for these):
  - nasopharyngeal swab for *C. trachomatis,* nasopharyngeal aspirate for *U. urealyticum,* CMV or BAL fluid for culture or antigen detection of all
- Fourfold ↑ in paired serum IgG or positive IgM also confirmatory
- *If conjunctivitis present:* scraping can also be cultured or sent for nonculture test (eg, ELISA or DFA) for chlamydia
- CMV can also be isolated from urine, blood buffy coat and tissue cultures
- Identification of any of three organisms in themselves not 100% proof they are cause of pneumonia

DIFFERENTIAL DIAGNOSIS

- Respiratory viruses (RSV)
- Adenovirus
- Parainfluenza virus
- *Pneumocystis carinii* pneumonia
- *Bordetella pertussis* (chest x ray usually normal, unless 2° bacterial infection)

TREATMENT

- Empiric treatment for infant suspected to have chlamydial or ureaplasmal infection:
  - erythromycin (40 mg/kg/d div qid) or
  - sulfisoxazole (150 mg/kg/d div qid) × 10–14 d

- Both chlamydia, ureaplasma also susceptible to tetracyclines, newer azalide antibiotics, clarithromycin and azithromycin. Tetracyclines contraindicated in children <8 yrs of age but azalides may become important second-line drugs
- Sick infants w/CMV isolated from bronchoalveolar lavage specimens probably should be treated (in consultation w/specialist) w/either ganciclovir (10 mg/kg/d q12h × 24 h, then 5 mg/kg/d q24h) or foscarnet (180 mg/kg/d q8h × 24 h, then 90 mg/kg/d q24h) and IV immunoglobulin

COMPLICATIONS

- Generally benign and self-limited, except for severe infections in immunocompromised pts
- Most treated pts clinically improve within 2–10 d (mean ~6 d) following start of treatment, esp if chlamydia is the cause

WHEN TO REFER

- Most pts need hospital admission at least initially to ensure proper oxygenation, to monitor for complications
- Prolonged or complicated illness should be referred early on to pediatric infectious diseases consultant or pulmonologist

PNEUMONIA, BACTERIAL (COMMUNITY ACQUIRED)

VAL G. HEMMING

BACKGROUND

- Common at any age, infancy through adolescence
- Only one-tenth of acute onset childhood pneumonias have bacterial etiology
- Most common agent in neonate perinatally acquired group B *Streptococcus*, rarely *L. monocytogenes;* >1 mo *S. pneumoniae*, less common *H. influenzae, S. aureus, S. pyogenes, L. pneumophilia,* rarely *N. meningitidis, B. pertussis, M. pneumoniae,* chlamydia, tuberculosis
- Highest incidence in very young/those w/underlying lung disease (ie, bronchopulmonary dysplasia, cystic fibrosis, asthma)

CLINICAL MANIFESTATIONS

- Antecedent/concurrent signs of URI
- Fever
- Cough
- ↑ respiratory rate, nasal flaring, retractions, distressed breathing, splinting, cyanosis
- Occasional chest/abdominal pain, headache, toxicity or prostration

LABORATORY FEATURES

- *Microbiologic evaluation:* blood culture, helpful if positive/majority negative. Sputum rarely available in infants/young children. Bronchoalveolar lavage (BAL), tracheal/lung aspirate culture occasionally useful if etiologic Dx important. Endotracheal aspirate culture useful only immediately after intubation
- *WBC counts:* >15,000 frequent but may be normal, <5,000 occurs w/overwhelming sepsis
- *Chest radiograph:* Dx pneumonia requires abnormal chest radiograph; however, radiograph/clinical symptoms correlate poorly—esp early in clinical course

DIFFERENTIAL DIAGNOSIS

- Nonbacterial pneumonia primarily viral but including fungal pneumonias such as *C. immitis, H. capsulatum* (geographic Hx important)
- Noninfectious disorders, including atelectasis, pulmonary sequestration, CHF, aspiration of gastric contents, foreign body, malignancy
- Empyema/pleural effusion: *S. aureus, S. pneumoniae,* malignancy, rarely other bacterial infection; tuberculosis must always be considered

INITIAL TREATMENT

- *Neonatal:* group B streptococcus, *S. aureus, L. monocytogenes* must be considered; hospitalize for parenteral treatment
- *Infants through adolescence: S. pneumoniae,* mycoplasma, *C. pneumoniae* most common; less common *H. influenzae, S. aureus, S. pyogenes.* Antimicrobial resistance of pneumococci serious problem requiring new strategies for Tx: cefotaxime, 150 mg/kg/24h q8h, or ceftriaxone, 50–75 mg/kg/24h q12h for empiric Tx when resistant strains are suspected/recovered; empiric oral Tx for young children remains ampicillin, 50–100 mg/kg/24h q6h, or amoxicillin/clavulanate, 40 mg/kg/24h q8h, or erythromycin, 30–50 mg/kg/24h q8h, or azithromycin, 10 mg/kg one dose first day/then 5 mg/kg days 2–5, or clarithromycin, 7.5 mg/kg/24h q12h in older children; parenteral Tx in older children, ceftriaxone; oral Tx where drug-resistant *S. pneumoniae* common, oral quinolones (levofloxacin [consultation recommended]) may be indicated
- Pleural fluid—if present—should be aspirated for characterization/culture

FOLLOW-UP TREATMENT

- Treatment must be individualized according to organisms recovered, local sensitivity patterns, severity of illness, underlying lung disease
- W/negative yield from cultures, empiric Tx should be continued if recovery continues/adjusted for poor, inadequate pt response

COMPLICATIONS

- Most pts recover; pulmonary function may be compromised for some time following pneumonia; pulmonary abscess formation uncommon; pleural effusions relatively common/may require needle/chest tube drainage
- Children w/underlying pulmonary disease frequently experience decrements in pulmonary function after bacterial pneumonia

WHEN TO REFER

- Most pts managed w/o hospitalization/referral
- W/complications such as effusion/empyema, abscess formation, serious extension to other parts of lung, failure to respond to Tx, consultation/hospitalization may be required; clinical responses often precede radiographic response. Persistence of pneumonia w/undetermined etiology requires reformulation of possible etiologies

BACKGROUND

- Three chlamydia species can cause pneumonia in humans: *Chlamydia trachomatis, C. pneumoniae, C. psittaci*
- Epidemiology distinct for each species

	C. trachomatis	C. pneumoniae	C. psittaci
Age	Infants 1–6 mos	All ages	Older children, adolescents
Transmission	Vertical mother-to-infant during delivery	Person-to-person via aerosol droplets	Bird-to-person via aerosolized fecal material

CLINICAL MANIFESTATIONS

- *C. trachomatis:*
  - infants afebrile, rales on auscultation
- *C. pneumoniae:*
  - presents as "atypical" pneumonia similar to *M. pneumoniae*
    - cough, wheezing frequent
    - pharyngitis
    - headache
- *C. psittaci:*
  - often presents as fever of unknown origin
    - high fevers, severe pneumonia
    - severe headache

LABORATORY FEATURES

- *C. trachomatis:*
  - chest x ray: hyperexpansion, interstitial alveolar infiltrates
  - WBC count and differential: normal to slightly ↑, eosinophilia (≥400 cells/cu min)
- *C. pneumoniae:*
  - chest x ray: variable infiltrates, lobar consolidation, pleural effusions may also occur
  - WBC count and differential: normal to >10,000 w/left shift
- *C. psittaci:*
  - chest x ray: variable infiltrates, pleural effusions
  - WBC count, differential usually normal, mild leukocytosis

- other: 50% of pts may have abnormal liver function tests including SGOT, alkaline phosphatase, bilirubin

DIAGNOSIS

- *C. trachomatis:* isolation of *C. trachomatis* or positive nonculture test (EIA, DFA, or PCR) from NP swab or aspirate
- *C. pneumoniae:* isolation of *C. pneumoniae* from NP swab, sputum or pleural fluid. No approved nonculture tests available at this time. Serology w/either CF test or microimmunofluorescence assay usually negative in children
- *C. psittaci:* fourfold rise of CF titer or single titer ≥1:32

DIFFERENTIAL DIAGNOSIS

- *C. trachomatis:*
  - viral pneumonia including RSV, parainfluenza, adenovirus
- *C. pneumoniae:*
  - *M. pneumoniae* infection
  - viral pneumonia
  - bacterial pneumonia, specifically pneumococcal infection
  - legionella
- *C. psittaci:*
  - same as for *C. pneumoniae*

TREATMENT

- *C. trachomatis:*
  - erythromycin ethyl succinate suspension: 50 mg/kg/d, po × 10 d–2 wks
- *C. pneumoniae:*
  - erythromycin, 50 mg/kg/d po × 10 d
  - clarithromycin, 15 mg/kg/d (max. daily dose, 1,000 g) × 10 d
  - azithromycin, 10 mg/kg po on day 1, 5, mg/kg/d on days 2–5 (max. 500 mg on day 1 and 250 mg/d, days 2–5). If >8 yrs, doxycycline, 100 mg bid po × 2–3 wks
- *C. psittaci:*
  - doxycycline 100 mg q12h po × 10–14 d,
  - tetracycline, 500 mg q6h po × 10–14 d
  - alternative: erythromycin, 2 g/d × 10–14 d; may be less effective
- Treatment should be continued for 10–14 d *after* fever remits

COMPLICATIONS

- Large pleural effusions or empyema may occur in small number of individuals w/ *C. pneumoniae* infection

WHEN TO REFER

- Most pts managed w/o referral
- Referral indicated for serious complications (large pleural effusions); when Dx in doubt; if disease fails to respond readily to initial antibiotic treatment

BACKGROUND

- Most common single cause of community-acquired pneumonia in children, young adults
- Highest incidence ages 6–18 w/peak 8–10
- Prototype for "atypical pneumonia" w/insidious onset, prolonged course, minimal complications
- Etiologic agent, *Mycoplasma pneumoniae,* strictly human pathogen; highest incidence in groups such as schoolchildren, children's homes, military, college campus
- Organisms lack cell walls; thus resistant to penicillins, cephalosporins

CLINICAL MANIFESTATIONS

- Indistinguishable from viral URI at onset
- Bronchitic cough, cardinal feature
- Pharyngitis, common early feature
- Physical findings of bronchopneumonia, variable
- X rays do not always correlate w/physical findings
- Failure to respond to penicillin or cephalosporin antibiotics

LABORATORY FEATURES

- WBC and differential in normal range (exception: sickle-cell anemia w/high PMNs)
- Culture of organism unavailable in routine labs
- Cold hemagglutinins (IgM) rise early (≥1:64)
- Complement fixing (CF) antibodies diagnostic if ≥4-fold change in titer
- Rapid antigen detection (PCR, etc) unreliable/unavailable

DIFFERENTIAL DIAGNOSIS

- *Chlamydia pneumoniae* pneumonia (indistinguishable)
- *Legionella pneumophila* pneumonia (rare in children)
- Pertussis (esp in teenagers, young adults)
- Viral respiratory infection w/or w/o reactive airways
- Rare bacterial, nonbacterial pneumonias including partially treated cases

TREATMENT

- Macrolide antibiotics drugs of choice for all ages. Erythromycin (7–10 d) cheapest but may cause GI distress. Azithromycin (5 d) expensive but cost effective
- Tetracyclines alternatives for ≥8 yr olds

COMPLICATIONS

- Rare but include extrapulmonary manifestations such as nonspecific skin rashes, erythema multiforme, mild encephalitis, cerebella ataxia, peripheral neuropathies, cardiomyopathy, myocitis, pancreatitis, hemolytic anemia. Rarely does pneumonitis progress to fatal adult respiratory distress syndrome

PREVENTION

- *None:* attempts to develop vaccines unproductive
- Prophylactic antibiotics treatment probably prolongs onset of disease; not indicated

WHEN TO REFER

- Unusual; most cases are mild, self-limited
- Infectious diseases consult for unusual manifestations or suspected complications

BACKGROUND

- Occurs almost exclusively in immuno-compromised host
- Infection limited to lung; rarely extra-pulmonary
- Bilateral diffuse alveolar disease
- Probably not contagious
- Affects all age groups but rare <1 mo of age
- Occurs worldwide

CLINICAL MANIFESTATIONS

- Tachypnea
- Dyspnea
- Fever
- Cough, nonproductive
- Intercostal retractions

LABORATORY FEATURES

- *Arterial O_2 tension (P_aO_2):* ↓; usually <90 mmHg, often <70 mmHg at room air in severe cases
- *Alveolar-arterial O_2 gradient* (A-A): ↑; >35 mmHg in moderate, severe cases
- *Chest radiograph:* typically bilateral diffuse pneumonitis w/air bronchograms; begins in perihilar area and spreads peripherally, often sparing apical areas: rarely, atypical cases may present w/solitary lesion, lobar pneumonia, cystic, other lesions
- *Lactic dehydrogenase:* ↑, but not specific
- *WBC count:* normal

DIAGNOSIS

- Requires demonstration of *P. carinii* in pulmonary tissue or secretion
- Specimens obtained by bronchoalveolar lavage, lung biopsy, or expectorated sputum stained w/Grocott-Gomori, Toludine blue, Giemsa, anti *P. carinii* fluorecein-labeled antibody methods. Sputum rarely available in infants, children; and, when obtained, reveals organism in only 25% of cases. Lung biopsy (open lung or transbronchial) most sensitive, specific specimen for Dx but most hazardous method. Bronchoalveolar lavage usually most appropriate diagnostic approach for most pts

DIFFERENTIAL DIAGNOSIS

- Cytomegalovirus pneumonia
- Acute diffuse bacterial pneumonia
- Lymphoid interstitial pnemonitis (in AIDS)
- *Mycobacterium avium complex* pneumonia, tuberculosis
- Respiratory viral pneumonitis (parainfluenza, influenza, advenovirus)

TREATMENT

- *Trimethoprim / sulfamethoxazole:* may be given IV for moderate, severe cases; orally for mild cases
  - IV dose: 15 mg trimethoprim, 75 mg sulfamethoxazole/kg/d in 4 div doses, each infused over 60 min
  - oral dose: 20 mg trimethoprim, 100 mg sulfamethoxazole/kg/d in 4 div doses q6h. Suspension, tablets available
- *O_2:* as needed to maintain P_aO_2 <70 mmHg. Keep fraction of inspired oxygen (F_iO_2) below 50 vol. % to avoid O_2 toxicity
- *Assisted ventilation:* indicated w/P_aO_2 <60 mmHg at F_iO_2 ≥50%
- *Prednisone:* indicated in moderate, severe cases (PaO_2 <70 mmHg). Initial adult dose: 40 mg prednisone 2×/d × 5 d, then 20 mg 2×/d × 5 d, followed, if needed, by 20 mg/d until recovery. Pediatric doses not established. Initial dose 2.0 mg/kg/d seems reasonable for children

ALTERNATIVE THERAPY

- For pts unable to take trimethoprim/sulfamethoxazole or who fail to respond:
  - pentamidine isethionate, 4.0 mg/kg as single IV (or IM) dose daily; or,
  - atovaquone, 30 mg/kg/d in 3 div doses as oral suspension. Adult dose: 750 mg 3×/d; or,
  - dapsone, 2.0 mg, trimethoprim, 20 mg/kg/d in 2 or 3 div doses

COMPLICATIONS

- *From P. carinii pneumonitis:* pneumothorax, adult respiratory distress syndrome (ARDS), 2° opportunistic infections
- *From trimethoprim / sulfamethoxazole:* rash, neutropenia, anemia, Stevens-Johnson syndrome, fever, vomiting, diarrhea, toxic nephrosis
- *From O_2 Tx:* ARDS

WHEN TO REFER

- Moderate–severe pneumonitis (P_aO_2 <70 mmHg: A-A O_2 >35 mmHg). Such pts may require assisted mechanical ventilation in ICUs
- Infants <2 yrs of age
- Concomitant infections
- Complications of 1° disease (cancer, AIDS, etc)

BACKGROUND

- Viral agents responsible for most lower respiratory infections in preschool children
- *Major pathogens:* respiratory syncytial virus (RSV), parainfluenza, influenza, adenovirus. RSV, influenza, parainfluenza types 1, 2 occur in seasonal outbreaks in temperature climates. Infections due to parainfluenza type 3, adenovirus occur sporadically throughout year. RSV most commonly identified cause of lower respiratory tract disease in children <2 yrs of age, accounts for 40–50% of hospitalizations for bronchiolitis, 25% of hospitalizations for pneumonia. Other viral pathogens more commonly associated w/other clinical syndromes (see table). Infants <6 mos of age, infants/children w/underlying conditions such as prematurity, congenital heart disease, immunodeficiency, bronchopulmonary dysplasia at ↑ risk for severe illness associated w/RSV infections. Although fewer studies have been done of other respiratory viruses, children in these high-risk groups presumably at ↑ risk for severe disease when infected with any of viral respiratory pathogens

CLINICAL MANIFESTATIONS

- Tachypnea, dyspnea, cough, fever, rhinorrhea
- GI symptoms may be associated w/these illnesses esp in young children
- Clinical features of viral pneumonia may not be significantly different from those of bacterial pneumonia, except for presence of wheezing (more common in children w/viral pneumonia)

LABORATORY FEATURES

- No specific laboratory features of viral pneumonia
- WBC counts, band forms may be ↑
- Chest x-ray abnormalities commonly seen in viral pneumonia include hyperinflation and bilateral, patchy alveolar or interstitial infiltrates. Lobar or segmental infiltrates, pleural effusions more likely associated w/bacterial etiologies
- Rapid diagnostic testing generally available for RSV; however, specific laboratory identification of viral pathogen not generally necessary for management of pts

DIFFERENTIAL DIAGNOSIS

- Viral pneumonia cannot be reliably distinguished from bacterial pneumonia by clinical or radiographic criteria
- Detection of virus or viral antigen does not exclude Dx bacterial infection because bacterial co-infection occurs in as many as 25% pts w/viral pneumonia
- *Other illnesses in differential Dx:* asthma, CHF, foreign body aspiration

TREATMENT

- Viral pneumonia in children generally treated only w/supportive care
- Aerosolized ribavirin approved for treatment of RSV pneumonia or bronchiolitis in high-risk infants but has minimal impact on clinical course of RSV disease. Drug delivered via continuous aerosol 12–18 h/d using small particle aerosol generator. Ribavirin may clog ventilator circuits; use w/caution in mechanically ventilated pts
- Influenza A infections may respond to amantadine hydrochloride or rimantadine hydrochloride. Start treatment with antiviral agent within 48 h of onset of illness at 5 mg/kg/d (for children <9 yrs) given in single daily dose and continued until 48 hrs after resolution of symptoms. These drugs *not* effective for treatment of infections caused by influenza B

COMPLICATIONS

- Bacterial superinfections have been recognized as complications of viral pneumonias, particularly influenza
- Bacteria may also serve as copathogens in up to 26% of children w/viral pneumonia
- Adenovirus occasionally results in severe, necrotizing pneumonitis, which may lead to chronic lung disease
- Viral pneumonia may lead to respiratory failure, esp in children w/risk factors as described above

PREVENTION

- Prophylactic measures available for influenza and RSV, recommended for certain high-risk pts
- Administer influenza vaccine yearly to children w/asthma or other chronic lung diseases, significant heart disease, sickle-cell anemia, or HIV, and consider for other children w/chronic diseases such as renal insufficiency or diabetes mellitus. Use split virus vaccine in children <12 yrs of age. Children <8 yrs of age who have not previously been immunized should receive 2 doses of vaccine, administered 1 mo apart. For unimmunized children, chemoprophylaxis w/amantadine or rimantadine may be given during influenza season. Dosage of these agents for prophylaxis same as treatment dose
- RSV immune globulin (RSVIG) preparation recently approved to prevent RSV illness in young premature infants, infants w/bronchopulmonary dysplasia. Safety and efficacy of RSVIG for prevention of serious illness in pts w/underlying cardiac disease not established. RSVIG administered IV monthly during RSV season

WHEN TO REFER

- Most pts managed w/o referral
- Referral for consultation may be needed in pts w/severe underlying disease or immunodeficiency

Agent	1° syndrome	Other syndromes	Season	Peak age
RSV	bronchiolitis	pneumonia, common cold	w, spr	2 mos–2 yrs
parainfluenza 1	croup		F	2–5 yrs
parainfluenza 2	croup		sporadic	2–5 yrs
parainfluenza 3	croup	bronchiolitis, pneumonia	sporadic	<3 yrs
influenza	pneumonia	pharyngitis, croup, common cold, bronchiolitis	w, spr	5–9 yrs
adenovirus	pharyngoconjunctival fever	bronchiolitis, pneumonia	sporadic	<2 yrs

PNEUMOTHORAX AND PNEUMOMEDIASTINUM   LELA W. BRINK AND LEWIS H. ROMER

BACKGROUND

- "Air leak syndromes" include pneumomediastinum, pneumothorax
- Syndromes may lead to respiratory failure, shock, sudden death
- Air collections in mediastinal or pleural spaces most commonly result from trauma or as complication of positive pressure ventilation. May be seen at any age
- Spontaneous pneumothorax, pneumomediastinum do occur
- Small collections of air may be asymptomatic and treatable w/conservative measures
- Some cases of pneumomediastinum evolve into pneumothoraces
- More dangerous and emergent presentations of air leak syndromes involve air collections under "tension." Air collection said to be under tension if heart and mediastinal structures shifted from midline and/or compressed by expanding air. *Tension* pneumothorax or pneumomediastinum is life-threatening emergency

CLINICAL MANIFESTATIONS

- Hx sudden onset of dyspnea and cyanosis
- Physical examination findings:
  – tachypnea, tachycardia, hypertension/hypotension, hypoxemia
- SubQ crepitations upon palpation of neck and/or anterior chest wall
- Asymmetric chest expansion, w/↓ air entry by auscultation, ↑ resonance by percussion on more distended side
- Muffled or displaced heart sounds
- Transillumination (utility limited to neonates, young infants) w/asymmetrically ↑ area of diffusion of light on affected side

LABORATORY FEATURES

- Chest radiograph demonstrates extrapulmonary hypolucency in mediastinum and/or apical, lateral, and/or subpulmonic pleural spaces. Heart, mediastinal structures shifted from midline in tension pneumothorax. SubQ air may be evident

DIFFERENTIAL DIAGNOSIS

- Etiology of air leak:
  – idiopathic (newborn)
  – traumatic (crush, blunt, penetrating mechanisms)
  – iatrogenic (resulting from manual or mechanical support for respiratory failure, or from surgical manipulation of airway)
  – mechanical (heterogeneous alveolar distension in asthma or foreign body aspiration)
  – congenital (cystic malformations, connective tissue disorders—eg, Marfan's)
  – acute inflammatory (staphylococcal pneumonia)
  – chronic inflammatory (cavitary tuberculosis, bronchiectasis w/cystic fibrosis)
  – oncologic (tumor-associated airway compression or erosion)
- Other pleural and mediastinal processes compressing lung and contiguous structures
  – hemothorax (traumatic)
  – hydrothorax or effusion (hydrostatic/cardiac vs. oncologic vs. anasarca w/hypoproteinemia)
  – chylothorax
  – mediastinal tumors
  – mediastinal adenopathy
  – pneumopericardium

TREATMENT

- All pts w/pneumomediastinum or pneumothorax at risk for respiratory failure and should be treated w/supplemental O_2. Even asymptomatic pts require cardiorespiratory and pulse oximetry monitoring. Small pleural air collections in asymptomatic children may be treated w/supplemental O_2 alone
- *Pneumomediastinum* not under tension rarely requires direct intervention. Identification of cause and prevention of further air collection indicated. Pneumomediastinum under tension requires referral for emergency needle decompression; rarely may require surgical placement of mediastinal drainage catheter
- *Pneumothoraces* may be decompressed and drained by needle aspiration or by thoracostomy:
  – needle aspiration: after aseptic preparation of site, 21 or 23 gauge butterfly-needle or catheter-over-needle device may be inserted over second rib lateral to nipple in supine pt. Air may be aspirated directly, or w/attachment of three-way stopcock. This may provide definitive treatment of pneumothorax not under tension in spontaneously breathing pt. Needle aspiration will also rapidly palliate tension pneumothorax, but will not prevent reaccumulation of pleural air and tension. Effectiveness of procedure assessed by immediate chest radiograph
  – thoracostomy: placement of tube or catheter in pleural space attached to water seal or continuous suction device required for stabilization, management of children w/ongoing or recurrent accumulations of air in pleural space, for tension pneumothoraces, in most children that develop pneumothoraces while receiving positive pressure ventilation. Thoracostomy tube may be placed by surgical or Seldinger technique; usually positioned in fourth or fifth intercostal space at anterior (or mid-) axillary line. In ambulatory pt, tube directed anteriorly and superiorly toward air collection. In supine, bedridden pt, tube directed anteriorly, medially. Thoracostomy tube position always secured w/skin sutures, confirmed by chest radiograph

COMPLICATIONS

- Progressive *respiratory failure* most common complication; seen in significant number of pneumothorax cases w/o tension; inevitable in cases of untreated tension pneumothorax. Children w/underlying pulmonary pathology should be treated aggressively due to ↑ risk for respiratory failure
- *Cardiac tamponade* may occur from tension pneumothorax w/mediastinal shift, or from large collections of air in pneumomediastinum, or from associated pneumopericardium
- *Pneumoperitoneum* may result from dissection of pneumothorax into peritoneal cavity
- Thoracostomy tube treatment may be complicated by hemothorax, pulmonary contusion, bronchopleural fistula, or cardiac perforation

PREVENTION

- Restriction of exertion indicated and may be preventive in pts at risk for spontaneous pneumothorax due to congenital connective tissue diseases or chronic bronchiectasis
- Asthmatics benefit from adequate control of bronchospasm and intensification of Tx in anticipation of exacerbations during intercurrent viral respiratory infections, seasonal allergen exposure
- Prevention of air leak syndromes major challenge during mechanical ventilation Tx of severe respiratory failure. Appropriate, monitored use of sedation and/or neuromuscular blockade ↓ risk of air lead syndromes in infants, children requiring mechanical ventilation for any reason. Poor pulmonary compliance and/or high airways resistance ↑ risk of these complications. Barotrauma may be avoided or minimized by limiting peak inspiratory pressure and positive end expiratory pressure when possible; by limiting rate of mechanical ventilation to allow completion of expiratory phase; and by permissive hypercapnia. Consider alternative Tx (including high-frequency oscillatory ventilation, partial liquid ventilation, extracorporeal membrane oxygenation) early in course in order to prevent air leak, improve survival in severe respiratory failure

WHEN TO REFER

- Newborns presenting w/asymptomatic, spontaneous pneumothorax may be managed w/o referral in settings equipped, staffed for, practiced in emergency needle aspiration of pleural air, treatment of babies w/respiratory failure
- In infants, children presenting w/spontaneous pneumothorax, referral may be necessary to screen for etiologic diagnoses
- Referral to pediatric intensive care unit indicated for most children who present w/pneumothorax or pneumomediastinum in setting of respiratory failure

BACKGROUND

- >1 million preschooler poisonings reported to US poison centers annually
- Incidence peaks at ages 18–36 mos
- For adolescent intentional overdoses (suicide attempts) females predominate 4:1
- Early childhood poisonings most commonly occur at home at mealtimes when medications open and in use, parents distracted by meal preparation

Highest Incidence Poisonings Among Children <6 Yrs Old

Top 5 Pharmaceuticals	Top 5 Nonpharmaceuticals
Analgesics	Cosmetic/personal care items
Cough/cold remedies	Household cleansers
Topical preparations	Plants
Vitamins	Foreign bodies
Antimicrobials	Pesticides

CLINICAL MANIFESTATIONS

- Many agents involved in childhood poisonings may cause typical constellation of Sx termed *toxidrome*
- Anti-cholinergic toxidrome (eg, antihistamines, phenothiazines, atropine, belladonna alkaloids, tricyclic antidepressants [early]):
  - dry skin
  - dry mouth
  - mydriasis
  - fever
  - delirium
  - constipation
  - flushing
- Cholinergic toxidrome (eg, carbamate or organophosphate pesticides):
  - sweating
  - fasciculations
  - weakness
  - coma
  - seizures
  - diarrhea
  - lacrimation
  - salivation
  - bradycardia
  - bronchorrhea
  - urination
  - respiratory failure
- Salicylism:
  - tinnitus
  - fever
  - lethargy
  - hyperpnea
  - tachypnea
  - metabolic acidosis
  - seizures

LABORATORY FEATURES

- *Toxic screen:* send both urine and blood (many drugs of abuse more likely detected in urine than in blood); do not bother to send gastric aspirate or emesis. Always check w/laboratory personnel if looking for particular toxin. Different hospital laboratories include different agents on toxic screens. A typical toxic screen might offer acetaminophen, barbiturates, some benzodiazepines (eg, diazepam or oxazepam, but not triazolam), diphenhydramine, ethanol, methanol, opiates, some hallucinogens, salicylate, stimulants (eg, amphetamine, cocaine)
- Osmolar gap:
  - calculated serum osmolarity (in metric system units):

$$\frac{2x\ Na}{(in\ mEq/L)} + \frac{Blood\ Glucose}{(in\ mg/dl)}\ 18 + \frac{BUN}{(in\ g/dl)}\ 2.8$$

  - measured osmolarity (by freezing point depression method only)
  - osmolar gap = measured – calculated. ↑ osmolar gap seen in poisoning by ethylene glycol, isopropyl alcohol, ethanol, methanol. Each milliosmole of difference in osmolar gap translated into blood alcohol level using following conversion table: methanol: 1 mOsm = 3.3 mg/dl, ethanol: 1 mOsm = 4.5 mg/dl, ethylene glycol: 1 mOsm = 5.3 mg/dl, isopropanol: 1 mOsm = 6.0 mg/dl
- Metabolic Acidosis + High Anion gap (AG > 16) = MUDPILES differential
  - *m*ethanol
  - *u*remia
  - *d*iabetic ketoacidosis
  - *p*henformin
  - *i*soniazid, iron
  - *l*actic acidemia
  - *e*thylene glycol
  - *s*alicylate

DIFFERENTIAL DIAGNOSIS

- For child w/unknown poisoning presenting w/delirium, seizures, or coma:
  - sepsis or septic shock
  - intracranial masses or bleeding
  - meningitis
  - encephalitis
  - major head trauma

TREATMENT

- Four basic principles of management for poisoning:
  - resuscitate and support the pt: advanced life support, fluid resuscitation, airway control, maintenance of adequate ventilation/blood circulation. Anticonvulsants, antihypertensive agents, vasopressors typical supportive pharmacotherapy required to treat severe poisoning
  - decontaminate pt: irrigate, wash, dilute pts w/dermal or eye exposures; pts w/toxic inhalations should be moved to fresh air or O_2 by mask. Do not attempt to decontaminate pts who have ingested nontoxic agents, caustics, hydrocarbons (exceptions exist for particularly noxious agents such as benzene, carbon tetrachloride)
    - induced emesis (ipecac) should be reserved for home use, only if overdose has occurred within last 30–60 min
    - orogastic lavage reserved for symptomatic pts who have ingested agents w/potential for moderate–severe toxicity, who present to medical attention within 60 min of overdose
    - activated charcoal (1 g/kg body weight) administered orally or by NG tube considered adequate decontamination for most toxic ingestions. Does not work well for some toxins (eg, alcohols, cyanide, heavy metals, pesticides), contraindicated for use in caustic or hydrocarbon ingestions
  - enhance elimination of toxin:
    - diuresis: promote good urinary flow (3–5 cc/kg/hr) to assure endogenous clearance of many drugs or chemicals
    - alkalinization: "ion trapping" by ↑ urinary pH above 7.5; works well for salicylate or phenobarbital poisoning
    - multiple dose activated charcoal (give activated charcoal q2–4 h): can enhance clearance of selected toxins (eg, salicylates, theophylline) by interfering w/biliary recirculation of parent compound or active metabolites or by enhancing GI dialysis of toxin down an osmotic gradient back into lumen of bowel
    - hemodialysis and/or hemoperfusion useful strategies for some pts severely affected by poisoning. Typical dialyzable toxins include ethylene glycol, lithium, methanol, salicylate, theophylline

    - whole bowel irrigation (oral administration of polyethylene glycol [PEG] solutions in amounts up to 6 L to effect clear rectal effluent): potentially useful for evacuating large doses of iron, ingested bags of heroin or cocaine, masses of enteric-coated or sustained-release tablets
  - administer antidote, if one exists:

Toxin	Antidote
Acetaminophen	N-acetylcysteine
Benzodiazepine	Flumazenil
Carbon monoxide	100% oxygen or hyperbaric oxygen
Cyanide	Lilly cyanide antidote kit
Digitalis	Anti-digoxin fab antibiotics
Heparin	Protamine solution
Iron	Deferoxamine
Isoniazid	Pyridoxine
Methanol	Ethanol or 4-methyl-pyrazole
Methemoglobin	Methylene blue
Opiates	Naloxone
Organophosphates	Atropine/pralidoxime
Phenothiazine (dystonia)	Diphenhydramine or benzotropine
Rattlesnake	Crotalid antivenin

PREVENTION

- *Child resistant packaging:* has prevented hundreds of child deaths from poisoning since implementation in the US in 1974
- *Emergency telephone number:* put sticker w/local or regional poison center's number on telephone or include telephone number of automatic redial feature
- Teach parents 4 R's of poison prevention:
  - *recognition:* know what items in child's environment may be toxic
  - *removal:* dispose of unnecessary household toxins (eg, old medications, used paints, used automotive products); lock all others away in shoulder-level or higher cabinets
  - *readiness:* have poison center's telephone number available and purchase ipecac for storage at home
  - *response:* parents should be familiar w/poisoning first aid: call poison center immediately for any suspected ingestion; wash off dermal exposures; flush eye exposures w/stream of water; move inhalation victims to fresh air

WHEN TO REFER

- Always notify local or regional poison center of any child w/acute or chronic symptomatic poisoning or potentially toxic overdose
- *Triage to ER:* children w/new onset of symptoms temporally related to toxic exposure and children becoming progressively more symptomatic w/passage of time
- *Keep at home:* children w/exposures to nontoxic agents or exposures to nontoxic doses of drug or chemical
- When calculating dose of poison to which child could have been exposed, assume worst case scenario (max. dose child could have theoretically obtained) using pill counts, container sizes, concentration of drug or chemical, in order to assess appropriate triage of poisoned child
- Be wary of parent's ability to estimate accurately how much of substance child might have swallowed
- Be skeptical or adolescent's account of how much of agent or what agent ingested in suicidal attempt! Obtain blood concentrations of both aspirin and acetaminophen in any adolescent suicidal overdose

POLIOMYELITIS

SAMUEL L. KATZ

BACKGROUND

- One syndrome of number caused by enterovirus family
- Usually follows nonspecific febrile illness/mild respiratory or GI upset
- Ranges from asymptomatic infection to paralytic illness 100–1,000:1
- Three different serotypes (polio 1, 2, 3); types 1, 3 most paralytogenic
- Most common in summer-autumn in temperate climates, although possible year-round
- Absent from Western Hemisphere but endemic in sub-Saharan Africa, India, other parts of southern Asia

CLINICAL MANIFESTATIONS

- Early-onset fever, fatigue, headache, stiff neck
- May remit for 48 hrs, then return more acutely
- Stiffness of legs, back
- Hyperesthesias of extremities
- Onset of paralysis usually beginning asymmetrically in lower limbs
- May progress to involve respiratory musculature, upper limbs
- Fever, muscle spasms may continue 6–10 d
- Variable spectrum of recovery over subsequent weeks, months
- Residual paralysis if significant will lead to atrophy of involved muscles
- Unusual bulbar form involves motor nuclei of cranial nerves, other medullary centers (5–10% of cases w/paralysis)

LABORATORY FEATURES

- WBC normal or modestly ↑
- Cerebrospinal fluid (CSF) pleocytosis w/20 to several hundred cells; initially polymorphonuclear predominance shifting rapidly to lymphocytic predominance
- Normal CSF glucose, modestly ↑ CSF protein
- Virus recovered readily from stool specimen

DIFFERENTIAL DIAGNOSIS

- Guillain-Barré syndrome
- Aseptic meningitis-encephalitis
- Infectious polyneuritis

TREATMENT

- New antienteroviral drug pleconaril possibly effective, but no clinical trials w/paralytic disease; available on compassionate release protocol
- Immunoglobulin for rare pts w/agammaglobulinemia
- Rest w/initial hot packs to involved muscles
- Graduated physical Tx after acute phase

COMPLICATIONS

- Respiratory failure if diaphragm and/or intercostal muscles paralyzed
- Respiratory failure and/or unstable BP w/bulbar involvement
- Swallowing difficulties w/lower cranial nerve involvement

WHEN TO REFER

- As soon as Dx suspected

POLYMYOSITIS AND DERMATOMYOSITIS

ANN M. REED

BACKGROUND

- Most frequently found 3–12 yrs of age w/peak incidence at 7
- Commonly follows viral illness
- *Infectious agents reported to be associated w/dermatomyositis/polymyositis:* enteroviral infections (eg, Coxsackie B), hepatitis B
- Predictors of:
  - best outcome:
    - early Dx
    - adequate dose, duration of Tx
  - adverse outcome:
    - rapid onset, extensive weakness
    - extensive cutaneous vasculitis, ulceration
    - GI vasculitis
    - infarct in muscle biopsy
- Recovery of normal–good function, 64–78%; minimal atrophy or contractures, 24%; wheel chair dependence, 5%
- *Mortality:* 5% from respiratory insufficiency and GI perforation

CLINICAL MANIFESTATIONS

- Constitutional symptoms
- Progressive limb girdle muscle weakness (eg, positive Gowers, difficulty climbing stairs, difficulty brushing hair, frequent falling)
- Skin rash (erythema and/or papules over extensor surfaces of elbows, knees, ankles, hands; eyelid telangiectasia, soft tissue calcifications, cutaneous vasculitis)
- Alopecia
- Arthritis
- Raynaud phenomenon
- Periungual erythema and telangiectasia

LABORATORY FEATURES

- ↑ muscle enzymes (CK ↑ in 85% of pts, AST in 87%, aldolase in 65%; LDH in 64%)
- CBC, ESR usually normal–mildly ↑ (may help differentiate noninflammatory disease)
- ANA + in 50–70% in speckled pattern
- EMG (electromyogram) AU insertional activity and classic spike and wave forms
- *Muscle biopsy:* usually of deltoids or quadriceps (or muscle clinically involved); disease may be focal w/inflammatory cell infiltrates, vasculitis, atrophy, focal necrosis
- MRI of muscle to localize inflamed area for biopsy

DIFFERENTIAL DIAGNOSIS

- Postinfectious myositis
- Neuromuscular diseases
- Myopathies
- Metabolic disorders
- Trauma/drugs
- Genetic disorders
- Inclusion body myositis
- Autoimmune disease

TREATMENT

- Drug treatment:
  - prednisone po, 2 mg/kg/d (div doses when more severe disease) w/gradual taper over 2 yrs
  - methylprednisolone IV, 30 mg/kg/d IV × 3 d for significant muscle weakness, if protection of airway a concern, or if concern over lack of proper GI absorption
  - hydroxychloroquine po, 6–7 mg/kg/d in addition to prednisone to control skin disease
- *Immunosuppressives:* 1° indication includes glucocorticoid resistance, dependence, or, more recently, as a steroid sparing agent at the onset of treatment
  - methotrexate po, IV, or SubQ, 0.35–0.65 mg/kg/wk
  - cyclophosphamide IV, 500–750 mg/m²/mo
  - cyclosporine po, 2.5–7.5 mg/kg/d
  - azathioprine po, 1–3 mg/kg/d
- *IV immunoglobulin:* 1° indication includes glucocorticoid resistance or dependence: 2 g/kg/mo (may be div into 2 doses over 2 consecutive d/mo)
- *Supportive care if needed:* airway and swallowing support, good skin care
- *Physical, occupational Tx:* provide early to prevent loss of ROM, later to normalize function, minimize contractures

COMPLICATIONS

- Contractures
- Pulmonary insufficiency/aspiration
- Calcinosis
- Ulcerations (cutaneous and GI)

WHEN TO REFER

- Always refer to pediatric rheumatologist/neurologist to assure adequate treatment plan and continued improvement

BACKGROUND

• Juvenile polyps most common polypoid lesion of colon in children, 90% of colorectal polyps
• Most frequently diagnosed 2–10 yrs of age
• >50% of pts have >1 polyp (but <5)
• Origin, genetic predisposition of juvenile polyps unknown. Etiology believed hamartomatous (arising as malformations from normal tissue) or inflammatory
• Juvenile *polyposis* syndromes considered rare and familial. Autosomal dominant inheritance suspected, but not proven; juvenile polyposis likely when ≥5 juvenile polyps discovered in colon (or presence of any number of juvenile polyps *plus* strong family Hx this polyposis syndrome)
 – juvenile polyposis of infancy: associated intestinal anomalies include malrotation, Meckel diverticulum; polyps may also be found in stomach, small intestine
 – generalized GI polyposis: multiple juvenile polyps throughout stomach, intestines, sometimes exclusively confined to stomach

CLINICAL MANIFESTATIONS

• *Asymptomatic hematochezia:* rectal bleeding usually mild but can be profuse
• Chronic blood loss may lead to anemia
• Occasionally presentation rectal prolapse or prolapse of rectal polyp
• Intussusception associated w/pedunculated juvenile polyps rare

LABORATORY FEATURES

• Hgb usually normal but hypochromic anemia not unusual
• Most juvenile polyps large (>0.5 cm), pedunculated
• *Histologically:* mucosal lesions consist of dilated, mucus-filled, tortuous cystic glands and inflammatory cells in lamina propria; not neoplastic, but focal adenomatous changes and epithelial dysplasia may be noted

DIFFERENTIAL DIAGNOSIS

• *Other causes of rectal bleeding:* anal fissures, infectious enterocolitis, peptic ulcer disease, inflammatory bowel disease, Meckel's diverticulum, esophageal varices, Henoch-Schönlein syndrome
• Lymphoid polyposis and associated overlying ulcers
• Peutz-Jeghers syndrome (polyposis w/mucocutaneous pigmentation)
• Inherited adenomatous polyposis syndromes (eg, Gardner syndrome)
• *Rarely, intestinal tumors:* neurofibroma, leiomyoma, carcinoid tumor, gastrinoma, non-Hodgkin lymphoma, multiple endocrine neoplasia

TREATMENT

• Colonoscopy to cecum prudent when polyps noted by barium contrast study or suspected because of prolapse of rectal mass or unexplained rectal bleeding

• Because of significant anemia, possibility of adenomatous polyps, removal of all juvenile polyps warranted
• After discovery, removal of isolated juvenile polyp(s), no further evaluation necessary (unless rectal bleeding recurs)
• Dx juvenile polyposis or mixed juvenile-adenomatous polyps requires regular colonoscopic surveillance, at least q2–3 yrs, or earlier for recurrence of rectal bleeding

COMPLICATIONS

• Focal adenomatous changes, epithelial dysplasia in pts w/juvenile polyps confer risk of carcinoma, even in children, *but* degree of association between juvenile polyps and GI carcinoma probably low
• Pts w/juvenile polyposis, and their relatives, at risk of developing cancer

WHEN TO REFER

• Most pts w/suspected polyps require referral to pediatric gastroenterologist for colonoscopy
• Referral indicated for complications, eg, polyp lead point for intussusception, when Dx in doubt, or for recurrence of rectal bleeding in any child w/Hx juvenile polyp(s)

BACKGROUND

- *Definition:* True (also known as central or complete) precocious puberty is sexual development (adrenarche and gonadal maturation) < age 8 in girls, 9 in boys 2° to premature activation within CNS of neuroendocrine pathways (the hypothalamic-pituitary-gonadal axis) involved in normal puberty
- *Pathogenesis:* in girls, ~75% true precocious puberty idiopathic, 25% neurogenic. In boys, ~33% idiopathic, 77% neurogenic
  - idiopathic: preponderance of females; M:F = 1:5
  - neurogenic: damage to CNS areas that normally inhibit neuroendocrine axis, 2° to:
    - ○ CNS tumors
    - ○ arrested hydrocephalus, other congenital structural lesions
    - ○ seizure disorder, mental retardation
    - ○ post–CNS infection
    - ○ post–CNS radiation
    - ○ perinatal asphyxia, cerebral palsy
    - ○ head trauma

CLINICAL MANIFESTATIONS

- *Signs of gonadal maturation:* breast development (thelarche), testicular enlargement
- *Signs of adrenal maturation (adrenarche):* axillary odor, axillary hair; pubic hair; oily facial skin
- Hx inappropriately rapid growth for age
- Later, vaginal mucus, menarche; muscle development, voice changes in boys

LABORATORY FEATURES

- FSH, LH in pubertal range, give pubertal response to testing w/hypothalamic gonadotropin-releasing hormone (GnRH)
- Testosterone, estradiol above normal for age, in pubertal range

- Bone age inappropriately advanced for chronological age
- Brain MRI, normal in idiopathic, shows lesion in neurogenic forms
- Pelvic ultrasound (females) shows maturing uterus, ovaries
- *Adrenal androgens:* dehydroepiandrosterone sulfate (DHEAS) pubertal, but other adrenal androgens normal

DIFFERENTIAL DIAGNOSIS

- *Normal variants of puberty:* by far most common types of precocious sexual development seen in general practice. *Premature thelarche* ("benign breast hypertrophy"), usually in toddlers: isolated breast development w/o adrenarche, growth spurt, or advanced bone age. *Premature adrenarche:* presence of pubic, axillary hair, odor, oily skin, w/o signs of thelarche in girls or testicular enlargement in boys, w/o growth spurt or advanced bone age
- *Incomplete or pseudo-precocious puberty:* sexual development 2° to abnormal secretion of, or ingestion of, sex hormones:
  - ovarian or testicular hormone-secreting tumors or ovarian follicular cysts
  - tumors (eg, hepatomas) in males that secrete human chorionic gonadotropin (HCG) (has LH-like effect)
  - virilizing congenital adrenal hyperplasia w/signs of adrenarche 2° to excessive adrenal androgens
  - ingestion of sex hormone–containing drugs; foods w/added estrogen content
  - exposure to estrogen-containing creams
- *Gonadotropin-independent precocious puberty:* rare, usually familial; activating mutations of LH receptor in ovaries and testes cause autonomous secretion of pubertal amounts of estrogen and testosterone

TREATMENT

- *Strongly recommended that Tx be prescribed, monitored by pediatric endocrinologist.* Progression of true precocious puberty may be very slow, not require treatment. Decision to treat based on evidence of potential compromise of final height 2° to premature epiphyseal closure of bones, and/or presence of significant emotional distress
- If decision made to treat, drugs of choice are long-acting analogues of hypothalamic GnRH, which suppress pituitary secretion of FSH, LH, thus prevent gonadal maturation, sex hormone secretion. Dosage based on body weight
- *Drugs used:* leuprolide acetate as IM injection q28d, *or* histrelin as SubQ injection daily, *or* nafarelin acetate as intranasal spray 2×/d

COMPLICATIONS

- Inadequate dosing will result in stimulation of puberty
- Leuprolide acetate may be associated w/irritation/sterile abscess at site of injection

WHEN TO REFER

- Variants of premature adrenarche, premature thelarche need not be referred so long as no signs of precocious puberty
- All suspected cases of precocious puberty (true, incomplete, independent) should be referred for Dx and initiation of, monitoring of treatment

PSORIASIS

BERNICE R. KRAFCHIK

BACKGROUND

- Common, chronic, inflammatory skin disease characterized clinically by scaly, erythematous lesions, pathogenetically by accelerated epidermal cell turnover
- Incidence in general population 1–3%, w/one-third presenting < age 20. Two percent present <2 yrs of age; condition rarely may occur at birth
- Slightly more common in females; F:M ratio: 1.5:1
- Genetic, environmental, infectious, immunologic factors all thought to play role in etiology and pathogenesis
- Family Hx psoriasis present in 35%. An association between psoriasis and HLA types, particularly Cw6, in children exists

CLINICAL MANIFESTATIONS

- In *infants,* diaper area primarily involved w/erythematous, scaly plaques that may not have typical silver scale seen in other areas
- Lesions common on scalp, w/plaques that are well demarcated, often w/thick silvery scale
- Other areas of body may be involved but typical adult lesions on elbows, knees unusual
- In *children* lesions often develop 2–6 wks after streptococcal infection w/small guttate (teardrop), scaly plaques commonly on trunk. Although this presentation common (up to 34% of cases in children), some reports describe typical adult presentation of plaques on elbows, knees, scalp, sacral area as more common presentation in children. Face more commonly involved than in adults
- Lesions may be pruritic or asymptomatic
- Typical finding in psoriatic pts is Koebner phenomenon or isomorphic response, which is reproduction of characteristic lesion in areas of trauma
- Nail involvement occurs in ~10% of children. Lesions affect nail plate w/irregular pits and yellow proximal onycholysis—"oil drop" sign. Whole nail may become dystrophic w/severe onycholysis, subungual keratosis
- Psoriatic arthritis occurs in small percentage of children. Occurs either concomitantly or prior to eruption of skin lesions
- Less common presentation in infants and children is sudden development of high fever associated w/appearance of sheets of pustules that may occur on normal skin, or studded peripherally on circinate or annular lesions. Other findings in this pattern of presentation include geographic tongue, sterile osteomyelitis, and, very rarely, lung involvement

LABORATORY FEATURES

- Biopsy diagnostic, consists of parakeratosis of stratum corneum, loss of granular layer, Monroe abscesses (accumulation of neutrophil in the epidermis), spongiform pustules of Kogoj. Lymphocytic perivascular infiltrate present in dermis

DIFFERENTIAL DIAGNOSIS

- Dx "napkin psoriasis" easily confused w/seborrheic dermatitis, as scalp and diaper area involved in both. In seborrheic dermatitis lesions are erythematous patches in the folds, particularly axillary. Scalp lesions diffuse w/cradle cap, whereas in psoriasis, lesions in scalp well demarcated, extensors rather than folds involved w/scale
- Langerhans cell histiocytosis common in diaper area, but lesions crusted, purpuric
- Most common differential of pustular psoriasis is widespread bacterial infection that can easily be excluded by bacterial cultures, biopsy findings

TREATMENT

- Guttate skin lesions of psoriasis usually respond well to application of mid-strength corticosteroid on body areas tid (Valisone or Aristocort) and mild preparation on face and folds (hydrocortisone 1%). If not sufficient, refined tar product may be added to steroid. Available in formulation of 5–10% liquor carbonis detergens (LCD)
- New vitamin D analogue (calcitriol) an alternative to steroids, used bid. May be irritating to skin
- More widespread lesions may require short stay or inpt hospital care, w/crude coal tar, anthralin, UV-B treatment
- Pustular eruptions often unresponsive to topical preparations, may require use of systemic steroids, methotrexate, cyclosporin

WHEN TO REFER

- Widespread eruptions, pustular lesions best managed by dermatologist

PSYCHOSOMATIC ILLNESS

DENNIS C. HARPER

BACKGROUND

- Psychosomatic illness characterized by physical symptoms (complaints) presumably "caused" by emotional factors involving single organ or organ systems
- Physiologic changes are normative that usually accompany emotional states, but more intense/sustained
- Individuals may not be aware of precipitating or concurrent upsets
- Childhood aches, pains represent functional symptoms as somatization
- *2–10% report somatic complaints:* headache, abdominal pain, constipation, irritable bowel, general fatigue
- May follow illnesses or exist concurrently as exaggeration of illness
- Negative life events w/child and family often present
- Multiple complaints (somatization) periodically move, abate, reappear
- Chronicity likely if persistent onset by age 6
- M:F: 1:1 ratio up to 10 yrs of age; 10 yrs of age females 2:1
- Recovery 90% 1 mo, much less for recurrent multiple complaints

CLINICAL MANIFESTATIONS

- The following can be viewed as checklist for clinical manifestations present in varying degree:
  - negative or minimal laboratory findings
  - periodic minor febrile episodes
  - intercurrent common illnesses may be present
  - 2° gain surrounds complaints
  - high frequency of minor complaints
  - parent/sibs have similar complaints, maybe other health problems as well
  - overconcern w/health/body issues
  - school absence >15 d annually
  - complaint exists 3 mos or more: chronicity
  - multiple complaints: abate, change, move, reappear
  - complaint/discomfort often not consistent w/functional impact
  - discordance between complaint and manifest affect (eg, positive, negative, bland)
  - high frequency of worries, fears, nervousness
  - picky eater
  - changes in mood concurrent w/complaint, increasing irritability
  - neurovegetative changes may be present
  - school avoidance, decrease in school performance
  - multiple medical contacts
  - rejection of stress-based interpretation of complaints by family, child

CLINICAL EVALUATION AND FINDINGS

- Pain/complaints/psychosomatic illness often contingent on stress-related responses that can become chronic
- Pain real, debilitating regardless of etiology
- Pain multiply determined
- Negative evidence for organic disease not sufficient to diagnose psychosomatic illness
- Positive evidence of emotional stress required for Dx of psychosomatic illness
- Clinical interview:
  - complaint status note:
    - location, quality, chronicity, intensity, intensifying circumstances
    - 2° gain analysis, functional impact of complaint
    - behavior/affect, neurovegetative status, moods, behavior, conduct

DIFFERENTIAL DIAGNOSIS

- Early prodrome of systemic, neoplastic, autoimmune diseases
- Psychiatric depression, anxiety, school phobic
- Somatoform disorder
- Sexual/physical abuse
- Chronic fatigue

TREATMENT

- What is significance of psychosomatic illness (pain) for this specific child and family? Clinical experience suggests pain complaints used in at least three general fashions:
  - avoidance behaviors (task avoidance)
  - reactions to conflict and stress (conflict response)
  - habitual coping style (multiple somatic)

TASK AVOIDANCE

- Child getting something identifiable out of being in "sick" role: out of school, home w/parent, exempted from chores, etc

Descriptive Characteristics

- Complaint acute rather than chronic
- Complaint lacks clarity and sophistication
- Situational stress coincides w/complaint
- Complaint prevents normal activity
- Complaint may follow illness; child extends recovery
- Child socially immature
- Child younger, <8 yrs of age
- Family Hx negative for similar complaints
- Few psychological problems in family

Treatment

- Review problem, acknowledge its reality as genuine; pain/complaints real
- Review findings, give reassurance
- Clarify role of emotions in precipitating complaint/pain; eg, may be caused by stress as well as disease
- What evidence led to identification of these factors
- Emphasize transitory nature of symptoms
- Parents use positive attitude, positive suggestions, focusing away from symptoms
- Emphasize return to normal activity

CONFLICT RESPONSE

- Complaint directly tied to identifiable conflict or stress problems at home, at school, or w/peers

Descriptive Characteristics

- Complaint has variable Hx
- Complaint occurred as reaction to stress
- Child appears upset, depressed, anxious—associated symptoms in appetite, weight, mood
- Complaint reduces normal activity but child often continues to try to function
- No clear gain associated w/complaint; pain adds to problems
- Complaint may serve some function in family
- Age variable
- Family health Hx negative for similar complaints
- Family under stress due to child's complaints and/or problems

Treatment

- Review problem, acknowledge its reality as genuine—pain/complaints real
- Review findings, give reassurances
- Clarify role of emotions in precipitating complaint/pain: eg, may be caused by stress as well as disease
- What evidence led to your identification of these factors
- Discuss particular stress behind child's pain response if known; solution: remove stress
- If referral needed to help remove stress, emphasize need for professional assistance
- If no referral warranted, discuss w/family how stress might be removed

MULTIPLE SOMATIC

- Multiple frequent complaints of long-standing nature present. Child displays habitual style of pain responding. Chronic series of complaints w/multiple physician contacts, w/many health concerns, overfocus on complaints, sensitivities to their interpretation

Descriptive Characteristics

- Child dramatic in expression of complaints; inconsistency of report of pain
- Child selective in activities to avoid
- Family Hx of many illnesses often w/other similar complaints
- Child displays rigid behavioral styles
- School absenteeism chronic
- Gains from complaints present but selective and variable
- Age usually >10
- Parent/child not psychologically minded
- Negative life problems in family, child, and/or siblings

Treatment

- Review problem, acknowledge its reality as genuine
- Review findings, give reassurances
- Clarify role of emotions in complaint/pain; eg, it may be caused by stress as well as disease
- Focus on child's stresses, upsets as suggested by clinical data collected; indicate concern that child seems to have developed habit, or style, of dealing w/stress through bodily symptoms
- Discuss identified personality characteristics of child in relation to symptom maintenance
- Referral often required

COMPLICATIONS

- If complaints persist, high risk of adults w/similar complaints, later psychiatric disorder

WHEN TO REFER

- Most young children w/simple task avoidance complaints managed w/o referral
- If psychosomatic illness linked to other psychosocial, emotional, learning, behavioral or family problems, referral for psychological/psychiatric assistance necessary

PULMONARY VALVE STENOSIS

DAN G. McNAMARA

BACKGROUND

- Domed type of pulmonary valve stenosis (PVS-D) comprises 7–12% of all congenital cardiovascular defects, among seven most common cardiac defects (others: ventricular septal defect, atrial septal defect, patent ductus arteriosus, transposition of great vessels, tetralogy of Fallot, coarctation of aorta)
- *Cause:* usually no known prenatal teratogen, anomaly seldom familial. Nondomed less common form of PVS is dysplastic type, which occurs in ~one-third of pts w/Noonan syndrome, often associated w/other congenital cardiac anomalies (pulmonary artery branch stenosis, supravalvular aortic stenosis)

PATHOLOGY

- PVS-D lacks distinct leaflets, resembles wind sock w/centrally placed opening from 2–3 mm up to 12–15 mm in diameter. Orifice diameter determines severity of defect
- One-fifth of all forms of PVS are of dysplastic type of valve (DYS-PVS), which consists of three thickened unfused redundant leaflets; obstruction relates to bulk of leaflets, to narrowed pulmonary valve annulus. Also may be narrowing of subpulmonary infundibulum as well as narrowing of pulmonary trunk just above valve. Other types of PVS classified according to number of identifiable cusps, group in which only narrow pulmonary annulus responsible for obstruction but w/relatively normal leaflets. None of these types truly qualifies as *isolated* pulmonary valve stenosis. Focus here on isolated PVS of domed type; however other types should be considered in differential diagnosis for definitive treatment and predicting likely natural course

CLINICAL MANIFESTATIONS

- Usually PVS-D seen in outpt setting in asymptomatic infant or child w/heart murmur whether stenosis mild, moderate, or severe. Growth of infant or child normal; high percentage of cases have height, weight well above 75% percentile, for both severe as well as mild form
- Rarely pts w/severe PVS-D develop right heart failure exhibiting exertional but usually no resting, fatigue, dyspnea. Liver may enlarge, peripheral edema can occur. Some very severe; long-standing cases develop protein-losing enteropathy. Because no left heart failure, no pulmonary edema, no orthopnea
- Murmur of some intensity invariably present in all levels of severity. Intensity of murmur gives good indication of severity of defect. In very mild cases, intensity of murmur only Grade I–II/VI; murmur in this type of case peaks in early or mid-systole, thus allows easy identification of clearly split second heart sound in pulmonary area. In more severe cases w/high-pressure gradient between right ventricle and pulmonary trunk, murmur louder, peaks late in systole obscuring second heart sound, which might be interpreted as absent second sound

- Distinctive auscultatory feature of PVS-D is early systolic ejection click. In mild cases, may be necessary to elicit click by creating condition of ↑ cardiac output such as might occur after exercise or feeding in an infant. Click best heard w/pt in supine position, during held expiration. In extremely severe cases w/reduced contractility (reduced dP/dT), click may be absent, murmur may become less intense. Pulmonary ejection click difficult to learn how to hear but once learned is very distinctive sign of PVS-D. Loud murmur may distract examiner, who has not yet learned how to search for, recognize click
- In moderately severe cases in which right ventricular hypertrophy invariably develops, clinician may feel parasternal tap, esp in young child w/thin chest wall, w/pt in supine position. In severe cases in which right ventricular dilatation as well as hypertrophy has developed, right ventricular or parasternal lift or heave can be felt w/palm of examiner's hand. Again, best detected when pt supine
- "Cyanosis" (arterial blood oxygen desaturation) may occur in severe, moderately severe pulmonary valve stenosis in which atrial communication (either open foramen ovale or gross defect in atrial septum) exists. If atrial septum intact, right-to-left shunting does not occur in isolated pulmonary valve stenosis no matter how severe the obstruction. If right-to-left shunt small, may require transcutaneous pulse oximetry to identify hypoxemia; may require exercise or sustained Valsalva maneuver in cooperative older child to bring this out. Right-to-left shunt may be most readily identified by color Doppler ultrasound
- *Neck vein pulsation:* when pt old enough to cooperate, prominent A-wave in neck vein w/pt sitting up, head slightly extended seen in more severe form of pulmonary valve stenosis, indicates ↑ right atrial pressure 2° to ↑ right ventricular end-diastolic pressure
- Liver enlargement occurs only in very severe cases w/critical reduction of right ventricular ejection fraction, CHF. Complication represents surgical emergency or at least plan for prompt definitive treatment
- Exceptionally good growth, lack of resting symptoms in pts w/severe pulmonary stenosis may distract many physicians from proper concern that ideal management of these pts w/severe stenosis calls for. Anomaly in its severe form has been cause of what superficially appears to be sudden unexpected death. On other end of spectrum of severity, mild cases usually allow lifetime free of exercise intolerance; these pts have no ↑ risk for sudden death

LABORATORY EVALUATION

- Cardiac ultrasound (echocardiography) provides definitive Dx, estimation of severity of defect (type of pulmonary valve stenosis; that is, motility, thickness, whether or not valve domed, mobile, measurement of velocity of jet across pulmonary valve for documentation of severity, and presence of atrial communication, whether or not inter-arterial right-to-left or left-to-right shunt exists). Echo obviates the need for cardiac catheterization for Dx, but catheterization needed to carry out balloon dilatation of pulmonary valve
- *Chest radiograph:* cardiac silhouette may appear normal in mild or even moderately severe pulmonary valve stenosis. In those severe cases in which right ventricular dilatation has occurred, cardiac silhouette ↑ w/prominence of right atrium, right ventricle. Prominent pulmonary trunk a common though not invariable radiographic feature. Both mild and severe cases may develop pulmonary trunk dilatation. Before advent of ultrasound, angiography was important in establishing Dx of pulmonary valve stenosis, but injection of large amount of radio-opaque dye in very severe cases of pulmonary stenosis unnecessary hazard

TREATMENT

- Surgical pulmonary valvulotomy first carried out by Sir Russell Brock, reported in 1949. Treatment of choice for PVS-D until balloon catheter dilatation accomplished first by Kan in 1982. Success of balloon dilatation for PVS-D such that place for surgical relief of domed type of valve stenosis no longer exists. However, direct vision surgery may still be required for severe form of dysplastic type of PVS as well as strictly annular stenosis
- *Indication for definitive balloon dilatation of pulmonary valve stenosis:* in mild cases w/gradient 20–50 mmHg est from Doppler echocardiogram, balloon dilatation not justified. In moderately severe cases w/right ventricular to pulmonary artery pressure gradient of 50–90 mmHg, balloon dilatation can effectively remove gradient. Severe cases w/pressure gradient across valve of 90 mmHg or near systemic arterial level require prompt relief by balloon valve dilatation. In very severe cases w/pressure gradient > peak systolic systemic arterial pressure, relief of stenosis urgent in view of possibility of sudden, unexpected cardiac death
- Closure of atrial communication may not always be necessary, would require direct vision open heart surgery; but if atrial communication only stretched foramen ovale, this type of defect usually taken care of by relief of pulmonary stenosis. Gross defect in atrial septum w/persistent postop right-to-left shunt may require subsequent surgical closure of atrial septal defect

BACKGROUND

- Most frequently found in infants 3–8 wks of age
- *M:F ratio:* 4:1
- *Overall incidence:* 1:500–1,000
- Thought more common in children of parents who once had pyloric stenosis, although association not proven
- Etiology unknown but suggested processes include ↓ ganglion cells, hypergastrinemia, dyscoordination between gastric peristalsis and pyloric relaxation, ↓ nitric oxide synthase in pyloric muscle wall

CLINICAL MANIFESTATIONS

- Nonbilious, projectile vomiting that usually occurs after feeding
- Infant usually hungry again after vomiting
- Abdominal protuberance may be present due to gastric distention
- Gastric peristaltic waves may be seen through abdominal wall
- Hypertrophied pylorus may be felt on physical exam; known as "olive sign"
- Infant must be very relaxed and stomach must be emptied to be able to feel hypertrophied pylorus
- Infants who have been vomiting for number of days may be significantly dehydrated

LABORATORY FEATURES

- *Electrolytes:* hypokalemic, hypochloremic, metabolic alkalosis may be present if vomiting prolonged
- *Glucose:* hypoglycemia may be present
- *UA:* paradoxical aciduria occurs if infant significantly dehydrated and hypokalemic
- *Bilirubin:* unconjugated hyperbilirubinemia may be present if infant significantly dehydrated
- *Ultrasound:* best diagnostic test. Pyloric stenosis present if pyloric channel ≥16–17 mm, muscular wall thickness ≥3.5–4 mm
- *Upper GI series:* may also be diagnostic w/ presence of "string sign," thin line of barium that passes through thickened pylorus which does not relax during gastric emptying

DIFFERENTIAL DIAGNOSIS

- Gastroesophageal reflux
- Food allergy
- Gastroenteritis
- Malrotation w/ or w/o volvulus
- Incarcerated hernia
- Duodenal stenosis

TREATMENT

- Assessment of hydration and electrolyte status must always be accomplished first when pyloric stenosis diagnosed. Rehydration can be undertaken w/ D5½ NS solution run at 1.5 × maintenance w/ 20–40 mEq KC1/L added as needed according to electrolyte resuscitation required
- Once infant adequately rehydrated, Ramstedt pyloromyotomy may be performed
- Infants can generally be started on graduated feeding schedule 4–6 hrs after surgery and usually discharged 24–48 hrs after surgery

COMPLICATIONS

- Complications rare
- If mucosa entered during surgery initial pyloromyotomy may be closed and pyloromyotomy may be performed on another part of muscle. Feeding usually delayed for 24 hrs after occurrence
- Rarely if pyloromyotomy not adequate, reoperation w/ further separation of muscle may be needed
- *Other rare complications:* wound infections and wound dehiscences

WHEN TO REFER

- Whenever infant vomiting to where cannot maintain adequate hydration by oral intake
- Vomiting that persists >48 hrs even if hydration adequate
- Any time vomiting is bilious; may be malrotation with volvulus
- Any time Dx made by physical exam, ultrasound, or upper GI exam in primary care setting

BACKGROUND

- Represents 0.5% of all childhood skin nodules
- Most frequently found in children <5 yrs of age w/subsequent frequency ↓ linearly w/↑ age
- ↑ incidence in pregnancy ("epulis" on gums during second or third trimester), oral contraceptive use, previous sites of trauma or surgery, areas of port-wine stains or other vascular malformations
- In childhood, M:F ratio 1:1
- Cause unknown but possible factors include hormonal influences, antecedent treatment and/or trauma, viral oncogenesis, infection, arteriovenous anastomoses, tumor angiogenic or other growth factors

CLINICAL MANIFESTATIONS

- Abrupt and spontaneous in onset
- Usually solitary sessile or pedunculated nontender, rapidly growing, friable vascular mass
- Glistening red or purple papule/nodule w/constricted "collarette" stalk
- Prone to ulceration, episodic hemorrhage
- Locations:

Solitary (most common)	Head and neck (62.5%) Oral cavity and nose (most common) Trunk (19.7%) Extremity (upper > lower) (17.9%)
Multiple (seen in unusual variants)	
Disseminated	Trunk (esp scapulae)
Multiple satellite nodules	Trunk (esp scapulae)
Intradermal/SubQ (including acquired tufted angioma)	Trunk (esp scapulae)
Pseudopyogenic granuloma (aka "angiolymphoid hyperplasia w/eosinophils" or "histiocytoid angioma")	Ear, scalp, face
Intravascular	Neck, upper extremities

- Natural course:
  - rapid growth: few millimeters–centimeters (average <1.0 cm) in diameter which stabilizes after several weeks to months; eventually shrinks to become fibrotic
  - destruction often curative
  - lesions during pregnancy often remit after parturition but can recur w/subsequent gestations

LABORATORY FEATURES

- Characteristic histopathology
- Lobular configuration of capillary vessels in dermis or submucosa w/constricted base or collarette
- Granulation tissue formation seen as newly formed capillaries w/plump endothelial cells
- 2° changes such as ulceration, edema, mixed inflammatory infiltrate may be present
- Fibrosis seen in later regression stage
- Special immunohistochemical markers may help distinguish from lymphoproliferative disorders if necessary

DIFFERENTIAL DIAGNOSIS

- Finding of friable vascular nodule in child most likely pyogenic granuloma
- Carcinomas and sarcomas usually not seen in children
- These entities and esp dermal and subcutaneous variants can be distinguished by distinctive biopsy findings:
  - molluscum contagiosum
  - verrucae (warts)
  - bacillary angiomatosis
  - amelanotic melanoma
  - pseudopyogenic granuloma
  - granulation tissue
  - Kaposi's sarcoma
  - angioendotheliomatosis
  - angiosarcoma
  - adnexal tumors (follicular in origin)
  - carcinomas (basal cell, squamous cell, or metastatic)

TREATMENT

- *Principal options:* no treatment; excision; destruction w/or w/o concomitant excision; adjunctive intralesional steroids
- *No treatment:* indicated for pts w/asymptomatic small classic lesions stable in size that do not bleed or have cosmetic concern or in pregnant pts where thought lesion may spontaneously remit postpartum
- *Excision (tangential shave or simple elliptical):* indicated for pts where possibility of malignant Dx has not been excluded, making biopsy confirmation necessary prior to destruction
- *Destruction w/or w/o concomitant shave or elliptical excision:* indicated for pts w/classic lesions either continuing to grow, symptomatic, and/or of cosmetic concern; options include destructive methods such as tangential shave excision, electrodesiccation of base to ↓ risk of recurrence, cryosurgery, chemical cauterization, laser Tx (pulsed dye, argon, or carbon dioxide) or simple elliptical excision; *biopsy should be obtained at time of excision/destruction for diagnostic confirmation*
- *Adjunctive intralesional steroid injections:* indicated for pts at times in conjunction w/destructive methods in recurrent, larger, or subcutaneous cases

COMPLICATIONS

- Scar formation
- Disfigurement

WHEN TO REFER

- Referral indicated when Dx in doubt or if lesion ether symptomatic or has not stabilized by Hx at time of initial evaluation and provider not comfortable w/evaluation and/or surgical management

BACKGROUND

- Rabies an infection of warm-blooded animals. Single animal species harbor majority of rabies in each geographical region
- Humans infected by saliva from bite or scratch of infected animals, through contact w/mucous membranes, or by infected aerosols
- 9/13 human cases in US 1980–90 from out-of-country animal exposures
- Most commonly rabies-infected animal vectors dogs and cats
- Two recent cases (1996) of rabies in US were from bat rabies virus strains; 19/34 cases in US since 1980 have been bat-related strains. Insignificant physical contact w/bats may result in viral transmission
- Most human rabies cases males <15 yrs of age

CLINICAL MANIFESTATIONS

- Clinical stages correlate w/disease physiology
- First phase asymptomatic incubation period, which reflects virus travel along nerves; generally 10–90 d
- Second, prodromal phase occurs w/virus invasion of CNS and lasts 2–10 d. Symptoms include respiratory, GI, behavior, emotional changes. Local pain, pruritus, paresthesia occur at inoculation site in half of cases
- Third phase results in neurologic signs from widespread brain infection. A furious clinical form results in altered behavior (biting, hitting, yelling, hallucinations). Half of these pts have hydrophobia when attempting to drink liquids
- Paralytic rabies including flaccid paralysis, weakness occurs in 20% of pts and more commonly after bat rabies virus infections
- Both clinical forms may be accompanied by fever, convulsions, hypersalivation, hyperventilation, fasciculations, nuchal rigidity
- Fourth phase is coma and death, usually within 7 d

LABORATORY FEATURES

- Virus can be cultured from skin punch biopsies from hair follicles at base of neck inoculated into mice or neuroblastoma cell lines in specialty. Virus can be detected from saliva, CSF, urine, respiratory specimens. Special reagents can determine strain types of rabies viruses for epidemiologic purposes
- Punch biopsy of skin preferred site for immunofluorescent rabid study using specific monoclonal antibodies. Specific fluorescent staining of brain tissue more sensitive than histology for Negri bodies
- Serum neutralizing antibodies can be detected by Rapid Fluorescent Focus Inhibition Test (RFFIT)
- CSF findings characteristic of viral meningitis, but may be normal early in illness. Only clinical rabies produces CSF antibodies to rabies virus
- EEG, CT may be normal early in illness

DIFFERENTIAL DIAGNOSIS

- For furious rabies, includes meningitis, epilepsy, drug toxicity, tetanus, encephalitis, inflammatory polyneuropathy
- For paralytic form, includes Guillain-Barré syndrome, Alzheimer's disease, transverse myelitis

TREATMENT

- Careful use of narcotic analgesics for pain control, sedation. No specific antiviral Tx available

COMPLICATIONS

- To prevent nosocomial transmission health-care givers w/direct contact should wear gowns, gloves, masks, goggles. Give prophylaxis to any health-care worker w/parenteral or mucous membrane exposure to saliva or tissue from suspected cases

PREVENTION

- Preexposure prophylaxis:
  - prophylax individuals w/↑ risk of exposure to animals w/rabies (veterinary workers, wildlife managers, spelunkers, workers in rabies virus laboratories)
  - give 3 doses inactivated rabies virus Human Diploid Cell Vaccine (HDCV) IM on days 0, 7, 21, 28 into deltoid muscle, or into anterolateral upper thigh of infants
  - measure antibody produced from vaccine at regular intervals of 6 mos–2 yrs for those w/ongoing risks. If antibody falls <0.5 IU, give booster dose
- Postexposure prophylaxis:
  - wash wound in soap or detergent and repeatedly flush. Avoid suturing, occlusive dressings
  - give hyperimmune serum and immunize those bitten after unprovoked attacks of wild animals or suspected rabid cats or dogs. Start immunization as soon as possible
  - give passive immunization w/Human Rabies Immune Globulin (HRIG) at dose 20 IU/kg, one-half into wound area, one-half IM into gluteal or anterolateral thigh muscle w/different syringe. Give HRIG within 7 d of first immunization
  - for unimmunized individuals, 1.0 mL HDCV IM into deltoid muscle on days 0, 3, 7, 14, 28
  - for those previously immunized, immunize on days 0, 3
  - stop immunization if brain of suspected rabid animal negative or if domestic cats or dogs healthy throughout 10 d observation period

WHEN TO REFER

- Consult public health officials regarding nature of infected animals in community, use of diagnostic tests, appropriate management of wounds, immune globulin and vaccine

RADIAL HEAD SUBLUXATION (NURSEMAID'S ELBOW) AND CONGENITAL DISLOCATIONS

WALTER W. HUURMAN

NURSEMAID'S (PULLED) ELBOW

BACKGROUND

- *Average age first presentation*: 2–3 yrs; has been reported as early as 2 mos; may occur rarely up to 7 yrs of age
- Slight predominance of girls; represents >25% injuries to elbow region
- Caused by forceful distraction of extended forearm; results in radial head being pulled distally, away from capitellum, allowing proximal portion of pulleylike orbicular ligament to be interposed; some dispute whether pronation/supination part of injury mechanism; because reduction occurs w/supination, pronation more likely position at time of displacement
- Not true dislocation; radial head does not completely lose contact w/capitellum of humerus; it slides slightly laterally, under proximal ligament margin
- Important to note that injury usually occurs inadvertently at hands of another, not uncommonly parent. Sensitivity to feelings of guilt important, assurance that long-term effects unlikely may be helpful

CLINICAL PRESENTATION

- Hx sudden, forceful pull on forearm, occasionally accompanied by audible snap
- Although acute pain transient, infant/child does not voluntarily use arm; attempts to move arm/rotate forearm result in pain. Localization of pain difficult; other specific findings frustratingly few
- X rays normal; proximal radius continues to point at capitellum; abundance of radiolucent cartilage obscures slight lateral displacement radial head

TREATMENT

- Gentle examination of extremity by palpation for sites of reproducible pain to r/o occult fracture. Pay particular attention to distal radius/distal humerus where undisplaced torus/supracondylar fracture may be source of complaints. Any evidence of swelling/joint effusion reason to obtain premanipulation x ray; Nursemaid's elbow not typically accompanied acutely by joint effusion; presence of such fluid should raise suspicion of fracture, bone/joint infection
- Single attempt at reduction may be attempted prior to obtaining x ray. Gently flex elbow w/forearm supinated (palm up) until palpable snap felt at lateral elbow. Flexion well past 100° necessary, will cause some moderate discomfort. With elbow passively held at 90°, pronation/supination should be relatively free w/o severe pain
- If passive pronation/supination not possible after one attempt at reduction, obtain elbow *and* forearm x rays to r/o fracture
- If subluxation recurrent, immobilization in long arm cast for 2 wks to allow soft tissue healing appropriate; slings, swaths, etc, not effective in immobilizing

CONGENITAL RADIAL HEAD DISLOCATION

BACKGROUND

- May occur w/o other accompanying musculoskeletal abnormalities
- Must be differentiated from acquired traumatic dislocations
- When congenital/isolated, usually exists bilaterally
- Abnormality which, if isolated entity, usually unrecognized by parents/medical personnel until incidentally discovered in late childhood/early teenage years. Frequently brought to light during investigation of acute traumatic episode
- Result of individual anatomic/functional adaptation; abnormality not source of significant disability

CLINICAL PRESENTATION

- Other than incidental finding, pt may present w/complaints of bony protrusion at elbow subject to direct trauma because of prominence/lack of full motion (flexion, extension, rotation) of forearm coming to light when involved in some athletic activity
- X-ray findings distinctive; differentiate between acquired vs. congenital dislocation; because radial head/capitellum have never articulated, complementary shape of these two structures does not overlap; typically proximal radius domed shaped; lies anterior, posterior, lateral to distal end of humerus where capitellum small/unrecognizable. If proximal radius lies anterior to capitellum, it articulates w/distal, anterior metaphysis of humerus. In this situation, groove develops in humerus to accommodate proximal radius

TREATMENT

- True, isolated congenital radial head dislocation requires no treatment
- Occasionally bony prominence may be symptomatic due to its exposure to direct trauma; if this occurs, resection of prominence *after* skeletal maturity may be considered; premature resection will result in wrist instability, attempts at reduction will result in additional stiffness; unwise given minor degree of disability

BACKGROUND

- Sexual assault in children, adolescents may involve stranger rape, acquaintance rape, incest
- Population-based studies indicate >700,000 rapes/yr in US, only 15% of which reported
- Half of all rapes occur to females <18 yrs old; one-third occur in adolescents age 11–17; approximately 5% reported rape victims are male
- Alcohol, other drug use risk factor strongly associated w/sexual assault. In studies of adolescent, young adult victims, approximately 75% of assailants, 50% of victims had used drugs, alcohol, or both immediately before sexual assault
- Being raped is a devastating experience w/serious physical, emotional effects long after event, including chronic pain syndromes, post-traumatic stress disorder (PTSD), depression, substance abuse, suicide
- Health-care providers should be familiar w/state laws defining rape, w/legal mandates for reporting suspected sexual assault, collecting medical evidence. This information available from most state medical associations

LEGAL DEFINITIONS

- Legal definition of rape varies by state. Traditionally rape has referred to forcible sexual penetration w/o person's consent. In current terms, penetration may involve any body orifice including mouth, anus, vulva, or vagina. Lack of consent may result from use of force, threat, intimidation, or from physical or mental limitations including age and intoxication, or from coercion by person in authority
- Most states have replaced term *rape* w/definitions of sexual assault
- *First-degree sexual assault:* sexual penetration by a part of perpetrator's body or an object into genital, anal, or oral openings, which occurs when there is force or coercion or mental or physical inability to consent
- *Second-degree sexual assault:* sexual contact w/o penetration, which could include intentional touching of victim's intimate parts or clothing covering these parts, when there is force or coercion or physical or mental inability to consent
- *Third-degree sexual assault (statutory rape):* sexual penetration by an adult ≥18 yrs of age of a minor < age of consent by state definition (usually < age 14–16)
- *Acquaintance (including date) rape:* sexual assault perpetrated by individual whom victim knows and had established some trust before intent to rape became apparent
- *Incest:* sexual assault perpetrated by family member

CLINICAL MANIFESTATIONS

- Rape is serious medical, psychological emergency. Child victims usually brought to ER or physician's office by family, police, other officials
- Adolescents may seek medical attention alone, have concerns about confidentiality, fear of parental reactions, guilt about associated behaviors such as underage drinking, lack of knowledge about legal rights
- Before assessment, counsel pt on value of reporting assault, need to collect forensic evidence if legal charges contemplated. If within state's designated time frame, forensic exam ("sexual assault kit") should be strongly encouraged to preserve victim's future legal options. *The forensic assessment must be performed exactly in accordance w/speci-fied procedures, reporting requirements. Meticulous documentation, an unbroken chain of medical evidence essential.* Information that follows generally appropriate for nonforensic assessment

- Hx, examination should be performed in private, quiet area, in presence of chaperone, supportive friend or family member if pt desires. In all cases, sensitive, nonjudgmental approach to victim, family essential
- Hx should include date, time of alleged assault, details of alleged assault, last menstrual period (for females), use of contraception, any actions such as showering or douching that might affect findings, date of last voluntary intercourse. Medical report forms for suspected sexual assault should be used if available
- Nonforensic examination usually includes general appearance, emotional state, examination of entire body for signs of trauma (seen in 25–45% of cases), careful abdominal exam to evaluate blunt trauma or abdominal bleeding, thorough examination of external genitalia, rectum (genital injuries found in 15–30% of cases). In prepubertal child, if external genital exam normal, internal exam rarely necessary
- Pelvic exam should be done last, w/warm, water-lubricated instruments, avoiding any further mental trauma. (Ask if this is pt's first pelvic.) Any signs of injury/trauma should be recorded, including secretions, lacerations, abrasions, bruising. Colposcopy enhances detection of genital trauma

LABORATORY FEATURES

- For forensic exam, extensive specimen collections required in strict adherence to specified procedures. DNA testing becoming standard
- For nonforensic evaluation, following tests recommended: chlamydia and gonorrhea cultures from appropriate sites; wet mount microscopy for sperm, bacterial infection, trichomoniasis; blood tests for syphilis serology, HIV antibody, hepatitis B surface antigen; baseline urine pregnancy test
- Follow-up testing for pregnancy (2 wks), syphilis, hepatitis B antigen (6–12 wks), HIV antibody (24 wks) should be done if indicated. Although risk low, victim, family often obtain significant psychological relief from negative test results

TREATMENT

- *Emergency assessment:* evaluate acute victim for life-threatening physical or emotional conditions; stabilize accordingly. Arrange for private, safe place for further evaluation
- *Acute care:* within 72 hrs of assault, protocols, procedures established by state should be followed for collection of forensic medical evidence, medical testing. Most states do not consider medical evidence collected after 72 hrs as admissible; hence prompt evaluation of victim necessary. After 72 hrs, nonforensic assessment can be done in office setting, w/careful attention to pt's medical, emotional needs
- *Prophylaxis for sexually transmitted diseases:* incidence of STDs acquired from sexual assault not known. Standard to offer victim prophylactic treatment against incubating chlamydia, gonorrhea, trichomoniasis, bacterial vaginosis: ceftriaxone, 125 mg IM in single dose; plus azithromycin, 1 g orally, in single dose; plus metronidazole, 2 g orally, in single dose. (For allergic pts requiring alternative treatments, see appropriate CDC guidelines.)

- *Pregnancy prevention:* in reproductive-age girls, risk of conception following sexual assault ~4%. If pt not using effective contraceptive method, emergency contraception (ECC) should be offered within 72 hrs using combined oral contraceptive pills (Nordette, Levlen, Lo/Ovral, Triphasil (yellow pills), or Tri-Levlen (yellow pills), 4 tablets orally stat, then 4 tablets orally 12 hrs later, or using as directed a commercially available prescription ECC kit *(Preven)*
- *Immunizations:* for lacerations/penetrating injuries, give tetanus booster if needed. Hepatitis B vaccination should be offered to adolescents not previously immunized (w/instructions to complete HBV series during follow-up care)
- *Psychological support:* both victim, family need emotional support, counseling about immediate, longer term feelings, reactions. Parents may feel anger, guilt, even blame victim for perceived contributory behavior. Victims may feel intense anxiety, shame, self-blame, irrational fears about body damage (infertility, infection, pregnancy). Immediate support from rape crisis team if available very helpful. Return visits should be scheduled for medical, counseling follow-up
- *Reporting:* sexual assaults should be reported in accordance w/state requirements, even if victim does not intend to file legal charges

COMPLICATIONS

- Medical sequellae may include recurrent psychosomatic complaints such as chronic abdominal pain, menstrual disorders, frequent gyn complaints
- Post-traumatic stress disorder (characterized by reliving the trauma in thoughts and dreams, loss of ability to enjoy activities, avoidance of setting where rape occurred, difficulties w/sleep, memory) may affect up to 80% of rape victims
- Other reactions include depression, substance abuse (often to self-medicate the depression), suicide, acting-out behaviors including running away, truancy, promiscuity

PREVENTION

- Educate pts, families about risk factors associated w/sexual assault, esp at vulnerable ages such as school entry, puberty, leaving for college
- Provide anticipatory guidance about acquaintance rape, its association w/alcohol, drug use as part of annual adolescent health visit
- Support school programs for middle school, high school students, and programs for out-of-school youth that offer similar educational, preventive advice
- Vigorous reporting, prosecution of perpetrators is strongest social deterrent

WHEN TO REFER

- Within 72 hrs of acute rape, referral to ER knowledgeable in forensic procedures recommended
- Majority of assault victims benefit from counseling by trained rape counselors; such referrals should be offered, encouraged
- Psychiatric referral indicated for serious mental health complications

REFRACTIVE ERRORS (NEARSIGHTEDNESS/FARSIGHTEDNESS/ASTIGMATISM)

JOHN M. DEVARO AND MILLICENT WINFREY PETERSEIM

BACKGROUND

- Newborn vision normally poor (~20/600 by preferential looking)
- Steady improvement to 20/20 levels occurs by 3–5 yrs of age
- *Farsightedness (hyperopia):* most children born farsighted
  - amount of hyperopia ↑ until 4–7 yrs of age, at which shift toward nearsightedness occurs/continues until adulthood
  - uncorrected high hyperopia can present as accommodative esotropia (crossed eyes) in preschool children (see *strabismus*)
- *Nearsightedness (myopia):* prevalence of myopia in US population ~20%
  - risk factors include prematurity, congenital glaucoma, family Hx
  - children who present w/ myopia <10 yrs of age at greater risk of progression to high myopia/associated retinal complications
- *Astigmatism (cylindrical refractive error):* common in infants but usually ↓ by age 1
  - high astigmatism requires spectacle correction
- *Note:* refractive errors can be associated w/ more serious underlying ocular disorders such as aphakia/orbital tumor (hyperopia); congenital glaucoma/coloboma (myopia); corneal forceps injury/dislocated lens (astigmatism); uncorrected high refractive error/anisometropia (large difference in refractive error between eyes) can lead to *amblyopia*

CLINICAL MANIFESTATIONS

- Reduced vision, squinting, eye rubbing, headaches, strabismus, sitting close to objects of interest, holding objects close to face, worsening performance in school

TREATMENT

- *Glasses* safe, easy, protective, effective Tx correcting refractive errors
- *Contact lens* wear in children raises concerns regarding hygiene/infection; helpful in conditions such as high refractive error in infants (high myopia, aphakia), anisometropia, cosmesis in older children
- *Refractive surgery* not recommended until adulthood, when refractive error has stabilized

PREVENTION

- Theories abound regarding environmental influences on induction of myopia
- Effectiveness of Tx such as atropinization, undercorrection, bifocals have not been shown to reduce progression of myopia

WHEN TO REFER

- Children w/ family Hx strabismus, amblyopia/high refractive error should be referred for ophthalmologic evaluation by age 3 yrs; Hx prematurity, ocular disease, surgery, injury may prompt earlier referral
- All children should have reliable visual screening w/ each eye covered by age 4–5 (or as early as possible); any ↓ vision or difference between eyes should be referred for ophthalmologic evaluation
- Photoscreeners increasingly accurate in detection of refractive errors, anisometropia, strabismus, media opacities

ROSS E. PETTY

DEFINITION

- Syndrome of reactive arthritis specific GI or GU infections w/triad of arthritis, conjunctivitis, urethritis, occurring simultaneously or sequentially
- Additional clinical features include anterior uveitis, keratoderma blenorrhagicum
- Arthritis w/o other components of Reiter triad may also occur following same infections; not fundamentally different than arthritis of Reiter syndrome

ETIOLOGY

- Occurs 7–12 d following genitourinary tract infection w/*Chlamydia trachomatis*, or GI tract infection w/*salmonella typhimurium, Salmonella enteritidis, Shigella flexneri, Campylobacter jejuni*, or *Yersinia enterocolitica*

PREDISPOSING FACTORS

- HLA B27 present in ~85%
- M:F ratio 4:1
- More common in older children, adolescents than in young children

PATHOGENESIS

- Immunologically mediated response to extraarticular bacterial infection. T lymphocytes that react w/components of bacterium, cross-react w/self-constituents believed to play central role. Although living bacteria not present in joints, fragments of bacteria or bacterial DNA present in inflamed joint

CLINICAL FEATURES

- Low-grade fever often present at onset
- Preceding GI symptoms (abdominal pain, diarrhea) mild–severe
- Acute arthritis in one or more joints following genitourinary or GI tract infection by 7–12 d, accompanied, preceded, or followed by dysuria w/sterile pyuria, and unilateral or bilateral symptomatic conjunctivitis (red painful eyes), often w/photophobia
  - joints usually hot, may be red, exquisitely painful
  - knees, ankles most commonly affected
- Enthesitis (inflammation of site of insertion of tendon, ligament, fascia, or capsule to bone) usually present around knee (2 o'-clock, 10 o'clock positions around patella and tibial tubercle), or foot (achilles tendon insertion, plantar fascia insertions to calcaneum, base of 5th metatarsal and heads of 1st and 5th metatarsals)
- Conjunctivitis present in two-thirds at onset:
  - grittiness, redness, or bulbar and palpebral conjunctivae
  - may have blepharitis and mucopurulent discharge
- Urethritis in one-third:
  - may be missed: dysuria often mild
  - balanitis in up to 50% of males
  - labial ulceration may occur in girls
- Mucocutaneous lesions:
  - painless lesions on palate, tongue, buccal mucosa
  - keratoderma blennorrhagicum on soles of feet (may resemble pustular psoriasis)

LABORATORY FEATURES

- ↑ WBC count, ESR
- ANA, RF negative
- Sterile pyuria, may be few erythrocytes, low-grade proteinuria
- Synovial fluid WBC ↑ (10,000–40,000), mostly neutrophils. Cultures negative
- Radiographs of affected joints normal or show only evidence of synovial effusions, osteoporosis
- Cultures of stool often negative by time arthritis has developed

DIFFERENTIAL DIAGNOSIS

- Septic arthritis (if monarticular)
- Oligoarticular juvenile rheumatoid arthritis
- Early ankylosing spondylitis if enthesitis present
- Arthritis w/inflammatory bowel disease
- Kawasaki disease (if child young, conjunctivitis nonpurulent)

TREATMENT

- NSAIDs:
  - naproxen, 15 mg/kg/d, 2×/d
  - tolmetin sodium, 30 mg/kg/d, 3×/d
- Glucocorticoids:
  - intraarticular triamcinolone hexacetonide (20–40 mg/joint) if response to NSAIDs poor
  - occasionally short course (1–3 wks) of oral prednisone (1 mg/kg/d) necessary
- Slow acting antirheumatic drugs seldom needed, except when syndrome prolonged or progresses to ankylosing spondylitis, in which case sulfasalazine (50 mg/kg to max 2.0 g/d) useful
- Custom-made orthotics useful to minimize foot pain caused by enthesitis, or inflammation of joints of ankle or foot
- Physiotherapy to regain lost ROM as soon as level of pain permits
- Antibiotics probably not indicated

PROGNOSIS

- May recover completely in several months. Others progress to develop sacroiliitis like that of ankylosing spondylitis. Recurrences may follow reinfection w/arthritogenic organism

BACKGROUND

- *Dysplasia:* histologic Dx—undifferentiated mesenchyme w/primitive tubules. Occasionally, islands of cartilage; may be partial or total
- *Multicystic dysplasia:* dysplastic kidney w/many large cysts resembling "bunch of grapes"
- *Autosomal recessive polycystic kidney disease (ARPKD):* formerly called "infantile." Caused by mutation on chromosome 6p; ectatic collecting ducts. Most frequent pre-sentation perinatal but can be in childhood, adolescence. *Always* accompanied by biliary dysgenesis ("congenital hepatic fibrosis")
- *Autosomal dominant polycystic kidney disease (ADPKD):* "adult polycystic kidney disease." Mutations on chromosome 16p, 4q, others. Globular cysts involve Bowman capsule or any segment of tubule. May present at any age, including identification by prenatal ultrasound, but most commonly symptomatic third–fifth decade
- *Juvenile nephronophthisis / uremic medullary cystic kidney disease (JD / UMCD complex):* mutation on chromosome 2q. Medullary tubule ectasia w/interstitial fibrosis, small kidneys. Presents in mid–late childhood. Severe forms in infancy
- *Medullary sponge kidney:* medullary duct ectasia. Presents in adolescence–early adulthood w/hematuria, stones, distal renal tubular acidosis

CLINICAL MANIFESTATIONS

Dysplasia	ARPKD	ADPKD	JN/UMCD
Unilat or bilat flank masses in nb; if bilat, no renal function; may accompany syndromes; usually no family Hx	Bilat flank masses; pulmonary hypoplasia; hypertension; biliary dysgenesis; hepatosplenomegaly; uncommon family Hx	Occ hematuria; occ hypertension; assoc. hepatic cysts, Berry aneurysms, mitral valve prolapse, diverticulosis; usually + family Hx	Short stature; salt wasting; polyuria; pallor; uncommon family Hx

LABORATORY FEATURES

Dysplasia	ARPKD	ADPKD	JN/UMCD
Bilat: ↑ BUN, creatinine	50%: ↑ BUN, creatinine; urine dilute; often ↑ renin, aldosterone	Occ ↑ renin, aldosterone; occ ↑ BUN, creatinine; urine dilute when older; ↑ FE_{Na}, U_{Ca}	↓ Hgb, Hct ↑ BUN, creat Occ ↓ Na; urine dilute; ↑ FE_{Na}
RUS: cysts, often contralateral hydronephrosis	RUS: bilat ↑ size, hyperechoic (later resolvable cysts)	RUS or CT: globular cysts, >3 bilat	RUS or CT: small, hyperechoic; may not have resolvable medullary cysts
Scintigraphy: no flow to affected kidney	IVU: mottled	IVU: later—↑ size, vessels stretched, cysts	

DIFFERENTIAL DIAGNOSIS

Dysplasia	ARPKD	ADPKD	JN/UMCD
Ureteric obstruction w/dilated calyces	ADPKD; bilateral Wilms; benign nephromegaly; infiltrative disease	ARPKD (esp w/later presentation); tuberous sclerosis	Reflux nephropathy; chronic interstitial nephritis

COMPLICATIONS

Dysplasia	ARPKD	ADPKD	JN/UMCD
Pulmonary hypoplasia common w/bilat; renal failure common w/bilat	↑ BP common; hypersplenism common; renal failure common by adolescence	Rupture of Berry aneurysms: 10% (adults); abdominal/flank pain/hepatomegaly common in adults; renal failure common in adulthood	Severe short stature common; renal failure common by adolescence

TREATMENT

- None of these has any cure, but progression of disease may be retarded by treatment of complications. Hypertension of ARPKD, ADPKD often best treated w/ACE inhibitors (in ADPKD, renin produced in tubular cells). Repletion of volume and Na losses may help preserve function
- As glomerular function falls, treatment for hyperparathyroidism, anemia, acidosis, growth failure should be instituted. Eventually dialysis and/or transplantation necessary for majority of ARPKD, ADPKD, JN/UMCD. These modes may be considered in bilateral dysplastic disease
- For those w/ARPKD, congenital hepatic fibrosis may lead to significant portal hypertension and varices that warrant treatment

PREVENTION

- Genetic counseling should be provided at appropriate time for decision making. Although dysplasia usually sporadic, association in syndromes may be inherited. Consideration must be given to at-risk parent/sibling who is asymptomatic in view of insurance and work vulnerability

WHEN TO REFER

- Dysplasia, for confirmation of Dx or if contralateral kidney obstructed
- ARPKD, JN-UMCD, when suspected
- ADPKD, for at-risk or diagnosed child w/abdominal pain, hypertension, and/or ↑ BUN, creatinine

JONATHAN D. HEILICZER

BACKGROUND

- Hemolytic uremic syndrome (HUS) most common form acute renal failure (ARF) requiring intervention
- Postinfectious glomerulonephritis (PIGN), usually poststreptococcal, most common form leading to renal dysfunction w/o need for acute intervention
- ARF can develop any age. Some etiologies age dependent
- Consider possibility of acute presentation of chronic renal disease
- *Drug intoxication:* chronic (antibiotics; IVP dye); acute (lead, mercury, antihypertensives)
- Acute UTI (even pyelonephritis) *not* cause of ARF by itself
- Etiologic classifications:
  - prerenal: severe dehydration (consider concentrating defect), sepsis (marked vasodilatation), nephrotic syndrome (marked intravascular depletion)
  - postrenal: congenital obstructive uropathy
  - renal: acute glomerulonephritis: HUS, PIGN, systemic lupus erythematosus (SLE); chronic renal failure acutely: focal segmental glomerulosclerosis (FSGS), membranoproliferative glomerulonephritis (MPGN), SLE, chronic pyelonephritis

CLINICAL MANIFESTATIONS

- *Edema:* may be insidious, "shifts" w/gravity. In am, periorbital; in pm, pretibial
- Diarrhea (bloody) prodrome in HUS
- Rash (SLE, Henoch-Schönlein purpura)
- Oliguria common; however, urine output may vary particularly in children w/concentrating defect
- Hematuria may not be present; proteinuria *always* present w/glomerulopathy
- Hypertension (may manifest as headache)
- *Respiratory difficulty:* sign of pulmonary edema/effusion or tachypnea compensating for metabolic acidosis

LABORATORY FEATURES

- Electrolyte imbalance, particularly hyperkalemia, requires immediate attention
- Metabolic acidosis
- Reverse calcium:phosphorus ratio more common in chronic renal failure
- Hypoalbuminemia more common in nephrosis than nephritis
- Anemia more likely found in chronic renal failure but acutely seen in HUS and SLE

DIFFERENTIAL DIAGNOSIS

- 4 etiologies of edema:
  - cardiac: can not "pump it"—CHF
  - oncotic: can not "retain it"—nephrosis, liver failure (both 2° to hypoalbuminemia)
  - glomerular: can not "filter it"—renal failure, acute vs. chronic
  - tubular: "overreabsorb it"—SIADH, hyperaldosteronism

TREATMENT

- Acute treatment immediately required for hyperkalemia:
  - K > 6: Kayexalate 1 g/kg pr (more rapid effect) or po (more efficient)
  - K > 7: above and IV D25W 2 mL/kg + regular insulin (0.1 µ/kg)
  - K > 7.5: above and IV NaHCO$_3$ 1–2 mEq/kg over 0.5 hrs
  - K > 8: above and IV 10% Ca gluconate 1 mL/kg over 0.5 hrs (monitor EKG)
- Consider placement of NG tube w/continuous suction; will remove potassium, hydrogen ions
- If PH < 7.25 consider NaHCO$_3$ infusion. Remember any Na delivers H$_2$O as well and can contribute to fluid overload
- Treat BP > diastolic of 95% for age w/nifedipine sublingually (0.25–0.5 mg/kg dose)
- Restrict fluids to insensible H$_2$O loss (400 mL/m^2/d); can add fluids to equal output only if euvolemic
- Review *all* pharmaceutical treatment; any renal-cleared drug will require adjustment of interval or dose
- No specific treatment (ie, steroids) w/o understanding specific etiology (usually requires renal biopsy)
- *Indications for dialysis:* marked fluid overload, persistence of significant hyperkalemia or acidosis

COMPLICATIONS

- Cardiac arrhythmia 2° to electrolyte imbalance
- Seizures 2° to electrolyte imbalance or hypertension
- CHF/pulmonary edema 2° to fluid overload

WHEN TO REFER

- Any child w/electrolyte imbalance, fluid overload not responding to Tx
- Any child w/significant hypertension
- Any child w/creatinine clearance <70 mL/min/1.73 m^2
- Children w/electrolyte imbalance/significant hypertension require inpt monitoring

BACKGROUND

• Persistent (>3 mos)/irreversible ↓ in glomerular filtration rate (GFR): ↑ in serum creatinine level >1.5 mg/dl in child <2 yrs of age/>2.0 mg/dl in child >2 yrs
• *Incidence:* 4–20 new cases/1 million <15 yrs of age
• Etiologies (in order of ↓ frequency):
  – chronic pyelonephritis: posterior urethral valves, ureteropelvic junction obstruction, vesicoureteral reflux)
  – glomerulonephritis: long-term complication of focal segmental glomerular sclerosis (FSGS)/membranoproliferative glomerulonephritis (MPGN)
  – hereditary disorders: polycystic kidney disease, hereditary nephritis (Alport syndrome)
  – hypoplastic (congenitally small kidneys)/dysplastic (congenitally malformed kidneys) kidneys)
  – hemolytic uremic syndrome: most common cause of acute renal failure in children (small number of these children develop CRF)
  – bilateral renal vein thrombosis, bilateral Wilms tumors

CLINICAL MANIFESTATIONS

• Anorexia, nausea/vomiting may be earliest manifestations of CRF
• Renal osteodystrophy manifests as skeletal pain in extremities/lower back, easily fractured bones that heal slowly and poorly
• Anemia of CRF results in ↓ exercise tolerance, easy fatiguability, ↓ appetite
• Hypertension often asymptomatic in CRF, but may have headaches, nosebleeds
• Easy bruising from platelet dysfunction (not thrombocytopenia) in uremic environment
• Itching may result from uremia/from 2° hyperparathyroidism
• Delay in sexual maturation occurs in CRF
• Fluid retention/edema variable findings

LABORATORY FINDINGS

• ↑ serum creatinine, blood urea nitrogen, uric acid
• Hyperphosphatemia, hypocalcemia, ↑ total/bone fraction of alkaline phosphatase, 2° hyperparathyroidism typical in CRF; may start seeing changes when 50% of GRF lost

• Normochromic, normocytic anemia after 60% of GFR lost
• Metabolic acidosis
• Hyperkalemia late finding, after >90% function of GFR lost
• Platelet count normal/platelets do not function properly, prolonged bleeding time
• *Variable findings:* hyponatremia, hypoalbuminemia, proteinuria, hematuria

RADIOGRAPHIC CHANGES

• *Renal ultrasound:* hydronephrosis (obstruction, reflux) or small kidneys w/abnormal architecture
• *Cortical imaging renal scans* (glucoheptonate, dimercaptosuccinic acid): diffuse renal scarring (chronic pyelonephritis) or small kidneys w/poor uptake
• *Osteomalacia/rickets:* generalized ↓ in bone mineralizations/widening of metaphyses of long bone, fraying of distal ends of long bones, cupping of distal ulna/radius
• Osteitis fibrosa rarely seen at present time/characterized by resorption of bone/cyst formation in distal femur, proximal tibia/distal radius
• Osteosclerosis (replacement of lamellar osteoid by woven osteoid, most noticeable in vertebrae (rugger jersey spine)

DIFFERENTIAL DIAGNOSIS

• *Acute renal failure:* reversible ↓ in GFR
• *Prerenal azotemia:* dehydration results in reversible axotemia, typically BUN out of proportion to any increase in serum creatinine

TREATMENT

• Metabolic acidosis treated w/bicarbonate/citrate (Bicitra, Polycitra)
• Hyperphosphatemia treated w/phosphate-binding calcium supplements, such as calcium bicarbonate/calcium acetate, administered w/each meal/snack; Sevelamer hydrochloride new calcium-free, aluminum-free phosphate binder; infants may require low-phosphate formula (human breast milk, Similac PM 60/40)
• Renal osteodystrophy treated w/biologically active vitamin D metabolites such as calcitriol/enantiomers of calcitriol (dihydrotachysterol)
• Anemia of chronic renal failure treated w/IV/SubQ injections of recombinant human erythroproietin w/iron supplementation

• Growth failure treated w/daily SubQ injections of recombinant human growth hormone
• Hypertension treated w/restriction of sodium intake, fluid restriction, antihypertensive medications
• Hyperkalemia treated by limiting foods high in potassium (bananas, tomatoes, fruit juices); severe hyperkalemia treated w/potassium-binding resins (sodium polystyrene sulfonate); persistent hyperkalemia indication for proceeding w/end-stage renal failure management such as dialysis/kidney transplantation

COMPLICATIONS

• ↓ exercise tolerance, poor oral intake, short stature, delay in sexual maturation, emotional problems related to above issues/need to take large numbers of medications, often several times each day
• Electrolyte abnormalities may lead to cardiac arrhythmias/may be life threatening if severe
• Hypertension may rarely cause seizures

PREVENTION

• Prenatal ultrasound finding of pelviectasis, family Hx vesicoureteral reflux in first-degree relative (parent, sibling)/occurrence of acute pyelonephritis in first 5 yrs of life indications for obtaining renal ultrasound/voiding cystourethrogram
• Prophylactic antibiotics administered to children w/obstruction/reflux (trimethoprim/sulfamethoxazole, nitrofurantoin); urologic consultation needed for posterior urethral valves, significant ureteropelvic junction obstruction, vesicoureteral reflux w/breakthrough UTIs
• Prompt recognition of acute glomerulonephritis/referral to center familiar w/Dx/treatment of childhood glomerulonephritis may ↓ incidence of CRF 2° to glomerulonephritis

WHEN TO REFER

• Hyperkalemia
• Metabolic acidosis refractory to alkali supplementation
• Moderate to severe hypertension
• Chronic renal failure of unknown etiology
• End-stage renal failure w/need for dialysis/transplantation

BACKGROUND

- Children generate 1–3 mEq/kg/d of acid from dietary protein, bone formation that must be excreted by kidneys
- Accomplished by secreting H^+ in distal nephron and forming H_2PO^- and NH_4^+
- Proximal nephron must reabsorb filtered load of HCO_3, ~1,600 mEq/d in 5 yr old
- *Proximal RTA:* ↓ ability to reabsorb completely normal filtered HCO_3 load
- *Distal RTA:* ↓ ability to secrete H^+
- *Hyperkalemia inhibits ammonia formation:* hyperkalemic RTA

CLINICAL MANIFESTATIONS

- Failure to thrive, esp w/proximal RTA
- Proximal RTA can be part of global proximal tubule disorder—Fanconi syndrome
- Severe acidosis more common in distal RTA
- Nephrocalcinosis/nephrolithiasis more common in distal RTA
- RTA can be inherited both as autosomal recessive or dominant trait
- Familial distal RTA associated w/deafness

LABORATORY FEATURES

- RTA associated w/normal serum anion gap $(Na - \{Cl + HCO_3\} = 12 \pm 4)$
- Urine pH > 6.0 associated w/RTA but not diagnostic
- ↑ fractional excretion (FE) of HCO_3, when serum HCO_3 22–24 mEg/L, diagnostic of proximal RTA (Type II) – FE HCO_3 = $(Urine_{bicarbonate} \times Serum_{creatinine}/Serum_{bicarbonate} \times Urine_{creatinine})$ (100%) FE HCO_3 > 15% in proximal RTA
- ↑ ammonia excretion most important response to acidosis, can be estimated from urine net charge (Urinary net charge = urine Cl – [urine Na + K]), positive value indicates normal ammonia response, no distal RTA; negative value indicates inadequate response and RTA
- Hypokalemia, negative urine net charge, urine pH > 6.0, significant acidosis typical findings of classic or secretory defect distal RTA (type I) w/absence of H^+ pumps
- Mild acidosis, failure to thrive w/normal ability to lower urine pH characteristic of rate-dependent distal RTA
- Rate-dependent distal RTA diagnosed by low urine pCO_2 when urine pH > 7.6 by bicarbonate loading
- Hyperkalemic distal RTA (type IV) associated w/obstructive uropathy, aldosterone deficiency, or aldosterone resistance

APPROACH TO THE DIAGNOSIS OF RTA

- First, determine anion gap. Consider other causes of acidosis if anion gap ↑ (organic acidoses, diabetic ketoacidosis, poisoning)
- Second, determine urine net charge. Positive value indicates either proximal RTA or bicarbonate loss from GI tract. Measure fractional HCO_3 excretion and look for other evidence of proximal tubule defect, such as glucosuria, to evaluate for proximal RTA
- Negative urine net charge indicates poor ammonia excretion and distal RTA
- Third, assess serum K:
  — hyperkalemia: evaluate for aldosterone problem or impaired tubular excretion of potassium
  — normal or low serum K:
    ○ inability to lower urine pH below 5.5 w/acute acid load indicative of secretory defect
    ○ low urine pH but low urine pCO_2 w/HCO_3 loading indicative of rate-dependent RTA

- Finally, review pt medication list. Amphotericin B associated w/mild, hypokalemic distal RTA; ifosfamide, acetazolamide w/proximal RTA

TREATMENT

- *Proximal RTA:* 5–20 mEq/kg/d of alkali to normalize serum HCO_3 because as serum HCO_3 rises, more HCO_3 excreted. Urinary potassium excretion also ↑ w/treatment, usually requires replacement
- Distal RTA in older children, adolescents corrected w/2–3 mEq/kg/d of alkali. Hypokalemia usually resolves w/correction of acidosis. Higher doses needed to maximize growth, prevent nephrocalcinosis/nephrolithiasis. Infants require larger doses, may need as much as 10 mEq/kg/d
- Hyperkalemic distal RTA responds to maneuvers that lower serum K such as mineralocorticoid supplementation, furosemide, Kayexalate administration

OUTCOME

- Infants w/proximal RTA w/o Fanconi syndrome thrive when supplemented w/alkali
- Proximal RTA may resolve w/time in infants
- Rate-dependent distal RTA in infants also may be transient
- Classic distal RTA usually lifelong problem
- Distal RTA can lead to chronic renal failure from nephrocalcinosis/nephrolithiasis
- Acidosis in distal RTA can be life threatening

WHEN TO REFER

- Referral indicated for pts w/Fanconi syndrome, severe acidosis, nephrocalcinosis/nephrolithiasis, renal insufficiency, unclear Dx

BACKGROUND

- First described in 1948 in association w/glomerular disease, nephrotic syndrome
- Now known to occur across wide spectrum of ages, clinical severity
- Neonatal incidence 1/1,000 live births
- Peak incidence in neonatal period, in older adults w/glomerular disease, in renal transplant population. Most cases associated w/inflammatory states, deficiency of physiologic anticoagulants, poor perfusion, or compression of renal vein
- Associated conditions in neonates:
  - volume depletion
  - maternal diabetes or hypertension
  - neonatal asphyxia or prematurity
  - occasionally occurs w/no associated disease
- Associated conditions in renal transplant recipients:
  - young donors (<6 yrs old)
  - young recipients (<2 yrs old)
  - use of OKT3 or cyclosporin A
  - technical compression of renal vein
  - postop hypotension
- Associated conditions in older children:
  - nephrotic syndrome
  - lupus, other inflammatory states
  - poor perfusion states

CLINICAL MANIFESTATIONS

- Sx depend on whether sudden or gradual in onset
- Acute onset usually associated w/more symptoms
- More gradual onset may lead to loss of renal function w/o overt symptoms
- *Acute symptoms:*
  - in neonatal period:
    - gross hematuria
    - flank mass
    - azotemia (if RVT bilateral)
    - hypertension
  - in renal transplant recipient:
    - graft enlargement

- ↓ urine volume, ↓ GFR, ↑ serum creatinine
    - hematuria
  - in older children or adults:
    - hypertension
    - flank pain or mass
    - hematuria
    - other deep vein thrombotic disease
- *Late-phase symptoms:*
  - ↓ renal function
  - hypertension

LABORATORY AND RADIOLOGIC FEATURES

- Acute phase:
  - enlarged affected kidney(s), w/↑ echogenicity by ultrasound, ↓ venous flow by Doppler
  - ↓ function in affected kidney(s) by nuclide renal scan, CT or IVP
  - hematuria, proteinuria
  - ↑ serum creatinine
  - thrombocytopenia—may be severe
  - ↓ AT III, Protein C, Protein S concentrations—transient or congenital
- Long term:
  - proteinuria
  - ↓ renal function
  - ↓ renal size
  - ↑ echogenicity

DIFFERENTIAL DIAGNOSIS

- Acute renal failure (acute tubular necrosis)
- Pyelonephritis
- Hemolytic uremic syndrome
- Wilms tumor or nephroblastoma
- Acute renal arterial occlusion

TREATMENT

- Reverse underlying cause (volume depletion, shock):
  - provide supportive care including normalizing BP
  - most important component of treatment

- *Surgery:* does not ↑ survival in acute phase:
  - nephrectomy may reverse hypertension in chronic, late phase
- *Anticoagulation:* prevents or slows thrombus extension:
  - dosages for children extrapolated from adult data
  - heparin, 75–100 U/kg bolus, then 20–28 U/h × 5–7 d
  - warfarin, 0.2 mg/kg/d, adjusted to INR = 2–3; treat for 3 mos
- Thrombolytic Tx: should be used only in bilateral massive RVT, where extension up IVC exists, or where concern about pulmonary embolus present:
  - streptokinase 2,000 U/kg load, then 1,000 U/kg/h × 6 h
  - TPA (dose not established for infants)
- Replacement of physiologic anticoagulant factors (when deficient):
  - antithrombin III (commercially available), Protein C, Protein S

COMPLICATIONS

- Renal scarring w/↓ function if scarring extensive (very common)
- Hypertension (moderately common)

WHEN TO REFER

- Late discovery after acute phase can often be managed w/o referral unless management of hypertension difficult
- If ↓ renal function or severe hypertension in acute phase, consultation may be required
- If indications for anticoagulation or for thrombolysis, referral recommended
- If serious complications or questions about Dx, referral indicated

BACKGROUND

- Retropharyngeal abscess (RPA):
  - described as abscess involving space behind posterior pharynx
  - true RPA spatially located off midline due to limitation by longitudinal midline raphe that divides fascial compartment
  - two lymph node chains contained within compartment, typically involute by 5 yrs of age. Suppuration of these lymph nodes thought to be etiology of RPA. These facts account for age of predilection of RPA for children <5 yrs of age (50% <3 yrs). RPA most frequently seen in infancy
- Peritonsillar abscess (PTA):
  - most common of head, neck abscesses to present at any age
  - occurs between tonsil and superior constrictor muscle
  - although, by definition, not truly "deep neck infection," it is frequent precursor
  - generally follows episode of tonsillitis
  - far more common in children >5 yrs of age
- Both RPA, PTA have recovery rates >95% w/appropriate Tx

CLINICAL MANIFESTATIONS

- RPA:
  - most frequent manifestations of RPA include fever, neck swelling, anorexia
  - most common physical finding: cervical adenopathy
  - pharyngeal bulge often present and may be detected depending on accuracy of physical examination. In infants oropharyngeal examination always challenging due to inherent limitations of size, secretions, lack of pt cooperation
  - torticollis, stridor, neck stiffness not infrequently seen in these pts
- PTA:
  - commonly present w/complaints of sore throat, fever, dysphagia, anorexia
  - physical findings include trismus, an *asymmetric* tonsillar bulge, and uvular edema and deviation to opposite side
  - due to the older age of pt population, these findings commonly visualized, rather sensitive
  - upper airway obstruction may be seen in advanced cases

LABORATORY FEATURES

- Laboratory findings in RPA, PTA similar, nonspecific, including fever, leukocytosis w/left shift
- Microbiologic results of culture reveal most commonly isolated pathogens *Streptococcus pyogenes* (18%), *Staphylococcus aureus* (18%). Other common isolates include anaerobe *Bacteroides melanogenicus* (17%), gram-negative microbe *Haemophilus parainfluenzae* (14%)
- Diagnostic radiology:
  - in pediatric population, diagnostic radiology frequently plays critical role due to difficulty of obtaining adequate oropharyngeal examination
  - lateral soft tissue neck radiographs often used to evaluate presence of retropharyngeal pathology. Dx made on basis of characteristic prevertebral soft tissue swelling, loss of cervical lordosis, presence of air within tissue seen in RPA. Lateral radiographs taken in *inspiration,* avoiding significant false positive results commonly encountered w/expiratory films. Normal measurements include soft tissue thickness up to 7 mm at level of C2 and 14 mm–22 mm (in adults) at C6. Up to 33% false negative rate reported for lateral soft tissue radiographs despite appropriate technique
  - detail provided by CT scan *w/ contrast* makes it superior modality for confirming not only presence or absence of abscess, but also for evaluating surrounding anatomic structures, important for surgical intervention. Contrast material mandatory for accurate detail of soft tissue, inflammatory, vascular elements. Reported sensitivity/specificity of CT scan for differentiating cellulitis/adenopathy from frank abscess 93%, 60%, respectively
  - ultrasound may be some help as 1° diagnostic modality in very limited circumstances

DIFFERENTIAL DIAGNOSIS

- Scope of differential for RPA, PTA may be as broad as differential of pediatric neck masses or that of occult infantile febrile illnesses, depending on presenting Sx
- In general, balance of physical evidence points to head, neck source. Initial clinical Dx supported by confirmatory radiographic studies

COMPLICATIONS

- Spectrum of potential complications of RPA, PTA includes both common sequelae such as anorexia, dehydration, as well as more devastating complications, potentially seen w/advanced RPA or w/spread of PTA to deep neck fascial compartments
- Airway compromise, empyema, meningitis, internal jugular vein thrombosis all recognized sequelae

TREATMENT

- Treatment or RPA, PTA bimodal; appropriate care includes both adequate drainage, antimicrobial Tx
- Routine Tx for PTA in children involves incision, drainage of abscess, in either office or OR, w/or w/o concurrent tonsillectomy (Quinsy tonsillectomy). Needle aspiration of PTA shown to be effective Tx; may be plausible in older children who can cooperate. In younger children or infants, may be technically difficult, potentially unsafe
- Adequate drainage of RPA generally requires operative management. Either intraoral or external transcervical approach may be necessary for full access to abscess cavity for drainage
- Antibiotics covering gram-positive, gram-negative, anaerobic, beta-lactamase-producing organisms should be selected for empiric antimicrobial Tx and then targeted toward results of culture and sensitivities. Requirements can be achieved by number of drug combinations. Penicillin plus beta-lactamase inhibitor, such as amoxicillin-clavulamate or ticarcillin-clavulamate, frequently recommended. Ampicillin/sulbactam, clindamycin both shown effective in anaerobic infections of head, neck. Additionally, combination of piperacillin, tozobactam effective in treating polymicrobial infection as single agent

WHEN TO REFER

- Most pts w/either PTA or RPA benefit from combined efforts of pediatrician and otolaryngologist
- Because adequate drainage of abscesses integral element of appropriate management, and because late complications can be catastrophic, early surgical consultation essential

EPIDEMIOLOGY

- Most frequent soft tissue sarcoma of childhood
- Arises in virtually any anatomic site from primitive mesenchymal cells located throughout body
- Seventh most common malignancy of childhood:
- 4.3 new cases per million white children annually; 3.3 per million among blacks; M:F ratio 1.4:1
- Median age at Dx 7 yrs; 65% pts <11 yrs, 4% <1 yr
- May be associated w/familial cancer syndrome of Li-Fraumeni (breast cancer, leukemia, brain tumors, adrenocortical carcinoma)

BIOLOGY/PATHOLOGY

- *Most common locations:* GU tract (23%), extremity (17%), cranial parameningeal area (16%), other head and neck excluding orbit (10%), orbit (8%), trunk (10%), retroperitoneum (11%), other sites (5%)
- Histologic variants:

Histologic Subtype	% of Pts	Common Sites	Prognostic Significance
Embryonal	54	Head, orbit, GU tract	Favorable
Botryoid subtype	6	Vagina, uterus	Favorable
Spindle cell	3	Paratestes	Favorable
Alveolar	21	Extremity, trunk	Unfavorable
Undifferentiated	8	Extremity, trunk	Unfavorable
Other	11	Extremity, trunk, other	Intermediate/Unfavorable

- Alveolar histology frequently has characteristic structural chromosomal rearrangement t(2;13)
- Up to 50% cases of both alveolar or embryonal tumors may have mutations in tumor suppressor gene p53
- Embryonal tumors have loss of heterozygosity at chromosome 11p15, often hyperdiploid
- Distant metastasis common and can occur early
- Frequent sites of metastatic disease include regional lymph nodes, lungs, bone marrow, bone, CNS, heart, liver, breast

CLINICAL MANIFESTATIONS

- Asymptomatic mass w/o constitutional symptoms unless widespread disease present
- *Symptoms depend on anatomic location:* orbital masses: proptosis or eyelid mass; cranial parameningeal sites: cranial nerve palsies or signs of ↑ intracranial pressure; nasopharynx lesions: purulent or sanguinous nasal discharge, epistaxis; GU sites: urinary obstruction, hematuria; extremity sites: palpable mass lesions; intra-abdominal tumors: palpable mass, pain, or obstruction of abdominal viscera

DIAGNOSTIC EVALUATION/STAGING

- Complete physical examination, attention to site of 1° tumor, surrounding structures, lymph node areas
- CBC, blood chemistry analysis, UA, bone marrow aspiration and/or biopsy
- Chest radiograph, bone scan, CT of chest to identify pulmonary and/or mediastinal metastasis, CT scan or MRI of abdomen-pelvis to evaluate viscera and retroperitoneal lymph nodes, CT scan and/or MRI of 1° lesion to determine extent of tumor, cranial MRI for parameningeal lesions
- Staging by Intergroup Rhabdomyosarcoma Study surgical and pathologic grouping classification system:
  - group I: localized disease completely resected:
    ○ confined to muscle or organ of origin
    ○ contiguous involvement—infiltration outside muscle or organ of origin
  - group II: total gross resection w/evidence of regional spread:
    ○ grossly resected tumor w/microscopic residual
    ○ regional disease w/involved nodes, completely resected w/no microscopic residual
    ○ regional disease w/involved nodes grossly resected, but w/evidence of microscopic residual and/or histologic involvement of most distal regional node in dissection
  - group III: incomplete resection or biopsy w/gross residual disease remaining, nonresectable
  - group IV: distant metastatic disease present at Dx
- Additionally, still under study is pretreatment TNM staging classification that categorizes tumors (stage 1–4) based on anatomic location, size (> or <5 cm), clinical evidence of regional node involvement, presence of distant metastasis

DIFFERENTIAL DIAGNOSIS

- *Orbital masses:* infection, metastatic neuroblastoma, leukemia (granulocytic sarcoma), lymphoma, optic nerve glioma, histiocytosis
- *Nasopharyngeal, sinus or neck masses:* benign: infection, branchial cleft cysts; malignant: lymphoma, leukemia, carcinoma, histiocytosis, nonrhabdomyosarcomatous soft tissue sarcomas
- *Abdominal masses:* benign: mesenteric cysts, duplications of the gut, renal or ovarian cysts, inflammatory masses; malignant: Wilms tumor, neuroblastoma, lymphoma, hepatoblastoma, germ cell tumors, nonrhabdomyosarcomatous soft tissue sarcomas
- *Extremity and trunk lesions:* other soft tissue sarcomas, bone tumors (Ewing or osteogenic sarcoma), neuroectodermal tumors
- *GU tract lesions:* neurofibromas, hemangiomas or other soft tissue sarcomas of the bladder; embryonal carcinoma, lymphoma and germ cell tumors of the testis/spermatic cord

TREATMENT

- Multidisciplinary approach coordinating surgery, chemotherapy, radiation Tx
- *Surgery:* complete resection, including adequate margins if technically feasible w/o unacceptable loss of function, otherwise open biopsy
  - clinical, pathologic evaluation of regional lymph nodes
- *Combination chemotherapy:* improves survival, indicated for all pts
  - may be used to reduce nonresectable tumors to resectable size
  - current front-line Tx consists of vincristine, actinomycin-D, cyclophosphamide w/hematopoietic growth factor support
  - achieves complete responses in 50–70% pts, partial responses in additional 20%
  - other active agents: doxorubicin, ifosfamide, etoposide, cisplatin, melphalan, topotecan, high-dose methotrexate, dacarbazine, mitomycin C
- Radiation Tx:
  - necessary for all pts except those w/group I lesions of nonalveolar histology
  - all other groups, stages require radiotherapy to 1° disease site and if feasible to areas of metastatic disease
  - doses of 4,000–5,500 cGy required to achieve durable local tumor control

PROGNOSIS

- Overall 5 yr survival varies according to disease group:

Group	5 Yr Survival %
I	90
II	80
III	70
IV	30

- Site of 1° tumor also conveys prognostic significance w/orbit and nonbladder or nonprostate GU sites more favorable than cranial parameningeal, bladder, prostate, trunk, extremity sites
- Other prognostic variables include tumor size (< 5 cm favorable), histologic subtype (nonalveolar cell type favorable), cytogenetic abnormalities (t[2;13] unfavorable)
- Any recurrence conveys poor prognosis

LATE EFFECTS OF THERAPY

- Long-term complications can arise 2° to Tx (surgery, radiation, chemotherapy):
  - neuroendocrine abnormalities such as growth hormone deficiency, thyroid dysfunction, delayed puberty, infertility
  - diminished growth of underlying or surrounding structures in radiation fields
  - cardiac, renal abnormalities
  - second malignancies such as acute myelogenous leukemia, several types of solid tumors

WHEN TO REFER

- Refer to specialist when diagnosis a serious consideration

RHEUMATIC FEVER

HUGH D. ALLEN

BACKGROUND

- Most frequently occurs 6–15 yrs of age: rare <5 yrs of age
- No gender difference in incidence
- Worldwide, most common cause of heart disease in children/young adults; most common in hot climates, developing countries
- US regional outbreaks in late 1980s, still seen most commonly in spring
- Onset 2–3 wks after group A streptococcal pharyngitis (no other sites)
- Limited to certain streptococcal subtypes, esp mucoid strains
- Immune response w/cross-reactive antibody attacking heart, joints, basal ganglia; occurs only in certain genetically susceptible individuals
- *Inflammatory reaction affects serosal surfaces:* pericardium, peritoneum, joint capsules; also basal ganglia, myocardium, endocardium (nearly always left sided, esp mitral valve), vascular tissue
- *Pathognomonic finding:* Aschoff body in myocardium

CLINICAL MANIFESTATIONS

- Jones criteria (see table) necessary for Dx; 2 major or 1 major plus 2 unrelated minor (softer/can lead to overdiagnosis); documentation of antecedent group A streptococcal pharyngitis absolutely necessary

Major Criteria

- *Arthritis: not* arthralgias associated w/streptococcal infections; migratory, polyarticular, esp large joints: elbow, wrist, knee, ankle; hot, red, swollen, extremely painful: mere touching elicits marked tenderness; exquisitely responsive to salicylates, even in low doses
- *Carditis:* if pericarditis, will have pancarditis
  - most common manifestation: mitral valve involvement, then mitral/aortic valve; uncommon aortic alone. Myocarditis reflected by cardiac enlargement, left ventricular failure; findings include cough, grunting, chest pain, orthopnea, anxiety, anorexia, wide pulse pressure, pulsus paradoxus, friction rub, arrhythmias, new onset apical holosystolic mitral regurgitation murmur (w/or w/o mid-diastolic murmur), and/or early diastolic aortic regurgitant murmur. CHF manifested by tachycardia, even while sleeping, dyspnea, wheezing, rales, hepatomegaly, laterally/downward displaced point of maximal impulse, apical S3/S4 (gallop)
- *Sydenham chorea (St. Vitus dance):* affects 15%; can appear late, 3 mos/more after pharyngitis; emotional lability, crying, frustrated, acting out, ↓ attention span, new onset poor school performance; flailing gross motor movements while awake/stressed; facial grimaces, tongue fasciculates, voice wavers, extended arms pronate, fingers writhe, fingers hyperextend, handwriting deteriorates (good way to follow improvement), pencil can fly from hand; persists wks to mos, even yrs
- *Erythema marginatum:* occurs in ≤5%; serpentine, erythematous border, macular, evanescent; usually on trunk, limbs, not face
- *SubQ nodules:* rarely seen; over extensor surfaces, esp elbow, knee, ankle, back of hand; sometimes scalp/back; measure 0.5–2 cm, movable, painless

Minor Criteria

- *Fever:* short duration; not w/Sydenham
- *Arthralgia:* pain, but no swelling, tenderness, heat, redness
  - not criteria, but often seen:
    - epistaxis
    - abdominal pain: some pts have undergone laparatomy

LABORATORY FEATURES

- *Acute phase reactants:* normal in Sydenham, otherwise, ↑ in proportion to severity:
  - WBC count: no longer minor criterion
  - ESR: can be in 70–80 range, low in CHF; good parameter to follow improvement if not in CHF
  - C-reactive protein: not affected by CHF
- Proof of streptococcal infection:
  - throat culture best, can be negative because of latency of RHF onset; need serum antibody tests for presence of streptococcal antigens (extracellular include anti-streptolysin O (ASO), anti-DNAse B, anti-hyaluronidase, anti-streptokinase, anti-NADase, anti-A carbohydrate; streptozyme incorporates all, but is variable in accuracy; cellular antibodies include type-specific antibody (against M protein)/anti-A carbohydrate; most peak at 1 mo, if valvular disease, anti-A stays ↑ × 2 yrs; remainder not diagnostic of RHF, only of streptococcal infection
- Laboratory evaluation of effects of RHF:
  - chest x-ray: may show basilar infiltrates, pericardial effusion, ↑ venous vascularity and/or pulmonary edema if CHF; useful for serial evaluation
  - *electrocardiogram:* may show tachycardia, prolonged P-R interval, first degree AV block, AV dissociation, nodal rhythm, ST-T changes, widened QRS, T wave inversion, occasional arrhythmias
  - Doppler echocardiogram: may show pericardial effusion, ↓ left ventricular function, mitral/aortic regurgitation; useful serial tool

DIFFERENTIAL DIAGNOSIS

- Myocardiopathy from other causes (most commonly viral)
- *Juvenile rheumatoid arthritis:* smaller joints, more chronic, not migratory, slow salicylate response
- Lupus erythematosis; ANA may help
- Postinfectious reactive arthritis (includes poststreptococcal)
- Serum sickness
- Kawasaki syndrome
- Bacterial endocarditis
- Sickle-cell disease
- Infectious arthritis, esp gonococcal (blood culture, and joint culture useful)
- Leukemia
- Coccidiomycosis
- Histoplasmosis
- Congenital choreoathetosis
- Brain tumors

TREATMENT

- Must eradicate/prevent future streptococcal pharyngitis:
  - benzathine/penicillin G, 1.2 million units IM, for pts >27 kg; 600,000 units IM for pts < 27 kg; phenoxymethyl penicillin, 250 mg qid × 10 d; erythromycin ethyl succinate, 40 mg/kg/d, max. 1 g/d, 3–4 doses/d × 10 d. Prophylaxis: benzathine penicillin G, 1.2 million units monthly, phenoxymethyl penicillin, 250 mg bid, sulfadiazine, 1.0 g daily, erythromycin ethyl succinate, 250 mg bid; duration debated; safest = lifetime, esp if had carditis; if only arthritis, many recommend giving for 5 yrs after attack, at least into early 20s
- *Arthritis:* if no carditis, salicylates, 50–75 mg/kg/d
  - continue 2 wks, taper × 2–3 wks; follow ESR
- *Carditis:* stop inflammation; controversy regarding salicylate vs. steroid Rx; most prefer steroids; salicylates, 50–100 mg/kg/d, in 4 div doses; follow serum salicylate level, keep at 25 mg/dl, do not exceed 30; continue 4–8 wks; steroids: oral prednisone, 2 mg/kg/d; give 2 wks, taper 2–3 wks; at last week, start salicylates to avoid rebound; to treat CHF: diuresis, acutely use dobutamine and/or dopamine, chronic use lanoxin; may need afterload-reducing agents such as enalapril; bed rest very useful acutely, slowly return to normal activity after acute phase
- *Sydenham chorea:* mild: bed rest, avoid stress, home tutor; severe: haloperidol, start low dose 0.5 mg, ↑ to 2.0 mg q8h; may need to go as high as 5.0 mg; some use phenobarbital, valproate also recently recommended

COMPLICATIONS

- Few occur after first attack
- Death
- Chronic myocardial scarring/CHF
- Chronic valvulitis requiring valve replacement

PREVENTION

- Avoid streptococcal pharyngitis! See Treatment

WHEN TO REFER

- Immediately upon suspecting Dx

Jones criteria for Dx Rheumatic Fever*

Major Criteria
Migratory polyarthritis
Carditis
Sydenham chorea
Erythema marginatum
SubQ nodules

Minor Criteria
Clinical: arthralgia, fever
Laboratory: ↑ sed rate, ↑ C-reactive protein, prolonged PR interval on EKG

Require 2 major; less desirable are 1 major, 2 unrelated minors (can't use prolonged PR interval if already have carditis).

*Proof of antecedent group A streptococcal pharyngitis required: culture or antibody titers.

Modified from Dajani AS, Ayoub EM, Bierman FZ, et al. Guidelines for the diagnosis of rheumatic fever: Jones criteria, updated 1992. Circulation 87: 302–307, 1992.

BACKGROUND

- Disorder of skeletal mineralization known since antiquity
- Acquired/inherited forms exist, generally result in ↓ supply of calcium/phosphate to skeleton, become manifest as mineralization defect
- Acquired rickets usually due to vitamin D deficiency; because minimal vitamin D found in breast milk/because also synthesized in skin w/sufficient UV light exposure, predominant setting in which rickets occurs is in breast-fed infants, not supplemented w/vitamins, in northern environments in winter; pigmented races appear to be at higher risk; calcium deficiency may complicate problem/be sole cause of rickets in rare situations
- Breast-fed premature infants may develop rickets due to dietary phosphorus deficiency as mineral demands of rapidly growing skeleton can exceed low phosphorus supply in breast milk
- Most common form of inherited rickets due to renal phosphate wasting, usually transmitted in X-linked dominant fashion (X-linked hypophosphatemia/[XLH]); incidence ~1/20,000
- Other rare forms of inherited rickets include defects in metabolism/action of vitamin D

CLINICAL MANIFESTATIONS

- Initial presentation may be short stature/decrement in rate of linear growth
- Progressive bow/sometimes knock-knee deformity of legs typical; in severe vitamin D deficiency craniotabes (Ping-Pong skull)/rachitic rosary may be evident
- Vitamin D deficiency/inactivity may also manifest hypocalcemic tetany, muscle weakness, ↑ frequency of infections
- Dental caries/abscesses may occur

RADIOGRAPHIC FEATURES

- Demineralization/coarse trabeculae of long bones; bow defects
- Loss of well-defined metaphyseal border w/fraying, metaphyseal flaring, cupping
- In XLH, legs more severely affected than other sites

LABORATORY FEATURES

- Alkaline phosphatase activity ↑ in almost all forms (↑ may be masked in malnutrition involving zinc)
- Serum levels/urinary excretion of calcium/phosphorus, parathyroid hormone (PTH), vitamin D levels vary with form of rickets (see table); single best test for vitamin D deficiency: circulating 25-hydroxyvitamin D level

Serum laboratory findings

	Calcium	Phosphorus	PTH	25-OH D	$1,25(OH)_2$ D
Vitamin D deficiency	Low, Nl	Low, Nl	High	Low	Low, Nl, High
Vitamin D dependency (pseudo deficiency)	Low	Low, Nl	High	Nl	Low, Nl
Hereditary resistance to vitamin D	Low	Low, Nl	High	Nl	Nl, High
Phosphate deficiency	Nl, High	Low	Low, Nl	Nl	Nl, High
XLH	Nl	Low	Nl, High	Nl	Nl

- Urinary calcium excretion usually ↓ in calciopenic rickets; urinary phosphorus excretion ↓ in phosphorus deficiency, ↑ in XLH

DIFFERENTIAL DIAGNOSIS

- In addition to above, similar bony lesions may be seen in other disorders, *underlying diagnoses may need to be looked for;* these include:
  - hypophosphatasia: inherited disorder of low alkaline phosphatase activity resulting in characteristic mineralization defects, only subtle changes in serum mineral levels
  - renal osteodystrophy: seen in chronic renal failure
  - bone disease induced by parenteral nutrition
  - fat-soluble vitamin malabsorption, as in cystic fibrosis, inflammatory bowel disease, severe liver dysfunction
  - osteopenia of prematurity
  - neoplastic causes of bone disease
  - osteoporosis, where mineralization normal, but ↓ bone mass throughout skeleton
  - metaphyseal dysplasias

PREVENTION

- Breast-fed infants should be given vitamin supplements; if dietary calcium clearly deficient, supplementation w/calcium-containing foods/medication helpful

TREATMENT

- Specific Tx depends on type of rickets. Common preparations:
  - vitamin D (Drisdol), 200 units/drop
  - $1,25(OH)_2$ vitamin D (calcitriol, Rocaltrol), 0.25 or 0.5 mcg/capsule
  - calcium glubionate (Neoclaglucon), 115 mg elemental calcium/5 ml
  - calcium carbonate (Tums), 200 mg elemental calcium/tablet
  - phosphate (K-Phos Neutral tablets, Neutra-Phos powder), 250 mg of elemental phosphorus per tablet, capsule, packet
- *Vitamin D deficiency:* 2,000 units oral vitamin D daily, until correction of alkaline phosphatase level, then 400–800 units daily as nutritional requirement; alternatively, in settings of poor follow-up, 600,000 units of vitamin D given in 2 div doses in one day po or IM; calcitriol should not be used routinely in vitamin D deficiency rickets; calcium should be provided such that total daily intake ~30–50 mg of elemental calcium/kg body weight/d
- *Vitamin D dependency:* calcitriol used in dosages of up to 2 mcg/d; required as chronic medication
- *Hereditary resistance to vitamin D:* spectrum of severity exists; some may respond to high-dose calcitriol; others may require long-term IV calcium; pts should be evaluated/treated at center w/experience in pediatric bone disease
- *XLH:* requires combination of calcitriol (0.25–2.0 mcg/d), phosphate (0.25–2.5 g/d of elemental phosphorus); balance in dosage of two medications required/management with direction of experienced center

COMPLICATIONS

- Progressive bow deformities may require corrective surgical osteotomy
- Severe hypocalcemia can lead to seizures, coma, even death
- Complications of treatment include vitamin D intoxication w/hypercalcemia/soft tissue calcification; in XLH, nephrocalcinosis common/chronic hyperparathyroidism may occur

WHEN TO REFER

- Most straightforward vitamin D deficiency rickets can be diagnosed/treated w/o referral to specialist; however, severe disease/failure to respond to Tx should prompt referral
- If Dx/laboratory findings do not appear to fit straightforward Dx referral necessary for more complex investigations
- Inherited/chronic forms should be referred for long-term management
- Pediatric orthopedic intervention may be required for irreversible deformities

BACKGROUND

- Known as familial hypophosphatemic rickets, renal phosphate rickets, phosphate diabetes, vitamin D resistant rickets, X-linked hypophosphatemic rickets (preferred nomenclature)
- Commonly presents 6 mos–3 yrs of age, although Dx often delayed into fourth year of life
- Most common inheritance X-linked dominant, due to defect in endopeptidase-like gene located on Xp22.1 chromosome. Spontaneous mutations common
- Basic defects in X-linked hypophosphatemia involve:
  - inappropriate phosphaturia w/resulting hypophosphatemia
  - in response to hypophosphatemia, subnormal blood level of the active vitamin D metabolite 1,25-dihydroxyvitamin D from lack of appropriate ↑ in activity of renal enzyme, 25-hydroxyvitamin D-1-alpha hydroxylase

CLINICAL MANIFESTATIONS

- Rachitic changes common in untreated infant or child:
  - palpable, visible enlargements of costochondral junctions, of ends of long bones (esp at wrists, ankles, knees)
  - bowing deformities of lower extremities, most commonly seen after weight bearing has occurred developmentally
  - occipital skull softness, sign of undermineralization, esp in infants <3 mos of age (craniotabes), enlarged sutures and fontanelles, occipital or parietal flattening in usually recumbent infant
- Diminished linear growth rates, short stature
- Dental abnormalities common:
  - delayed tooth eruption (but w/o enamel hypoplasia seen in hypocalcemic varieties of rickets (see Laboratory Features)
  - pulp abscesses

- Less common abnormalities include:
  - delayed motor development w/mild hypotonia
    - umbilical hernia, protuberant abdomen
    - bone pain
    - waddling gait
    - muscle fatigue

LABORATORY FEATURES (IN UNTREATED PT)

- Normocalcemia (important finding in differential Dx) w/normal serum intact parathyroid hormone (iPTH) level
- Severe hypophosphatemia, w/concomitant phosphaturia (measured simply as tubular reabsorption of phosphate, or TRP, <70%)[1]
- Normal/slightly ↑ serum level of 25-hydroxyvitamin D; normal or slightly ↓ serum level of 1,25-dihydroxyvitamin D
- ↑ serum level of bone-specific alkaline phosphatase activity

---

[1]% TRP = 100 ×

$$\left(1 - \frac{\text{random urine [phosphorus} \times \text{serum [creatinine]}}{\text{serum [phosphorus]} \times \text{random urine [creatinine]}}\right)$$

RADIOGRAPHIC FEATURES

- W/active rickets, typical findings include cupping, fraying/widening of metaphyses in long bones
- Early in course of disease, generally before any Tx, absence of radiologic signs of hyperparathyroidism
- After growth has ceased, ossification of ligaments, tendons, synovia (enthesopathy); may result in spinal cord compression, consequent neurologic deficits

DIFFERENTIAL DIAGNOSIS

- Other rachitic disorders, including vitamin D deficiency, malabsorption, impaired hepatic synthetic capacity, disruption of enterohepatic circulation, renal Fanconi syndrome, renal osteodystrophy, hereditary hypophosphatemia w/hypercalciuria, tumor-induced hypophosphatemia, postrenal transplantation tubulopathy w/hypophosphatemia
- Jansen metaphyseal chondrodystrophy (recently shown to be due to one of several mutations in PTH/PTH-rp receptor, which leads to auto-activation of receptor in absence of ligand)

TREATMENT

- Most commonly used treatment protocols involve frequent administration (5–6×/d) of phosphate salts, 1–3×/d administration of oral 1,25-dihydroxyvitamin D
  - phosphate salts, 30–50 mg/kg/d
  - 1,25-dihydroxyvitamin D, 10–50 ng/kg/d
- Recombinant human growth hormone in experimental trials

COMPLICATIONS

- Acute risk of induction of hypercalcemia w/use of potent vitamin D metabolites real, or if continued in absence of concomitant oral phosphate Tx
- Radiographic nephrocalcinosis, often seen as complication of Tx w/phosphate, vitamin D metabolite itself
- Hypercalciuria, 2° hyperparathyroidism, often seen as complication of Tx w/phosphate, vitamin D metabolite itself
- Impaired renal function, from both hypercalcemia and nephrocalcinosis

WHEN TO REFER

- All pts in whom Dx of X-linked hypophosphatemia entertained should be referred to pediatric specialist interested in bone, mineral disorders. Complex algorithms for initial care and subsequent monitoring and changing of therapies removes this Dx from practice of general pediatrician or family practice physician

EUGENE D. SHAPIRO

BACKGROUND

- Most common of potentially fatal tick-borne diseases in US
- Caused by *Rickettsia rickettsii,* obligate intracellular bacterium
- Transmitted primarily by *Dermacentor variabilis* (dog tick)/*Amblyomma americanum* (lone star tick)
- Most cases occur in southern/south-central states, although cases may occur in virtually any area in US
- Incidence highest during period of peak activity of ticks (spring–fall)/among children
- Nearly 50% pts report tick bite in preceding 2 wks; no evidence to support antimicrobial prophylaxis for persons bitten by potential vectors
- Mortality ~5%; delay in beginning treatment important risk factor for more severe/fatal illness

CLINICAL MANIFESTATIONS

- *Common clinical manifestations:* fever, headache, rash (80–90%), myalgia, hyponatrimia, pleocytosis, hepatitis
- Onset often abrupt/heralded by fever, headache, myalgia
- Characteristic rash (80–90% of cases) begins on wrists/ankles, spreads to trunk; palms/soles usually involved; face often spared; begins as erythematous, maculopapular rash, often becomes petechial/purpuric
- Severe headache/disorientation may progress to coma
- Generalized vasculitis can lead to involvement of virtually any organ, occasionally, to disseminated intravascular coagulation; damage to vessels leads to edema/abnormalities in electrolytes

LABORATORY FEATURES

- Laboratory findings nonspecific; WBC count may be normal, ↑, ↓; mild thrombocytopenia/hyponatremia common, rarely may be severe; mild CSF pleocytosis common; hepatic transaminases usually ↑
- Early Dx made by detection intracellular *R. rickettsii* by fluorescein-conjugated antibody in biopsies of skin lesions; in most Dx based on results of serologic tests that detect antibodies which appear after first week of illness; tests for specific antibody to *R. rickettsii,* such as indirect hemagglutination, microimmunofluorescence, latex agglutination, enzyme-linked immunosorbent assays, complement-fixation tests have largely replaced less specific Weil-Felix test

DIFFERENTIAL DIAGNOSIS

- Meningococcemia as well as purpura fulminans from other causes (eg, *S. pneumoniae*), noninfectious vasculitis including erythema multiforme, collagen vascular disease, Kawasaki syndrome, measles, other rickettsial infections, enteroviral infections

TREATMENT

- Tetracycline, doxycycline, or chloramphenicol × 7–10 d
- Although tetracycline/doxycycline usually not recommended for children <9 yrs, effect on teeth of relatively short courses of treatment negligible/potential benefits of treatment probably outweigh small risk
- Critical to begin treatment early if Rocky Mountain spotted fever suspected

COMPLICATIONS

- CNS sequelae occur in small proportion of pts, occasionally, amputation of fingers, toes/other tissues may be necessary because of gangrene; complications more likely if delay before antimicrobial treatment begun

PREVENTION

- In endemic areas minimize exposure to ticks, check for/remove ticks daily

WHEN TO REFER

- Pts w/severe disease may need supportive care

ROSEOLA (EXANTHEM SUBITUM) AND OTHER HUMAN HERPESVIRUS 6/7 INFECTIONS

JAY H. MAYEFSKY

BACKGROUND

• 80% of roseola caused by human herpesvirus (HHV)-6; 10% by HHV-7; 10% by enteroviruses, adenoviruses, parainfluenza viruses
• HHV-6/HHV-7 enveloped, double-stranded DNA virus members of family *Herpesviridae*
• Both viruses ubiquitous; by adolescence almost all children have been infected
• Peak incidence HHV-6 infection 6–12 mos of age; infection rare <3 mos/>4 yrs
• HHV-7 infection occurs slightly later in life; 70% 7 yr old children seropositive
• Full spectrum HHV-6/HHV-7 infection still unknown
• 1° infection followed by persistent asymptomatic infection; site of latency not known
• Viral transmission probably via oral secretions; requires close contact; greatest during febrile phase of illness
• No seasonal variation

CLINICAL MANIFESTATIONS

• Roseola:
– fever: sudden onset of high fever (39–41°C); lasts 3–4 d, then falls rapidly
– general appearance: child looks well despite fever
– rash: appears after fever falls; macular/maculopapular; lesions discrete, 2–5 mm diameter, blanch on pressure, nonpruritic; start on trunk, spread to arms, neck, occasionally to face/legs; lasts for few hours–2 d; no desquamation/pigmentation

– other Sx: seizures during febrile stage; bulging fontanelle; injection of tympanic membranes, pharynx; maculopapular lesions on soft palate; cough/coryza; abdominal pain; headache; vomiting; diarrhea; occipital/cervical adenopathy, upper respiratory symptoms; edematous eyelids
• *Other manifestations of HHV-6/HHV-7 infection:* asymptomatic infection (most common); febrile illness w/o localizing signs; febrile illness w/ respiratory/GI complaints
• *Other diseases possibly related to HHV-6/HHV-7 infection:* mononucleosislike syndrome; intussusception; idiopathic thrombocytopenic purpura; hemophagocytic syndrome; hepatitis; chronic fatigue syndrome; pneumonitis, marrow suppression; multiple sclerosis; lymphoproliferative disorders; autoimmune diseases; Gianotti-Crosti syndrome
• Manifestations of reactivation in healthy persons unknown; in immunosuppressed persons may cause fever, hepatitis, marrow suppression, pneumonia

LABORATORY FEATURES

• WBC count/differential: during first 2 d, leukocytosis w/↑ neutrophils; subsequently WBC ↓ (mean 6,000/mm³) w/lymphocytosis (to 90%), occasionally monocytosis
• *CSF:* usually normal
• *IgM antibody:* detectable 5 d after onset of disease; persists 2–3 wks; also present during reactivation
• *IgG antibody:* appears at 1 wk; remains ↑ at least 2 mos; persists indefinitely
• *Viral isolation:* from peripheral blood lymphocytes during 1° infection

DIFFERENTIAL DIAGNOSIS

• Rubella
• Measles
• Other causes of fever in infants (otitis media, urinary tract infection, etc)
• Fever w/o focus
• Enteroviral/adenoviral infections
• Allergic reaction to antibiotic prescribed for febrile illness

TREATMENT

• Supportive

COMPLICATIONS

• *Seizures:* 30% of febrile seizures associated w/HHV-6 infections
• Persistent seizures
• Encephalitis
• Meningitis
• ↑ intracranial pressure
• Fatal disseminated disease
• Thrombocytopenic purpura
• Death

PREVENTION

• None known

WHEN TO REFER

• Referral indicated only for severe complications

DAVID O. MATSON

BACKGROUND

- Most common cause of severe gastroenteritis in children worldwide
- Causes ~4% of hospitalizations among children in US
- Causes ~3.0 million illnesses, 775,000 physician visits, 75,000 hospitalizations, 100 deaths in US each year
- More common in winter
- Serious illness most common 3–24 mos of age
- Causes ~10% of diarrhea episodes seen in office setting/50% of diarrhea episodes resulting in hospitalization in children
- Feces while symptomatic contains ~10^{10} infectious particles/g; infectious dose ~100 particles

CLINICAL MANIFESTATIONS

- Diarrhea, vomiting, fever (not specific to rotavirus); up to 20 diarrhea/vomiting episodes in 24 hrs not unusual; anorexia, cramps, myalgias can occur in adults/older children/difficult to evaluate in young children
- Dehydration/acidosis usually normonatremic
- Virus replication in liver/kidney of few pts w/severe immunocompromise, including AIDS, SCIDS, DiGeorge syndrome, documented; clinical implications uncertain
- Febrile seizures may occur w/fever

LABORATORY FEATURES

- Acidosis common w/severe symptoms. ↑/↓ serum Na^+, ↑/AD K^+, prerenal azotemia may occur
- Transient ↑ in liver enzymes 1–2 × normal in first few days in ~ one-third pts

DIFFERENTIAL DIAGNOSIS

- Many viral, bacterial, parasitic pathogens cause gastroenteritis
- Rotavirus suspected on basis of seasonality, age distribution, severity, lack of stool blood/mucus
- Absence of WBCs visualized by Wright stain indicates fecal lack of colitis/supports Dx rotavirus
- Specific Dx established by detection of viral particles in stool specimen, usually using commercial latex/enzyme-based assay; electron microscopy/research methods also available
- Fresh bulk stool unfrozen to laboratory (may be sent as soiled diaper); <0.1 g stool needed

TREATMENT

- No specific antirotavirus treatment recommended for otherwise healthy child; in immunocompromised infant/infant w/protracted/severe episode, immunoglobulin/human milk intestine/modification of intestinal milieu w/lactobacillus/similar preparation may be indicated; antidiarrheal agents not recommended
- *Dehydration and acidosis:* treatment directed toward correction of dehydration/acidosis, restoration of electrolytes by rehydration solutions; preferred route enteric, po/NG tube (permits regulation of transport of solute/water across intestinal wall, permitting normalization w/o "overshooting"/too rapidly changing fluid/solute status in different body compartments
- *Refeeding:* start as soon as possible; if dehydration <10%, begin as soon as fluid deficit corrected; if ≥10%, refeeding delayed until recovery from shock

COMPLICATIONS

- Death due to delayed/inappropriate Tx of dehydration
- Myelinolysis/cerebral edema from rapid drops in serum Na^+/solute concentration w/rehydration
- Potential morbidity from shock
- Evaluation for neurologic disease when febrile seizures occur

PREVENTION

- Good hand washing, by parent/child, esp after changing diapers, may ↓ spread of virus
- Ill children should be cohorted from susceptibles
- Diapering/food preparation areas should be separate
- Soiled diapers should be bagged before moving/not disposed of in kitchen waste
- A wipe-down solution at diaper changing area should be used after each diaper change

WHEN TO REFER

- Decision to refer guided by practitioner's experience w/treatment of often severe dehydration/metabolic imbalance
- Prolonged diarrhea (>7 d) w/no response to usual treatment
- Severe dehydration
- Hypernatremic dehydration
- Immunocompromised pt
- For additional information, see http://rotavirus.com or elsewhere on the Internet

BACKGROUND

• Infestations w/round worms present interesting study of relationship of parasite to host/variations of life cycle of different worms required to attain infections in human host

• In some cases, human not final/definitive host; parasite finds itself at dead end

• In others parasite may require another intermediate host before it matures enough to settle in humans as its final/definitive host

• In others parasite lives in human/no need for immediate host to complete its life cycle

CLASSIFICATION

• Phylum Nematohelminth includes class Nematode (roundworms); Trematode (flukes/Cestodes). Tape worm belong to phylum Platyhelminthes

• Nematodes may be completely parasitic (eg, Ascaris spends life in human intestine); others free living in soil/water like Ancylostoma, Nectar, Strongyloides, larva of which penetrate human skin/ultimately reach intestine, develop into adults; larvae of other species (not those of humans) do not reach intestine but produce local irritation as in creeping eruptions

• Parasites that produce cutaneous lesions listed in table

Disease	Agent
Ascariasis	*Ascaris lumbricoides*
Enterobiasis	*Enterobius vermicularis*
Ancylostomiasis (hookworm disease)	*Nectar americanus*
Ancylostoma duodenale	
Strongyloidiasis (larva currens)	*Strongyloides stercoralis*
Trichinosis	*Tricenella spiralis*
Gnathostomiasis	*Gnathostoma spinigerum*
	Gnathostoma hispedium
	Gnathostoma nipponicum
Angiostrongyloides	*Angiostrongylus cantonensis*
Dracunculosis	*Dracunculus medinensis*
Fiiriasis	
Onchocerciasis	*Onchocerca volvulus*
Loaisis	Loa loa
Lymphatic filiriasis	*Wuchereria bancrofti*
	Brugia malayi
	Brugia timori
Cutaneous larva migrans	*Ancylostoma brasiliensis, A. caninum, A. ceylonicum, Uncinaria stenocephala and Bubostomum phlebotomum*
Visceral larva migrans	*Toxicara canis, T. cati, T. leonensis*
Streptocerciasis	*Mausorella streptocerca*

RUBELLA

STANLEY A. PLOTKIN

BACKGROUND

- Previously common infection in school-age children/young adults; now relatively rare because of vaccination
- Agent an RNA-containing enveloped virus
- *Transmission by respiratory droplets:* nasopharynx quite susceptible to viral implantation
- Incubation period 14–21 d, w/16 d most common; in unvaccinated populations, seasonal peak of disease in spring
- Major factor in pathogenesis sustained viremia that starts ~1 wk before onset of rash/ends at ~ time of rash; viremia leads to complications of acquired disease
- If pt pregnant, virus may infect placenta/fetus

CLINICAL MANIFESTATIONS: ACQUIRED

- Silent period ~1 wk
- Lymphadenopathy (often occipital) in week 2; may persist for wks
- Maculopapular rash in wk 3, first on face/neck, descending rapidly to involve entire body; many infections inapparent
- Rash fades in 1–3 d
- Fever (usually low grade), conjunctivitis/malaise common

COMPLICATIONS OF ACQUIRED INFECTION

- *Arthralgia/arthritis:* vastly more common in adults (incidence may be 30%); development of chronic arthritis not proven
- *Encephalitis:* 1/6,000 cases; chronic progressive rubella panencephalitis rare
- *Thrombocytopenia:* ↓ platelets common; symptoms in ~1/3,000 cases

CONGENITAL RUBELLA SYNDROME

- Result of fetal infection, almost always during first 16 wks of gestation
- Chronic infection involves many organs but does not always kill fetus
- When virologic confirmation of rubella positive, >50% of fetuses exposed during first 10 wks of pregnancy damaged; risk falls rapidly during next 6 wks/generally absent thereafter, except for mild deafness
- At birth/mos thereafter, infant may still excrete rubella virus, should be isolated until culture negative
- Characteristic clinical signs in table. Triad of ocular, cardiac, aural disease pathognomonic, typically associated cataracts, patent ductus arteriosus or peripheral pulmonic stenosis, central deafness; chorinoretinitis/metaphyseal rarefactions helpful in clinical Dx

Prominent clinical findings in congenital Rubella Syndrome

General	CNS	Ocular	Cardiac	Aural	Bone	Pulmonary	Blood, RE System	Late
• Intrauterine growth retardation	• Encephalitis • Microcephaly • Mental retardation • Autism	• Retinitis • Cataracts • Microphthalmia • Glaucoma	• Patent ductus arteriosus • Peripheral pulmonic artery stenosis	• Cochlear deafness • Central auditory imperception	• Metaphyseal rarefactions	• Interstitial pneumonitis	• Hepatosplenomegaly • Thrombocytopenic purpura	• Diabetes • Hypothyroidism

LABORATORY DIAGNOSIS

- Acquired disease:
  - rise in IgG antibodies (acute/convalescent)
  - presence of IgM antibodies
  - isolation of virus (not usually done)
- Congenital disease:
  - presence of IgM antibodies
  - isolation or PCR of virus from nasopharynx/urine
  - persistence of IgG antibodies longer than expected from passive transplacental transfer
- Clinical laboratory findings:
  - leukopenia/thrombocytopenia common during acute disease, otherwise not helpful

DIFFERENTIAL DIAGNOSIS

- *Acquired infection:* large number of infections (eg, enteroviruses, parvovirus B19)

mimic rubella; Dx important, as in pregnancy, laboratory confirmation should be sought
- *Congenital infection:* above abnormalities frequently permit clinical Dx/laboratory confirmation should always be sought for prognostic/public health reasons; cytomegalovirus/toxoplasmosis infections may be confused

TREATMENT

- No antiviral for rubella virus available

PREVENTION

- *Immune serum globulins:* no hyperimmune globulin now available; ordinary IgG given in enormous volume (20–30 ml to pregnant woman)/effect doubtful; rash may be avoided, but fetal infection not always prevented
- *Vaccination:* live attenuated virus (strain RA 27/3) used both in infants/adults:

  - 1st dose of rubella vaccine given at 12–15 mos (part of MMR); 2nd recommended 6–12 yrs (also as MMR)
  - universal vaccination of children has led to virtual disappearance of rubella/CRS in US
  - adults in certain categories may also be vaccinated (see table). Vaccination of pregnant women not recommended (although vaccine virus not teratogenic)
  - vaccine induces long-lasting antibodies/protection, sharply ↓ risk of fetal infection
  - adverse reactions to vaccine: mild rash, fever, arthralgia/arthritis; uncommon in childhood, higher in adult women (25%)

WHEN TO REFER/REPORT

- All cases must be reported to public health authorities
- Infants w/CRS require referral to ophthalmologists, cardiologists, audiologists, other specialists according to clinical manifestations

Indications and contraindications for Rubella Vaccination

Indications

Children ≥12 mos (w/measles and mumps vaccines [as MMR]) in 2 dose schedule

Susceptible individuals in the following groups:
  Prepubertal girls, boys
  Adults, esp premarital or postpartum women
  College students
  Child-care personnel
  Health-care personnel
  Military personnel

Contraindications

Pregnancy
Immunodeficiency or immunocompromised condition
Recipient of IG or blood in past 3 mos

BACKGROUND

- W/routine immunization, rate of measles infection fell to 0.6 cases/100,000 in 1983. However, 1989–1991, marked ↑ in measles in children <5 yrs of age w/55,622 measles cases reported, 125 deaths. Reason for resurgence was low vaccination coverage, esp in urban areas
- After 1° inoculation of epithelium of nose or conjunctivae via airborne infectious droplets, measles virus replicates 2–3 d after which viremia occurs. Reticuloendothelial system infected. Second wave of viremia occurs 3–4 d later

CLINICAL MANIFESTATIONS

- Incubation period 8–12 d from exposure to onset of symptoms, 14 d to rash
- Prodrome lasts 2–4 d (range 1–7); notable for fever, malaise, conjunctivitis w/photophobia, cough, coryza (runny nose)
- Koplik spots (white spots on erythematous base on buccal mucosa) appear 1–2 d prior to onset of rash, are pathognomonic
- Macular-papular rash appears first at nape of neck, then progresses to face, next to neck and trunk, last to extremities, hands and feet, over 3 d period. May become confluent
- By day 4–5, rash begins to clear, leaving brownish discoloration, fine scaling
- Fever always present at time of prodrome and rash, but resolves usually by day 4–5 of rash
- Pharyngitis, cervical lymphadenopathy, splenomegaly may be noted on exam in uncomplicated course of illness

LABORATORY FEATURES

- Because measles relatively rare infection, important to confirm Dx in what may be beginning of outbreak
- Virus can be cultured, detected w/rapid immunofluorescence test from nasal secretions. Isolation/detection of virus best within 24 hrs of rash
- Measles-specific IgM titers confirm acute infection but do not appear until 5 d after rash. Specific IgG ↑ documented w/acute and convalescent titers drawn 7–10 d apart

DIFFERENTIAL DIAGNOSIS

- RMSF
- Erhlichiosis
- Steven-Johnson syndrome
- Kawasaki disease
- Viral exanthem

TREATMENT

- No specific antiviral Tx for measles. Anecdotal reports of IV or aerosolized ribavirin used in critically ill or immunocompromised pts w/measles; treatment not approved by FDA
- Vitamin A Tx should be considered for children 6 mos–2 yrs of age who are hospitalized/are recent immigrants from areas of high mortality from measles

Vitamin A therapy for children hospitalized with Measles

Age	Vitamin A Dosage	
6 mos–1 yr	100,000 IU*	Repeat in 24 hrs
>1 yr	200,000 IU*	Repeat in 24 hrs+

*Water-miscible vitamin A, concentration 50,000 IU/ml.
+Third dose should be given at 4 wks for children w/ophthalmologic evidence of vitamin A deficiency

COMPLICATIONS

- In 1989–90 outbreak, 23% of pts had complication of measles infection including:

Hospitalization	20%	
Diarrhea	9%	
Otitis media	7%	
Pneumonia	6%	Pneumonia, either viral or 2° bacterial, most common cause of death
Seizures	0.6%	
Encephalitis	0.1%	Encephalitis occurred on average 6 d *after* rash w/symptoms of meningitis, mental status changes
Death	0.1%	

- Subacute sclerosing panencephalitis occurs 1/100,000 children w/naturally occurring measles. Mean incubation period 10 yrs. Symptoms include progressive encephalopathy w/seizures

PREVENTION

- Routine vaccination at 12–15 mos of age (combined vaccine against measles, mumps, rubella [MMR]) w/second dose at 4–6 yrs of age
- During outbreaks of measles, susceptible household, day-care center contacts should be vaccinated beginning 6 mos of age
- Infection may be prevented after exposure:
  – w/immunoglobulin, 0.25 ml/kg
  – IM if given within 6 d of exposure or w/vaccine if given within 3 d of exposure
- Infection control measures for hospitalized children should include placement in negative pressure isolation room until 5 d after rash has appeared
- Immunocompromised pts require isolation for length of illness

WHEN TO REFER

- Children w/measles should be followed closely (by phone) if possible, stressing fluid intake, watching for signs of respiratory distress
- *Report all suspected measles cases to the Health Department*

SALMONELLA AND SALMONELLA TYPHI

KAREN L. KOTLOFF

EPIDEMIOLOGY IN US

	Nontyphoidal *Salmonella*	*Salmonella typhi*
Major serotypes	*S. enteritidis, typhimurium*	S. typhi, paratyphi
Reported cases	50,000/y	<500/y
Reservoirs	Domestic/wild animals	Humans
	Pets (eg, turtles, chicks, cats, dogs)	
	Humans	
Transmission	Food from infected animals (eg, poultry, red meat); grade A shell eggs (intact, disinfected) implicated in >80% of outbreaks	Food/water contaminated by human feces/urine; common vehicles are raw fruits/vegetables, shellfish, milk products
	Contaminated food/water	
	Fecal–oral contact	
	Contaminated medical equipment/drug	
Peak age	<5, >70 yrs; peak 0–3 mos	5–19 yrs
Incubation	6 hrs–10 d; usually 6–48 hrs	3 d–3 mos; usually 1–3 wks
Risk factors	Age <3 mos	Travel to endemic area
	Hemolytic anemia	Laboratory exposure
	Malignancy	Contact w/carrier
	Immunodeficiency	
	GI pathology (ulcerative colitis, achlorhydria, antacid Tx, rapid gastric emptying (neonates, after gastrectomy/gastroenterostomy)	
	Recent broad-spectrum antibiotic Tx	

CLINICAL MANIFESTATIONS

Syndrome	Manifestations
Simple enterocolitis	*Onset:* usually abrupt
	Nausea, vomiting, abdominal cramps, fever (70%), headache, watery/dysenteric diarrhea, often contains blood, mucus, WBC
	Recovery: 1 wk; diarrhea occasionally persistent
	Bacteremia in 5–45% of infants <3 mos (infants w/, w/o bacteremia generally cannot be distinguished clinically)
Extraintestinal infection	Sepsis and/or focal infection (eg, meningitis, osteomyelitis, pneumonia)
	Most common in high-risk pts. Seeds sites w/anatomic abnormality (eg, tumor, polycystic kidney). Prolonged diarrhea, weight loss, persistent/recurrent bacteremia, disseminated infection seen in HIV-infected pts. Most common cause of osteomyelitis in sickle-cell anemia
Enteric (typhoid) fever	Classically associated w/*S. typhi;* occasionally other serotypes
	Symptoms: headache, malaise, anorexia, constipation (early) diarrhea (wk 2), abdominal discomfort, cough
	Signs: fever, relative bradycardia, abdominal tenderness, rose spots, hepatosplenomegaly, mental status changes. Sustained/intermittent bacteremia

LABORATORY FEATURES

- Nontyphoidal *Salmonella:*
  - Dx established by culture/sensitivity of following:
    - stool (preferred)/rectal swab (positive for ~5 wks; 5% excrete >1 yr)
    - blood/material from foci of infection if indicated
- *S. typhi* (culture of multiple sites necessary):
  - Dx established by culture/sensitivity of following:
    - blood (40–50% positive)
    - urine (<10% positive)
    - stool (30–40% positive; found during first week through convalescence
    - rose spots (60–70% positive)
    - duodenal string capsule (50–60% positive)
    - bone marrow (80–90% positive after first week of illness)
  - serology (Widal test): some value in unvaccinated travelers from nonendemic areas/in children <10 yrs old from endemic area

DIFFERENTIAL DIAGNOSIS

- Nontyphoidal *Salmonella:*
  - infectious enterocolitis: *Shigella, Campylobacter, Yersinia,* enterohemorrhagic/enteroinvasive *Escherichia coli,* amebiasis, *Clostridium difficile* toxin
  - Hirschsprung disease-associated enterocolitis
  - necrotizing enterocolitis
  - rectal fissure
  - allergic proctocolitis
  - ischemic bowel from intussusception, incarcerated hernia, midgut volvulus
  - inflammatory bowel disease
  - Meckel diverticulum
  - colonic polyp
- Typhoid fever:
  - infectious mononucleosis
  - disseminated histoplasmosis
  - ehrlichiosis
  - brucellosis
  - tularemia
  - plague
  - typhus

PREVENTION

- Avoid consuming raw eggs/food containing raw eggs (including cake batter)
- Thoroughly cook eggs/other foods of animal origin
- Sanitize hands, utensils, surfaces after contact w/raw/partially cooked food of animal origin
- Avoid high-risk pets
- Hand washing to prevent fecal–oral/person-to-person transmission via food
- Exclude fecal excreters from occupational food handling/child care
- Exclude infected children from day care if symptomatic/if adequate hygiene cannot be ensured
- Typhoid fever vaccines:
  - indications in children:
    - travel to endemic area
    - intimate contact w/chronic carrier

Vaccine	Age	Route	Adverse Reactions
Ty21a (Vivotif Berna)	>6 yrs	PO	Rare: GI upset, rash
Vi polysaccharide (Typhim Vi)	≥2 yrs	IM	Local reaction (14%), fever (3%)
Heat-phenol-inactivated	≥6 mos	SubQ	Severe local reaction (30%), fever, headache

TREATMENT

- Antibiotics *not* indicated to treat asymptomatic carriage/simple enterocolitis in normal host
- *Indications for antibiotics:* all children w/typhoid fever, children w/nontyphoidal salmonellosis who have any of following:
  - age <3 mos
  - conditions that predispose to disseminated infection: hemolytic anemia, malignancy, immunodeficiency, chronic colitis
  - "ill" or "toxic" appearance
  - documented bacteremia
  - extraintestinal focus of infection
- Regimens (choice should be guided by susceptibility data):
  - ampicillin, 200–300 mg/kg/d IV div q4–6h, max. 8 g/d (if proven susceptible)
  - amoxicillin, 40–100 mg/kg/d po div q8h (if proven susceptible)
  - trimethoprim (10 mg/kg/d) plus sulfamethoxazole (50 mg/kg/d) po or IV div q12h
  - chloramphenicol, 75 mg/kg/d po or 100 mg/kg/d IV div q6h, max. 3 g/d
  - cefotaxime, 200 mg/kg/d IV div q6h, max. 12 g/d
  - ceftriaxone, 100–150 mg/kg/d IM or IV div q12–24h, max. 4 g/d
- Duration and route:
  - bacteremia: 14 d
  - osteomyelitis: 4–6 wks
  - meningitis: 4 wks
  - typhoid fever: 2–3 wks; shorter courses (5 d) of ceftriaxone may be efficacious
  - HIV-infected pts w/bacteremia: consider chronic suppressive Tx w/oral agents such as ampicillin/amoxicillin
  - consider parenteral route for infants <3 mos/children at high risk for invasive infection if they have suspected, proven sepsis/for those appearing "ill" w/focal infection
  - eradication of chronic typhoid carriage: high-dose parenteral ampicillin, high-dose oral amoxicillin, or ciprofloxacin (in adults); if unsuccessful/cholelithiasis, cholecystitis present, cholescystectomy may eliminate carriage
- Pts w/typhoid fever who develop delirium, obtundation, stupor, coma, shock should receive dexamethasone, 3 mg/kg followed by 1 mg/kg q6h × 48 hrs
- Pts w/intestinal perforation should receive broad-spectrum antibiotics

COMPLICATIONS

- Nontyphoidal *Salmonella:*
  - persistent diarrhea
  - failure to thrive
  - chronic carriage (weeks to months)
  - meningitis associated w/high mortality (50%)/neurologic sequelae, even w/prolonged antibiotic Tx
  - disseminated infection may persist/recur
  - reactive arthritis follows 2% of *Salmonella* infections, usually in HLA-B27 positive adults
- Typhoid fever:
  - chronic carriers for >1 y (3–5%, most often elderly females)
  - relapse (5–20%)
  - intestinal hemorrhage/perforation (0.5–1%)
  - myocarditis
  - cerebral dysfunction, delirium, shock
  - focal infection (eg, meningitis, pneumonia)
  - death: case fatality rate <1% w/prompt antibiotic Tx

SCABIES

SONALI G. HANSON AND MOISE L. LEVY

BACKGROUND

- Caused by burrowing mite *Sarcoptes scabies*
- Transmitted by close personal contact
- Mite burrows into/lays eggs within stratum corneum of epidermis
- Dermatitis/pruritus due to cell-mediated immunity directed against mite
- Clinical manifestations may take days–weeks to evolve
- If reinfection occurs, clinical findings tend to develop in hours/days because pt already sensitized

CLINICAL MANIFESTATIONS

- Pruritus prominent/may take 4–6 wks to develop
- 1° lesions pruritic papules, vesicles, linear burrows, often w/2° changes
- Indurated, skin-colored, tan–brown, reddish scabetic nodules, have smooth surface, but w/scratching develop 2° changes of scale/crust
- Nodules most commonly seen on covered areas of body, such as upper trunk/proximal arms, esp near axillae; occasionally found on legs, esp about ankles
- In infants/young children, palms, soles, head, neck, face more typically involved
- In adults/older children lesions typically seen in finger webs, axillae, flexures of arms/wrists, belt line, areas around nipples, genitals, lower buttocks
- Burrows, rarely seen clinically, curvilinear red, gray, skin-colored tracts 1–2 mm wide; represent path along which mite has tunneled through epidermis
- *Crusted (Norwegian) scabies:* distinctive form characterized by extensive heavily crusted skin lesions, thick hyperkeratotic areas on scalp, elbows, knees, palms, soles, buttocks; highly contagious because of vast mite numbers in exfoliating scales

LABORATORY FEATURES

- Microscopic examination of mineral oil/potassium hydroxide (KOH) preparation of skin scraping w/#15 blade from end of intact burrow/papule, vesicle, area of inflammation found under nails, in finger webs, wrists, palms, soles, elbows, axillae reveals mite, its ova, feces
- *Technique for scraping:* apply mineral oil/H_2O to lesion to be scraped, to allow abraded skin to adhere to blade/be easily deposited on microscope slide; then hold blade edge perpendicular to skin surface until scale, vesicle, other evidence of inflammation removed along w/superficial epidermis
- Place drop of mineral oil/KOH on slide to cover specimen, cover w/cover slip
- Examine slide under low-power microscopic magnification, w/hand lens, handheld microscope

DIFFERENTIAL DIAGNOSIS

- Atopic, contact, irritant dermatitis
- Letterer-Siwe disease
- Seborrheic dermatitis
- Dermatitis herpetiformis
- Papular urticaria

TREATMENT

- Drug of choice is permethrin (5% cream: Elimite, 1% cream rinse: Nix)
- Thoroughly massage into skin from head to soles of feet, paying particular attention to intertrigenous areas; then remove by washing after 8–14 h
- Because in teenagers/adults scalp rarely infested, it need not be treated; in infants scalp, forehead, temples should be treated
- All members of household/other close contacts should be treated
- Because mites remain in epidermis for days–weeks after no longer viable, hyper-sensitivity/symptoms continue even after use of effective scabicide; topical corticosteroids/oral antihistamines used to relieve ongoing symptoms
- Nodules persist ≥6 mos in spite of eradication of viable mites, ova
- Permethrin can safely be repeated, if necessary, 2 wks after initial treatment
- Lindane no longer drug of choice because of reports of possible drug resistance/potential toxicity, esp in infants, young children; but still effective Tx

COMPLICATIONS

- Eczematous changes due to scratching, rubbing of involved areas/to topical therapeutic agents
- Urticaria
- Empiric corticosteroid treatment, either topical/systemic, may mask symptoms; frequently results in unusual clinical presentations, atypical distributions, unusual extents of involvement
- *2° infection:* consider treatment w/appropriate systemic antibiotics, since scabetic lesions may be favorable to growth of nephritogenic strains of streptococci; consider UAs in pts suspected of being secondarily infected
- Extensive involvement in infants may result in poor feeding/irritability

PREVENTION

- Undergarments/other items of clothing worn against skin, along w/bedding, towels, should be laundered in warm/hot H_2O, machine dried at highest feasible temperature to eradicate mites, to prevent reinfestation

WHEN TO REFER

- Referral is not usually necessary

SCALDED SKIN SYNDROME, STAPHYLOCOCCAL

STEVEN D. RESNICK

BACKGROUND

- Staphylococcal scalded skin syndrome (SSSS) encompasses spectrum mild–severe blistering skin disease
- Ranges in severity from localized bullous impetigo to syndrome w/widespread blistering/superficial denudation; latter, sometimes known as Ritter disease, clinical situation usually thought of in reference to SSSS
- Caused by toxigenic *Staphylococcus aureus,* usually belonging to phage group 2, producing epidermolytic toxins (ET) ET-A/ET-B
- Separate/distinct disorder from toxic epidermal necrolysis (TEN)
- Children <5 yrs of age, esp neonates, most commonly affected
- Older children/adults may also develop SSSS (renal insufficiency/immunodeficiency appear to explain susceptibility to toxins in these cases)
- Unlike most cases in young children, teenagers/adults w/SSSS often have positive blood cultures for toxigenic *S. aureus;* mortality can be significant in these age groups

CLINICAL MANIFESTATIONS

- Generalized form (Ritter disease):
  - early findings:
    - faint, orange-red macular exanthem
    - purulent conjunctivitis, otitis media, occult nasopharyngeal infection
    - cutaneous tenderness often apparent
    - periorificial/flexural accentuation may be observed
  - within 24–48 hrs:
    - rash progresses from scarlatiniform to blistering eruption, w/tissue paper–like wrinkling of epidermis followed by flaccid bullae in flexures/around body orifices
    - subsequent generalized involvement, but spares mucous membranes
    - as sheets of epidermis shed, moist "scalded" base revealed

  - despite worrisome appearance, eruption typically dries w/superficial desquamation; healing usually complete within 5–7 d
  - cultures obtained from intact bullae usually sterile, consistent w/hematogenous dissemination of toxin produced at distant focus of staphylococcal infection
  - healing phase characterized by extensive desquamation w/marked perioral crusting
- Localized forms:
  - bullous impetigo: localized manifestation of toxigenic staphylococcal skin infection, w/o hematogenous dissemination of toxin
  - bullous impetigo predominantly disease of children; adult cases also occur
  - early lesions: cloudy vesicles surrounded by red rim; shiny, superficial erosions w/minimal crusting more commonly seen
  - in contrast to generalized SSSS, both Gram stain/cultures of blisters reveal staphylococci; cutaneous tenderness absent
  - rarely, localized bullous impetigo can progress to generalized SSSS

LABORATORY FEATURES

- Skin biopsy generally demonstrates characteristic histopathology
- Routine biopsies/frozen sections can be utilized; latter offers rapid Dx
- All forms of SSSS characterized by intraepidermal cleavage w/splitting occurring beneath/within stratum granulosum (granular layer of epidermis)

DIFFERENTIAL DIAGNOSIS (GENERALIZED SSSS)

- Toxic epidermal necrolysis (TEN) (in contrast to SSSS, TEN represents disorder of full-thickness epidermal necrosis, most commonly caused by medications/graft vs. host disease)
- Scarlet fever (could be confused w/SSSS prior to blistering)

- Toxic shock syndrome (could be confused w/SSSS prior to blistering)

TREATMENT

- Eradication of staphylococci from foci of infection (generally requires IV penicillinase-resistant antistaphylococcal antibiotics for generalized SSSS)
- Usually, oral antibiotic Tx can be substituted within several days/sooner
- Antibiotics, supportive skin care, attention to fluid/electrolyte management in presence of disrupted barrier function usually ensures rapid recovery

COMPLICATIONS (GENERALIZED SSSS)

- Staphylococcal sepsis, pneumonia, cellulitis
- *Mortality:* 2–3%
- Teenagers/adults more likely to have staphylococcal bacteremia; prognosis poorer

PREVENTION

- Potential for epidemic disease in neonatal care units
- Identification of health care workers colonized/infected w/toxigenic *S. aureus* integral part of managing problem
- Control measures should be applied, including strict enforcement of chlorhexidine hand washing, oral antibiotic Tx for infected workers, application of mupirocin ointment to nares for eradication of *S. aureus* in persistent nasal carriers

WHEN TO REFER (GENERALIZED SSSS)

- Refer if you are unable to perform a skin biopsy/get rapid results
- Most cases managed w/o referral, but failure to distinguish/diagnose TEN can lead to loss of life; virtually all cases of TEN require ICU/burn unit management

SCALP SWELLING, POST-TRAUMATIC
David M. McKalip and Steven K. Gudeman

BACKGROUND

- Swelling of scalp after trauma may be seen in neonates or children <~2 yrs of age, depending on etiology
- Four major sources identified (see table)
- Each has distinct clinical features, underlying pathologies, management strategies (see table)

CLINICAL MANIFESTATIONS

- On palpation, cephalohematomas may give false impression of depressed skull fracture
- Pts presenting acutely w/scalp-associated hemorrhages should be evaluated for signs of head injury. If no source of trauma obvious, child abuse or coagulopathy should be suspected
- Scalp hematomas should not be aspirated because this may introduce infection, unlikely to remove all of hematoma. Most resolve over time (see table)

LABORATORY EVALUATION

- Radiologic evaluation recommended in pts presenting w/cephalohematomas, subgaleal hematomas to r/o underlying skull fractures (which could progress to "growing skull fracture")
- Following linear skull fracture, radiologic evaluation should occur 2–3 mos following injury to r/o growing skull fracture

WHEN TO REFER

- All pts w/blunt head injury or skull fracture should undergo neurologic evaluation preferably by specialist experienced in dealing w/head injury

	Caput succedaneum	Cephalohematoma	Subgaleal hemorrhage	Leptomeningeal cyst
Extent	Diffuse	Focal	Diffuse	Focal
Suture lines	Crossed	Respected	Crossed	Variable
Transillumination	↑	↓	↓	↑
Features	• Edematous scalp • Possible ecchymosis	• Initially soft, fluctuant, nonpulsatile • May harden if calcifies	• Soft, fluctuant • May be bilateral	• Soft • May be pulsatile • May transiently ↑ w/valsalva
Source	Scalp edema	Subperiosteal hemorrhage	Bleeding under Galea aponeurotica	Growing skull fracture
Using timing of injury	Perinatal	Perinatal, infants (<2 yrs of age)	Perinatal, infants (<2 yrs of age)	Infants
Length to resolution or appearance	Resolves over days	• May appear in hours or days • Resolves over 2–6 wks • May calcify, remain for months	Resolves over days–weeks	Appears after wks–yrs
Possible associated conditions	Normal (vertex vaginal delivery)	• Traumatic labor • Child abuse	• Coagulopathy (w/birth trauma) • Child abuse	• Hydrocephalus • Arachnoid cyst, progressive porencephaly • Child abuse
Possible sequelae	None	• Hyperbilirubinemia • Anemia • Hemorrhagic shock	• Hyperbilirubinemia • Anemia • Hemorrhagic shock	• Seizures • Developmental delay • Neurologic deficits
Treatment	Expectant	• Expectant • Rarely: surgery if disfiguring calcification fails to regress	Expectant	Surgical

BACKGROUND

- Common accompaniment of group A streptococcal infections–most frequently pharyngitis
- Can follow streptococcal pyoderma (impetigo), erysipelas, soft tissue infections
- Most common in school-age children (5–12 yrs); unusual in infants
- Caused by hypersensitivity to streptococcal pyrogenic exotoxins A, B, C (erythrogenic toxins)
- Incubation period 1–5 d, usually 2–3 d
- Usually mild illness but recently some cases severe

CLINICAL MANIFESTATIONS

- Streptococcal pharyngitis usually present
- *Rash:* red, finely papular (sandpaper); starts axilla, neck, groin, generalized in 24 hrs
- Hyperpigmented areas in deep skin creases (Pastia lines); strawberry tongue; circumoral pallor
- Generalized disquamation starts in ~1 wk; varies due to severity of illness

LABORATORY FEATURES

- Required: demonstration of group A streptococcus or antigen:
  – throat culture on sheep blood agar "gold standard"; 90 + % sensitive; less specific
  – rapid strep test on throat swab; almost 100% specific but less sensitive than throat culture
  – standard practice: do rapid strep test first; if positive no need for throat culture; if negative, do throat culture
  – if scarlet fever due to an infection other than pharyngitis, culture infection site
- Optional:
  – WBC count: usually ↑ in streptococcal pharyngitis; not helpful in most cases

  – determination of streptococcal antibody (usually ASO) in acute/convalescent blood samples; rise makes retrospective Dx

DIFFERENTIAL DIAGNOSIS

- Staphylococcal scalded skin syndrome
- Kawaski disease
- *Arcanobacterium hemolyticum* pharyngitis
- Drug reactions, serum sickness

TREATMENT

- Pencillin:
  – drug of choice except in pts w/penicillin allergy; no resistant organisms
  – adequate treatment of streptococcal pharyngitis prevents spread to contacts/acute rheumatic fever
  – oral penicillins:
    ○ penicillin V: 250 mg 2–3 ×/d in most children; adolescents, 500 mg 3×/d; take 10 full d
    ○ ampicillin/amoxicillin; satisfactory treatment but offers no microbiologic advantage
  – IM benzathine penicillin G: preferred in pts unlikely to complete 10 d course of oral Tx; 600,000 U IM for pts weighing ≤27 kg/1,200,000 U for heavier children; combination of 900,000 U benzathine penicillin G/300,000 U procaine penicillin G satisfactory for most children; less painful
- Other antimicrobial agents:
  – macrolides:
    ○ oral erythromycin × 10 d acceptable for pts allergic to penicillin
    ○ erythromycin estolate, 20–40 mg/kg/d in 2–4 doses; erythromycin ethyl succinate, 40 mg/kg/d in 2–4 doses; max dose erythromycin 1 g/day
  – oral cephalosporins:
    ○ 10-day course of oral, narrow-spectrum cephalosporin acceptable alternative

  – clindamycin:
    ○ 10-day course of oral clindamycin also acceptable alternative
- Unacceptable antimicrobial drugs for treatment:
  – tetracyclines, sulfonamides, trimethoprim-sulfamethoxazole

COMPLICATIONS

- Recurrence of disease; retreat only symptomatic relapses
- Suppurative complications such as otitis media, sinusitis, cervical adenitis
- Development of streptococcal toxic shock syndrome (STSS)
- Acute rheumatic fever/acute glomerulonephritis

PREVENTION

- Early treatment w/eradication of streptococcus prevents spread; pts considered noninfectious 24 hrs after treatment started
- Sulfomamides/penicillin effective prophylactic measures but infrequently used except in pts who have had rheumatic fever/in unusual circumstances such as in military populations

WHEN TO REFER

- Most pts managed w/o referral
- Pts w/streptococcal toxic shock syndrome should be hospitalized immediately/referred if adequate acute care cannot be assured
- Pts w/severe complications such as cellulitis/necrotizing fasciitis should be hospitalized immediately/referred if adequate acute care, surgical consultation not available

DENNIS C. HARPER

BACKGROUND

- Defined by variable array of underlying/associated problems
- Features include oppositional behaviors, aggression, violation of school rules
- 3–4× more common in males
- Often associated w/familial dysfunction
- Learning problems often associated
- Problems present in early years (<8 yrs of age); predict chronicity/more severe behavioral disorders (eg, delinquency)
- Familial patterns reflect genetic/environmental predispositions

CLINICAL MANIFESTATIONS

- Breaks school rules
- May steal, be truant
- Displays antisocial behaviors in multiple settings
- Learning disorder (LD)/developmental disorder may coexist
- Anger
- Coexisting impulsive, inattentive distractible behaviors often overlaps w/ADHD disorder

CLINICAL EVALUATION

- Parental Hx reveals inconsistent limit setting
- School reports acting-out/noncompliance
- Low self-esteem of child
- Demonstrates impulsive behavior
- Unaware of consequences of misbehaviors
- Similar behaviors in sibs
- Inappropriate family models
- Low frustration tolerance
- May share indicators associated w/ADHD/LD disorders
- Low average cognitive level more common
- Incidence of CNS insult/injury higher—comorbidity versus consequence?

DIFFERENTIAL DIAGNOSIS

- 1° ADHD
- 1° cognitive disorder (eg, mental retardation/major developmental disorders)
- 1°/comorbid adjustment disorder (eg, depression/psychosis)
- Organic/head injury/CNS
- Concurrent substance use/abuse
- Physical/sexual abuse

TREATMENT

- Family-based counseling w/practical, behaviorally based strategies
- Address school deficits/LD concerns
- Address social skills
- Treat associated disorders (eg, ADHD, LD)
- Coordinate community resources

WHEN TO REFER

- To coordinate school/home behaviorally based treatments
- For medication w/associated comorbid disorders (eg, ADHD, depression)
- For educational tutors for associated LD

BACKGROUND

- Children w/school avoidance repeatedly stay home from school/sent home from school for physical symptoms of emotional origin
- School avoidance most common cause of vague physical symptoms in school-aged children
- Terms *school refusal, school avoidance, school phobia* often used interchangeably
- 5% elementary school children/2% junior high school children have this disorder; peak age 5–10 yrs; F:M ratio 2:1
- Incidence ↓ because of ↑ need for mothers to work outside home, which requires most children to master their separation fears long before entering kindergarten

CLINICAL MANIFESTATIONS

- Child complains of recurrent vague, mysterious physical symptoms; most common symptoms: recurrent abdominal pains, headaches, vomiting, sore throats
- No physical cause found on careful evaluation, including physical examination/appropriate laboratory tests; discrepancy between how sick child sounds/how well child looks one hallmark of disorder
- Physical symptoms predominate in am/accentuated when family tries to send child to school; often symptoms clear by 10 am
- Child has missed ≥5 d of school because of these vague physical symptoms

LABORATORY FEATURES

- Each specific physical symptom determines which laboratory studies (if any) appropriate
- All test results normal

DIFFERENTIAL DIAGNOSIS

- School stressors (eg, new school, loss of school friend, teasing, bus/playground stress, academic stress, bathroom restrictions)
- Overresponse to minor illnesses
- Chronic physical disease w/poor adaptation
- Learning disability w/poor adaptation
- Truancy
- Panic reaction
- Substance abuse
- Depression
- Family dysfunction

TREATMENT

- Convince parents child in excellent physical health
- Convince parents child has school avoidance; explain school avoidance/stress can cause real physical symptoms; explain difference between physical symptoms/physical disease; explain pain real, even when it has emotional origin; point out everyone's body has certain physical way of responding to emotional stress
- Return child to full-time school attendance; insist on immediate return to school; being in school intrinsically therapeutic/ breaks vicious cycle that occurs when child gets out of step with schoolwork/friendships; parents need to be firm in am for several weeks; on any am "child has to stay home for illness," reassess child/send him, her to school if condition minor/new psychosomatic symptom
- Contact school staff; school staff can also help to make return to school as nontraumatic as possible (eg, canceling some make-up work)
- Treat contributory stressors; most school stressors can be dealt w/by parent, school principal, special education teacher, primary care clinician; correction of most of these factors alone may improve/not cure school attendance problems, because they only partially account for child's preference for staying home
- Provide follow-up visits; follow-up visits essential for monitoring attendance; children w/school avoidance should have return visits in ~1 wk, 1 mo, again ~2 wks into following school year

COMPLICATIONS

- None

WHEN TO REFER

- Severe emotional problem
- Pts unresponsive to pediatric counseling
- Most pts managed w/o referral to mental health services

SCLERODERMA

BACKGROUND

- Rare autoimmune disease of unknown etiology characterized by indurated skin
- Classification:
  - localized scleroderma: confined to skin/SubQ tissues:
    - morphea (plaque, guttate, keloidal)
    - generalized morphea
    - linear scleroderma (extremity/face, *en coup de sabre*)
  - systemic sclerosis (SSc):
    - diffuse cutaneous SSc
    - limited cutaneous SSc (CREST syndrome)
    - overlap syndrome (SSc w/features of dermatomyositis, systemic lupus erythematosus, rheumatoid arthritis)
- Localized scleroderma much more common in children than SSc (10:1)
- Localized scleroderma affects girls more frequently than boys (3–4:1)

CLINICAL MANIFESTATIONS

- Morphea characterized by one/more circumscribed patches of indurated skin w/violaceous/erythematous border during active phase
- Morphea more common on trunk than on extremities
- Linear scleroderma affects extremities more commonly than trunk
- Linear scleroderma characterized by hyperpigmentation/skin induration in band-like distribution
- *En coup de sabre:* linear scleroderma of face/scalp w/ivorylike depressed appearance
- Morphea/linear scleroderma may coexist
- SSc characterized by acrosclerosis w/or w/o truncal skin induration, Raynaud phenomenon, telangiectasia, esophageal dysmotility, pulmonary fibrosis, cardiac involvement, hypertension, scleroderma renal crisis

LABORATORY FEATURES

- *Antinuclear antibody (ANA):* present in 25–75% of children w/localized scleroderma/>90% of children w/SSc; nonspecific
- *Scleroderma-specific autoantibodies:* anticentromere antibody (ACA)/anti-topoisomerase 1 (Scl-70) detected less frequently in children w/SSc than in adults w/SSc
- *Anti-ss DNA antibodies:* seen in localized scleroderma/may correlate w/extensive skin disease, prolonged disease duration; nonspecific
- *Blood eosinophilia:* may be seen in localized scleroderma; correlates w/disease activity
- *Polyclonal ↑ of serum IgG and IgM:* occurs in nearly 50% of localized scleroderma cases w/widespread cutaneous involvement; may be useful marker of disease activity
- *Serum sIL-2R levels:* marker of active localized scleroderma; still investigational
- *Skin biopsy:* early lesions contain inflammatory cell infiltrate composed of lymphocytes, plasma cells, macrophages, eosinophils, mast cells; later lesions consist of dermal collagen deposits that entrap skin appendages; rarely indicated for Dx
- *Other:* ESR/RF may be abnormal but nonspecific; abnormal barium swallow, pulmonary function tests, chest radiographs, electrocardiogram, UA, nailfold capillary morphology in SSc

DIFFERENTIAL DIAGNOSIS

- Eosinophilic fasciitis
- Scleredema of Buschke
- Scleromyxedema
- Phenylketonuria (PKU)
- Graft-versus-host disease following bone marrow transplantation
- Lichen sclerosis et atrophicus
- Atrophoderma of Pasini and Pierini
- Acrodermatitis chronica atrophicans
- Diabetic cheiroarthropathy
- Porphyria cutanea tarda
- Syndromes of premature aging

TREATMENT

- *No proven effective treatment* for scleroderma
- *Localized scleroderma* may require only emollient, eg, Eucerin creme bid/topical steroid cream, eg, hydrocortisome valerate, 0.2% bid to facial lesions/fluocinomide, 0.05% bid to truncal, extremity lesions; topical steroids may cause hypopigmentation, telangiectasia, skin atrophy; observe carefully/discontinue topical steroids if any of these signs appear
- *Systemic sclerosis* complications treated symptomatically:
  - *vasodilators* for Raynaud phenomenon, eg, procardia, 5–10 mg tid; side effects: hypotension, peripheral edema, headache
  - *H₂ blockers* for gastroesophageal reflux, eg, ranitidine, 75–150 mg bid
  - *antihypertensives* (ACE inhibitor) for SSc renal crisis, eg, captopril, 6.25–25 mg tid
  - *corticosteroids,* eg, prednisone, 1 mg/kg/d/*immunosuppressive agents,* eg, cyclophosphamide, 1–2 mg/kg/d used to treat SSc interstitial lung disease, but experience lacking in children

COMPLICATIONS

- Rare complications of localized scleroderma include seizures, encephalitis, brain calcifications, uveitis
- Limb length discrepancy/flexion contracture may occur in linear scleroderma
- Very rarely localized scleroderma may progress to SSc
- SSc may be complicated by esophageal stricture, pulmonary insufficiency, cardiac arrhythmia, CHF, renal failure

PREVENTION OF COMPLICATIONS

- *Physical Tx* important to prevent joint contractures in cases where skin induration crosses joint
- Carefully *monitor BP*/aggressively treat any ↑ w/ACE inhibitor to prevent SSc renal crisis
- *Antireflux* precautions, eg, elevation of head of bed/H₂ blockers, to prevent esophageal stricture in SSc

WHEN TO REFER

- Refer all pts w/localized scleroderma to dermatologist to confirm Dx/rheumatologist to exclude SSc
- Refer all pts w/SSc to rheumatologist for complete evaluation, monitoring

BACKGROUND

- 5–10% of adolescents may have detectable spinal curvatures; progression to significant curvatures (>15°) only occur in <0.5%
- Although incidence of curvatures <20° has only slight female predominance, likelihood of further progression significantly > in females; F:M ratio of curves >30° 7:1
- Familial predisposition; children w/positive family Hx should be screened carefully; however, most cases have no family Hx
- May be 2° (see differential Dx); vast majority have no specific identifiable cause/classified as idiopathic
- Appears in early adolescence/may show significant progression during adolescent growth period
- Goal of treatment to maintain curvatures <40° at time of skeletal maturity; curves of lesser magnitude not likely to show further progression/cause symptoms; curves >45° likely to continue to show slow progression (1–2°/y)/cause symptoms in adult life
- No currently available lab test that predicts progression; children skeletally immature should be followed through puberty to assess for progression
- School screening most effective when done in grades 6–8 to detect progressive curves early
- Thoracic curves usually convex to right/lumbar curves usually convex to left; other patterns may be indicative of nonidiopathic etiology

CLINICAL MANIFESTATIONS

- Curvatures can be detected by physical examination/should be part of routine physical examination of child/adolescent; done by visually assessing uncovered back from shoulders to hips; following areas should be specifically noted:
  - shoulder height asymmetry: (mild shoulder asymmetry common)
  - scapular asymmetry w/prominence of right scapula
  - loss of thoracic kyphosis, ie, flattening of back in thoracic area
  - flank asymmetry: look at triangular space defined by arm/body contours at waist; asymmetry indicative of lumbar/thoraco-lumbar curve
  - deviation of spinous processes from midline may occur/may also be absent due to fact that as curvature develops, posterior spinous processes rotate toward midline; therefore, absence of deviation of spinous processes does *not* r/o significant curvature
  - most important test: forward bend test wherein pt bends at waist until chest horizontal/examiner looks at posterior thorax tangentially from both cranially as well as caudally noting asymmetry in height of

thorax on either side of midline; asymmetry most sensitive indicator of scoliosis
  - thoracic asymmetry may be quantitated w/a scoliometer, simple handheld device adapted from boating trim gauge; measures ATR (angle of trunk rotation), which is inclination of posterior thorax relative to horizontal w/pt in forward bend position; pts w/ATR >5° should be referred for x-ray study

LABORATORY FEATURES

- Pts w/significant asymmetry in chest/flanks, those w/scoliometer measurement >5° should have single, standing, P-A radiograph of entire spine from C7 to S1 (x rays taken P-A to ↓ breast radiation): full "scoliosis series" unnecessary for screening purposes
- Scoliosis measured by Cobb method, which measures angle described by line drawn along superior end plate of most tilted vertebra at cranial end of curve w/line drawn along inferior end plate of most tilted vertebra at inferior end of curve; care must be taken to ensure proper end vertebra chosen; most common source of error: choice of improper levels
- Atypical curves (rapidly progressive, painful, unusual patterns, those w/associated neurologic abnormalities, particularly asymmetric abdominal reflexes) may require MRI of entire spine to r/o tethered cord, diastometamyelia syrinx/other underlying problems

DIFFERENTIAL DIAGNOSIS

- Scoliosis may be 2° manifestation of wide variety of other 1° problems; curves w/no identifiable cause constitute bulk of adolescent scoliosis/classified as "idiopathic"; pts w/atypical curvatures should be carefully screened for other underlying causes
- Other causes of scoliosis include:
  - congenital: 2° to vertebral anomalies
  - neuromuscular: conditions such as Duchenne muscular dystrophy, Charcot-Marie-Tooth disease, cerebral palsy
  - osteoid osteoma/other irritative lesion
  - other: neurofibromatosis, Rett syndrome, Prader-Willi, dysautonomia, structural neurologic abnormalities such as tethered cord/diastometamyelia

TREATMENT

- Curvatures <20° Cobb angle in skeletally immature children should be followed w/clinical examination including scoliometer assessment until 1–2 yrs following menarche in girls/voice change in boys; curves >20° should be x-rayed at 6 mo intervals w/single standing P-A x ray; if no progression less frequent radiologic evaluation indicated; if progression more close follow-up needed

- Curvatures 25–45° should be treated by scoliosis specialist, usually w/custom-fitted brace until skeletal maturity; max. progression of curves occurs during adolescent growth period, if curves maintained at <40° progression unlikely following achievement of skeletal maturity; goal of bracing: prevention of progression, although in ~ one-third of cases some degree of correction may be achieved/maintained; bracing shown to significantly ↓ risk of curve progression/successful in >75% of pts
- Brace options include:
  - Milwaukee brace: brace w/plastic girdle/metallic superstructure extending to shoulder level, usually worn 16–23 hrs/d
  - TLSO: underarm brace custom molded/modular, custom fitted (Boston); worn 16–23 hrs/d
  - extended TLSO (Charleston bending brace): worn for sleep only
- Curvatures >45° require corrective surgery w/segmental instrumentation/fusion, such curves will continue to progress throughout adult life; curves <40° usually do not progress following skeletal maturity; curves >70°/those in premenarcheal females/skeletally immature males should also have anterior spinal discectomy/fusion to prevent further anterior spinal growth/↑ deformity
- No other modalities, including physical Tx, spinal manipulation, electrical stimulation, acupuncture, etc, have been shown in any scientific study to retard curve progression

COMPLICATIONS

- W/↑ magnitude, curvatures lead to severe cosmetic deformity/painful spinal osteoarthritis later in life; curvatures involving thoracic spine may restrict pulmonary function/reduce exercise tolerance; scoliosis alone rarely if ever causes neurologic dysfunction

PREVENTION

- Early detection of pts w/spinal curvatures/appropriate bracing can prevent development of more severe curvatures in many pts

WHEN TO REFER

- Pts w/<25° may be followed by 1° healthcare provider if competent/experienced in curve measurement
- Pts w/curves >25° who have not reached skeletal maturity should be referred to orthopedic surgeon who specializes in scoliosis management/should be fitted for brace by orthotist experienced in orthotic treatment of scoliosis pts

SEBORRHEIC DERMATITIS, INFANTILE

HOWARD B. PRIDE

BACKGROUND

- Name misnomer as sebum does not play role in pathogenesis
- Cause unknown, although occurrence in some siblings suggests genetic component
- Yeast *Pityrosporum ovale* may play role in some infants
- Appears in first several weeks of life/generally gone by 8–12 mos, even if untreated
- Some ↑ tendency toward later development of adult seborrheic dermatitis, atopic dermatitis, psoriasis

CLINICAL MANIFESTATIONS

- *Typically occurs in "seborrheic" areas:* scalp, face, postauricular region, eyebrows, flexures, trunk, diaper region
- Itch uncommon/if present, suggests Dx atopic dermatitis
- Thick, greasy, yellow scale (cradle cap) may encase entire scalp
- Hair loss should not be present
- Other areas have greasy, scaly, red–salmon colored, sharply marginated plaques

LABORATORY FEATURES

- Laboratory studies rarely needed/clinical Dx usually easily made
- Biopsy not diagnostic/may r/o entities in differential Dx

DIFFERENTIAL DIAGNOSIS

- Atopic dermatitis (two may coexist)
- Psoriasis
- Scabies
- *Candida* infection
- Tinea capitis
- Congenital syphilis
- Congenital HIV infection
- Acrodermatitis enteropathica/zinc deficiency
- Essential fatty acid deficiency (may be only manifestation of undiagnosed cystic fibrosis)
- Biotin deficiency
- Langerhans cell histiocytosis (histiocytosis X)
- Inherited ichthyosis

TREATMENT

- *Reassurance:* parents need to know not serious/will go away, even if left untreated; reinforce that rash not indication of poor parenting
- *Oils:* warm (not hot) mineral oil, P and S oil (mixture of liquid paraffin oil, sodium chloride, phenol), Aveno oil, other similar products may be applied to scalp several hours prior to tubbing; occlusion w/warm moist towel helpful
- *Shampoos:* should be done daily; any of large number of adult antiseborrheic shampoos may be used safely in infants if eye irritation avoided; tars (eg, T-gel, Tarsum), selenium sulfide (eg, Selsun), zinc pyrithrione (eg, Head and Shoulders), salicylic acid (eg, T-Sal, P and S shampoo) all effective; should be left on scalp long enough to loosen adherent scale
- *Low-potency steroids:* solution best for scalp (eg, fluocinolone acetonide .01%)/cream, ointment used for other areas (eg, hydrocortisone 1%, triamcinolone .025%); use 2–3 ×/d; stop when clear
- *Topical yeast Tx:* ketoconazole 2% cream/other azole antifungals to target *Pityrosporon ovale*/2° *Candida*
- *Antibiotics:* antistaphylococcal antibiotics such as erythromycin, cephalexin, dicloxacillin to treat 2° bacterial infection if present

COMPLICATIONS

- 2° bacterial/candidal infection; check culture w/or w/o KOH preparation

WHEN TO REFER

- Referral seldom necessary for typical cases
- Referral indicated when no response to usual treatments, Dx in doubt, child ill/has systemic findings along w/skin lesions/if biopsy needed

SEIZURES: ABSENCE (PETIT MAL)
FRITZ DREIFUSS AND MICHAEL B. TENNISON

BACKGROUND

• Absence seizures occur in a variety of epileptic syndromes that include childhood absence epilepsy (petit mal), juvenile absence epilepsy, juvenile myoclonic epilepsy. All represent 1° generalized epilepsies. In addition, seen as one of several seizure types in Lennox-Gastaut syndrome and in epilepsy w/myoclonic absence
• Childhood absence epilepsy occurs most frequently 5–15 yrs of age (peak 6–7 yrs); girls predominate. Strong genetic predisposition w/autosomal dominant trait. Gene locus not established
• Juvenile absence epilepsy predominates in teenage girls
• Juvenile myoclonic epilepsy occurs in adolescence in both sexes
• Epilepsy w/myoclonic absence has onset ~7 yrs; males predominate

CLINICAL MANIFESTATIONS

• Frequent seizures (in childhood absence epilepsy many times/d; in other syndromes much less frequently
• Onset sudden w/blank stare, cessation of ongoing activities, brief upward rotation of eyes
• May be mild jerking of eyelids or hands; if prolonged, may be automatisms
• Pupils dilate
• After few seconds, sudden return to consciousness, resumption of ongoing activities
• Patients frequently deny event has occurred

LABORATORY FEATURES

• EEG shows bilateral, synchronous symmetrical 3 cycles/sec spike waves on normal background activity. In Lennox-Gastaut syndrome background very abnormal and spike wave irregular and slow. In juvenile myoclonic epilepsy rhythm faster than 3 cycles/sec and short bursts of polyspike/wave activity seen
• Hyperventilation for 2–3 min may provoke a spell, especially if patient untreated

DIFFERENTIAL DIAGNOSIS

• Daydreaming in children
• Other seizure types characterized by staring such as complex partial seizures of temporal or frontal lobe origin
• Inattention as may occur in ADHD

TREATMENT

• *Principal drug options:* ethosuximide or valproic acid
• *Ethosuximide:* preparations include 250 mg capsules or liquid preparation 250 per 5 mL. Dose 15–40 mg/kg to achieve therapeutic blood level concentration 40–100 mcg/mL. Side effects may include GI disturbance, hiccups, headache, rarely skin rash, Stevens-Johnson syndrome or drug-induced lupus can occur. Hematologic complications rare, include neutropenia or aplastic anemia
• *Valproate (valproic acid, divalproex sodium):* preparations include sodium valproate 250 mg capsules, 250 mg per 5 mL syrup, Depakote 125, 250, 500 mg enteric-coated tablets, 125 mg sprinkles. Recommended dose 15–60 mg/kg to achieve blood levels of 50–120 mcg/ml. Side effects include GI disturbances, occasional weight gain, transient alopecia, transient ↑ liver enzymes, rarely hepatic failure, which occurs more in children <3 yrs and receiving polytherapy. Pancreatitis rare complication, as is reversible emotional disturbance
• Ethosuximide generally considered drug of choice where absence only seizure type and valproate where other seizure forms including generalized tonic-clonic seizures, myoclonic seizures, etc, complicate picture
• Monotherapy preferred and successful in 75% except where seizures complicate more serious encephalopathy as in Lennox-Gastaut syndrome, myoclonic absence, or where absence seizure manifestation of 2° bilateral synchrony from unrecognized focus

EVOLUTION

• Three main outcomes:
  – remission usually ~ time of puberty
  – rare persistence of absence seizures
  – tonic-clonic seizures during adolescence or later

WHEN TO REFER

• Most pts managed w/o referral
• EEG performed for initial diagnostic evaluation. Performed again if seizures do not remit with Tx and prior to consideration of discontinuation of medication, which should be by 12 yrs of age or when pt has been seizure free for 2–4 yr
• Imaging studies not often necessary in this form of seizure unless indications of focality
• If seizures do not respond favorably, further diagnostic evaluation, drug trials indicated

SEIZURES, COMPLEX PARTIAL (PSYCHOMOTOR, LIMBIC)

COLIN ROBERTS AND
AMY R. BROOKS-KAYAL

BACKGROUND

- Involuntary paroxysm of behavior, motor activity, sensation, autonomic function arising from abnormal focal brain activity
- Consciousness may be preserved (simple partial)/impaired (complex partial)
- May secondarily generalize, resulting in whole body tonic-clonic movements
- Usually brief (<1 min)/self-limited; may become prolonged/continuous (status epilepticus)
- 4–6% of all children have ≥1 seizure <age 16 (>50% will be partial in onset)
- *Risk factors:* previous seizure (febrile/afebrile), recent withdrawal of anticonvulsant Tx, CNS neoplasm, neurodegenerative disease, Hx remote CNS insult (stroke, hemorrhage, head trauma, meningitis), family Hx seizures

CLINICAL MANIFESTATIONS

- May begin w/aura (unusual smell/abdominal discomfort)
- Arrest of normal activity signals onset of impaired consciousness in complex partial seizure
- Ictal features may include:
  - *motor* automatisms, focal tonic/tonic-clonic movements
  - *vocalizations*
  - *sensory* disturbances, paresthesias, pain, visual disturbances, hallucinations
  - *affective* disturbance
- 2° generalization may be rapid, obscure partial features of onset
- Commonly followed by period of postictal confusion/somnolence
- Hx: previous seizure/CNS abnormality; preceding illness/neurologic disturbance (headaches, weakness, lethargy, emesis); recent head trauma, ingestion, alteration of medications (including anticonvulsants); birth, developmental, family Hx for risk factors
- Physical findings:
  - evidence of *systemic/CNS infection:* meningismus
  - evidence of ↑ *intracranial pressure:* papilledema, bulging fontanelle, Cushing's triad of erratic respirations, ↓ HR, ↑ BP
  - evidence of *head trauma:* Battle's sign, raccoon eyes, CSF rhinorrhea, retinal hemorrhages
  - evidence of *neurocutaneous disorder* (café-au-lait spots, hypopigmented macules, port-wine hemangiomas)
  - Evidence of *focal neurologic dysfunction:* asymmetric pupils, tonic eye deviation, focal weakness

LABORATORY FEATURES/STUDIES

- Metabolic derangement (glucose, Na, K, Ca, Mg)
- Anticonvulsant levels (if applicable)
- Toxicology screen
- CSF:
  - glucose, protein, cytology, cultures, if child <2 yrs of age/suspect infection (may need CT/MRI prior to LP if evidence of ↑ ICP/focal lesion)
- CNS:
  - Imaging indicated in nearly all pts w/new onset partial seizures
  - CT: rapid for medically unstable pt
  - MRI: preferred due to better resolution
  - Pre-/postcontrast images should be obtained
- *EEG:* immediately for persistent convulsions/prolonged impairment of consciousness; indicated at soonest opportunity for all children w/new onset seizures, first atypical febrile seizure, those w/known epilepsy who have significant change in clinical status

DIFFERENTIAL DIAGNOSIS

- Idiopathic
- *Remote symptomatic:* perinatal asphyxia, Hx prior stroke, intracranial hemorrhage, head trauma, meningitis/encephalitis, AVM, cortical dysplasia
- *Acute symptomatic:* CNS infection, metabolic derangement, anoxia, head trauma, stroke/hemorrhage, intoxication, AED withdrawal
- Neurodegenerative disorder
- CNS neoplasm
- Neurocutaneous syndromes: tuberous sclerosis, Sturge-Weber, neurofibromatosis
- Nonepileptic event: syncope, night terrors, breath-holding spells, tics, shuddering spells, psychogenic

TREATMENT

- *None:* most w/single partial seizure do not require anticonvulsant Tx, esp if precipitating factor clear/transient; if significant risk of future seizures (eg, structural brain lesions, ≥2 unprovoked seizures, focally abnormal EEG/exam, prior epilepsy w/recurrence), consider medication
- Anticonvulsant Tx:

Starting Dose	Maintenance	Therapeutic Levels	Potential Side Effects
Carbamazepine 5–10 mg/kg/d div bid–tid	20–30 mg/kg/d (advance 5 mg/kg/wk)	8–12 mcg/dl	aplastic anemia, hepatotoxicity
Phenytoin 15–20 mg/kg load IV fosphenytoin or div oral doses	5–7 mg/kg/d div bid–tid infants require more	10–20 mcg/dl	hirsuitism, gum hypertrophy
Valproic acid 5–10 mg/kg/d div bid–tid	20–50 mg/kg/d (advance 5 mg/kg/wk)	50–120 mcg/dl	hepatotoxicity, alopecia, weight gain

- Agents currently available but not yet FDA approved for partial seizures in children include lamotrigine, topiramate, tiagabine, gabapentin

COMPLICATIONS

- Dependent on precipitating etiology (eg, tumor, CNS infection, neurodegenerative disease, etc)
- Persistent status epilepticus, whether partial/generalized, can result in permanent brain injury

WHEN TO REFER

- All pts should have EEGs/CNS imaging reviewed by qualified clinicians w/experience in pediatric neurologic disease
- Children w/abnormal neurologic exam, EEG, CNS imaging/recurrent unprovoked partial seizures should be evaluated by pediatric neurologist

MARY ANNE GUGGENHEIM

BACKGROUND

- Febrile seizures (FS) related to fever, not associated w/any specific illness, not associated w/either metabolic disturbance or 1° CNS infection; considered one of many developmentally determined seizure syndromes. Despite frequently repeated opinion that more likely to occur if rate of rise of child's fever rapid, actually more closely related to actual degree of temperature elevation and individual child's threshhold for FS (related to developmental state of brain)
- Occur in 2–4% of all children, generally 6 mos–5 yrs of age; peak incidence ~18 mos; FS can occur outside of these arbitrary age ranges
- Genetic predisposition w/positive family Hx in close relative in 25% of cases
- Dx implies child has not had prior nonfebrile seizure or identified brain disease

CLINICAL MANIFESTATIONS

- *Simple febrile seizures:* last <15 min, manifest generalized tonic-clonic activity
- *Complex febrile seizures:* may be focal, and/or last >15 min or be multiple within same illness; occur in ~25 % of FS

LABORATORY FEATURES

- No required or diagnostic laboratory abnormalities
- CBC may show leukocytosis, either from seizure itself or from underlying illness
- EEG done *during* actual seizure (rarely done) shows electrical pattern of seizure activity; EEG done *after* seizure may be normal, or slow, or epileptiform, but not helpful either for Dx or prognosis
- CSF if checked, normal; indications for doing lumbar puncture include young age (infants may not manifest physical signs of meningeal irritation), excessive and/or persistent lethargy, or any other suspicion of meningitis; always better to do normal LP than miss 1° CNS infection (roughly 1/1,000 children who present w/FS have an underlying 1° CNS infection
- Metabolic abnormalities may reflect underlying illness (low blood sugar, hyper- or hyponatremia, hypocalcemia); if such found, then not FS; seizure itself may cause *transient hyperglycemia*

DIFFERENTIAL DIAGNOSIS

- 1° CNS infection
- Toxin, esp those agents that may cause both fever and seizures (anticholinergics, theophylline, salicylates, amphetamines, cocaine)
- Metabolic disturbance (hypoglycemia, electrolyte imbalances, hypocalcemia)
- Underlying brain disease (neurodegenerative, tuberous sclerosis, vascular malformation, epilepsy, etc)

TREATMENT

- If seizure activity prolonged (>10 min), use IV antiepileptic drugs in this order to stop seizure:
  – lorezepam, 0.05–0.1 mg/kg
  – diazepam, 0.2–0.4 mg/kg
  – phenobarbital, 20 mg/kg
  – phenytoin, 20 mg/kg
- Combination of benzodiazepine, phenobarbital may cause respiratory depression; if using these drugs, be prepared to support respiration
- Antipyretic measures:
  – acetaminophen, 10–15 mg/kg per rectum or po q4–6h
  – remove clothes, cool environment
- Treat specific underlying infection, dehydration, respiratory distress, etc, on individual basis
- Reassure family, esp if child's first FS; most parents think child will either die or have permanent brain damage

COMPLICATIONS

- None (except for either iatrogenic or psychological); FS does not cause epilepsy, brain damage, neurologic deficits, mental retardation, or learning disorders

PREVENTION

- No indication for prophylaxis w/antiepileptic drugs, since FS benign, use of prophylactic drugs carries w/it risks for allergic or idiosyncratic drug reactions as well as financial burden of obtaining, monitoring medication
- Anticipatory advice for antipyretic measures during future febrile illnesses
- Education of family about FS crucial. They should understand FS benign, often inherited trait, child likely to "outgrow" FS by 4–5 yrs of age, if not sooner
- Recurrence risk ~35% over child's lifetime, ~25% over next 12 mos (thus ~60% have single FS)

WHEN TO REFER

- If child has neurologic deficits or developmental retardation apparent after recovery from seizure, further neurodiagnostic tests may be indicated. Usually more cost effective to have evaluation by specialist (pediatric neurologist) to determine which tests, if any, may be indicated (EEG, neuroimaging, neurometabolic, genetic) rather than start w/expensive battery of tests
- If parents seem unduly frightened or insist on prophylactic antiseizure medications, referral to specialist may help them better understand, deal w/concerns

SEIZURES, GENERALIZED, MYOCLONIC

SARIT RAVID AND JOSEPH MAYTAL

BACKGROUND

- Myoclonus is sudden, brief, involuntary, lightning-like movements of muscle/muscles unassociated w/obvious disturbance of consciousness
- Myoclonic jerks may be focal/generalized, may affect one or several groups of muscles. No common etiology, or common anatomic/physiologic features for all types of myoclonus
- May be totally normal phenomena such as hypnic jerks or sleep starts, but also associated w/severe insult to brain whether toxic metabolic, infectious, traumatic, degenerative. Myoclonus also reported in association w/lesions in spinal cord, brain stem, cerebellum, cortex
- Some types of myoclonus nonepileptic, classified as movement disorder such as tics, chorea, or tremors; other types epileptic phenomena
- Myoclonus termed epileptic when it occurs in combination w/cortical epileptiform discharges on EEG; in nonepileptic myoclonus EEG normal

CLINICAL MANIFESTATIONS

- In generalized myoclonic seizures, myoclonic jerk usually bilateral, massive or minor; consists of one or few muscle contractions
- Consciousness preserved during myoclonic episode, although level of awareness may ↓ slightly
- Myoclonus can be single or repetitive, rhythmic or arrhythmic, w/low or high amplitude
- Other types of seizures such as absences or generalized tonic-clonic seizures may be combined
- Clinical manifestations depend greatly on specific etiology or syndrome (see later)
- In epileptic myoclonus 2° to infectious etiologies, myoclonus part of acute illness (ie, viral encephalitis), 2° to subacute (ie, subacute sclerosing panencephalitis), or 2° to more slowly progressive encephalopathy (ie, Jakob-Creutzfeldt disease)
- Myoclonus 2° to hypoxic-ischemic injury may be very massive, involving many muscles
- In benign myoclonic epilepsies such as juvenile myoclonic epilepsy (JME) or benign myoclonic epilepsy of infancy, myoclonic seizures can be only clinical manifestation; pts respond well to antiepileptic drugs
- In progressive myoclonic epilepsies such as juvenile ceroid lipofuscinosis, Lafora disease, or myoclonic epilepsy w/ragged red fibers, severe developmental delay, deterio-

ration in cognitive functions associated w/myoclonic seizures
- Abdominal examination may be abnormal in opsoclonus-myoclonus syndrome (neuroblastoma), or in one of storage diseases such as Gaucher or Neimann-Pick
- In progressive myoclonic epilepsy 2° to lysosomal enzymes deficiencies such as Tay-Sachs or sialidosis, cherry red spots can be found on fundoscopic examination
- In generalized myoclonic epilepsies EEG shows diffuse bilateral synchronous symmetric discharges of high-amplitude polyspike or spike wave usually w/higher amplitude over fronto-central regions

DIFFERENTIAL DIAGNOSIS

- Infections:
  - subacute sclerosing panencephalitis (SSPE)
  - Jakob-Creutzfeldt disease
  - encephalitis
- *Metabolic:* uremia, hepatic failure
- Postanoxic
- *Toxins:* lead, bismuth, mercury, strychnine, etc
- Component of familial progressive neurologic disease:
  - Lafora disease
  - ceroid lipofuscinosis: juvenile or adult type
  - Unverricht-Lundborg syndrome
  - myoclonus epilepsy w/ragged red fibers
  - lysosomal storage diseases
  - mitochondrial disorders (MELAS)
- 1° generalized epileptic syndromes:
  - infantile spasms
  - benign myoclonic epilepsy in infancy
  - juvenile myoclonic epilepsy of Janz
- As a component of other seizure types:
  - absence w/clonic component
  - component of generalized tonic-clonic seizures
  - Lennox-Gastaut syndrome

LABORATORY FEATURES

- *Serum:* glucose, calcium, nitrogen, electrolytes, amino acids, lysosomal enzymes, to r/o metabolic disease, errors of metabolism, lysosomal enzyme defects
- Urine studies for toxic screen, including heavy metal screen if Hx intoxication suggested
- CSF for protein, glucose, cell count if infectious, inflammatory, or degenerative diseases suspected
- EEG should differ between epileptic and nonepileptic myoclonus. Special attention should be given to background activity, and

any slowing should raise question of progressive condition
- MRI of brain may show tumor, congenital brain malformation, or atrophy in degenerative disorders
- Biopsy of skin liver or muscle may be necessary if Lafora disease, ceroid lipofuscinosis, or mitochondrial disease suspected

TREATMENT

- Treatment of myoclonic seizures depends greatly on specific syndrome
- *Current drugs of choice:* valproic acid, benzodiazepines. Myoclonic seizures usually refractory to phenytoin, barbiturates, carbamazepine
- *Vaproic acid:* 75% of pts improve, usually w/no change in alertness/behavior. In addition, effective in controlling generalized tonic-clonic and absence seizures that may accompany
- *Clonazepam:* major problem side effects such as hypotonia, lethargy, behavioral changes. Some pts may develop tolerance w/seizure recurrence
- Ketogenic diet often helpful in controlling myoclonic seizures when medical treatment fails
- ACTH, steroids have been used primarily in infantile spasms, less frequently in other types of myoclonic seizures

COMPLICATIONS

- Long-term prognosis, response to treatment depend on specific etiology of myoclonic seizures. Excellent in benign myoclonic epilepsies (ie, juvenile myoclonic epilepsy), and poor in pts w/progressive myoclonic epilepsies (ie, Lafora disease, lysosomal enzyme deficiencies) or in pts w/2° etiology such as postanoxic. In the latter, seizures may be intractable, require multiple drug Tx

WHEN TO REFER

- All pts w/myoclonic seizures need to be referred for consultation w/neurologist for diagnostic workup, treatment. Genetic consultation may be needed
- Pts w/1° generalized myoclonic seizures who respond well to medications may continue care w/1° physician; more intractable cases need to be followed by neurologist
- If developmental delay suspected, child should be referred for early intervention Tx

SEIZURES, GENERALIZED TONIC-CLONIC (GRAND MAL)

FRITZ DREIFUSS AND MICHAEL B. TENNISON

BACKGROUND

• Generalized tonic-clonic seizures are either generalized from beginning or become generalized after focal onset (partial seizure becoming secondarily generalized). Important distinction from etiologic, subsequent management point of view. Generalized tonic-clonic seizures may begin w/tonic phase, which subsequently gives way to clonic contractions prior to cessation of seizure, or may begin w/clonic contractions then becoming tonic, then reverting to clonic, as seen in juvenile myoclonic epilepsy. Partial seizure becoming secondarily generalized has subjective or objective finding, signature of which depends on location prior to becoming generalized, although objective phenomena may become lost in amnesia associated w/generalized attack

• 1° or idiopathic generalized tonic-clonic seizures begin most often in childhood or adolescence. Partial seizures becoming secondarily generalized may present at any age, may occasionally be idiopathic, but more often symptomatic of underlying focal disturbance

• Early-onset generalized tonic-clonic seizures have strong genetic predisposition, no sex preference

CLINICAL MANIFESTATIONS

• Following account adapted from International League Against Epilepsy Classification of Epileptic Seizures: "Some pts experience vague ill-described warning, but majority lose consciousness w/o any premonitory symptoms. There is a sudden sharp tonic contraction of muscles; when this involves respiratory muscles there is stridor, cry or moan, and pt falls to ground in tonic state, occasionally injuring self in falling. Pt lies rigid; during this stage tonic contraction inhibits respiration and cyanosis may occur. Tongue may be bitten; urine may be passed involuntarily. Tonic state then gives way to clonic convulsive movements lasting for variable periods of time. During this stage small gusts of grunting respiration may occur between convulsive movements, but usually pt remains cyanotic and salvia may froth from mouth. At end of this stage, deep respiration occurs and all muscles relax, after which pt remains unconscious for variable period of time and often awakens feeling stiff and sore all over. Pt then frequently goes into deep sleep and upon awakening feels quite well, apart from soreness and frequent headache. Generalized tonic-clonic convulsions may occur in childhood and in adult life; not as frequent as absence seizures, but vary from 1×/d–1 q3/mos, occasionally to 1 every few years."

LABORATORY FEATURES

• EEG shows bilateral synchronous symmetrical 2–4 cycles/sec spike and wave or multiple spike and wave discharges. During seizure ictal phase obscured by muscle artifact; after seizure over flattening of EEG for variable period of time. In case of partial seizures secondarily generalized, focality may be electrographically evident at onset

DIFFERENTIAL DIAGNOSIS

• Generalized tonic-clonic seizure usually very evident; chief differential Dx between primarily and secondarily generalized episodes. Accompanying features may indicate syndrome responsible for generalized tonic-clonic seizure such as juvenile myoclonic epilepsy, epilepsy on awakening, febrile convulsions, progressive myoclonic epilepsy, etc

• Any aura other than a vague rising feeling implies secondary generalization from a focal onset.

TREATMENT

• Because a number of antiepileptic drugs are available for management of generalized tonic-clonic convulsions, choice of agent determined by other factors such as tendency to cognitive disruptions, cosmetic side effects, breadth of spectrum of antiepileptic activity, or cost of long-term treatments. Phenytoin, carbamazepine, or valproate all enter contest for drug of choice in any particular case. Any of these efficacious in secondarily generalized; valproate preferred for primarily generalized seizures

• Monotherapy usually successful

• Attention to underlying or precipitating factors, when known, important. Sleep deprivation, under certain circumstances, photic stimulation such as strobe lights, emotional stress or alcohol should be avoided. Attention to regularity of treatment necessary. Avoidance of driving for period of time prescribed by law, which varies in different states, should be observed

WHEN TO REFER

• If seizures persist despite maximally tolerated doses of two primary antiepileptic drugs, referral should be considered

SEIZURES, INFANTILE SPASMS
(MASSIVE SPASMS, EPILEPTIC SPASMS)

FRITZ DREIFUSS AND MICHAEL B. TENNISON

BACKGROUND

- Spasms symptom of variety of epilepsies occurring usually in first year of life, including idiopathic West syndrome, Ohtahara syndrome of early infantile epileptic encephalopathy, glycine encephalopathy, Aicardi syndrome, tuberous sclerosis, among others
- Condition usually occurs during first year of life; boys predominate 60% in idiopathic West syndrome; Aicardi syndrome involves only girls, characterized by severe retardation, cystic retinal degeneration, absence of corpus callosum

CLINICAL MANIFESTATIONS

- Condition characterized by frequent seizures of massive flexion (salaam attacks) or tonic extension (cheerleader seizures) occurring in *clusters,* usually near time of awakening several times/d. The recurrent clusters may last several minutes, the spasms 1–2 sec. In tuberous sclerosis, neuronal migration disorders may be focal or unilateral occurrence. Individual spasms may be associated w/cry, grimacing. Consciousness may be impaired

LABORATORY FEATURES

- EEG characterized by hypsarrhythmia, irregular high-voltage slow wave disorder intermixed w/diffuse asynchronous in both hemispheres. Ictal pattern frequently high-amplitude slow wave followed by diffuse fast rhythms or period of voltage decrement

flattening of EEG. Immediately after seizure hypsarrhythmic pattern returns. In tuberous sclerosis or cortical malformations pattern may be asymmetrical or even unilateral. Because of absent corpus callosum, in Aicardi syndrome hypsarrhythmic pattern may be quite asynchronous in two hemispheres

- In symptomatic West syndrome due to cortical dysgenesis or heterotopias PET scan may be required for Dx. Here abnormal area demonstrates cerebral hypometabolism. Major malformations (eg, lissencephaly or hemimegalencephaly) demonstrated by MRI

DIFFERENTIAL DIAGNOSIS

- Early-onset myoclonic epilepsies both benign and progressive
- Other paroxysmal spasms such as caused by gastroesophageal reflux (Sandifer syndrome), intestinal colic may be confused

TREATMENT

- *Principal drug option:* ACTH or prednisone administration; ACTH IM as ACTHAR gel, 30–60 U; prednisone, 1–2 mg/kg po. In either case pay close attention to BP, which may ↑; steroids contraindicated where active infection w/CMV present
- Benzodiazepines such as clonazepam, 0.05–0.2 mg/kg, or sodium valproate, 15–60 mg/kg, may be employed but w/less confidence of success in abolishing spasms. In valproate, transient ↑ liver enzymes, rarely

hepatic failure may occur in children who suffer from severe neurologic disturbances

- Although not currently approved in US, vigabatrin highly recommended elsewhere as emerging drug of choice, particularly where etiology tuberous sclerosis
- In cases of localized cerebral dysgenesis or in massive cases of hemimegaloencephaly, focal cortical excision or even hemispherectomy may result in favorable outcome, should be considered under appropriate circumstances

EVOLUTION

- Main outcomes include complete remission following treatment; most likely to occur w/idiopathic West syndrome, which accounts for ~≤25% pts presenting w/infantile spasms
- Evolution to Lennox-Gastaut syndrome frequent w/pts w/symptomatic West syndrome; significant mental retardation the rule, which accounts for largest proportion of pts
- Mortality 5–20% depending on etiology; may be considerably higher in pts w/early infantile epileptic encephalopathy

WHEN TO REFER

- This is catastrophic disorder; referral to specialized center indicated w/some urgency; evidence that early treatment may result in salvage of significant proportion of pts whose outlook favorable

SEIZURES, STATUS EPILEPTICUS

MICHAEL B. TENNISON AND FRITZ DREIFUSS

BACKGROUND

- *Definition:* A single seizure lasting greater than 30 min or serial seizures lasting 30 min without regaining consciousness between. In practice, any seizure lasting longer than 10 min should be approached as if it were status.
- Status may occur as first indication of epilepsy (60–80%) or occur in a patient already under treatment for seizures
- May indicate a serious cerebral disturbance such as head injury, drug intoxication, CNS infection
- 85% of status occurs in children <5 yr and 25% in those <1 yr
- Roughly ¼ in each category: acute encephalopathy (such as CNS infection), long-standing encephalopathy (e.g. Chronic CP), idiopathic febrile (~5% of all those with febrile seizures), afebrile idiopathic
- Etiology depends on age
  - Neonates—hypoxia/ischemia or metabolic
  - Infants—CNS infection or metabolic (especially hyponatremia)
  - Second year of life—idiopathic febrile status

CLINICAL MANIFESTATIONS

- Generally divided into convulsive (tonic-clonic) and noconvulsive (partial complex or petit mal) forms
- Nonconvulsive status may mimic a psychiatric state and stupor or coma
- Convulsive status requires most urgent intervention

LABORATORY EVALUATION

- Sodium, creatinine, calcium, glucose, CBC in everyone
- Antiepileptic drug levels if appropriate
- Imaging with CT or MRI in most
- LP if indicated (unknown etiology, fever, meningeal signs)
- EEG monitoring in some patients—especially nonconvulsive status or to confirm cessation of electrical status

TREATMENT

- First the ABCs, including place on side, start oxygen, and protect from harm such as falls or flailing against bed rails
- Cardiac and pulse oximetry monitoring
- Obtain IV access if possible and draw lab studies
- Check bedside blood sugar and administer glucose if needed (2cc/kg of D25)
- At time 0
  - Lorazepam 0.1 mg/kg up to 2–4 mg in adult-sized patient given IV as slow push over 3–5 min. Can be given IM or IO if IV access not available.
  - Fosphenytoin 18 phenytoin equivalents/kg in small volume of IV fluid given over 10 minutes
- At 20 min if seizures not controlled
  - Repeat lorazepam dose
- At 30 min if seizures not controlled
  - Arrange for intubation to control airway
  - Phenobarbital 20–30 mg/kg infused over 20–30 min
- At 60 min if seizures not controlled
  - Induce anesthesia with pentobarbital 10–20 mg/kg load followed by 1–3 mg/kg/h as continuous infusion (watch for hypotension)

PROGNOSIS

- Etiology most important factor in prognosis. Duration also important, with most morbidity and mortality occurring after 1 h
- Prolonged status may produce permanent neuronal death
- Stopping clinical seizures without suppressing electrical status (as seen on EEG) may still allow permanent sequelae

DIFFERENTIAL DIAGNOSIS

- Acute repetitive seizures (cluster seizures or serial seizures) crescendo type events, may result in status
- Nonconvulsive status may be confused w/psychiatric disorders
- Psychiatric disorders may present as nonepileptic status, may precipitate status in those w/adequate predisposition

WHEN TO REFER

- Most should have neurologic consultation unless seizures easily stopped and etiology clear

BACKGROUND

- Sepsis/septic shock most common cause of death in medical, surgical pediatric ICUs
- Incidence ↑ in last decade as result of improved, more prolonged survival rates from cancer, leukemias, severe traumas and burns, prematurity
- For children 1–4 yrs of age, sepsis 9th leading cause of death in US. In infants <1 yr of age, incidence of sepsis, its associated mortality higher, peaking in premature infants (mortality rates ~50%)

DEFINITIONS

- *Infection:* microbial phenomenon characterized by inflammatory response to presence of microorganisms or their invasion of normally sterile host tissues
- *Bacteremia:* presence of viable bacteria in blood
- *Systemic inflammatory response syndrome (SIRS):* systemic host response to variety of severe clinical insults (infection, trauma, burns, asphyxia, etc)
- *Sepsis:* SIRS plus infection: systemic host response to documented infection
- *Severe sepsis:* sepsis associated w/hypoperfusion or hypotension, which respond rapidly to adequate fluid resuscitation
- *Septic shock:* severe sepsis that persists despite vigorous fluid replacement, requires use of inotropic or vasopressor agents
- *Multiple organ dysfunction syndrome (MODS):* presence of altered organ function in acutely ill pt so severe that homeostasis cannot be maintained w/o intervention

CLINICAL MANIFESTATIONS

- Fever or hypothermia
- Persistent tachycardia (>2 SD above age normal)
- Persistent tachypnea (>2 SD above age normal)
- Irritability (inability to console pt), somnolence or lethargy
- Hypoperfusion (poor capillary refill, cold, clammy extremities, weak pulse, peripheral cyanosis, oliguria <0.5 mL/kg/h) or hypotension (BP <2 SD below age normal)
- *Other findings:* feeding difficulties, vomiting, abdominal distention, diarrhea, jaundice, hepatosplenomegaly, cutaneous manifestations (rash, petechiae, purpura, bullous lesions, cellulitis, ecthyma), meningeal signs (simultaneous meningitis)

LABORATORY FEATURES

- Leukocytosis (>15,000 cells/mm^3) or leukopenia (<4,000 cells/mm^3) or >10% band forms (>20–30% in neonates and young infants)
- ↑ *acute-phase reactants:* ESR >30 mm/h (>15–20 mm/h in neonates): usually takes 24–48 h to ↑ after sepsis onset; C-reactive protein (CRP) >20 mg/L: usually ↑ after 6–12 h of sepsis onset
- Positive cultures (blood, CSF, urine, normally sterile sites, abscesses, IV catheters)
- Hypoxemia, ↑ serum lactic acid, metabolic acidosis w/initial compensation by respiratory alkalosis (findings indicative of hypoperfusion)
- Prolongation of prothrombin, thromboplastin coagulation times, ↓ fibrinogen concentrations, presence of fibrin degradation products (indicative of disseminated intravascular coagulation)
- *Other findings:* anemia, thrombocytopenia, hyperglycemia, hypoglycemia, hyponatremia, hypocalcemia, ↑ concentrations of transaminases, urea nitrogen or creatinine

MANAGEMENT

- Antimicrobial Tx: drainage of abscesses and removal of infected foreign bodies should accompany adequate antimicrobial Tx:
  - 0–3 mos of age: ampicillin (150–300 mg/kg/d) + amikacin (15–30 mg/kg/d) or cefotaxime (150–200 mg/kg/d)
  - >3 mos–adolescence: ceftriaxone (75–100 mg/kg/d) or cefotaxime or cefuroxime (if meningitis has been excluded)
  - special situations:
    ○ addition of clindamycin or metronidazole if anaerobic etiology likely (abdominal source of infection)
    ○ addition of nafcillin (150 mg/kg/d) or oxacillin (200 mg/kg/d) if staphylococcal infection likely
    ○ replace vancomycin (40 mg/kg/d) for nafcillin/oxacillin if methicillin-resistant staphylococci likely (catheter-related infection)
    ○ addition of ceftazidime (150 mg/kg/d) if pseudomonas infection likely (hospital-acquired infection or immunosuppression); also consider use of amphotericin B
- Supportive Tx:
  - O$_2$ (some pts require mechanical ventilation to achieve >95% arterial O$_2$ saturation). Pts w/anemia may benefit w/transfusion of packed RBCs (10–15 mL/kg)
  - parenteral fluids: loading doses (20 mL/kg) isotonic crystalloid solutions (normal saline or Ringer lactate); maintenance doses (100–150 mL/kg/d) of D$_5$W/NS. Pts w/hypoalbuminemia or ↓ oncotic pressure may benefit w/use of colloid solutions (plasma, albumin, or dextran)
  - bicarbonate (0.3 × base deficit × weight in kg): to correct acidosis if pH <7.2
  - vasoactive/inotropic support: dopamine (1–20 μg/kg/min), dobutamine (1–20 μg/kg/min), norepinephrine/epinephrine (0.05–1.0 μg/kg/min), nitroprusside (0.05–8.0 μg/kg/min), amrinone (1–10 μg/kg/min)
  - steroids: efficacy still not established in septic children (if bacterial meningitis present, give dexamethasone, 0.4 mg/kg q12h × 2 d, the first dose administered 15–20 min before antibiotics)

WHEN TO REFER

- All infants, children w/sepsis should be managed in hospital, preferably in ICU. Before transferring, hemodynamic stabilization, O$_2$ Tx crucial. Good vascular (intraosseus if IV fails) access critical for adequate fluid replacement. Initial antimicrobial Tx can aggravate hemodynamic status, esp in some pts w/hypovolemia or hypoperfusion
- Pediatric pts w/bacteremia (w/o signs of sepsis) can be managed on outpt basis, provided they are followed closely

SHELDON L. KAPLAN

BACKGROUND

- Bacteria spread hematogenously to vascular synovium of joint space
- Bacteria may reach joint space in osteomyelitis by direct extension in young children because joint capsule of hip, shoulder extend past metaphysis of femur, humerus, respectively
- *Peak incidence:* children <3 yrs of age

MANIFESTATIONS

- Acute-onset fever; refusal to walk/limp
- Large joints (knee, hip, ankle) most common
- Swelling, warmth, erythema of joint w/↓ mobility
- Abduction, external rotation typical w/hip
- In neonate, systemic symptoms may be minimal
- In neonate, multiple joints, contiguous osteomyelitis common
- Small joints tend to be involved w/gonococcal infection

ETIOLOGY

Organism	Neonate	Months 2–36	>36
S. aureus	+++	+++	+++
S. pneumoniae	––	++	++
S. pyogenes	––	+	+
Group B streptococcus	+++	––	––
N. gonorrhoeae	+	––	+ (adolescent)
Candida sp.	++	––	––
H. influenzae (immunized)	––	––	––
(unimmunized)	––	+++	+
Salmonella (SSA)	––	++	++
Kingella kingae	––	++	––

LABORATORY FEATURES

- Blood cultures positive ~40% of cases
- Synovial fluid culture and Gram stain

	WBC count/mm³	%PMN	Fluid: blood glucose
Septic arthritis	>50,000	90%	↓↓↓ (30%)
JRA	<15–20,000	60%	normal to ↓ (75%)

- Vaginal or urethral culture, if appropriate
- *Plain radiograph:* soft tissue swelling, joint space widening, osteomyelitis
- Ultrasound of hip detects effusion more readily than plain radiographs
- Bone-joint scan may be helpful in unusual cases such as sacroiliitis

DIFFERENTIAL DIAGNOSIS

- *Nonbacterial infection:* virus, hepatitis, tuberculosis, fungi, Lyme disease
- JRA, other collagen vascular disease
- Acute rheumatic fever
- Inflammatory bowel disease
- Leukemia
- Toxic synovitis, psoas abscess, pelvic osteomyelitis when unable to bear weight
- Reactive arthritis (shigella, yersinia, salmonella; endocarditis)
- Trauma (hemarthrosis)
- Cellulitis

TREATMENT

Age	Agents	Duration
Neonate	nafcillin/vancomycin + aminoglycoside/cefotaxime	3 wks
Infant or child	nafcillin/oxacillin*; add cefotaxime/ceftriaxone if no Hib vaccine (cefuroxime)	3 wks for *S. aureus;* 2 wks for *H. influenzae* type B, *S. pneumoniae*
Adolescent w/presumed GC	ceftriaxone	7 d
Immunocompromised child	nafcillin/oxacillin + aminoglycoside or extended-spectrum cephalosporin	3 wks

*Criteria for oral Tx same as for osteomyelitis.

INDICATIONS FOR SURGERY

- Joint remains swollen, erythematous after repeat needle aspiration
- Remove foreign material 2° to penetrating injury
- Hips should be drained surgically
- In neonate surgical drainage of most joints indicated
- Arthroscopic lavage of knee or hip alternative to arthrotomy

COMPLICATIONS

- Young age <6–12 mos (esp neonate)
- Prolonged duration of symptoms prior to treatment
- Hip, shoulder infection (esp w/ *S. aureus*)
- *Sequelae:* cartilage damage, stiff joint w/poor mobility, abnormal bone growth if epiphysis involved, unstable joint, chronic dislocation

WHEN TO REFER

- Usually orthopedic surgeon w/pediatric experience consulted
- Unusual organism, antibiotic susceptibility, or site
- Underlying illness or condition
- Pt has allergy to beta-lactam antibiotic

BACKGROUND

- Clinical syndrome consisting of cutaneous eruption, arthralgia/arthritis, fever, lymphadenopathy
- *Most common causes at present:* antibiotics; recently esp cefaclor, but also penicillin, sulfa, others. Esp common after multiple exposures to antibiotics
- Originally described w/heterologous antiserum; currently rarely used except for transplantation, envenomations
- Infrequent causes include allergy injection Tx, bee stings, IVIG, during prodrome of infections, esp hepatitis B
- Serum sickness–like syndrome w/marked eosinophilia; atypically hepatic dysfunction may occur w/anticonvulsant Tx (phenytoin)
- Onset of symptoms typically 7–10 d after exposure to causative agents. Accelerated form may develop when presensitization to inciting agent has occurred
- Symptoms may persist 1–2 wks

PATHOGENESIS

- Circulating immune complexes in presence of mild antigen excess deposited in vascular endothelium. Complement activation results in inflammatory changes. IgE antibodies often participate, may ↑ deposition of immune complex, may cause some allergiclike symptoms

CLINICAL MANIFESTATIONS

- Malaise, fever may precede other symptoms by 1–2 d and occur in almost all cases
- Other findings include:
  - cutaneous eruption (may include erythema, urticaria, and/or morbilliform eruption)
  - of arthralgia/arthritis (pain often in excess of objective findings)
  - lymphadenopathy
  - GI symptoms
  - cephalgia
  - myalgia
  - dyspnea or wheezing
  - hoarseness or upper airway congestion

LABORATORY FEATURES

- Usually nonspecific, suggesting inflammatory process
- *Only pathognomonic finding:* presence of circulating plasma cells
- Other findings variable, but may include:
  - leukopenia/leukocytosis
  - ↑ ESR
  - eosinophilia
  - evidence of complement activation
  - immune complexes
  - presence of IgE antibody vs. inciting antigen
  - mild proteinuria

DIFFERENTIAL DIAGNOSIS

- Association of cutaneous findings, arthralgias w/fever may suggest Dx serum sickness in presence of:
  - Stevens-Johnson syndrome
  - Henoch-Schönlein purpura
  - Kawasaki disease
  - infection w/hepatitis B or C, CMV, EBV
  - lymphoma
  - Lyme disease
  - collagen vascular disease (eg, SLE) w/urticaria
  - rheumatic fever
  - leukocytoclastic vasculitis—urticaria syndrome
  - allergic vasculitides

TREATMENT

- If causative agent being administered at time serum-sickness syndrome, should be discontinued
- Tx empirical, directed primarily at alleviating symptoms
- NSAIDs (eg, ibuprofen, acetylsalicylic acid, etc) to relieve fever, myalgia, arthralgias/arthritis
- *Antihistamine Tx:* sedating agent (eg, hydroxyzine or diphenhydramine) may have advantage of alleviating some discomfort by adding sedation to antihistaminic activity. For milder symptoms, consider age-related use of nonsedating antihistamine such as cetirizine, fexofenadine, or loratadine. Ongoing antihistamine Tx thought to be more effective than as-needed use
- As significant morbidity infrequent, use of corticosteroid Tx should be guided on basis of symptom severity. When used, 1–2 mg/kg/d of prednisone or methylprednisolone div doses could be considered. Duration of Tx necessary to control symptoms has not been evaluated; can be determined by clinical response, but Tx probably should be continued for at least 7 d

PREVENTION

- Avoid subsequent administration of antibiotics or other drugs associated w/serum sickness. Because IgE antibodies usually participate in serum sickness reactions, possibility of anaphylacticlike response should be kept in mind. Whether or not pretreatment w/antihistamine and/or systemic steroids may preclude subsequent reactions unclear, but in few cases where this has been tested, results have been disappointing

WHEN TO REFER

- Failure to respond to treatment/duration >2–3 wks
- If diagnosis in doubt

SEX CHROMOSOME ABNORMALITIES
(OTHER THAN TURNER SYNDROME)

PETER A. LEE

BACKGROUND

- Discovered when phenotype includes problems of sexual differentiation, lack of pubertal development, in assessment for multiple congenital anomalies, as unexpected finding after chromosomal determinations (eg, prenatal karyotype)
- Loss/redundancy of either X or Y chromosome suggests gonadal dysgenesis/abnormalities of sexual differentiation
- Variety of somatic findings, shown/presumed to be related to specific gene mutations/deletions located on X/Y chromosome
- Phenotype does not predict karyotype (eg, phenotypic male w/karyotype of 46,XX)
- Once entire genome/its properties known phenotype/genotype should be predictable (crucial genes for sexual differentiation may be present/not detectable by karyotype)
- *Practical approach:* categorize pts by classically described syndromes to determine appropriate diagnostic/therapeutic measures

CLINICAL MANIFESTATIONS

Female Phenotype
- *47,XXX syndrome (may include 48,XXXX, 49,XXXX w/X mosaicism):* differs from Turner syndrome (may have abnormal mental development, normal physical growth, normal but delayed menarche, ovulation, pregnancy carries risk of children w/extra X, premature menopause)
- *46,XX ovarian dysgenesis:* normal karyotype w/bilateral streak gonads, no pubertal development, normal height, eunuchoid proportions
- *46,XY complete gonadal dysgenesis (may include Yp-deletions):* mild clitoromegaly, normal uterus/tubes but streak gonads, no male internal ducts, usually normal stature, Turner stigmata may be present, present w/delayed puberty/1° amenorrhea
- *45,X; 46,XY-mosaicism:* 25% have female phenotype/most have ambiguous genitalia

Male Phenotype
- *47,XXY (Klinefelter) also 48,XXXY, 49,XXXXY:* small testes, generally normal puberty, tall w/eunuchoid proportions, gynecomastia, may have impaired mental development
- *48,XXYY; 49,XXXYY syndromes:* similar to Klinefelter w/frequent antisocial behavior
- *47,XYY:* does not present w/clinical syndrome; possible association w/antisocial behavior
- *46,XY true hermaphrodistism:* (rarely external male differentiation) ovarian as well as testicular differentiation, internally both male and female w/internal ducts partially developed
- *45,X; 46,XY mosaicism:* most present w/ambiguous genitalia, some w/male phenotype/most cases identified prenatally male phenotype
- *46,XX sex reversal (also 45,X or 45,X marker Y):* features of Klinefelter syndrome, during puberty seminiferous tubule degeneration occurs, may have other congenital anomalies, Y chromosome deletions spare testicular-determining factor (TDF)/sex-determining region (SRy)

Ambiguous Phenotype
- *45,X; 46,XY mixed gonadal dysgenesis (also 45,X/47,XYY; 45,X/46,XY/47,XYY):* ambiguous genitalia, often asymmetric w/more scrotal-like development on side w/dysgenetic testis, w/streak gonad on other side, male ducts may be partially developed on former side, w/variable development of uterus/tubes; some have Turner stigmata
- *46,XY partial gonadal dysgenesis (dysgenetic male pseudohermaphroditism):* dysgenetic testes
- *46,XX sex reversal:* may present w/hypospadius
- *46,XX; 46,XY; 46,XY/47,XXY; 46,XY/47,XXY:* true hermaphroditism: have differentiated ovarian tissue w/follicles/testicular tissue w/seminiferous tubules; may involve ovotestis (may present w/male genitalia)
- *46,XY gonadal dysgenesis/multiple congenital anomalies—(WAGR [Wilms tumor, aniridia, gonadal dysgenesis, mental retardation] syndrome, camptomelic dwarfism)* – ambiguous genitalia, well-developed Mullerian ducts and testes, or complete gonadal dysgenesis

LABORATORY FEATURES

- Gonadotropins (LH/FSH): ↑ in infancy/pubertal age indicates gonadal failure
- *Estradiol:* low levels, w/high LH/FSH, in infancy/puberty indicative of ovarian failure
- *Testosterone:* useful assessment of testicular function in infancy/approaching puberty
- *Inhibin B/Müllerian-inhibiting hormone:* assess testicular development, not readily available
- *Specific DNA analyses:* based on clinical findings

DIFFERENTIAL DIAGNOSIS OF AMBIGUOUS GENITALIA

- Adrenal (adrenal hyperplasia in 46,XX)/embryonal tumor source of abnormal sex steroids
- Maternal androgen excess

TREATMENT

- Ambiguous genitalia cases require sex of rearing assessment/multidisciplinary approach
- Ongoing education of parents (pt when age appropriate) concerning medical, physical, social, psychological issues/multidisciplinary approach useful
- Age-appropriate hormonal Tx/surgical correction

COMPLICATIONS

- Risk of gonadal tumors when abnormal differentiation and Y chromosome; prophylactic gonadectomy may be indicated/considered

WHEN TO REFER

- Endocrine/genetic consultation indicated for all cases/surgical where indicated

BACKGROUND

- Sexual abuse of children common, rates ↑. Third national incidence study of child abuse (1993) showed 4.5/1,000. Best estimates: at least 20% women, 5–10% men sexually abused as children in US
- Children most vulnerable ages 7–13
- Most perpetrators of sexual abuse men, persons known to child. Risk factors for sexual abuse include nonbiologic father figure and/or drug or alcohol abuse in home, social isolation of family
- No social class spared nor at ↑ risk of child sexual abuse

EVALUATION

- In taking Hx, child should be interviewed alone, parents should be interviewed alone
- Child interview should be conducted in calm, nonjudgmental manner, include opportunity for rapport building, assessment of child's own names for genitalia/anus, credibility, open-ended questions geared to elicit spontaneous narrative statements, description of abuse, respect for resistant children, closure—including description of physical examination to follow
- Physical examination should be performed in presence of support person(s) child chooses; includes complete examination to normalize experience for child. Ade-

quate visualization of genitalia enhanced by good light source, relaxed, cooperative child. Child should not be held down or forced to be examined (consider return visit or sedation). Speculum, digital examination *not* indicated

CLINICAL MANIFESTATIONS

- Dx sexual abuse made on basis of assessment of behavioral, historical, physical manifestations

Behavioral,
may include none or several of following:

- Sexualized behavior including excessive masturbation, victimization of others, promiscuity
- Fear/anxiety/anger, may manifest as regression
- Somatic problems including abdominal or genitourinary complaints, eating/bowel/sleep disturbance
- Depression
- Poor school performance, truancy
- Use of illegal drugs/alcohol
- Withdrawal from friends/family, running away from home

Historical

- Child, family member, or concerned citizen may relate concerning behavior, physical findings, or disclosure
- Disclosure of abuse a process that often evolves over time. Sexually abused children may give no, partial, or full disclosure of experience
- Recanting some/all of disclosure common in sexually abused children
- Note as many of child's own words as possible. Attention to contextual details, idiosyncratic language used by child important (helps confirm veracity)
- Clear, consistent disclosure of abuse can be diagnostic, even in absence of other manifestations

Physical

- Findings indicative of prior trauma include:
  - marked diminution of hymenal tissue
  - hymenal notches, particularly in lower hymen
  - very enlarged hymenal opening
  - scarring—seen as changes in elasticity, color, or vasularity of genital or anal mucosa
  - abrasions, bruises, fissures
  - spontaneous anal dilation >2 cm, w/no stool in vault
- Findings concerning for possible STDs:
  - genital discharge
  - lesions consistent w/ulcers, warts, vesicles
  - history of genital-genital or oral-genital contact (including anus as genital here)
  - findings indicative of prior anal or genital trauma
- *Normal exam* consistent w/any type of sexual abuse

LABORATORY FEATURES

- If findings raise concern of possible STDs, obtain appropriate specimens (paying attention to incubation periods for different organisms) to assess infection from *Chlamydia trachomatis, Neisseria gonorrhea, Trichomonas vaginalis, Herpes simplex,* condyloma acuminata, HIV, syphilis
- Although immunofluorescent, DNA techniques available for chlamydia, gonorrhea, culture mandatory for forensic documentation, should be done prior to treatment
- Consider pregnancy test for all postmenarchal females

DIFFERENTIAL DIAGNOSIS

- Differential Dx dependent on clinical manifestations observed. For example, for vaginal discharge differential Dx: vaginal foreign body, bacterial infection of nonsexual origin, pinworms; for behavioral manifestations: multiple etiologies for psychosocial stress or trauma

TREATMENT

- Child, family should be counseled about findings, conclusions made about likelihood of sexual abuse, reassured (as possible) that child physically healthy or healing
- Usually, referral to mental health professional indicated to facilitate disclosure and/or initiate mental health Tx. Other resources, such as groups for parents, may be available in community
- Report suspicion of sexual abuse to state social service agency, after explaining to parents legal obligation to do so
- Help ensure safety of this child, other children by making/facilitating police report, social service report, and/or helping family think through protective measures

COMPLICATIONS

- Sequelae of sexual abuse can include those listed above, and other psychopathology including cognitive distortions such as guilt or self-blame; post-traumatic stress; interpersonal problems such as fear of intimacy or revictimization; self-injurious behavior such as suicide; borderline personality disorder; chronic psychoses; multiple personality disorder

PREVENTION

- Promising home visitation, school-based, community-based programs exist for prevention of abuse
- Sexual abuse prevention programs have been shown to improve knowledge, skills, but evaluation of efficacy for prevention, usefulness in assault situation still needed

WHEN TO REFER

- Most pts do not need referral for 1° evaluation. Timely referral should be made for the 1° evaluation if clinician does not have skills to carry out the medical evaluation, so multiple exams may be avoided
- Referral for colposcopic evaluation *not* usually helpful, if initial exam has been performed adequately
- Referral to mental health and social services usually indicated for treatment and 2° prevention (see above)

BACKGROUND

- Found at all ages
- Pure human pathogen spread by direct person-to-person contact, contaminated food
- Infectious dose small, hence highly contagious
- Causes 1° invasive colitis, proctitis
- Capable of producing small bowel watery diarrhea
- Occasionally bacteremic in small children, who may have atypical disease
- Of four species, *Shigella dysenteriae* (Shiga bacillus) produces systemic cytotoxin that causes prostration, encephalopathy
- Associated neurologic symptoms frequent
- Infection w/*S. dysenteriae* may cause hemolytic-uremic syndrome
- Ampicillin resistance common

CLINICAL MANIFESTATIONS

- Incubation period 12–48 h
- Abrupt onset of fever, toxicity, abdominal pain, followed by diarrhea
- Colitic stool (blood, mucus, frequent small volume) in >50% cases
- High-volume, watery diarrhea may occur alone or preceding colitis
- *Younger infants may have atypical disease:* less fever, less colitis, more dehydration, more bacteremia
- *Extraintestinal manifestations in 50% of severe infections:* seizures, lethargy, confusion, meningismus
- Hemolytic-uremic syndrome may complicate *S. dysenteriae* infection
- Bacteremia 4–12% of young children; mortality may be high
- Shigella causes bloody vaginitis in prepubertal females
- Reactive arthritis or Reiter syndrome seen in HLA B27 positive pts

LABORATORY FEATURES

- Stool w/fecal leukocytes, occult blood
- CBC w/normal total leukocyte count but excessive band forms
- *Recovery from stool culture difficult:* rapid inoculation, processing of specimen optimizes recovery (20% false negative stool cultures)
- Blood culture in young infants appropriate

DIFFERENTIAL DIAGNOSIS

- Other bacterial colitis (salmonella, *E. coli,* campylobacter, *C. difficile)*
- Amebic colitis
- Inflammatory bowel disease

TREATMENT

- *Fluid resuscitation:* po vs. IV
- Oral trimethoprim/sulfamethoxazole (10 mg/kg/d trimethoprim component div bid) first-line Tx
- Nalidixic acid (55 mg/kg/d div qid) or ciprofloxicin (20–30 mg/kg/d div bid) available for resistant strains
- Ceftriaxone (50 mg/kg/d single dose) alternative for resistance or severe disease
- Efficacy of oral cephalosporins unproven
- Duration Tx for uncomplicated infection 5 d
- Bacteremic disease or complex *S. dysenteriae* infection treated as long as clinical signs persist

COMPLICATIONS

- Seizures, other neurologic manifestations
- Hemolytic-uremic syndrome
- Leukemoid reaction
- Reactive arthritis, Reiter syndrome

WHEN TO REFER

- Ambulatory management usually sufficient
- Toxic children, those w/neurologic findings or suspected hemolytic-uremic syndrome should be referred to pediatric center

BACKGROUND

- Early Dx/treatment of organic causes important if child to reach full genetic potential
- *Concern about short stature usually voiced:* during infancy (when the child's growth pattern fails to maintain expected rate); when child enters preschool/kindergarten (size compared w/other children); at puberty (when delay in onset may cause child to fall behind peers)
- Rather than evaluating relative stature such as below 5th percentile, think in terms of growth failure

CLINICAL MANIFESTATIONS

- Is child significantly short? Minus 2 standard deviations (SD) equals the 2.5th percentile; minus 2.5 SD equals 0.5th percentile; likelihood of pathology ↑ if minus 2 SD criterion used
- Is height velocity (cm/yr) ↓, consistently <25th percentile? If so, child's height percentile will ↓
- Is child short in relation to parents' heights? Estimate of genetic target zone obtained by plotting both parents' height *percentile* on child's growth chart, then calculating midparental height: genetic target lies within ~10 cm of midparental height
- Is there evidence of intestinal malabsorption, nutritional deficiency, chronic infection, inflammatory bowel disease, psychosocial dwarfism?
- Is there family Hx of delayed puberty?
- Is there evidence of syndrome associated w/short stature (Turner syndrome, Noonan syndrome, pseudohypoparathyroidism)?
- Does child have normal body proportions? If not, consider a skeletal dysplasia

LABORATORY FEATURES

- Screen for nonendocrine causes (CBC, sed rate, BUN, creatinine, calcium, phosphorus, electrolytes, albumin, UA) endomysial antibodies, IgA
- X-ray hand/wrist for bone age (significantly delayed bone age associated w/nonendocrine disease, endocrine disease, delayed puberty; normal bone age favors genetic short stature

- Look for endocrine causes:
  - thyroid deficiency: low T4/T3 uptake, high TSH confirms 1° hypothyroidism; w/a low TSH may indicate pituitary deficiency
  - growth hormone deficiency: random growth hormone levels generally low/not useful; growth hormone-dependent growth factor constant throughout day/can assess growth hormone function (IGF-I/IGFBP-3 suitable for assessing growth hormone); ↓ IGF-I/IGFBP-3 suggest growth hormone deficiency, confirm by growth hormone provocation test
  - gonadal dysgenesis (Turner syndrome): chromosomal analysis needed in *all* short girls >2.5 SD below mean for age
  - delayed puberty: ↑ LH/FSH suggest 1° gonadal dysfunction; LH/FSH ↓ in delayed puberty/pituitary deficiency (may not respond to gonadotropin-releasing hormone (GnRH) provocative test); exclude hyperprolactinemia
  - MRI in pts w/pituitary deficiency/hyperprolactinemia to exclude intracranial lesion

DIFFERENTIAL DIAGNOSIS

- *Genetic short stature:* height percentile appropriate for family background; bone age consistent w/chronologic age; height velocity normal
- Constitutional delay of puberty (lack of pubic hair/testicular enlargement in boys by 14 yrs of age, lack of breast development in girls by 12½): bone age delayed; predicted adult height appropriate for family background; often family Hx of delayed puberty; height velocity prior to pubertal onset may fall to levels consistent w/organic causes of growth failure; Dx of exclusion

TREATMENT

- *Nonendocrine organic causes:* controlling disease should lead to resumption of normal growth
- *Hypothyroidism:* levothyroxine, 0.1 mg/m²/d po (beyond infancy dosage)
- *Growth hormone deficiency:* somatropin, 0.3 mg/kg/wk SubQ in 6–7 div doses
- *Delayed puberty:* explain to pt/family when to expect puberty to start, predict adult height; usually sufficient/treatment is

not required; if pt emotionally upset about lack of sexual maturation, sex steroids prescribed to induce 2° sexual characteristics (in girls, use conjugated estrogens, 0.3 mg q0d × 6 mos, then 0.3 mg/d × 6 mos, then 0.625 mg/d × 6 mos; medroxyprogesterone acetate added then for menstrual cycling; in boys, testosterone enanthate, 50 mg IM (6 mos sufficient to induce pubic hair; if desired, ↑ dose in 50 mg increments q6mos to max. 200 mg monthly); assess pts periodically to determine if spontaneous puberty has started/treatment can be stopped
- *Turner syndrome:* adult height improved w/somatropin; monitor for thyroid disease; sex steroids to induce breast development
- *Genetic short stature:* only experimental protocols available

COMPLICATIONS

- *Levothyroxine:* rarely, benign intracranial hypertension; iatrogenic hyperthyroidism 2° excessive dosage; monitor T4, total T3, TSH to avoid over/undertreatment; to avoid adrenocortical insufficiency, delay levothyroxine in pts w/suspected hypopituitarism until tests confirm normal ACTH/adrenocortical function
- *Somatropin:* benign intracranial hypertension, peripheral edema; pts w/pituitary deficiencies due to previous tumors/cranial radiation at ↑ risk for leukemia; become familiar w/precautions in package insert
- *Conjugated estrogens/medroxyprogesterone acetate:* same as for oral contraceptive agents
- *Testosterone enanthate:* peripheral edema, erections, gynecomastia
- Pts w/pituitary hormone deficiency may develop multiple pituitary hormone deficiencies

WHEN TO REFER

- Referral based on experience of 1° care physician; refer for growth hormone provocation testing, treatment of growth hormone deficiency, of girls w/Turner syndrome, of pituitary deficiency, use of sex steroids to induce 2° sexual characteristics in children w/delayed puberty

BACKGROUND

- Short stature common complaint
- Short children w/normal growth rate (>5 cm/y) generally fall into one of two normal growth patterns:
  - familial short stature (short parents, normal bone age/normal onset of puberty)
  - constitutional delay in growth/development w/delayed onset of puberty (delayed bone age, delayed onset of puberty, parent who may have experienced delayed onset of puberty)
- Children who have growth rate <5 cm/y require careful evaluation

DIFFERENTIAL DIAGNOSIS

- Systemic disorders causing growth failure include psychosocial growth retardation, nutritional deficiencies (eg, zinc/iron deficiency), GI disease (eg, regional enteritis), congenital heart disease (eg, tetralogy of Fallot), pulmonary disease (eg, cystic fibrosis), renal disease (eg, renal tubular acidosis, renal insufficiency), endocrine disease (eg, hypothyroidism), other chronic disease (eg, sickle-cell anemia)
- Syndromic disorders associated w/short stature/growth failure (eg, Turner, Down syndromes)

CLINICAL EVALUATION

History

- Always short vs. recent onset of growth failure
- Nocturia (diabetes insipidus)
- Morning headaches (↑ intracranial pressure)
- Abdominal complaints (inflammatory bowel disease): frequent diarrhea, mucus/blood in stool
- Kidney disease, recurrent UTIs
- Brain injury, birth trauma, CNS infection, tumor
- Radiation Tx to head or neck; may cause pituitary/thyroid injury

Physical Exam

- Proportionality of limbs to trunk (possible chondrodysplasias/spondylodysplasias)
- Midline facial deformities (associated w/pituitary disease)
- Peripheral vision (bitemporal vision loss associated w/pituitary/hypothalamic tumors)
- Pubertal status

LABORATORY EVALUATION

- Urine analysis
- Chemistry profile
- CBC/ESR
- T_4, TSH
- *Karyotype:* must be done in all girls w/unexplained growth failure; girls w/mosaic Turner syndrome may have normal pubertal development, even menstruate
- *Bone age x ray*
- *Insulinlike growth factor I:* below normal in children w/growth hormone deficiency; IGF-I level ↓ w/poor nutrition
- *Exercise-stimulated growth hormone level:* random growth hormone levels worthless; >15 min aerobic exercise should cause growth hormone level to rise >7 ng/ml
- *Head MRI:* only required if Sx suggestive of brain tumor

WHEN TO REFER FOR POSSIBLE GROWTH HORMONE THERAPY

- Growth failure/Hx brain injury
- Growth failure/chronic renal insufficiency
- Known/suspected Turner syndrome
- Growth failure/no obvious systemic disorder as cause
- Growth failure/no obvious syndromic disorder associated w/short stature, such as achondroplasia; some children w/syndromic disorders associated w/short stature (Aarskog, Prader Willi) may actually have growth hormone deficiency/benefit from growth hormone Tx

TREATMENT FOR GROWTH HORMONE DEFICIENCY

- Must be documented by lack of growth hormone ↑ in response to two stimulation tests, except in case of renal insufficiency/Turner syndrome
- Treatment should start w/growth hormone (0.02 mg/kg given SubQ each night)
- Dosage may be ↑ to 0.04 mg/kg/night for classical growth hormone deficient children/0.05 mg/kg/night for children w/chronic renal insufficiency/Turner syndrome

COMPLICATIONS OF GROWTH HORMONE THERAPY

- Slipped capital femoral epiphysis
- Pseudo tumor cerebri
- Generalized edema
- Glucose intolerance
- Rapid growth of nevi
- Progression of scoliosis
- ↑ risk of transplant (kidney) rejection
- Acute pancreatitis; usually occurs in association w/valproic acid usage
- Arthralgia

BACKGROUND

- In recent years, incidence 1.8–12.9%, > two-thirds occurring within 1 mo of operation
- ↑ rate of infections in pts w/external shunts for posthemorrhagic hydrocephalus, infants <2 yrs of age, those w/revision of infected shunt
- Pathogens isolated from two-thirds infected shunts identical to organisms cultured from pt's skin; other pathogenic mechanisms: skin breakdown along shunt, ascending infection following shunt perforation of gut, direct hematogenous spread
- 60–85% of shunt infections caused by staphylococci, majority coagulase-negative (ie, *S. epidermidis, S. capitis, S. hominis*), commonly methicillin resistant; gram-negative bacilli cause 5–20% of infections (*E. coli* most common), streptococcal species 6–15%, other organisms 1–14%

CLINICAL MANIFESTATIONS

- 50% w/nonspecific Sx, result of shunt malfunction or other systemic disease (ie, URI or GI infection); therefore, high index of suspicion needed
- >50% present w/fever, changes in mental status, irritability, nausea, vomiting. Meningismus, headache occur in 10–25%. Overt signs of ↑ intracranial pressure (eg, cranial nerve palsies, hypertension, bradycardia) rare

LABORATORY FEATURES

- *Radiographic studies:* CT scan of head to exclude ↑ intracranial pressure, ventricular enlargement; abdominal ultrasound to exclude peritoneal cyst
- CSF:
  – *protein level:* of no value in determining infection
  – *glucose level:* usually normal to mildly ↓; significantly ↓ in gram-negative compared to gram-positive infections
  – *WBC:* if high, correlates w/infection (usually higher in gram-negative infections), but may be normal (<10 cells) in many cases; predominance of polymorphonuclears common; mononuclear cells less often present
  – *Gram stain:* positive in only small percentage of gram-positive infections but in 90% of gram-negative infections; positive gram stain, very low CSF glucose suggest prolonged positive CSF culture, even w/appropriate Tx
  – *culture:* vital that results interpreted in relation to clinical manifestations, other laboratory findings

DIFFERENTIAL DIAGNOSIS

- For ventricular involvement:
  – shunt obstruction or malfunction
  – meningitis (eg, viral, bacterial, fungal, chemical)
  – brain abscess, epidural abscess
  – malignancy
  – subdural empyema
  – protozoal infections (eg, cysticercosis)
- For distal part infection of ventriculoperitoneal (VP) shunt:
  – peritonitis
  – bowel obstruction
  – bowel perforation
- For distal part infection of ventriculoatrial (VA) shunt:
  – bacteremia or sepsis
  – immune complex nephritis
  – pulmonary emboli
  – endocarditis
- Nonspecific symptoms:
  – URI
  – GI infection
  – UTI

TREATMENT

- Variety of suggested medical, surgical Tx for shunt infection
- *Treatment of choice, w/>95% cure rate:* complete removal of infected shunt w/insertion of external ventricular drain (EVD), w/systemic antibiotics
- *Avoid other options:* immediate replacement w/new shunt, partial removal of infected shunt (ie, only distal portion), or systemic antibiotics alone—much lower cure rate
- Mildly sick children w/minimal CSF changes, negative gram stain, antistaphylococcal antibiotic initially; drug of choice vancomycin (60 mg/kg/d q6h), until established sensitivity of isolate to oxacillin; if sensitive to oxacillin, replace vancomycin w/oxacillin (200 mg/kg/d q6h)
- *Moderately to severely sick children:* add third-generation cephalosporin (ie, ceftriaxone, 100 mg/kg/d q12h or cefotaxime, 200 mg/kg/d q6h) to antistaphylococcal Tx
- *Duration of Tx:* for mild infection (ie, nearly normal CSF) where only first culture positive, 4 d. If CSF shows pleocytosis and/or abnormal chemistry, continue Tx 7 d
- Cultures positive >1 d after appropriate Tx should be followed by 10 d negative cultures before reinternalizing shunt. If pathogen *S. aureus* or gram negative, always continue Tx until CSF culture negative for 10 d

COMPLICATIONS

- ↑ morbidity, mortality
- Lower IQ scores

PREVENTION

- Efficacy of antimicrobial prophylaxis undetermined

WHEN TO REFER

- Consider referral to qualified neurosurgeon whenever shunt infection suspected or proven
- If CSF cultures remain positive for >2–3 d, suggesting failure of initial Tx

SICKLE-CELL DISEASE ANEMIA

WILLIAM REED AND ELLIOTT P. VICHINSKY

BACKGROUND

- *Systemic* disease characterized by chronic hemolytic anemia, high susceptibility to bacterial infection, intermittent vaso-occlusion due to sickling of RBCs
- Inherited abnormality of hemoglobin structure (beta 6: glutamine to valine)
- Intracellular polymerization of hemoglobin S contributes to membrane damage leading to hemolysis, altered endothelial adherence
- Chronic small vessel ischemia produces chronic organ damage
- Clinical features *highly variable* among pts
- 1/400 (~70,000) African Americans affected: 1/12 unaffected carrier
- SCD common in other regions: Middle East, Mediterranian, South and Central America, Africa
- Homozygous SS genotype most common; all anemic
- Sickle-hemoglobin C, sickle-beta thalassemia compound heterozygous forms of SCD. Pts often lack anemia, may be less severely affected (for most complications)
- Presymptomatic Dx through newborn screening in 44 states, plus DC
- Pts entirely well at birth; may become symptomatic w/the switch from fetal to adult hemoglobin occurring gradually over first year of life
- Pts acquire functional asplenia early in first year of life; they are immunocompromised, *highly* susceptible to bacterial infection

CLINICAL MANIFESTATIONS

- SCD may affect all organ systems. Pain syndromes, pulmonary disease, acute anemic events, suspicion of sepsis most common serious complications in young children. Most clinical manifestations relate to chronic hemolysis, vaso-occlusion
- Chronic hemolysis:
  - anemia
  - pigment gallstones
  - aplastic episodes (parvovirus B19)
  - jaundice
  - delayed growth and puberty
- Vaso-occlusion:
  - pain syndromes
  - acute chest syndrome
  - stroke
  - priapism
  - retinopathy
  - avascular hip necrosis
  - splenic sequestration
  - acquired asplenia
  - leg ulcers
  - hyposthenuria and enuresis
  - chronic nephropathy

LABORATORY FEATURES

- *Hemoglobin:* 6–9 g/dl at clinical steady state for SS pts. S-C, S-thal pts may not be anemic when well
- *Reticulocyte count:* increased in SS, nearly normal in pts w/SC, S-beta-thalassemia
- *Red cell indices:* usually normal. Microcytosis characteristic w/co-existing iron deficiency or S-beta-thalassemia
- *WBC count and differential:* normal or elevated at baseline
- *Sedementation rate:* low due to decreased tendency for sickle red cells to form rouleaux
- *Peripheral blood smear:* sickled forms, target cells, nucleated RBCs, thrombocytosis, leukocytosis may be present. W/S-C and S-thal, smear can be nearly normal
- *Chemistries:* mild indirect hyperbilirubinemia, elevated LDH common due to hemolysis
- *Urinalysis:* hyposthenuria, bilirubin metabolites usually present; urine specific gravity not reliable guide to hydration status
- *Sickle prep:* ("solubility test") almost never appropriate for Dx. Test does not distinguish carrier from disease state; may give false negative result. Sometimes used to confirm identity of electrophoretic band suspected of being Hgb SS
- *Hemoglobin electrophoresis:* separates and identifies hemoglobins according to their migration in electric field. Standard for Dx and monitoring sickle hemoglobin levels following transfusion
- *Chest x ray:* most SS pts develop mild cardiomegaly due to chronic anemia

DIFFERENTIAL DIAGNOSIS

- Most pts (since 1987) presymptomatically identified through newborn screening. Cases missed if born abroad, in state having absent or nonuniversal newborn screening, transfused w/red cells in neonatal period or if infant born very premature
- Differential diagnoses concern the *complications* cited above rather than underlying hemoglobinopathy. Examples:
  - sepsis may be mistaken for uncomplicated febrile illness
  - acute chest syndrome may be mistaken for simple infectious pneumonia
  - stroke or osteomyelitis, w/diminished use of extremity (particularly in preverbal child) may be mistaken for simple pain syndrome involving extremity
  - delayed hemolytic transfusion reaction, w/back pain, increasing jaundice, falling hemoglobin, may be mistaken for simple pain syndrome

TREATMENT

- *Prevention:* newborn Dx, family participation, daily prophylactic penicillin pivotal.

With these plus comprehensive care, childhood mortality reduced from 20% to <2%
- *Pain:* many pts manage pain at home using relaxation, local warmth, oral analgesics. When these measures fail, or pain involves head, chest, abdomen, pt should seek care. NSAIDs (including toradol), narcotic analgesics indicated; should be given *together*. Morphine narcotic of choice; most effective when given by pt-controlled analgesia device (PCA)
- *Fever:* SCD pt immunocompromised. Parenteral antibiotics (cefuroxime 50 mg/kg) administered at *beginning* of thorough laboratory evaluation *whenever temperature exceeds* 101 °F. Bacterial sepsis and meningitis, resistant pneumococcal infections, salmonella osteomyelitis, pyelonephritis, pneumonia all *common and carry excess morbidity* in SCD pt
- *Transfusion:* preferred product: leukofiltered PRBCs, w/limited phenotypic match for minor red cell antigens. Events that may require transfusion include acute chest syndrome, stroke, priapism, general anesthesia, acute anemic events due to sequestration or transient erythroid aplasia
- *Newer treatments:* hydroxyurea is antisickling agent promising in clinical trials. Carefully selected pts cured of SCD by stem cell transplantation. Pts at high risk for stroke now identified prospectively by transcranial Doppler. Access to these and other clinical trials available through regional sickle-cell centers

COMPLICATIONS

- List of clinical manifestations above serves as partial list of complications
- Additional complications include alloimmunizations, iron overload from red cell transfusion, depressive symptoms amplified by recurrent pain episodes, morbid pregnancy, need for dialysis, subclinical CNS lesions occurring in up to third of pts and detectable by MRI. Subtle, progressive cognitive impairment results.

WHEN TO REFER

- Where possible, all pts should have periodic contact w/comprehensive care center
- Early consultation appropriate w/this complex, rapidly changing systemic disease
- NIH publication *Management and Therapy of Sickle Cell Disease* (#95–2117) available without charge (703-821-8955, ext. 254). Delineates standards of care, contains an invitation for telephone consultation from authors, including phone numbers

BACKGROUND

- *Most common risk factors:* viral URIs, allergic inflammation
- Complicates ~5% of viral URIs
- Most frequently observed in children <7 yrs of age
- Mucosal inflammation initiated by virus infection or allergy causes obstruction of osteomeatal complex. Negative pressure within paranasal sinuses in concert w/sniffing, nose blowing leads to aspiration of secretions from densely colonized nasopharynx into paranasal sinuses. Multiplication of bacterial agents occurs. Most common bacterial species causing infection: *Streptococcus pneumoniae, Haemophilus influenzae, Moraxella catarrhalis*

MANIFESTATIONS

- Acute sinusitis distinguished from uncomplicated URI, chronic sinusitis by respiratory symptoms that are either "persistent" or "severe"
- "Persistent" respiratory symptoms last >10, <30 d:
  - nasal discharge of any quality (thin or thick, serous, mucoid or purulent)
  - or daytime cough (wet or dry)
  - or both
  - low-grade or no fever
- "Severe" respiratory symptoms:
  - purulent nasal discharge, *and*
  - fever >38.5° (for 3–4 consecutive d)

LABORATORY FEATURES

- Plain sinus radiographs may confirm Dx suspected on clinical grounds:
  - significant radiographic findings: complete opacification, mucosal thickness ≥5 mm or an air-fluid level
  - radiographs not necessary in children <6 yrs of age w/persistent symptoms (significant abnormalities found in ~90%)
  - radiographs useful in children >6 yrs of age w/persistent symptoms and in children >2 ys w/"severe" symptoms
  - WBC counts, ESR, Hgb levels not necessary

DIFFERENTIAL DIAGNOSIS

- Nasal discharge:
  - viral URI
  - allergic rhinitis
  - nonallergic rhinitis
  - streptococcal infection in children <5 yrs of age
- Cough:
  - viral URI
  - *Bordetella pertussis*
  - *Mycoplasma pneumoniae*
  - reactive airways disease
  - gastroesophageal reflux

TREATMENT

- Amoxicillin, 60 mg/kg/d in 2 div doses
- Amoxicillin, 40–45 mg/kg/d in 2 div doses plus Amoxicillin/clavulanate, 40–45 mg/kg/d in 2 div doses
- Cefuroxime, 30 mg/kg/d in 2 div doses
- Cefpodoxime, 9 mg/kg/d in 1–2 div doses

COMPLICATIONS

- CNS:
  - cavernous sinus thrombosis
  - subdural empyema
  - epidural empyema
  - brain abscess
- Other:
  - inflammatory edema, most common
  - orbital:
    - subperiosteal abscess
    - orbital abscess
    - orbital cellulitis
  - osteitis:
    - Pott puffy tumor

WHEN TO REFER

- Symptoms unresponsive to 2 courses of antibiotics
- Patient presents with orbital or CNS complications

BACKGROUND

- Most common hip disorder w/ onset during adolescence
- *Etiology:* weakening of growth plate and surrounding structures (perichondrial ring) of proximal end of femur during adolescent growth spurt
- "Slip" is displacement of proximal femoral epiphysis (capital femoral epiphysis) relative to femoral neck
- Severity graded by percentage of displacement of epiphysis relative to femoral neck: grade I (mild), <30%; grade II (moderate), 30–50%; grade III (severe), >50%
- Average age at onset: 10–13 yrs, females; 12–15 yrs, males
- Twice as common in males as females
- May be associated w/ endocrine abnormality (hypothyroidism, growth hormone excess), or end-stage renal disease
- Obese individuals, those of African descent more likely involved

CLINICAL MANIFESTATIONS

- Painful limp
- Pain most commonly in hip but may be referred to knee or thigh
- External rotation of involved extremity
- Limb shortening up to 2 cm may be present
- Considered chronic if symptoms present >3 wks
- 50% report traumatic incident
- Thigh atrophy possible if slip chronic

LABORATORY FEATURES

- Laboratory values are normal unless associated w/ end-stage renal disease or endocrine abnormalities. Thyroid function tests or growth hormone levels necessary only if appropriate Hx, physical findings present
- *Radiographic features:* earliest finding may be widening of growth plate w/o true "slip." Slip most commonly seen on lateral view. Single AP view of hip or pelvis inadequate. Epiphysis displaces inferiorly and posteriorly

DIFFERENTIAL DIAGNOSIS

- Legg-Calvé-Perthes disease
- Proximal femur or pelvic fracture
- Tumor
- Osteomyelitis or pyarthrosis
- If pain referred to knee or thigh it may be confused w/ any pathology about knee

TREATMENT

- Immediate non-weight-bearing status on the limb once Dx made
- In situ fixation of epiphysis to femoral neck w/ screw(s) or pin(s)
- Cast immobilization w/o pinning may be warranted in younger patients
- May be able to reduce slip in early, acute (<48 hrs) cases
- Late osteotomy for severe residual deformity

COMPLICATIONS

- *Leg length discrepancy:* usually not clinically significant
- *Chondrolysis (destruction of hip articular cartilage):* more common w/ nonoperative (Spica casting) treatment and in black pts (3×)
- *Avascular necrosis:* most common in pts whose slips reduced w/ manipulation or traction, and after osteotomy of femoral neck
- Early arthrosis

PREVENTION

- Close monitoring for bilaterality following initial slip, esp in younger (<10 yrs) pt
- Unclear whether weight loss would have any effect on incidence

WHEN TO REFER

- All pts w/ suspected or diagnosed SCFE should be made non–weight bearing on involved extremity and immediately referred to orthopedist

BACKGROUND

- Smoke inhalation leading to asphyxia, CO poisoning, respiratory failure, severe neurologic injury must be suspected in any child exposed to fire or fumes in enclosed space, any unconscious burn victim, or burn pts w/large surface area involvement
- ~50,000 children/y hospitalized for burn injuries
- Burns second only to motor vehicle accidents as cause of trauma death
- Major cause of death, neurologic morbidity in burn injury is smoke inhalation. House fires most common setting for smoke inhalation

PATHOPHYSIOLOGY

- Injury to respiratory system from smoke inhalation occurs by several mechanisms
  - asphyxia: fire in enclosed space rapidly consumes available O_2, most victims succumb to hypoxia
  - thermal injury: direct thermal injury generally confined to upper airway. Air is poor heat conductor, airway mucosa effectively dissipates heat
  - CO component of almost all smoke. Because of its affinity for Hgb and heme-containing protein (cytochrome oxidases), CO displaces O_2, interferes w/O_2 uptake, transport, delivery
  - cyanide: similar to CO, cyanide common component of smoke, uncouples oxidative metabolism
  - aldehydes, acids, other irritants: other combustion products produce tracheobronchial injury, may cause mucosal sloughing, severe inflammation, respiratory failure
- Although lung, upper airway are usual sites of 1° injury, resultant inadequate O_2 uptake and/or delivery can impair function of every organ system. Neurologic injury from prolonged hypoxia may be severe, irreversible

CLINICAL HISTORY, SYMPTOMS AND SIGNS

- Hx exposure to flame, fire, or fumes in enclosed space, unconscious pt, or large surface area burns should prompt evaluation even in absence of clinical Sx
- Neurologic symptoms range from nonspecific headache or dizziness to disorientation, visual disturbances, coma
- Respiratory symptoms of dyspnea, tachypnea, or stridor may be delayed but can progress rapidly
- Burns around face, edema, erythema, soot or charring of oropharyngeal mucosa suggests inhalational injury, requires evaluation

DIAGNOSIS

- Suspected thermal injury to airway should prompt direct bronchoscopic inspection and/or establishment of artificial airway
- Chest x ray may be normal (80%) but diffuse "ground glass" appearance suggests significant inhalational injury
- Both pulse oximetry, arterial blood glass derived O_2 saturation may be normal in CO poisoning! CO-oximeter direct measurement of oxy- and carboxy-hemoglobin must be performed

TREATMENT

- Stridor, respiratory distress, any suggestion of airway edema, or depressed LOC should prompt rapid airway evaluation, possible endotracheal intubation. Airway edema can progress rapidly to complete obstruction, complicate intubation
- 100% O_2 by tight-fitting nonrebreather mask should be administered until Dx confirmed. O_2 displaces CO by mass action and significantly reduces half-life of CO. Hyperbaric O_2 Tx may be helpful in CO poisoning even if delayed, should be considered in child w/evidence of neurologic dysfunction
- Note that carboxyhemoglobin represents only fraction of total body CO, as CO is bound to other heme-containing proteins including myoglobin and cytochrome oxidases. O_2 administration should be continued until CO levels <5%
- Establish IV access, proceed w/fluid resuscitation/treatment of other burns or injuries

COMPLICATIONS

- Respiratory failure from upper airway thermal injury, direct injury to tracheobronchial mucosa, aspiration, neurologic injury
- In one series 12% pts hospitalized w/CO poisoning had neurologic sequelae including personality change, memory impairment, behavioral difficulties. Delayed recovery from deficits in children possible
- Blindness, hearing deficits, other cranial nerve deficits, other organ system injuries due to prolonged hypoxia

WHEN TO REFER

- Imperative that resuscitation including evaluation, possible control of airway, O_2 administration, fluid resuscitation be started immediately before referral
- After stabilization, referral to burn or 3° care center should be dictated by presence of respiratory failure or impending failure, significant neurologic symptoms, or presence of burns that are threat to life or complete recovery of function or appearance (eg, face, hands, genitalia, or across major joints)
- Absolute levels of CO mandating referral cannot be given, as blood constitutes only part of the "reservoir," impacted by previous O_2 administration, time since exposure

SPEECH DISORDERS OTHER THAN STUTTERING JAMES COPLAN

BACKGROUND

- Most common symptom of developmental disability in preschool children
- *Prevalence:* 5–10%; M:F ratio: >2:1

MANIFESTATIONS

- Reduced/delayed cooing, babbling ("quiet baby"), delayed appearance of single words, 2 words phrases, sentences
- Intelligibility (clarity of speech) may be normal, proportionately delayed, or disproportionately delayed, relative to expressive language level
- *Rule of thumb:* (child's age in years)/4 = approx proportion of child's speech that should be understandable to examiner (ie, 1/4 @ 1 yr, 2/4 @ 2 yrs, etc.)
- Examiner must distinguish between isolated *speech* delay, vs. global display in *language,* including auditory comprehension, visual language

DIFFERENTIAL DIAGNOSIS

- *Developmental language disorder (DLD):* prevalence ~5%. Expressive delay, impaired intelligibility predominate initially. Auditory comprehension within normal limits, although auditory processing problems and/or reading difficulty often surface during elementary school. General intelligence, social skills normal. Often familial
- *Mental retardation (MR):* prevalence ~3%. Auditory expressive, auditory receptive, visual language delay all present. Parents may claim child "understands everything," but even ability to follow infinite number of 1 step commands (as opposed to multistep commands) no better than 18 mo receptive language level
- *Hearing loss (HL):* prevalence of permanent HL ~0.3%. Amount, intelligibility of speech affected first. Receptive language relatively well preserved unless severe HL present. Even severe–profound HL can be nearly impossible to detect by routine office examination. All children w/speech or language delay should be seen by audiologist, no matter how well child seems to hear. Anomalies of the external ear or mandible (1st and 2nd branchial arch) associated w/anomalies of ossicles, and moderate–severe conductive HL. Neural crest abnormalities (widely spaced eyes, albinism, iris bicolor, or heterochromia) associated w/sensorineural HL. Approx 33.3–50% congenital HL genetic; even w/negative family Hx
- *Autism:* prevalence ~0.1%, including milder forms (pervasive developmental disorder, Asperger syndrome). Deviant language development (echolalia, noncommunicative utterances); impaired visual language (absence of pointing to desired objects or participation in gesture games). Impaired social skills. Repetitious behaviors. Degree of autism may vary from mild to profound; may be accompanied by any level of intelligence from profound MR to genius IQ
- *Dysarthria:* prevalence ~0.1%. Usually seen as one component of generalized upper motor neuron dysfunction ("cerebral palsy"). Often preceded by Hx feeding problems. Receptive language normal, unless MR also present

TREATMENT

- Special education, amplification (HL), sign language, or computer-assisted speech (DLD, dysarthria)

WHEN TO REFER

- Parental concern, clinician concern, or persistent delays on standardized screening test. Do not wait to see if child "outgrows problem"

BACKGROUND

- Inherited hemolytic anemia
- Most common inherited hemolytic anemia in people of northern European extraction. Prevalence in US 1/5,000; evidence that if milder forms of disease included, may be 5 times more common
- Far less common in other ethnic groups
- Disease inherited as autosomal dominant characteristic in 75% pts. Remaining 25% autosomal recessive, new spontaneous mutation
- Disorder of red cell membrane. Majority of pts have defect in one or both of red cell membrane proteins spectrin and ankyrin

MANIFESTATIONS

- Clinical manifestations variable
- Triad of anemia, jaundice, splenomegaly major clinical manifestations
- Newborn jaundice occurs in 50% pts but controlled w/phototherapy in most pts, usually presents in first 48 hrs but can be delayed until after first week in 20% pts. Severe neonatal jaundice can require exchange transfusions
- Anemia (hemoglobin <15 g/dl) also common in newborn. Severe anemia rare but can occur. Some infants may require transfusions during newborn period. No evidence that symptomatic newborns have more severe form of disease
- Can present at any age but usually presents in childhood
- *Presenting Sx:* anemia (50%), jaundice (15%), splenomegaly (15%), family Hx (10%)
- Jaundice seen at one time or another in 50% pts
- Spleen palpable in ~50% children but in 75–90% adults

LABORATORY FEATURES

- Anemia, reticulocytosis, hyperbilirubinemia w/peripheral blood smear showing spherocytes hallmark of spherocytosis
- Osmotic fragility test used for Dx, although other tests have been used. Always use incubated osmotic fragility test (more sensitive)
- Newborn red cells are resistant to osmotic challenge and mask results of osmotic fragility test. However, if age-appropriate controls used, test can be done reliably in newborn

Laboratory classification of spherocytosis

Laboratory	Mild	Moderate	Severe
hemoglobin (g/dl)	>10 or normal for age	>8	6–8
bilirubin (mg/dl)	1–2	>2	<3
reticulocytes (%)	3–6	>6	<10
spectrin/red cell (% of normal)	80–100	50–80	40–60
osmotic fragility			
(fresh)	normal or slight increase	increased	increased
(incubated)	increased	increased	increased

Adapted from Eber et al: J Pediatr 117:409–416, 1990.

DIFFERENTIAL DIAGNOSIS

- Spherocytes commonly seen in poorly made smears; good smear very important in determining presence of spherocytes
- Spherocytes seen in oxidant injury of red cells like in G6PD deficiency crisis; hemolytic transfusion reactions; clostridial sepsis; severe burns; spider, bee, snake venoms; severe hypophosphatemia; hypersplenism. However, spherocytosis rare in these conditions
- True differential Dx between ABO incompatibility in newborn, autoimmune hemolytic anemia in older child, hereditary spherocytosis
- Coombs' test should be positive in both ABO incompatibility, autoimmune hemolytic anemia
- Iron and/or folate deficient red cells resistant to osmotic challenge, may mask spherocytosis. Incubated osmotic fragility test still should be positive

COMPLICATIONS

- Hemolytic crises usually occur w/viral illness. Pts develop mild increases in jaundice, mild anemia; spleen size may increase. Rise in reticulocyte count but crisis rarely produces severe anemia. Rarely severe hemolytic crisis occurs w/jaundice, anemia, tender splenomegaly, left-sided abdominal pain, pallor, malaise, fever, nausea, vomiting
- Aplastic crises more serious complication.

Less frequent, can cause severe anemia, even death. Characterized by pallor, anemia, low reticulocyte count. Typically follows viral illness w/fever, abdominal pain. Causative agent parvovirus B19 in most patients. Bilirubin levels may fall during aplastic crisis. Number of spherocytes in peripheral smear increase. Pts w/aplastic crisis should be placed in isolation, represent risk to pregnant women and immunocompromised pts
- Folic acid deficiency develops in pts w/hereditary spherocytosis because of increased red cell formation. All pts w/hereditary spherocytosis should be on folic acid supplements
- Gallstones occur in pts w/spherocytosis. Usually occur >10 yrs of age but can occur earlier. Incidence rises during second and third decade of life
- Growth may be retarded during puberty in pts w/severe spherocytosis
- Decreased exercise tolerance, fatigue may be seen in severe and moderate spherocytosis
- Rare complications include leg ulcers, extramedullary hematopoiesis, neurochromatons, variants of spherocytosis w/degenerative disease of CNS

TREATMENT

- All pts should be on folic acid 1 mg po qd to prevent folic acid deficiency
- Severe anemia may require transfusion therapy. Particularly pts w/aplastic crisis w/hemoglobin concentration of 4–5 g/dl and no reticulocytes or symptomatic anemia require transfusion Tx w/leukocyte-poor, filtered

packed red cells. Transfusion of 10 mL/kg of body weight (divided in 2 aliquots of 5 mL/kg of body weight when severe or symptomatic anemia is present) should be enough. Repeat as needed until pt recovers. Rarely pts w/spherocytosis have severe anemia that requires chronic transfusion Tx
- Treat symptomatic gallbladder disease or obstructive jaundice w/cholecystectomy
- Treat asymptomatic gallstones medically or by cholecystectomy
- Splenectomy can avert most symptoms and complications of spherocytosis, but risks, benefits of splenectomy must be weighed. Risk of infection postsplenectomy is greatest in infants and small children; splenectomy should be postponed until > age 6 if possible
- Pts w/mild spherocytosis rarely need splenectomy
- Splenectomy indicated in most pts w/severe spherocytosis
- Pts w/moderate spherocytosis may or may not need splenectomy; Tx should be tailored to specific pt's needs, symptoms

WHEN TO REFER

- Primary care physician usually can care for pts w/hereditary spherocytosis
- Pts referred once Dx confirmed so proper education, careful baseline evaluation carried out by center specializing in red cell disorders
- Pts referred if Dx in question
- Pts referred during severe crises
- Pts referred when splenectomy considered

THOMAS S. RENSHAW

BACKGROUND

- Defect in pars interarticularis of a vertebra (narrow bone bridge joining the facet joints)
- Defects develop most often 2–10 yrs of age
- Usually stress fracture; rarely acute trauma
- Can be unilateral
- Commonly at L5 (97%), then L4, rarely cephalad to L3
- Found in ~5% of population
- Great majority asymptomatic
- More common in young gymnasts, football linemen, divers, weight lifters
- Fewer than half develop spondylolisthesis (forward slipping on caudal vertebra)

CLINICAL MANIFESTATIONS

- Insidious or abrupt onset of persistent low back pain, usually in 2nd decade
- Often Hx completely negative
- Pain may radiate to buttocks, thighs; rarely more caudally
- Absence of weakness, hypesthesia, reflex asymmetry, other neurologic signs
- Often find tight hamstrings, ↓ lumbar spine mobility

RADIOGRAPHIC FEATURES

- Lytic, bandlike lesion in pars interarticularis on plain radiograph
- Seen on coned lateral view in >80% of cases
- Oblique views detect most of remainder ("Scotty dog collar" sign)
- CT scan should identify almost 100% if plain films inconclusive

DIFFERENTIAL DIAGNOSIS

- Nonspecific myalgia
- Acute, chronic low back strain
- Spondylolisthesis w/or w/o spondylolysis
- Herniated disc
- Bone, soft tissue neoplasm
- Bone, soft tissue infection
- Inflammatory spondyloarthropathy

TREATMENT

- *Restrict activities:* no running, sports, heavy lifting 4–6 wks
- *Daily exercises:* lumbar *flexion* program 4–6 wks
- Brace (Boston Overlap TLSO or equivalent) full time 3–6 mos (skillfully applied cast may be substituted)
- *Surgery:* one-level, in situ, bilateral, posterolateral transverse process fusion indicated for:
  - pain persistent >6 mos despite appropriate medical treatment
  - multiple recurrent episodes of pain
  - spondylolisthesis of >50% slipping
- If symptoms present <3 mos or specific Hx trauma, a technetium, SPECT, or CT scan may indicate acute fracture. If fracture present, treatment w/brace or cast often results in healing of pars defects
- Sports participation when asymptomatic

COMPLICATIONS

- Spondylolisthesis in up to half the cases. Tx same, unless slip >50%. Surgical fusion is indicated if further slipping, likely failure w/medical treatment

WHEN TO REFER

- Acute fracture detected
- Failure activities restriction, lumbar flexion program
- Spondylolisthesis >50%
- Multiple recurrences of symptoms
- Atypical Sx

BACKGROUND

- Relatively rare infection in children
- *Etiologic agent: Sporothrix schenckii,* a dimorphic fungus
- Distribution worldwide, primarily temperate, tropical zones
- Fungus commonly found in soil, on vegetation
- Human infection results from traumatic inoculation of skin from contaminated thorns, barbs, splinters, other objects
- Large outbreaks have occurred from contact w/highly contaminated sphagnum moss, bales of hay, packing straw for pottery, mine timbers
- Transmission from domestic cats w/ulcerating or draining sporothrix lesions to humans has occurred
- Human-to-human transmission unlikely because of small numbers of organisms in lesions

CLINICAL MANIFESTATIONS

- Lymphocutaneous form of disease most common presentation (80–90%). Initial lesion appears as SubQ nodule, then spreads along path of lymphatics w/multiple nodules appearing. Lesions may enlarge, ulcerate or suppurate
- Fixed cutaneous form of disease less frequent presentation; lesions identical to lymphocutaneous form but do not spread from inoculation site
- *Most commonly involved area:* hand in adults, face in children

LABORATORY FEATURES

- ESR usually normal in cutaneous disease; frequently ↑ in extracutaneous disease; serves as useful marker of disease activity
- Serum antibodies of little value in making Dx cutaneous sporotrichosis; when positive, highly specific indicators of disease activity; titers higher in extracutaneous infection than for cutaneous disease; negative or falling titer does not ensure resolution of infection; latex

agglutination, immunodiffusion, EIA test the more sensitive tests available
- Culture of tissue biopsy from lesion most sensitive means of making specific Dx; most grow in 3–5 d; mycelial phase grows on fungal media at 25–35°C; yeast phase grows at 37°C; growth of organism inhibited at 38.5°C
- Histopathology of minimal value except to r/o other potential etiologies because paucity of organisms found in tissue sections

DIFFERENTIAL DIAGNOSIS

- *Bacterial:* cutaneous nocardiosis, cat scratch disease, cutaneous anthrax, cutaneous mycobacterial infections, ulceroglandular tularemia
- *Other deep fungal infections:* blastomycosis, chromoblastomycosis, mycetoma, granulomatous trichophytosis, *Pseudoallescheria boydii* infections, *Scedosporium apiospermum* infections
- *Parasitic:* cutaneous leishmaniasis

TREATMENT

- Saturated solution of potassium iodide (SSKI) treatment of choice; starting dose 1–2 drops/yr of age given 3×/d
- Doses ↑ 1–2 drops/dose to max 10 drops 3×/d for child, 20–40 drops 3×/d for teenager. Can be given w/fruit juice or milk to disguise bitter taste
- Healing usually occurs in 2–4 wks; Tx continued 4–6 wks after healing
- Relapses rare but may respond to second course of SSKI or can use alternative Tx
- Itraconazole currently preferred alternative Tx for those pts intolerant to SSKI, have serious iodide sensitivity, or fail Tx w/SSKI
- Adult dosage 100–200 mg/d; for children oral suspension available (10 mg/ml), dosage 5 mg/kg/day once daily; duration of Tx, 3–6 mos
- Amphotericin B used in past as alternative agent for treatment of pts w/cutaneous sporotrichosis, but should now be reserved for rare treatment failures w/itraconazole or

for extracutaneous sporotrichosis; dosage 0.5 mg/kg/day × 6–12 wks
- Local heat (42°C) may accelerate healing of cutaneous disease; heat applied as moist compresses or heating pad for 30 min 2×/d
- Pts should be followed for 12 mos to ensure cure or detect relapses

COMPLICATIONS

- Rare dissemination results from hematogenous spread from 1° site; involves almost any organ system of body
- Bone and joints most common sites
- Pulmonary disease usually results from inhalation of spores, not from disseminated disease
- Rarely CNS involved
- Impaired cell-mediated immunity associated w/disseminated infection; risk factors include HIV infection, diabetes, prolonged corticosteroid Tx, chronic alcoholism, immunosuppressive drug Tx, malignancies

PREVENTION

- Wearing protective gloves, clothing when gardening or handling potentially contaminated materials such as soil, sphagnum moss, hay, straw
- Avoid direct contact w/skin lesions of cats
- Identify source of outbreaks because avoidance, decontamination, or destruction of involved material can abort epidemic

WHEN TO REFER

- Most children can be managed by primary physician
- Children w/evidence of disseminated sporotrichosis should be referred; fever, bone pain, joint swelling, or evidence of CNS symptoms are associated clinical evidence for possible dissemination
- ↑ ESR, high-serum antibody titers, abnormal CSF values are laboratory findings that correlate w/dissemination

BACKGROUND

- Previously thought to be uncommon in pediatric/adolescent pt
- Exact incidence of meniscal, ACL injury still unknown
- Injuries result from direct contact/non-contact rotational, deceleration mechanisms

CLINICAL MANIFESTATIONS

- Hx:
  - sudden pain, effusion, giving way
  - inability to bear weight/continue activity; limp
  - may have previous Hx injury w/ ACL, patellar instability
- Exam:
  - focal tenderness (joint line, patella, tibial tubercle, femoral/tibial physes, collateral ligaments)
    - effusion
    - ROM (active, passive)
- stability
- valgus, varus, anterior/posterior (Lackman, Drawer), rotational (pivot shift)
- distal sensory, vascular and motor status
- hip motion (r/o slipped epiphysis)

IMAGING

- Radiographs:
  - 4 views: AP, lateral, skyline, tunnel
  - usually normal
  - r/o tibial eminence fracture, avulsion fracture ACL/PCL, patellar position, osteochondral loose body, physeal morphology
  - comparison views unnecessary except when question of undisplaced physeal injury
  - stress views not indicated because do not affect physeal fracture management/ may cause further physeal damage
- MRI:
  - overused/often inaccurate
  - thorough clinical exam by experienced surgeon has equal accuracy
  - should be ordered (if indicated) by person involved w/ definitive care
  - MRI should not be used as screening test

DIFFERENTIAL DIAGNOSIS

- Acute patellar dislocation
- Meniscal tear
- ACL tear
- Collateral ligament injury
- Physeal fracture
- Tibial eminence fracture
- Tibial tubercle avulsion fracture

TREATMENT

- Initial:
  - make specific provisional Dx
  - ice, immobilize (knee immobilizer splint)
  - pain meds (npo w/ displaced fracture w/ expectant surgery)
  - crutch-protected partial weight-bearing touch-down gait
- 2°:
  - specific to Dx
  - meniscus: arthroscopic repair if criteria met
  - ACL: operative vs. nonoperative dependant on maturity, activity level (*not* an emergency)
  - patellar dislocation: reduce w/pt relaxed to prevent articular injury w/reduction
  - fractures: dependant on location, stability, need for reduction/fixation; assess distal neuro and circulatory status

COMPLICATIONS

- Uncommon if correct Dx made/treatment instituted
- Physeal fractures may cause distal neuro/ vascular compromise, physeal growth arrest w/ 2° deformity, even w/ type II femoral fractures; long-term follow-up required
- Recurrent patellar instability may occur postdislocation
- If ACL deficiency persists, meniscal/articular damage ensues w/ attempts to return to high-demand sports

PREVENTION

- Provide satisfactory playing surfaces, equipment, training techniques, rehabilitation postinjury
- "Prophylactic" knee braces not documented to prevent knee injuries

WHEN TO REFER

- At time of initial injury

SPORTS INJURIES/SPRAINS, ANKLE AND FOOT
BRYAN W. SMITH AND KELLY M. WAICUS

BACKGROUND

- Foot and ankle injuries ~12% adolescent injuries
- Lateral ankle sprains ~85% of ankle sprains
- Children, early adolescents more likely to sustain ankle fractures because of open growth plates
- Ankle sprains more likely in older adolescents
- Most fractures in physeal area in pts w/open growth plates
- Salter-Harris I, II fractures of distal fibula most common fractures in children

CLINICAL MANIFESTATIONS

- Usually present soon after injury
- 80–90% from inversion injury resulting in sprain of lateral ligament(s)—anterior talofibular (ATF), calcaneofibular, posterior talofibular (PTF), usually in that order
- Usually exhibits pain, swelling, sometimes followed by ecchymosis about ankle, foot
- May have severe limp or inability to bear weight
- Area of maximal tenderness over injured ligaments (usually anterior, inferior to malleolus) if examined shortly after injury occurs
- Diffuse edema, ecchymosis after 24–48 hrs may make it difficult to pinpoint injured structures
- Pain over distal fibular physis (at level of anterior ankle joint) or distal tibial physis (1–2 cm above anterior ankle joint) more likely associated w/growth plate fracture
- Fracture should be suspected w/findings of isolated, acute medial ankle pain

EVALUATION

- Palpation for ligamentous, bony tenderness
- Evaluation of gait, functional strength
- Anterior drawer test (pulling foot forward while anchoring ankle) detects instability from sprain of anterior talofibular ligament
- Talar tilt test (talus tilted into adduction/inversion w/knee flexed, foot in neutral/anatomic position) detects sprains of calcaneofibular ligament
- Both anterior drawer, talar tilt tests most helpful when compared to noninjured ankle
- Evaluation of neurovascular status
- *X rays:* AP, lateral, mortise views
- Radiographs likely appear normal immediately following Salter-Harris I fracture
- Comparison to films of uninjured ankle may help detect growth plate widening on injured side
- Pain at growth plate, soft tissue swelling following injury sufficient to make Dx of Salter-Harris I fracture even w/normal radiographs

DIFFERENTIAL DIAGNOSIS

- Ankle sprain
- Syndesmotic (high ankle) sprain
- Distal fibula fracture
- Fifth metatarsal avulsion fracture
- Distal tibia fracture
- Anterior/posterior impingement syndromes
- Peroneal tendon subluxation (rare)
- Osteochondritis dissecans of talus (rare)

TREATMENT

- Rest, ice, compression, elevation (RICE) to ↓ swelling in first 24–48 hrs
- NSAIDs for pain control
- Ambulate early—w/brace/air splint if needed
- Begin rehabilitation w/range of motion exercises progressing to strengthening, proprioception exercises
- Return to play when pain-free functional testing demonstrated
- Salter-Harris I fracture of distal fibula—air splint w/partial weight bearing, usually 3–4 wks healing time

COMPLICATIONS

- Recurrent ankle sprains may result in chronic ankle instability if return to play occurs before full functional recovery achieved
- Chronic ankle instability due to deficient ligaments may give sensation of ankle giving way, may sprain more easily
- Stress view radiographs may be helpful in determining chronic instability—particularly helpful when compared to stress views of uninjured ankle
- Arrest of growth due to growth plate injury—rare w/Salter-Harris I or II

WHEN TO REFER

- Following acute injury, if access to rehabilitation program unavailable in 1° care setting, early referral to physical therapy essential
- Severe sprains, particularly syndesmotic, may require orthopedic referral
- Chronic ankle instability that persists despite full rehabilitation may be referred for further evaluation, definitive treatment
- Orthopedic referral should be considered for any fracture beyond Salter-Harris I
- Salter-Harris I injuries have minimal risk for growth disturbance, do not necessarily need referral if close follow-up can be provided by 1° care physician

OTHER SPORTS-RELATED ANKLE INJURIES

- Injury to ankle syndesmosis ("high ankle sprain"):
  - occurs w/more severe ankle sprains
  - tenderness to palpation between distal tibia and fibula
  - compression of proximal tibia and fibula elicits pain over syndesmosis (between distal tibia and fibula)
  - passive external rotation of ankle w/foot in dorsiflexion elicits pain if syndesmosis involved
  - recovery time for injury may be much longer than w/isolated lateral sprain
- Avulsion fracture—base of fifth metatarsal:
  - occurs w/inversion injury, may be confused w/lateral ankle sprain
  - pop or crack may be heard or felt at time of injury
  - pain, edema usually over base of fifth metatarsal or over peroneus brevis tendon just proximal to its insertion
  - radiographs essential to r/o Jones' fracture (proximal diaphyseal fracture at base of fifth metatarsal) that usually requires surgical intervention
  - avulsion fracture may be treated w/RICE, hard sole shoe, early mobilization and rehabilitation
- Impingement syndromes:
  - posterior capsular impingement:
    ○ seen in dancers from prolonged maintenance of plantarflexion, also in soccer players
    ○ pain deep to Achilles tendon, ↑ by forced plantarflexion (Achilles tendinitis pain ↑ w/dorsiflexion)
    ○ treatment includes NSAIDs, ice, activity modification
    ○ felt pad strapped to back of heel may help prevent forced plantarflexion and impingement
  - anterior capsular impingement:
    ○ acute or gradually ↑ pain over anterior aspect of ankle
    ○ no associated effusion
    ○ often in gymnasts w/repeated marked dorsiflexion associated w/short landings
    ○ treatment includes ice, NSAIDs, activity modification
    ○ felt pad taped anteriorly may prevent forced dorsiflexion as well as provide athlete w/sense of correct position, stance
- Peroneal tendon subluxation:
  - lateral ankle pain due to anterior subluxation of peroneal tendons from posterior fibular groove w/tearing of peroneal retinaculum
  - occurs w/peroneal muscle contraction while foot plantar-flexed inverted
  - activities requiring repetitive equinus position (ie, ballet dancing) may predispose to peroneal tendon pathology
  - pt may report snapping or slipping sensation over lateral malleolus
  - discomfort localized to posterior fibula ~2 cm proximal to distal tip
  - edema, ecchymosis may be seen posterior to fibula
  - examiner may elicit subluxation by observing active eversion or resisting eversion
  - if not diagnosed initially, recurrent dislocations may occur w/minimal trauma
  - treatment usually involves casting for 4–6 wks to prevent recurrence
  - chronic dislocations usually treated surgically
- Osteochondritis dissecans of talus:
  - osteochondral injury from inversion mechanism similar to forces resulting in ankle sprain
  - should be considered in pts w/persistent pain and/or swelling in injured, stable ankle
  - may see osteochondral fracture on initial radiographs
  - most often on anterolateral or posteromedial aspect of talar dome
  - lateral lesions caused by impaction of talus on fibula during inversion and dorsiflexion
  - posteromedial lesions caused by external rotation of tibia on talus due to inversion and plantar flexion
  - OCD lesion should prompt orthopedic referral
  - displaced fragments may require surgical intervention

BACKGROUND

- 10% all athletic injuries in adolescents involve wrist
- Serious ligamentous injury to wrist rare in children
- Fractures, growth plate injuries more common than serious ligamentous injury in youth-age athlete
- *Most common mechanism of injury:* fall onto outstretched hand
- *Sports w/highest injury rates:* football, wrestling, basketball, gymnastics
- More total injuries occur in practice, but rate of injury higher in competition
- Chronic growth plate abnormalities seen in young gymnasts, weight lifters from overuse injury to wrist

CLINICAL MANIFESTATIONS

- Soft tissue edema
- Point tenderness (soft tissue vs. bony), depending on structure(s) injured
- ↓ ROM
- Mild–moderate loss of strength
- Normal sensation, vascularity
- *Snuffbox tenderness:* suspect scaphoid fracture
- *Ulnar grind test:* positive, suspect triangular fibrocartilage complex (TFCC) injury

LABORATORY FEATURES

- AP, lateral, oblique radiographic views of wrist recommended
- Comparison views of uninjured wrist may clarify Dx
- Special views may be required for specific injuries:
    - scaphoid fracture: scaphoid series
    - hook of the hamate fracture: carpal tunnel view
    - scapholunate dissociation: clenched fist view

DIFFERENTIAL DIAGNOSIS

- Fracture:
    - growth plate (radius, ulna)
    - scaphoid
    - triquetrum
    - hamate
- Kienbock disease (osteonecrosis of lunate)
- TFCC injury
- Scapholunate dissociation
- Tendonitis
- Stress-related injury to the distal radial physis

TREATMENT

- *Initial treatment:* rest, ice, compression, elevation (RICE)
- Wrist splinting for comfort
- OTC NSAIDs for pain prn
- Early mobilization, stretching, hand strengthening exercises
- Some scaphoid fractures not apparent on initial radiographs, so thumb spica casting w/repeat radiographs usually 2 wks following injury recommended in questionable cases

COMPLICATIONS

- Unrecognized fractures and/or resultant instability can result in permanent wrist disability; however, rare w/proper recognition, management

PREVENTION

- Wrist guards for inline skating
- Proper sport technique, conditioning

WHEN TO REFER

- Displaced fractures or fractures that provider uncomfortable w/managing
- Scapholunate dissociation
- Kienbock disease
- TFCC injury
- Symptoms that do not substantially improve w/conservative care within 2 wks

BACKGROUND

- *Definition:* congenital anomaly consisting of undescended, small, medially rotated scapula
- Most common congenital anomaly of shoulder girdle
- Associated in 30–50% of cases w/*omovertebral* bone—fibrous, cartilaginous, or osseous bar bridging scapula to posterior spine
- Scapulothoracic motion ↓, but glenohumeral motion remains intact
- Shoulder function compromised, esp in abduction
- May involve neurovascular deficit as result of compression of brachial plexus, subclavian vessels

ASSOCIATED ANOMALIES (SEEN IN TWO-THIRDS OF PTS)

- Failure of cervical spine segmentation (Klippel-Feil syndrome)
- Scoliosis
- Hemivertebra
- Spina bifida
- Renal anomalies
- Muscular hypoplasia (trapezius, serratus anterior, rhomboids, latissimus dorsi)
- Upper extremity/shoulder girdle congenital anomalies

DIAGNOSIS

- Deformity readily recognized on physical examination
- Adjunctive modalities (CT, MRI) may indicate presence of omovertebral bone

SURGICAL TREATMENT

- Not indicated before 3–4 yrs of age
- Only indicated in pts w/significant deformity, disability; best performed in children 4–8 yrs of age
- Simple excision of superior angle of scapula indicated in pts w/mild deformity
- For those w/severe deformity, surgical reposition of scapula, excision of omovertebral bone can be successful in restoring function, improving cosmesis

WHEN TO REFER

- Refer when diagnosis made if significant deformity, disability exists

STEVENS-JOHNSON SYNDROME
WILLIAM L. WESTON

BACKGROUND

- Very uncommon
- Incidence ~0.8 cases/million
- Commonly follows respiratory illness
- Spring/summer prevalence observed
- Hundreds of precipitating factors implicated; drugs predominate

Precipitating factors in SJS

Drugs (NSAIDs, sulfonamides, anticonvulsants, penicillins, doxycycline, tetracycline, others)
Mycoplasma pneumoniae infections
Yersinia infections
Many viruses (enteroviruses, adenoviruses, measles, mumps, influenza, etc)
Many bacteria (streptococcus, typhoid fever, pneumococcus enterobacteria)
Mycobacterium tuberculosis, BCG
Syphilis
Deep fungal infections
X-irradiation
Inflammatory bowel disease

CLINICAL MANIFESTATIONS

- *Distinct prodrome:* URI w/fever, cough, rhinitis, sore throat, headache, vomiting, diarrhea, malaise followed by abrupt onset of extensive areas of epidermal/mucosal necrosis
- Hemorrhagic crusts on lips/purulent conjunctivitis w/photophobia/pseudomembrane formation
- Skin involvement limited to few target-like lesions extensive
- Some develop widespread tender, red/dusky macules (rapidly enlarge/may become confluent)
- Unable to eat/drink; dehydration possible

- Generalized lymphadenopathy usually present, hepatosplenomegaly may be found
- *Genital involvement:* pain, redness, erosions accompanied by bleeding; occasional anal erosions; uncommonly, esophagus respiratory epithelium, nasal mucosa involved

LABORATORY FEATURES

- *Skin biopsy:* large sheets of epidermal necrosis
- Fluid, electrolyte imbalances
- ↑ ESR in 100%
- Leukocytosis in 60%
- Eosinophilia in 20%, leukopenia in 10%
- Anemia in 15%
- ↑ liver enzymes in 15%
- Proteinuria/microscopic hematuria in 5%

DIFFERENTIAL DIAGNOSIS

- Kawasaki disease
- Paraneoplastic pemphigus

TREATMENT

- Severe illness requiring prolonged hospitalization in pediatric ICU/burn center
- Managed as if a burn from inside out
- If an offending drug suspected, discontinue
- Correction of fluid/electrolyte imbalance, monitor urinary output, serum osmolality, electrolytes
- Protect from 2° infection
- Good ophthalmologic care
- Pulmonary toilet to include postural drainage
- Sputum cultures/prompt treatment of pulmonary infections
- Periodic cultures of skin, eyes, mucosal sites

- Caloric replacement
- Early skin grafting of large denuded areas/use of biologic dressings
- Physical Tx to prevent contractures
- Use of antacids/mouth rinses

COMPLICATIONS

- Protracted course 4–6 wks; mortality up to 30%/significant morbidity if child survives
- Frequently complicated by dehydration, electrolyte imbalance, 2° bacterial infection of skin, mucosa, lungs; cutaneous scarring/dyspigmentation
- Extensive areas of denuded skin may scar w/contractures if over joints
- Ocular sequelae serious; include pseudomembrane formation w/immobility of eyelids, symblepharon, entropion, trichiasis, corneal scarring, blindness; lacrimal scarring w/subsequent excessive tearing, anterior uveitis, panophthalmos: rare complications
- Mouth/lip lesions usually heal w/o sequelae; esophageal strictures, anal strictures, vaginal stenosis, urethral mental stenosis may occur
- Severe pneumonitis/pneumothorax may develop 2 wks or later
- Shedding of nails may result in permanent anonychia

WHEN TO REFER

- Child should be admitted to pediatric ICU/burn center where skilled nursing care/multidiscipline team available
- Ophthalmologic, pulmonary, dermatologic consultation obtained

BACKGROUND

- *Definition:* any misalignment or deviation of the two eyes (actually the two visual axes)
- *Prevalence:* up to 5% of children in North America
- Onset birth–6 mos in congenital cases, commonly 2–6 yrs of age in acquired cases
- *Risk factors:* family Hx, cerebral palsy/neurologic disease, structural abnormality affecting vision in one or both eyes
- Amblyopia ("lazy eye") commonly presents either as direct cause of, or as result of untreated strabismus

CLINICAL MANIFESTATIONS

- Esotropia:
  - most common form of strabismus in children
  - may result from one or more factors: accommodative (most common), innervational, mechanical, refractive, genetic
  - often associated w/amblyopia
  - acquired cases often associated w/uncorrected hyperopia (farsightedness)
  - may be worse when child views near targets
- Exotropia:
  - most cases develop during first 4 yrs of life
  - amblyopia uncommon but may occur
  - often starts as intermittent strabismus, then may become constant
  - may initially present when child views distant targets or is fatigued
- Vertical strabismus:
  - may be isolated, or may accompany horizontal strabismus in children
  - most common causes: 1° inferior oblique overaction, dissociated vertical deviation, congenital superior oblique palsy

CLINICAL TESTING

- *Corneal light reflex test (Hirschberg test):* suspect strabismus if light reflex falls on asymmetric portions of cornea of each eye
- *Cover/uncover test:* manifest strabismus (tropia) present if, when fixating eye covered, other (nonfixating) eye moves to pick up fixation. Latent strabismus (phoria) present if no movement of either eye occurs when other covered, but movement seen only when cover removed from either eye (ie, eye drifts while *under* cover)

DIFFERENTIAL DIAGNOSIS

- Pseudoesotropia:
  - eyes appear esotropic
  - no movement of either eye on cover/uncover test
  - typically seen in infants w/wide, flat nasal bridge, epicanthal folds
  - r/o coexisting true strabismus
- Pseudoexotropia:
  - eyes appear exotropic
  - no movement of either eye on cover/uncover testing
  - typically seen w/wide interpupillary distance, or temporal displacement of macula (visual, pupillary axis do not correspond)

TREATMENT

- Complete ophthalmologic examination in all cases
- Neurologic examination including neuroimaging in unusual, esp acquired, nonconcomitant strabismus
- Correction of any contributing structural lesion of eye (eg, congenital cataract, severe ptosis)
- Spectacle correction of any significant refractive error (eg, hyperopia, astigmatism, myopia)
- Vigorous treatment of amblyopia when present (usually patching of better seeing eye)
- Surgery on one or more of extraocular muscles
- Observation, careful follow-up in selected cases of intermittent strabismus

COMPLICATIONS

- Permanent loss of vision from amblyopia, esp if Dx made late (after 4 or 5 yrs of age)
- Failure to achieve or maintain binocularity (use of two eyes together)
- Persistence or reoccurrence of strabismus despite appropriate treatment

WHEN TO REFER

- Any child w/documented or suspected strabismus >2 mos of age
- Any child w/complaint of diplopia (double vision)
- Any pt w/documented risk factors by age 3 yrs, if adequate screening examination inconclusive or not possible
- Preventing, reversing amblyopia, maintaining or gaining binocular vision major reasons for early referral of children w/strabismus

Classification schemes for strabismus

Based on constancy of ocular deviation	Based on age of onset of ocular deviation	Based on relative positions of visual axes of both eyes (usually describes position of nonfixing eye relative to fixing eye)	Based on variation of ocular deviation w/direction of gaze
Manifest strabismus (tropia): deviation always present	Congenital/infantile strabismus: deviation documented <6 mos of age	Esotropia or -phoria: inward or nasal deviation, "cross-eyed"	Comitant (concomitant) strabismus: deviation does not vary w/direction of gaze; most common type
Latent strabismus (phoria): deviation kept under control when both eyes able to fixate a target (fusion)	Acquired strabismus: deviation w/onset documented >6 mos of age	Exotropia or -phoria: outward or temporal deviation, "wall-eyed"	Incomitant (noncomitant) strabismus: deviation varies w/direction of gaze; may be paralytic or restrictive
Intermittent strabismus: deviation sometimes present		Hypertropia or -phoria: upward deviation Hypotropia or -phoria: downward deviation	

STREPTOCERCIASIS

BACKGROUND

- Filarial nematode *Mansonella streptocerca* causative agent
- Occurs mainly in West/Central Africa; may affect chimpanzees
- Transmitted by blood-sucking gnats (Culicoides)
- Microfilaria reside in dermis/epidermis

CLINICAL MANIFESTATIONS

- Mostly asymptomatic
- Pruritus, papular rash, pigmentary changes may occur

DIAGNOSIS

- Recovering microfilaria from skin snips

TREATMENT

- Diethylcarbamazine as for bancrofti filariasis

CUTANEOUS LARVA MIGRANS (CREEPING ERUPTION)

BACKGROUND

- Many parasites causative agents including *Ancylostoma caninum*, *A. ceylonicum*, *A. brasileinses*, *Uncinaria stenocephalia*, *B. phlebotomum;* other parasites may produce same clinical picture including *A. caninum*, *S. stercorales*, *G. spinigerum*
- *A. brasiliensis* infects dogs/cats; adult reaches maturity in hosts; larvae discharged in feces, become filariform/can penetrate human skin

CLINICAL MANIFESTATIONS

- Nonspecific dermatitis at site of penetration usually hands, feet, buttocks
- Creeping begins immediately/weeks/months later
- Threadlike erythematous itchy linear lesions appear at times vesicular
- Parasites travel few millimeters to few centimeters daily; may attain length of 20 cm
- Disease self-limited/usually larvae die in ~4 wks
- Loeffler syndrome may develop ~50% of cases

DIAGNOSIS

- Clinical presentation typical/easily recognized
- Larva currens/migratory myasis/gnathostomiasis must be distinguished

TREATMENT

- Topical 10% thiabendazole effective, avoids use of systemic Tx; applied 2×/d × 1 wk
- Oral thiabendazole as suggested for hookworm
- Albendazole, 400 mg/d × 3 d effective/safe
- 2° bacterial infections should be treated appropriately

VISCERAL LARVA MIGRANS

BACKGROUND

- Roundworms of dogs, cats, carnivores, *Toxicara canis, T. cati, T. leonensis* causative agents
- High incidence of dog infections, particularly in puppies through transplacental/milk transmission
- Humans infected by ingesting eggs from soil/contaminated food, water; children esp susceptible
- Second-stage larvae migrate from intestine to muscle, lung, liver, brain mostly; any part of body can be involved
- Larvae ultimately die/contained in eosinophilic granuloma

CLINICAL MANIFESTATIONS

- Most infections not symptomatic
- Eosinophilia, cough, dyspnea, muscle pains, fever may develop
- Pruritus, urticaria, papular rash of legs/trunk may occur
- Ocular granulomas reported

DIAGNOSIS

- Biopsy of nodule/liver
- Fluorescent antibody/ELISA laboratory studies helpful

TREATMENT

- Thiabendazole/diethylcarbamazine helpful but cures not common

BACKGROUND

- *Pathogen: Streptococcus pyogenes,* also known as group A beta-hemolytic streptococci (GABHS), "strep throat" streptococcus. Causes pharyngitis, impetigo, erysipelas, nonsuppurative sequelae rheumatic fever, glomerulonephritis. Subgroup of strains that produce streptococcal pyrogenic exotoxins (particularly SPE A) more associated w/invasive disease
- *Host:* these infections generally occur in previously healthy children. Predisposing factors may include varicella, minor trauma or penetrating injuries, surgical procedures, burns

CLINICAL SYNDROMES

Soft Tissue/Osteoarticular Infection

- Cellulitis, abscess:
  – commonly occurs as 2° infection of varicella lesions. Suspect in pt w/varicella w/:
    ○ recurrent fever after initial defervescence
    ○ fever continuing >3 d or ↑ fever
    ○ tenderness or large (>2 cm) area of erythema around ≥1 lesions
  – pts often have positive blood cultures
  – may be accompanied by streptococcal toxic shock syndrome (see later)
- Necrotizing fasciitis, deep-seated infection of SubQ tissue w/progressive destruction of fat and fascia; medical, surgical emergency, should be suspected in toxic-appearing pts w/diffuse swelling of body region. Bullae may be apparent, gangrene may eventually appear
- Septic arthritis or osteomyelitis can present alone or in combination w/soft tissue infection
- *Myositis/pyomyositis:* comparatively rare

Pneumonia

- Occurs w/or w/o bacteremia
- Often w/prolonged fever despite antibiotic Tx
- Occurs w/or w/o empyema

Streptococcal Toxic Shock Syndrome

- Presents w/fever, localized pain, flulike symptoms, signs of soft tissue infection
- Probably more common in adults than in children

- Case definition:
  – clinical signs: hypotension *and* multi-organ involvement (at least 2):
    ○ renal dysfunction
    ○ coagulopathy
    ○ liver involvement
    ○ erythroderma
    ○ soft tissue necrosis
  – isolation of GABHS (from normally sterile site = definitive case or from nonsterile site w/o another etiology = probable case)
    ○ may or may not have positive blood culture
    ○ possible association w/ibuprofen usage (in adults)

Bacteremia/Sepsis

- May include purpura fulminans

LABORATORY EVALUATION

- All cases:
  – Gram stain, bacterial culture of lesion drainage or aspirate
  – blood culture (frequently positive in pts w/streptococcal toxic shock syndrome in contrast to pts w/staphylococcal toxic shock syndrome)
  – Gram stain of tissue biopsy
  – anti-streptolysin-O (ASLO) titer
  – in selected cases: analysis of isolate for DNA-encoding pyrogenic exotoxin or pyrogenic exotoxin production (in referral laboratories)
- Toxic shock syndrome:
  – typically leukocytosis, anemia exist; may be hyponatremia
  – organ system dysfunction: abnormalities in liver function tests, serum creatinine, laboratory evidence of disseminated intravascular coagulation

DIFFERENTIAL DIAGNOSIS

- Soft tissue infection:
  – infection due to *Staphylococcus aureus* (particularly in pts w/varicella)
  – necrotizing fasciitis due to anaerobic bacteria or mixed infection w/anaerobic and aerobic bacteria
- *Pneumonia:* based on clinical features, chest radiographic findings, difficult to distinguish from pneumonia due to pneumococcus or *S. aureus.* Prolonged fever common in GABHS pneumonia

- Shock and sepsis:
  – septic shock caused by gram-negative organisms, particularly *Neisseria meningitidis*
  – toxic shock syndrome due to *S. aureus*

MANAGEMENT

- *Antibiotic Tx:*
  – systemic antibiotic Tx: oral antibiotic w/activity against GABHS, *S. aureus* should be administered to any child w/varicella, evidence of 2° bacterial infection or 2° persistent fever
  – pts who appear toxic or have extensive area of cellulitis should be assessed for shock, admitted to hospital for monitoring, IV clindamycin or penicillin (nafcillin). Experimental data, anecdotal reports indicate possible superiority of clindamycin (inhibits protein synthesis, may ↓ toxin production). Some experts use both clindamycin and nafcillin in combination. Empiric antibiotic Tx should also be effective against *S. aureus* (clindamycin or nafcillin). Duration of fever and/or drainage may be prolonged, requiring long-term antibiotic Tx
- *Surgical intervention:*
  – cellulitis can be managed conservatively
  – fasciitis requires aggressive, sometimes extensive surgical debridement in addition to medical Tx
  – if distinguishing between these two entities difficult, biopsy w/frozen section can be performed to determine if extensive surgical debridement necessary
  – CT or MRI may be helpful to assess depth of infection
  – multiple debridements may be required
- IV IgG (IVIG) has resulted in clinical improvement in some cases of streptococcal toxic shock syndrome but not considered standard Tx

PROGNOSIS

- Necrotizing fasciitis has high mortality rate in adults; w/appropriate management, mortality rate in children probably <10%
- Survivors of necrotizing fasciitis frequently require skin grafting
- *Mortality of streptococcal toxic shock syndrome: 30–70%*

BACKGROUND

- *Stuttering:* movement disorder of speech-motor control, characterized by involuntary, audible or silent repetition, or prolongation of sounds, syllables, or words
- Most children experience transient periods of disfluency as they learn to speak. Normal or developmental disfluency persists >6 mos in 4% of children; ~1% of adult population stutter

- M:F ratio equal early in course of disorder, 4:1 by school age
- Stuttering has significant genetic component. Individuals w/neurologic disorders such as stroke have high prevalence of stuttering. Stuttering associated w/other communication problems
- Verbal fluency requires efficient integration of linguistic, motor, cognitive processes. Stuttering may result from anomalous cerebral dominance, atypical interhemispheric connectivity, aberrant subcortical organization, or spasms of articulators. Anxiety exacerbates stuttering but not 1° cause

CLINICAL MANIFESTATIONS

- Physician must differentiate normal or developmental disfluency from stuttering

Characteristics	Normal Disfluency	Mild Stuttering	Severe Stuttering
Age of onset	18 mos–7 yrs; typically resolves by 5 yrs	18 mos–7 yrs; occasionally later onset	18 mos–7 yrs; occasionally later onset
Frequency	<1/10 sentences	≥3% speech	≥10% speech
Duration of disfluency	Brief (<0.5 sec)	Long (0.5–1 sec)	Very long (>1 sec)
Characteristics of repetitions	Repetition of sounds, syllables, or words; word repetition most common	Repetition of sounds, syllables, or words; occasional prolongation of sounds	Repetition of sounds, syllables, or words; frequent prolongation of sounds or blockages
Associated behaviors	Hesitations, pauses, or fillers such as "uh" or "um"	Eyelid closing, blinking, averting eyes, physical tension	Distracting sounds, facial grimaces, head/extremity movements, extra words used to start
Child reactions	None	Little frustration or embarrassment	Embarrassment, fear of speaking, social phobia

Based on Guitar B, Conture EG. The child who stutters: To the pediatrician. Stuttering Foundation of America (1-800-992-9392; www.stutterSFA.org) 1991:1–16

DIFFERENTIAL DIAGNOSIS

- Receptive and/or expressive language disorder, dyslexia, articulation or phonological disorder
- Tic disorder or Tourette syndrome

TREATMENT

- Mainstay of treatment is Tx by qualified speech clinician w/expertise in stuttering
- Treatment improves fluency. Max effects occur in first 6 mos. Relapse common.

Treatment requires three phases: establishment of beneficial techniques, transfer to everyday situations, and maintenance. Impact of treatment related to intensity of program. For adults, establishment and transfer require at least 80–100 hrs

Approach	Description	Effectiveness	Comments
Prolonged speech	Decrease rate of speaking through prolongation of sounds	Effective, short and long term	Delayed auditory feedback may reduce rate further
Rhythm	Use of steady rhythm to pace speech such as w/metronomes	Effective short term	Many individuals abandon technique
Gentle onset speech	Gentle pronunciation of words; less effort in speaking	Improves speaker's, listener's reactions	May not ↓ frequency of stuttering
Gradual increase in length/complexity	Fluency in single syllables, then in longer phrases, sentences	May incorporate other methods to achieve goals	
Anxiety reduction or desensitization	Reduce anxiety, avoidance	Less effective than other traditional techniques	May be used w/other techniques
Operant techniques	Positive, negative reinforcement	Less effective than other traditional techniques	May be used w/other techniques

- Psychopharmacologic approaches have rarely been tested in rigorous double-blind, placebo-controlled trials. No medications restore normal fluency. Haloperidol shown to be effective in reducing frequency, severity of stuttering in >1 double-blind study; however, most subjects discontinued its use because of intolerable side effects. Other agents currently under investigation or producing variable results include clomipramine, serotonin reuptake inhibitor, that reduces unwanted repetitive behavior; bethanechol, acetylcholine analogue; tiapride, dopamine D_2-receptor antagonist that has central and anxiolytic effects; verapamil, calcium channel blocker that relaxes striated muscles of articulators; laryngeal botulinum toxin that reduces spasm of larynx

COMPLICATIONS

- Limited verbal output, anxiety w/speaking, generalized social phobia, chronic trait anxiety
- High absenteeism from school; ↑ grade retention, special schools or classes; ↑ use of medical services

PREVENTION

- Recommendations to parents, teachers may reduce severity, complications: reduce rate of speech to children w/stuttering, remain calm during disfluency, allow child to complete utterance w/o interruption, avoid criticizing or making suggestions such as "Slow down"

WHEN TO REFER

- Observe normal disfluency w/o referral unless parents (or child) become extremely concerned
- Observe mild stuttering for at least 6–8 wks to determine if it will be persistent
- Refer child of any age w/severe stuttering to qualified, experienced speech clinician as soon as possible. Early intervention better than delayed treatment for persistent, severe stuttering

SUBDURAL AND EPIDURAL HEMATOMAS
DAVID M. McKALIP AND STEVEN K. GUDEMAN

BACKGROUND

- Post-traumatic hemorrhages usually subdural or epidural, w/epidural being most common, often after minor head injury
- Possibility of child abuse may be investigated in infants w/intracranial hematomas
- Manifestations of subdural hematoma, epidural hematomas may be similar
- Acute subdural hematomas, epidural hematomas usually have dramatic presentation; chronic subdural hematomas often less dramatic
- Any child should improve 24–84 hrs following minor head injury
- Glasgow coma scale (GCS) should be used to grade level of consciousness (3 worst, 15 best)
- Children's (<4 yrs of age) coma scale (same as for adults, except for verbal score)

Points	Best eye opening	Best verbal response	Best motor response
6	—	—	obeys
5	—	oriented	localizes pain
4	spontaneous	confused	normal flexion
3	to speech	inappropriate words	abnormal flexion (decorticate)
2	to pain	incomprehensible sounds	extension (decerebrate)
1	none	none	none

Points	Best Verbal Response	
5	smiles, oriented to sound, follows objects, interacts	
	If crying:	*If interacting:*
4	consolable	inappropriate
3	inconsistently consolable	moaning
2	inconsolable	restless
1	none	none

CLINICAL MANIFESTATIONS

- Acute subdural and epidural hematomas:
  - Hx direct head injury or acceleration/deceleration injury
  - symptoms: headache, persistent vomiting, ↓ LOC, seizures, hemiparesis
  - possible signs: GCS <15, unilaterally dilated pupil, hemiparesis, sign of basal skull fracture (raccoon's eyes, Battle sign, CSF rhino- or otorrhea)
- Chronic subdural hematomas:
  - may present as above, but often less dramatic
  - usually seen in infants, not older children
  - Hx: child abuse (shaken baby), falls, blows to head, remote Hx meningitis
  - symptoms: megalencephaly, lethargy, seizures
  - possible signs: abnormal ↑ head circumference, GCS <15, anisocoria, hemiparesis

LABORATORY FEATURES

- When to scan:
  - any child w/clinical manifestations or skull fracture following head injury should undergo CT scan to r/o intracranial hemorrhage
  - high index of suspicion warranted in children w/coagulation disorders, CSF shunts, or congenital cerebral malformations, even if head injury minor
- Radiographic features:
  - *common to all:* possible midline shift, compressed ventricle, herniation, compressed sulci (mass effect). Intracerebral hemorrhages of cerebral edema may be present
  - *acute subdural:* usually unilateral. Hyperdense (brighter than brain), concave extraaxial collection, crosses suture lines
  - *chronic subdural:* may be bilateral. As w/acute, but hypodense (darker than brain). Isodense blood (same as brain) may be present if hematoma subacute (7–21 d old)
  - *epidural hematoma:* usually unilateral. Hyperdense, convex mass, respecting suture lines

DIFFERENTIAL DIAGNOSIS

- Consistent w/features of acute subdural or epidural hematoma:
  - seizure, contusion, intracerebral, hemorrhage, intracranial tumor, acute hydrocephalus, metabolic abnormality, drug overdose/poisoning, meningitis
- Consistent w/features of chronic subdural hematoma:
  - hydrocephalus, intracranial tumor, seizures, meningitis

MANAGEMENT

- In all cases, evaluation by neurosurgeon required
- Acute subdural and epidural hematomas:
  - nearly all require immediate, surgical evacuation by craniotomy and postop monitoring in ICU
  - small hematomas, w/mild clinical signs, no significant mass effect on CT may merely warrant close monitoring, may resolve
- Chronic subdural hematomas:
  - larger hematomas require drainage through burr holes
  - in stable pts w/no symptoms other than megalencephaly, percutaneous needle drainage may be performed
  - may require subdural to peritoneal shunt
  - fluid should be sent for culture to r/o infection

WHEN TO REFER

- If extraaxial hematoma diagnosed, neurosurgical evaluation required
- If CT scanner not available, pt should be transferred to center w/scanner

SUDDEN INFANT DEATH SYNDROME (SIDS)

ALAN R. SPITZER

BACKGROUND

- Sudden infant death syndrome (SIDS) refers to sudden, unexpected death of infant 1 mo–1 yr of age not explained by postmortem examination of child, by review of medical Hx, or from investigation of scene of death
- Leading cause of death 1 mo–1 yr of age (postneonatal mortality)
- Produces ~3,000–6,000 deaths/y in US, or ~0.8 deaths/1,000 live births
- Most frequently occurs 2–4 mos postnatal age in term infants, w/peak incidence ~52 wks postconceptional age for premature babies
- Usually occurs during sleep; most deaths unobserved by caretakers

EPIDEMIOLOGY

- Following epidemiologic factors appear to ↑ risk:
  - low birth weight
  - low Apgar scores
  - maternal factors: young maternal age; maternal smoking; lack of prenatal care; low education level; unmarried mothers; maternal substance abuse (in some studies)
  - cold-weather months in temperate climates
  - viral illnesses, minor infections in week prior to death
  - bottle feeding
  - ethnicity: more common in Native American, Native Alaskan, African American, Hispanic populations than in Caucasian or Asian American populations
  - siblings of SIDS victims
  - children w/apparent life-threatening events (ALTE)

PROPOSED MECHANISMS

- By definition, SIDS has no "cause." If death can be explained, not "SIDS death"
- Possible mechanisms for SIDS (none substantiated) include:
  - abnormal brain stem anatomy and/or function
  - apnea of infancy
  - defects in thermoregulation
  - gastroesophageal reflux
  - cardiovascular disorders (prolonged Q-T interval)
  - inborn errors of metabolism (medium chain acyl-CoA dehydrogenase deficiency)
  - altered chemoreceptor sensitivity
  - abnormal airway anatomy or obstruction
  - chronic hypoxemia
  - inadequate arousal mechanism

POSTMORTEM/DEATH SCENE FINDINGS

- Face-down position
- Usually well nourished
- Normal weight gain for age
- Stool or urine in diaper
- Cyanosis, pallor
- Blood-tinged oral secretions
- Pulmonary congestion
- Intrathoracic petechiae
- Laryngeal fibrinoid necrosis
- Prominent lymph nodes
- Apparent thermal stress (overbundling, high room heat) in some cases
- Soft bedding (polystyrene pillows) may prevent airway clearance

DIFFERENTIAL DIAGNOSIS

- Sepsis
- Pneumonia
- Congenital heart disease/cardiac arrhythmia
- Accidental suffocation
- Child abuse/neglect/homicide
- Shaken baby syndrome
- Poisoning

MANAGEMENT

- Obviously no treatment once child has died from SIDS. Prevention everything
- Management of family who has lost child to SIDS extremely important because overwhelming grief, guilt common. Appropriate counseling, Tx extremely helpful. Parent support groups may be valuable in providing comfort, reassurance to families. In addition, older siblings of deceased infant may require special counseling in order to cope w/death of brother or sister
- Physician who cares for these families should consider referring to center that evaluates children for ALTE or subsequent siblings of SIDS victims; questions often arise about risk to future offspring
- Value of home cardiorespiratory monitoring of subsequent siblings has not been established, but may have medical importance for certain infants, psychological value for parents of SIDS victims. Evaluation of subsequent siblings, treatment w/monitoring, however, best carried out within well-defined program of care
- Apparent measure of greatest value for SIDS prevention places normal newborn infants in supine, not prone, position for sleep. Numerous studies from around world indicate this approach significantly ↓ incidence. Elimination of smoking during pregnancy, in home environment also appears to have additional benefits

WHEN TO REFER

- If living child has had ALTE
- For evaluation of subsequent siblings and possible home monitoring
- For parental counseling and support

BACKGROUND

- Suicide third leading cause of death in persons aged 15–24 yrs, accounting for 1/7 deaths
- Since 1950, rate of suicide ↑ 400% for persons 15–19 yrs of age, nearly 600% for persons 10–14 yrs of age
- Ratio of attempted to complete youth suicides reported from 50:1 to 200:1
- Although only 1/8,000 youths complete suicide each year, among high school students, 1/10–1/20 report attempting suicide, 1/5 report serious consideration of suicide, almost half report thinking about suicide

CLINICAL MANIFESTATIONS

- Completed suicide infrequent to rare in individual practice but all providers of pediatric, adolescent health care will have:
  - pts who have attempted suicide
  - pts at significant risk for suicidal behavior
  - pts w/relative or friend who has committed suicide
  - requests for assistance when school or community experiences youth suicide
- Completed suicide 5× more often in boys, attempted suicide 5× more often in girls
- Completed suicide most often involves firearms; attempted suicide most often involves ingestion of drugs, other harmful products
- Hanging, jumping from heights, running into traffic are other methods, esp in younger children

ASSESSMENT OF RISK FOR SUICIDAL BEHAVIOR

- Associated risk factors and signals:
  - any previous suicide attempts
  - direct communication of intent—verbal, written
  - indirect communication—writing a will, giving away possessions
  - symptoms of depression—sleep problems, appetite problems, somatic symptoms, withdrawal from activities and people
  - substance abuse
  - conduct disorder
  - psychotic disorders
  - multiple, chronic stressors
  - family Hx suicide
- Specific vulnerabilities:
  - sexually abused youth
  - delinquent/incarcerated youth
  - sexual-minority youth (eg, gay/lesbian/bisexual
  - Native American youth
  - runaway/homeless youth
  - very high-achieving youth
  - impulsive youth
- Precipitating events:
  - loss of loved one—death, abandonment, moving away
  - breakup of relationship
  - interpersonal or family conflict
  - school problems
  - anniversary of a loss
  - recent media coverage of a suicide—prominent person, youth
- Protective factors:
  - willingness/ability to seek help
  - commitment to abstain from self-harm (contract)
  - ability to identify, express feelings
  - identification of alternative means of coping w/problems
  - availability of supportive, supervisory adults
  - nonavailability of methods (no guns, no dangerous drugs, no blades)

INTERVENTION BASED ON RISK PROFILE

- *Low risk:* enlist support of family, consider professional counseling, follow-up w/health-care provider weekly to resolution:
  - ambivalence about desire to die, no plan
  - no prior attempts
  - no substance abuse or other major psychiatric illness
- *Moderate risk:* timely referral to mental health provider, follow-through:
  - Hx suicide attempt(s)
  - psychiatric Hx, substance abuse
  - plan vague, limited feasibility, method unavailable
- *High risk:* immediate psychiatric evaluation, possibly at ER or crisis center; consider hospitalization for evaluation:
  - psychotic thinking, hallucinations
  - major depression
  - unremitting crisis
  - clear plan, methods readily available
  - lack or rejection of family support or other resources

SUNBURN

BERNARD A. COHEN

BACKGROUND

- Represents delayed inflammatory reaction from ultraviolet light injury to skin
- UVB (290–320 nm) primarily involved
- Light-complected individuals burn at temperate latitudes in midday summer sun in 15–20 min, quicker in south
- Risk ↑ w/low humidity, wind, ↑ elevation, reflection from snow, sand, water

MANIFESTATIONS

- Sun-exposed sites only
- Bright red erythema appears in 3–5 h, peak in 12–24 h, subsides in 3–4 d
- Occasionally blistering
- Initial tenderness, then pruritus, healing w/hyperpigmentation (tan), desquamation
- Headache, fever, chills, abdominal pain, dehydration in severe widespread burns

LABORATORY FEATURES

- Nonspecific findings; similar for thermal burns in severe cases
- Epidermal spongiosis, sunburn cells, dermal vasodilatation; edema, mixed infiltrate on skin biopsy

DIFFERENTIAL DIAGNOSIS

- Staphylococcal scalded skin syndrome
- Toxic epidermal necrolysis
- Drug-induced erythroderma (generalized erythema, scale)
- Drug-induced phototoxicity (exaggerated sunburn reaction)
- Photo-contact dermatitis (eg, PABA hypersensitivity)
- Photo-sensitivity disorders (polymorphous light eruption, subacute cutaneous lupus erythematosus, porphyria)
- Photo-exacerbated dermatoses (eg, some atopics)

TREATMENT

- Sun avoidance
- Symptomatic treatment: cool tap water compresses, baths; NSAIDs, oral fluids, topical steroids in nonblistered areas, topical antibiotics in blistered areas
- Burn unit management for severe widespread cases

COMPLICATIONS

- *Acute burns:* infection, occasionally scarring, altered pigmentation
- *Chronic, recurrent burning:* melanoma, nonmelamona skin cancers
- Freckles, lentigines, pigmented nevi, wrinkling, other actinic skin changes

PREVENTION

- Sunscreens, sunblocks

$$\text{SPF:} \quad \frac{\text{Time in sun to burn w/sunscreen}}{\text{Time in sun to burn w/o sunscreen}}$$

- SPF 15–30 esp for light-complected individuals
- *Sun-protective clothing:* hats, tightly woven fabrics
- Avoid midday sun esp in summer
- Suntan parlor tan, chemical-induced tan, oral vitamins, PABA of little value

WHEN TO REFER

- Severe, extensive burns
- Persistent sunburn reaction

SUPRAVENTRICULAR TACHYCARDIA

JAMES P. LOEHR

BACKGROUND

- Most common symptomatic tachycardia in childhood
- Predisposing factors (myocarditis, congenital heart disease, hyperthyroidism) more common if initial episode >9 mos of age

CLINICAL MANIFESTATIONS

- Infants may have CHF or shock
- Complaints in infancy often nonspecific (poor feeding, irritability)
- Children, young adults present w/palpitations, pallor, or dizziness, or may have no symptoms

LABORATORY FEATURES

- Paroxysmal in onset and termination
- Rate 160–350 bpm
- QRS complex usually narrow (if QRS complex wide, strongly consider ventricular tachycardia)

- P waves may not be visible; P axis usually abnormal if present

DIFFERENTIAL DIAGNOSIS

- *Sinus tachycardia:* QRS complex usually narrow, rate usually <230/min but may be as rapid as 260/min. P waves w/normal axis present. Rate slows gradually (nonparoxysmal). 1° concern in neonate w/rapid sinus tachycardia is sepsis; fever, dehydration also causative
- *Ventricular tachycardia:* QRS complex usually wide; atrioventricular dissociation present
- *Atrial flutter:* QRS complex usually narrow. Atrial rate rapid w/variable degree of atrioventricular block, producing beat-to-beat variation in QRS rhythm. Flutter waves seen on 12 lead electrocardiogram
- *Atrial fibrillation, atrial ectopic tachycardia, junctional ectopic tachycardia:* rare in childhood ambulatory setting

TREATMENT

- *Acute:* treat cardiogenic shock if present; perform 12 lead electrocardiogram
- Chronic:
  - high frequency of recurrence after acute conversion of SVT
  - obtain 12 lead electrocardiogram after conversion to sinus rhythm
  - examine for precipitating factors; consider chest x ray, echocardiogram
  - if Wolff-Parkinson-White syndrome not present, use digoxin:
- Give one-half digitalizing dose × 1 followed by one-quarter digitalizing dose q8–12h × 2. Maintenance dose div bid. If given IV, reduce dose 20–25%; administer over 10 min. Use w/caution in myocarditis, renal failure
- Verapamil, 3–6 mg/kg/day po, can ↑ digoxin level
- If Wolff-Parkinson-White syndrome present, propranolol, 2–6 mg/kg/day po div tid–qid

Treatment	Dose	Comments
Vagal maneuvers	Ice bag to face, gag reflex, rectal stimulation	Use only if shock not present, or if use will not delay other Tx
Adenosine	35–70 µg/kg IV; repeat q1–2min increasing to max 200–300 µg/kg (max adult dose 12 mg)	*Rapid* IV bolus through well-functioning IV; may exacerbate asthma; prolonged asystole possible
Synchronized cardioversion	0.25–2 joules/kg; sedation recommended	Hazardous in digoxin toxicity (hazard may be reduced by prior administration of lidocaine)
Verapamil	0.075 mg/kg IV; may repeat 1× in 15 min	Contraindicated in infants <1 yr of age (hypotension); use w/caution or not at all after beta blocker Tx

Digoxin Administration

Age	PO Digitalizing Dose (µg/kg/day) (max 1.25 mg)	PO Maintenance Dose (µg/kg/day) (max 0.25 mg/d)
Premature infant	20	5
<2 mos	30	8–10
2 mos–2 yrs	40–50	10–12
>2 yrs	30–40	8–10

COMPLICATIONS

- Cardiogenic shock in infants
- Drugs used for treatment have proarrhythmic effects
- Recurrent episodes common

PREVENTION

- Chronic drug Tx as described above
- Older pts can improve control of tachycardia w/vagal maneuvers
- Invasive electrophysiologic procedures often effective in preventing further episodes, eliminating need for drug Tx

WHEN TO REFER

- Consult pediatric cardiologist for all new pts w/SVT to confirm Dx, r/o underlying disorders
- Hospitalize pts w/Hx cardiovascular instability (shock, hypotension, syncope, presyncope) for observation, inpt consultation

BACKGROUND

- Infection caused by spirochete, *Treponema pallidum*
- Highest incidence in urban areas
- Risk factors include cocaine use during pregnancy, poor prenatal care, low socioeconomic status
- Highest risk in infants born to mothers w/1°, 2° syphilis
- Transmission from infected mother to unborn fetus occurs anytime during pregnancy; primarily occurs hematogenously/transplacentally. Rarely, transmission may occur at time of delivery through birth canal from contact w/infectious lesions
- Neonates should be considered infected if mother inadequately treated, mother adequately treated but antibody titers have not declined by fourfold (ie, two tube dilution), mother treated <30 d prior to delivery, and/or if infant's serum titer at least 4× higher than mother's titer

CLINICAL MANIFESTATIONS

- Frequently asymptomatic (60%)
- Low birth weight
- Prematurity
- Mucocutaneous lesions, loss of hair, fissures in lips/nares/anus
- *Snuffles:* profuse, persistent, nasal drainage
- Tachypnea should raise suspicion of associated pneumonia
- Hepatosplenomegaly; may see jaundice
- Lymphadenopathy, generalized
- Maculopapular rash
- Periostitis, osteochondritis
- Late findings, typically occurring after 2 yrs:
  – rhagades, mulberry molars, Clutton joints, Hutchinson triad (Hutchison teeth—notched upper central incisors, interstitial keratitis, eighth nerve deafness), saber shins, saddle nose, Higouménakis sign

LABORATORY FEATURES

- Hemolytic, Coombs negative anemia
- Thrombocytopenia
- Abnormal liver function tests

- Serum rapid plasma reagin (RPR) test/ Venereal Disease Research Laboratory test (VDRL):
  – typically positive in mother, confirmed by positive treponemal test (MHATP: microhemagglutinin assay for antibiotics to *T. pallidum*); if maternal infection occurred late in pregnancy, RPR/VDRL (often obtained early in pregnancy) may be negative. RPR/VDRLs obtained late in pregnancy or at time of delivery most useful
  – variable in newborn; therefore, must interpret w/maternal results. Neonate may not have mounted antibody response, and/or placental transfer of antibodies may have been incomplete
- *Cord rapid plasma reagin (cRPR) test:* false positive (up to 10%), false negative (up to 5%) results occur. RPR should be performed on infant's serum when syphilis suspected
- *VDRL test on CSF:* should be performed in all neonates w/suspected syphilis infection; high specificity, poor sensitivity. Other nontreponemal, treponemal tests should not be used on CSF
- May see mononuclear pleocytosis, ↑ protein on CSF analysis
- Darkfield microscopy, direct fluorescent antibody testing may be performed on specimens from skin lesions, lymph nodes, placenta, umbilical cord
- Chest radiographs should be obtained when pneumonia suspected
- Long-bone radiographs (abnormal in up to 20% of asymptomatic neonates, 65% of symptomatic neonates) help r/o bony manifestations, including metaphyseal osteochondritis, diaphyseal periostitis

DIFFERENTIAL DIAGNOSIS

- *Herpes simplex* virus infection
- Toxoplasmosis
- CMV infection
- Congenital rubella infection
- Bacterial sepsis

TREATMENT

- Treat all neonates w/suspected syphilis and/or if infant's CSF abnormal

- *Aqueous crystalline penicillin G:* 100,000–150,000 U/kg/d IV div bid or tid 10–14 d; 200,000–300,000 U/kg/d div qid for neonates >4 wks of age
- Repeat serologic tests in positive neonates at age 3, 6, 12 mos until test nonreactive. If no ↓ in titers by 3 mos of age, consider retreatment
- Repeat CSF evaluation q6mos for neonates w/neurosyphilis

COMPLICATIONS

- Stillbirth, spontaneous abortion, perinatal death (40% of pregnancies in untreated women)
- Hydrops fetalis
- Intrauterine growth retardation
- Nephrosis
- Disseminated intravascular coagulation
- Pseudoparalysis of Parrot
- Cranial nerve palsies
- Hearing loss (may not be apparent until 10–40 yrs of age)
- Interstitial keratitis (may not be apparent until 5–20 yrs of age)
- Cerebral infarction
- Seizure disorder
- Mental retardation

PREVENTION

- Perform prenatal screening for syphilis early in pregnancy and at 28 wks gestation, time of delivery in high-risk pts
- Treat infected, pregnant women
- Counsel on safe sex practices, STDs in women of childbearing age, pregnant women
- Report cases to the local Department of Health
- Avoid discharging newborns from hospital w/o knowing mother's serologic status for syphilis

WHEN TO REFER

- Consultation w/infectious disease specialist recommended for neurosyphilis, or when results of maternal or infant sera difficult to interpret

BACKGROUND

• Acquired syphilis an infection caused by spirochete *Treponema pallidum,* acquired by sexual contact w/open moist cutaneous or mucocutaneous ulcerations, or the rash, usually in first year of infection. Rare in children; more common in sexually active adolescents and adults

CLINICAL MANIFESTATIONS

• Syphilis has stages:
– 1° syphilis: 10–90 d after exposure:
  ○ ≥1 painless macule that progresses to papule, then painless ulcer (chancre) at site of sexual contact, often in genital or rectal area that heals w/o treatment in 3–6 wks
    ○ painless regional lymphadenopathy
– 2° syphilis: 3–6 wks after chancre; may be recurrent. May have some of following:
  ○ almost any type of rash, esp palms, soles (7–100%)
  ○ generalized lymphadenopathy (50–80%)
  ○ mucosal ulceration (6–30%)
  ○ fever
  ○ malaise
  ○ headache
  ○ arthralgia
  ○ sore throat
  ○ patchy hair loss
  ○ thinning of the hair
  ○ loss of outer half of eyebrows, eyelashes, or beard
    ○ mucous patches in mouth
    ○ moist fleshy smooth or warty papules (condyloma lata)
– latent syphilis: for many years asymptomatic
– 3° syphilis: ~15 yrs after 2° syphilis:
  ○ aortitis
  ○ gumma of skin, bone, viscera
  ○ neurosyphilis
• Other considerations: stages may progress much faster in HIV-infected pts

DIFFERENTIAL DIAGNOSIS

• 1° syphilis:
– genital ulcers, anorectal lesions
– herpes simplex, trauma, scabies
– 2° syphilis, furuncles, herpes zoster
– erosive balantitis, drug eruption
– chancroid, Reiter syndrome, Stevens-Johnson syndrome, Behcet syndrome
• 2° syphilis:
– viral, drug rashes
– pityriasis rosea, EBV, CMV, HIV infections
– Hodgkin disease, lymphoma

LABORATORY FEATURES

• Dark field examination of serum from abraded chancres for spirochetes in 1° syphilis
• Nontreponemal serum antibody [rapid plasma reagin RPR, or venereal disease research laboratory (VDRL) test]. Positive 14 d after chancre seen. False positives in TB, EBV infection, endocarditis, parenteral drug use, collagen disease. Use VDRL on CSF
• Treponemal antibody test (if nontreponemal antibody test positive). Use fluorescent treponemal antibody absorbed (FTA-ABS), microhemagglutination-treponema pallidum (MHA-TP), or treponema pallidum immobilization test (TPI). Positive at time of chancre. False positives: leptospirosis, Lyme disease, rat bite fever
• CSF examination, CSF VDRL if syphilis >1 y or symptoms of neurologic involvement

TREATMENT

• 1°, 2°, or latent syphilis <1 y:
– benzathine penicillin G, 50,000 U/kg IM (not >2.4 million U) once
– if penicillin allergic (except in pregnancy), doxycycline, 100 mg bid po × 14 d
– if penicillin allergic in pregnancy, desensitize, treat w/penicillin: 4 mg/kg/day (maximum 200 mg) given orally bisd × 14 days. Consult expert

• Latent syphilis >1 yr (if CSF normal):
– benzathine penicillin G as above, but give weekly ×3 or doxycycline as above but for 4 wks
• 3° syphilis, neurosyphilis, or syphilis in AIDS pt:
– consult expert
• Follow-up of treatment:
– 1°, 2°, or latent syphilis <1 yr:
  ○ if pregnant, repeat serum RPR or VDRL monthly
  ○ if not pregnant, repeat serum RPR or VDRL at 3, 6, 12 mos
– latent syphilis >1 y:
  ○ if CSF normal, repeat above tests at 3, 6, 9, 12, 24 mos
  ○ if CSF abnormal, repeat above tests q6mos; reevaluate CSF for at least 3 y if abnormal or until normal
• Retreat as for syphilis >1 yr if:
– symptoms recur or persist
– RPR or VDRL titer ↑ fourfold, esp if pregnant
– RPR or VDRL titer does not ↓ fourfold in 1y
– RPR or VDRL titer does not ↓ fourfold in 3 mos if pregnant w/1° or 2° syphilis, or 6 mos if latent syphilis
• Other considerations:
– report, evaluate sexual contacts
– in children w/syphilis, evaluate for sexual abuse
– evaluate all pts w/syphilis for HIV

PREVENTION

• Abstinence or condoms

WHEN TO REFER

• Consultation with infectious disease expert often useful

BACKGROUND

- *Definition:* episodic multisystem autoimmune disease characterized by inflammation of blood vessels, connective tissue
- ~ incidence 0.53–0.6/100,000 in children, rare <5 yrs of age (except in neonatal lupus) w/↑ incidence throughout adolescence to reach peak incidence in early 20s, F:M ratio 4.5:1 in childhood onset, most common in children of black, Hispanic, Asian origin
- Etiology unknown except in drug-induced cases. Studies suggest role for genetic susceptibility, immune dysregulation, hormonal factors, environmental factors such as infection, photosensitivity

CLINICAL MANIFESTATIONS

- American College of Rheumatology outlined 11 criteria for classification of disease, classification used for inclusion into studies (see table)
- Most common clinical manifestations at Dx: nephritis (84%), arthritis (72%), dermatitis (70%), constitutional symptoms: fever, malaise, weight loss (90%)
- Disease course can range from insidious and chronic to acute, rapidly fatal
- Skin involvement varied, ranges from butterfly rash occurring from malar eminencies over bridge of nose (33%), generalized dermatitis, photosensitivity, oral ulcers, Raynaud phenomena to chronic, scaring discoid lupus lesions on the scalp, face
- Arthritis can involve all joints but commonly involves small joints of hand, feet. Nondeforming
- Nephritis characterized by proteinuria, nephrotic syndrome, hematuria, casts, ↓ renal function
- Cardiopulmonary disease results in serosistis w/pericardial/pleural effusions, pneumonitis, cardiomegaly, myocarditis
- CNS disease most often manifested by psychosis, seizures, headaches
- Vasculitis of small (palpable purpura, cytoid bodies in retina) and medium (coronary arteries, stroke) vessels occurs
- Neonatal lupus manifested by complete heart block, rash, thrombocytopenia in infant born to affected but often asymptomatic mother

LABORATORY FEATURES

- *Hematologic (40–50%):* anemia (normocytic, hypochromic), leukopenia (<4.5 WBC/mm^3), thrombocytopenia (<150,000 platelets/mm^3)
- Low CH_{50}, C_3, C_4 often represent active disease
- Antinuclear antibodies present in sera of majority of cases but not diagnostic (see table). Results reported as titer and pattern. Patterns reported are related to distinct antigens found in cell nucleus being recognized by antibodies in pt's serum
- Antinative DNA antibody, anti-smith antibody or Sm (30%) are marker antibodies but not seen in all cases
- Anti Ro (SSA) and anti La (SSB) antibodies present in neonatal lupus; also seen in pediatric lupus, other connective tissue diseases
- UA abnormal w/proteinuria, RBCs and other casts

DIFFERENTIAL DIAGNOSIS

- Lupus can mimic many diseases such as infections, malignancy, other connective tissue diseases
- Drug-induced lupus in childhood commonly seen in association w/antiseizure medications

TREATMENT

- Varies according to severity of organ involvement
- NSAIDs for musculoskeletal involvement
- Hydroxychloroquinine (6 mg/kg) for cutaneous disease, adjunct to corticosteroid use for systemic disease
- *Corticosteroids:* po up to 1–2 mg/kg/d or IV depending on severity of situation
- *Immunosuppressives:* azathiaprine, methotrexate for steroid-sparing effect and IV cyclophosphamide, 500–1,000 mg/m²/mo for diffuse proliferative nephritis

COMPLICATIONS

- Nephritis major long-term determinant of outcome; ~80% 10 yr survival
- Mortality 2° to renal failure, unusual infections in immunocompromised host, vascular disease, encephalopathy
- *Morbidity:* dialysis, transplantation, neuropsychiatric dysfunction, atherosclerosis, recurrent infections, malignancy, osteoporosis, cataracts, infertility, fetal wastage, avascular necrosis

ACR criteria for Systemic Lupus Erythematosus*

Malar (butterfly rash)
Discoid rash
Photosensitivity
Oral or nasal mucocutaneous ulcerations
Nonerosive arthritis
Nephritis (proteinuria >0.5 g/d; cellular cast)
Encephalopathy (seizures, psychosis)
Pleuritis/pericarditis
Cytopenia
Positive serology (antibodies to native DNA, Sm, phospholipid and false positive tests for syphilis)
Positive antinuclear antibody test

*Four of 11 criteria provide sensitivity of 96% and specificity of 96%.
Adapted from Tan EM, Cohen AS, Fries JF, et al: The 1982 revised criteria for the classification of systemic lupus erythematosus. Arthritis Rheum 25(11): 1271–1277, 1982

Causes for positive antinuclear antibody

Normal healthy children (low titer, relative of person w/SLE, ↑ w/age)
Infectious (viral, bacterial, TB, parasite)
Malignancy (lymphoma, leukemia)
Hematologic (ITP, autoimmune hemolytic anemia)
Hepatic (chronic active hepatitis, 1° biliary cirrhosis)
Pulmonary (idiopathic pulmonary fibrosis)
Miscellaneous (diabetes, thyroiditis)
Drug induced
Rheumatic disease (SLE, JRA, myositis, Sjögren syndrome, scleroderma vasculitis)

WHEN TO REFER

- Referral indicated if Dx not clear for management of major organ involvement or if steroids and/or immunosuppressives to be used as part of management

BACKGROUND

- Congenital foot deformity, w/dislocation of navicular dorsally onto dorsal neck of talus; also known as convex pes valgus
- Etiology unknown
- May be isolated deformity; 40–50% of pts in all reported series have associated abnormality—cerebral palsy, arthrogryposis, myelomeningocele, or other musculoskeletal problems

CLINICAL MANIFESTATIONS

- "Rocker-bottom" foot, w/abducted, dorsiflexed forefoot, equinus hindfoot, and bony prominence in plantar aspect of midfoot; not clinically reducible
- Usually apparent at birth, but may be obscured by usual infant fat pad in longitudinal arch area

LABORATORY FEATURES

- Dx made by lateral radiograph taken w/foot plantar flexed; forefoot (axis of first metatarsal [MT]) should align w/hindfoot (axis of talus)
- Dorsiflexion view confirms usual equinus position of hindfoot (which may vary in severity), but not diagnostic alone

DIFFERENTIAL DIAGNOSIS

- Can be confused at birth w/calcaneovalgus foot, which lies in dorsiflexion, often apposing anterior tibia, but has flexible midfoot, demonstrable or palpable longitudinal arch w/o midfoot plantar prominence. If pt has active plantar flexors, calcaneovalgus foot almost always spontaneously resolves
- In older children, esp those w/neuromuscular disorder, CVT can be confused w/flexible flat foot, or w/foot w/oblique talus, which may appear "vertical" on weight-bearing lateral radiograph; in oblique talus plantar-flexion lateral x ray demonstrates complete reduction of forefoot, w/alignment of first MT and talar longitudinal axes. (Pts w/oblique talus may also have tight Achilles tendon, producing less flexible foot, and may need Achilles lengthening, but lateral plantar-flexion x ray remains diagnostic key)

TREATMENT

- Surgical reduction necessary for correction; usually done age 6–12 mos
- Manipulation, serial casting (weekly until 2 mos old, then q2 wks) can stretch skin, prepare for operation, but only very rare instances of true vertical talus reduce fully w/casting alone

COMPLICATIONS

- Untreated CVT not usually painful in young children, but becomes uncomfortable or painful when pt large enough to produce sufficient weight per square inch on small weight-bearing prominence in midfoot
- Footwear difficult to fit, deforms, or wears out rapidly
- Delayed correction may require fusion in addition to reduction, producing less flexible foot w/some risk of persistent or recurring long-term symptoms

WHEN TO REFER

- When condition suspected, refer to orthopedic surgeon (preferably pediatric). If necessary, obtain x rays first, but be sure to include plantar- and dorsiflexion lateral views, as well as weight-bearing AP and lateral, and send w/pt

BACKGROUND

- General:
  - oldest recognized affliction of humans
  - sizes: 2 cm–25–30 m in length
  - consist of scolex, multiple proglottid segments
  - adult worms lumenal parasites; well tolerated w/minimal symptoms
  - infection w/larval stage often causes serious disease
- Diphyllobothriasis (*D. latum*):
  - infection due to eating raw, insufficiently cooked, or lightly pickled fish containing plerocercoid larval stage
  - common in many ethnic groups where raw or lightly pickled fish considered delicacy
  - 9–10 million people infected worldwide
  - worm has high avidity for B_{12} (absorbs 80% of administered oral dose)
  - large tapeworm: 3–12 m long, w/3,000–4,000 proglottid segments
- Hymenolepiasis:
  - *H. nana*:
    - occurs most frequently in children
    - ↑ prevalence in institutions for mentally retarded, chronic care psychiatric hospitals
    - infection by ingestion of eggs from feces of infected individuals
    - smallest adult tapeworm, 25–30 mm long w/175 proglottid segments
  - *H. dimunata*:
    - rarely infects humans; usually parasite of rodents
    - of 200 reported human cases most have been in children <3 yrs of age
    - infection by ingestion of cysticercoid (larval) stage in insects (rat fleas, mealworms, cockroaches) found in dry grains, cereals, flour
    - size 10–60 cm w/80–1,000 proglottid segments
- Dipylidiasis (*D. caninum*):
  - parasite of dogs, cats, wild carnivores that occasionally infects humans
  - most infections have occurred in children <8 yrs of age, one-third in children <6 mos of age; believed to be due to close association of children and pets
  - infection by ingestion of cysticercoid (larval) stage in fleas
  - size 15–20 cm w/60–175 proglottid segments
- Taeniasis (*T. solium, T. saginata*):
  - infection by ingestion of cysticercoid larva in beef (*T. saginata*) or pork (*T. solium*)
  - *T. saginata* 4–12 m w/1,000–2,000 proglottid segments
  - *T. solium* 2–8 m w/1,000 proglottid segments
- Cysticercosis (*T. solium*):
  - infection by ingestion of eggs of *T. solium* in food or water contaminated w/feces of humans harboring adult worms
  - larva encyst in muscle, brain of infected humans
  - larva can persist 10–20 yrs
- Echinococcus (*E. granulosus*):
  - parasite of dogs (adult worm), herbivores such as sheep (larval stage)
  - infection in humans by ingestion of eggs contaminating food, water
  - adult worms not seen in humans, only larval stage
  - larva develop into hydatid cysts usually in liver
  - *E. multilocularis* or *E. vogeli* can also infect humans

CLINICAL MANIFESTATIONS

- Diphyllobothriasis (*D. latum*):
  - most pts asymptomatic
  - rarely: vague abdominal pain, bloating sore tongue or gums, hives, headache, change in appetite (↑ or ↓)
  - passage of large segments or worm
  - low B_{12} levels in serum (40% of pts)
  - megaloblastic anemia in 2% of pts due to B_{12} deficiency
  - neurologic symptoms due to B_{12} deficiency: weakness, numbness, paresthesias, disturbances of mobility/coordination
- Hymenolepiasis:
  - *H. nana*:
    - often asymptomatic
    - young children most commonly complain of diffuse abdominal pain
    - other reported symptoms include diarrhea w/mucus, pruritus ani and nasi, urticaria, loose bowel movements
  - *H. dimunata*:
    - most asymptomatic

- occasional vague abdominal pain
- Dipylidiasis (*D. caninum*):
  - often asymptomatic
  - occasional abdominal pain, diarrhea, urticaria, pruritus ani
- Taeniasis (*T. solium, T. saginata*):
  - often asymptomatic
  - occasional abdominal pain, diarrhea, urticaria
  - spontaneous passage of proglottid segments can give sensation of fecal incontinence
- Cysticercosis (*T. solium*):
  - 50% of infected humans asymptomatic
  - seizures most common presenting symptom
  - other neurologic findings include headache, encephalitis, focal deficits, obstructive hydrocephalus, arachnoiditis, visual changes, intracranial hypertension, positional syncope (Brun syndrome), psychiatric illness
  - rarely: inflammatory myositis or cardiac conduction defects
- Echinococcus (*E. granulosus*):
  - majority of infected pts asymptomatic, most cysts discovered incidentally by sonography/radiology
  - occasionally obstructive symptoms seen due to pressure excreted by growing cyst
  - in hepatic cysts one can see hepatomegaly, obstructive jaundice, abdominal pain
  - leaking cysts can be associated w/fever, hepatitis
  - cyst rupture can cause anaphylactic shock

LABORATORY FINDINGS

- Diphyllobothriasis (*D. latum*):
  - 40% of infected individuals have reduced vitamin B_{12} levels
  - 2% have megaloblastic anemia
  - reduced folate level due to ↓ absorption
- Hymenolepiasis (*H. nana, H. dimunata*), Dipylidiasis (*D. caninum*), Taeniasis (*T. solium, T. saginata*):
  - eosinophilia in 5–15% of pts
- Cysticercosis (*T. solium*):
  - CSF abnormalities: ↑ in total protein, low glucose, ↑ eosinophiles, ↑ cell count, antibody to *T. solium*
  - eosinophilia in 5–15% of pts
  - cystic lesion on CT or MRI of CNS
  - calcified cysticerci may be present in x rays of musculature
- Echinococcus (*E. granulosus*):
  - eosinophilia esp when leakage of cyst contents occurring
  - ↑ liver function tests may be present
  - space-occupying lesions evident on CT scanning or sonography
  - calcified cysts can be seen on plain x rays

DIAGNOSIS

- Diphyllobothriasis (*D. latum*), Hymenolepiasis (*H. nana, H. dimunata*), Dipylidiasis (*D. caninum*), Taeniasis (*T. solium, T. saginata*):
  - characteristic ova found in feces of infected individuals
  - proglottid segments in stool also used for identification
  - serology not useful
- Cysticercosis (*T. solium*):
  - characteristic cystic lesions on CT or MRI
  - serology (western blot) positive in 75% of cases w/solitary cyst, >98% of pts w/multiple cysts
  - biopsy of lesion reveals characteristic microscopic morphology. Careful skin examination may reveal SubQ cysts that can be biopsied easily for Dx
- Echinococcus (*E. granulosus*):
  - characteristic multiloculated cystic lesion in *E. granulosus*
  - serology (by western blot) positive in >95% of cases
  - examination of fluid in cyst reveals characteristic hydatid sand (scoleces, hooks)

DIFFERENTIAL DIAGNOSIS

- Diphyllobothriasis (*D. latum*), Dipylidiasis (*D. caninum*), Taeniasis (*T. solium, T. saginata*), Hymenolepiasis (*H. nana, H. dimunata*):
  - none
- Cysticercosis (*T. solium*):
  - Sx vary greatly because cysticerci produce single or multiple space occupying lesions in any part of brain, eye, musculature. Neurologic diseases w/similar manifestations to exclude include tuberculosis, coccidiomycosis, cry-

tococcosis, neurosyphilis, sarcoidosis, 1°/metastatic malignancy
- Echinococcus (*E. granulosus*):
  - Parasite produces cystic mass lesions. Diseases w/similar radiographic appearance include simple cysts, abscesses, 1°/metastatic malignancies

TREATMENT

- Diphyllobothriasis (*D. latum*), Dipylidiasis (*D. caninum*), or Taeniasis (*T. solium, T. saginata*):
  - praziquantal, 10 mg/kg as single dose
  - alternative: niclosamide, also effective, no longer available in US
  - in addition, for diphylidiasis, household pets should be examined for tapeworms, treated w/insecticides to remove fleas. Treatment of house for flea infestation also reasonable
- Hymenolepiasis (*H. nana, H. dimunata*):
  - praziquantil, 25 mg/kg as single dose
- Cysticercosis (*T. solium*):
  - solitary cysts do not require treatment
  - multiple parenchymal cysts should be treated w/:
    - steroids to suppress inflammation around degenerating cysts (prednisone, 2 mg/kg w/taper over 3 wks) and
    - albendazole, 15 mg/kg (max. dose 800 mg/d) div 2×/d × 8–28 d
  - alternative: steroids w/praziquantal, 50 mg/kg/d in 3 div doses × 14 d
  - surgical removal of cysticerci such as those in fourth ventricle, eye may be necessary before medical treatment
  - seizure control w/anticonvulsants
- Echinococcus (*E. granulosus*):
  - medical treatment w/albendazole, 15 mg/kg/d div 2 ×/d (max. dose 800 mg/d) × 28 d. Should be repeated 2–3× w/each course separated by 2 wks. Response ascertained by radiographic follow-up
  - surgical resection indicated for symptomatic or leaking lesions. Pts should receive at least one course of albendazole prior to surgery. Start 2–3 d before surgery on praziquantal, 50 mg/kg/d div 3 daily doses, albendazole, 15 mg/d div 2 ×/d. Praziquantal should be continued × 7–14 d, albendazole × 28 d. Many surgeons instill hyperosmotic saline or other scolecidal agents (such as 0.1% cetrimide) into cyst at time of surgery prior to resection

SIDE EFFECTS OF TREATMENT

- *Praziquantel:* reported side effects include headache, dizziness, nausea, urticaria, myalgias, arthralgias, abdominal pain. These appear within hours of ingestion and disappear by 48 hrs
- *Albendazole:* reported side effects include reversible reductions in WBC count (<1%), mild ↑ in liver function tests (10–15% of pts), nausea, headache (11% of pts w/neurocysticercosis), occasional alopecia

COMPLICATIONS

- Diphyllobothriasis (*D. latum*), Dipylidiasis (*D. caninum*), Taeniasis (*T. solium, T. saginata*), Hymenolepiasis (*H. nana, H. dimunata*):
  - rarely seen
- Cysticercosis (*T. solium*):
  - headache, seizures, ↑ intracranial pressure during treatment due to death of parasites
  - rare fatalities have occurred due to parasite death in pts w/large cyst burdens
  - endopthalmitis can occur in ocular cysticercosis
- Echinococcus (*E. granulosus*):
  - acute Sx associated w/traumatic or surgical rupture of cysts, can include anaphylactic shock, urticaria, edema, dyspnea, peritonitis, even death
  - leakage of cyst fluid containing germinal epithelium can generate new cysts

WHEN TO REFER

- Diphyllobothriasis (*D. latum*), Dipylidiasis (*D. caninum*), Taeniasis (*T. solium, T. saginata*), Hymenolepiasis (*H. nana, H. dimunata*):
  - can be managed w/o referral
- Cysticercosis (*T. solium*), Echinococcus (*E. granulosus*):
  - referral and consultation w/infectious diseases/tropical medicine specialist indicated for management

BACKGROUND

- *Tarsal coalition:* congenital bony, cartilaginous, or fibrous connection between two tarsal bones. Coalition generally fibrous or cartilaginous early in life; later becomes solid bony bar
- Most common coalitions between calcaneus and navicular (calcaneonavicular), between talus and calcaneus (talocalcaneal)
- May cause foot pain, deformity when coalition starts to ossify (generally 8–16 yrs of age)
- M:F ratio: 2:1
- Occurs in <1% of general population
- ~50% bilateral

CLINICAL MANIFESTATIONS

- Many coalitions asymptomatic
- If symptomatic, usually hindfoot pain; primarily medial w/talocalcaneal coalitions and lateral w/calcaneonavicular coalitions
- ↓ subtalar motion (inversion, eversion)
- May be associated w/hindfoot valgus, flat feet, or peroneal spasm (peroneal spastic flat foot)
- Symptoms usually aggravated w/activity, relieved w/rest

RADIOGRAPHIC FEATURES

- Coalitions not easily detected on AP, lateral x rays of foot. Lateral x ray may demonstrate talar neck beaking as 2° sign
- Calcaneonavicular coalitions usually seen on oblique x rays of foot as connection between anterior end of calcaneus and lateral aspect of navicular
- Talocalcaneal coalitions may be seen on Harris (axial) view of calcaneus, but usually require CT scan of hindfoot to confirm Dx

DIFFERENTIAL DIAGNOSIS

- Trauma-fracture, sprain, or osteochondral injury
- Arthritic conditions of foot, ankle
- Idiopathic flexible flatfoot (rarely symptomatic)
- Idiopathic peroneal spastic flatfoot

TREATMENT

- No treatment. For mild symptoms, may include activity modification
- Soft shoe inserts for mild–moderate symptoms
- Short leg cast for 4–6 wks if symptoms do not resolve w/other conservative methods
- *Surgery:* for moderate–severe symptoms that do not respond to conservative treatment. Includes coalition excision vs. hindfoot arthrodesis

COMPLICATIONS

- No significant complications to nonop treatment
- Small percentage of pts do not get relief w/coalition excision
- If hindfoot arthrodesis necessary, ↑ chance of arthritic changes in adjacent joints later in life exists

WHEN TO REFER

- Moderate–severe symptoms that do not respond to nonop treatment

BACKGROUND

- Germ cell tumors (GCTs) are diverse group of neoplasms that arise from primordial cells of gametogenesis
- Occur at varied 1° sites, w/range of benign, transitional, malignant histologic subtypes in fetus, infants, children, adults
- Pure benign histology (teratoma) occurs in 55%, pure transitional histologies (immature teratoma) in 10%, malignant histologies (yolk sac/endodermal sinus, embryonal carcinoma, germinoma, choriocarcinoma, mixed) in 35% of cases
- Teratomas of sacrococcygeal area, common presentation of pediatric GCTs, occur in 1/35,000 live births; usually recognized in early infancy
- Malignant GCTs have annual incidence 3.9 cases/million children <15 yrs of age: 2.4 cases at gonadal sites (ovary, testis), 1.5 cases at extragonadal sites (sacrococcyx, brain, mediastinum, retroperitoneum, other); represent 2–4% of childhood cancers
- Typical age of presentation varies by 1° site: sacrococcyx (neonates), ovary (≥4 yrs), testis (<4 yrs, >13 yrs), mediastinum (≥10 yrs), brain (≥2 yrs)
- Typically arise at midline anatomic sites, explained by aberrations in normal caudad to cephalad migration of primitive germ cells in developing embryo
- Genetic factors, including Klinefilter syndrome and gonadal dysgenesis (Swyer syndrome), and anatomic factors, such as cryptorchidism, ↑ risk

CLINICAL MANIFESTATIONS

- *Visible mass:* sacrococcyx, testis, head/neck
- *Tumor compression:* pain, constipation, urinary obstruction, respiratory embarrassment, neurologic dysfunction
- *Gonadal torsion:* ovary (may mimic appendicitis), testis
- *Metastases:* lung, lymph nodes, liver, bone, brain
- *Paraneoplastic syndromes:* precocious puberty, gynecomastia
- Pelvic masses producing beta-HCG may mimic pregnancy in adolescent females
- May present prenatally w/abnormal obstetrical ultrasound, polyhydramnios, hydrops, and/or birth dystocia

LABORATORY STUDIES

- Serum tumor markers:
  - *alpha-fetoprotein* (AFP; ↑ in yolk sac tumors; physiologically ↑ in children <9 mos of age; also ↑ in hepatoblastoma, nonneoplastic liver diseases; $T_{1/2}$ = 7 d)
  - *human chorionic gonadotropin* (beta-HCG; ↑ in choriocarcinomas; also ↑ in pregnancy, liver tumors; $T_{1/2}$ = 30 hrs)
  - draw baseline serum markers prior to initial surgery, then follow to assess response to Tx

  - physiologic ↑ of AFP during infancy makes use of this marker difficult in children <9 mos of age
  - elaboration of serum tumor markers varies according to tumor histology

Histology	Serum AFP	Serum beta-HCG
Yolk sac tumor (Endodermal sinus tumor)	++++	—
Choriocarcinoma	—	++++
Embryonal carcinoma	+/–	+/–
Germinoma	—	—
Teratoma		
Benign	—	—
Immature	+/–	—

- Diagnostic imaging:
  - 1° tumor: CT, ultrasound, and/or MRI; *note:* external sacrococcygeal lesions may include internal presacral component; therefore, imaging required for surgical planning
  - if tumor contains malignant elements, r/o metastases: chest CT, liver/abdominal CT, bone scan, brain CT (dependent on neurologic findings)
- Surgical pathology:
  - frequently large tumors w/mixed histologies; require extensive sampling to detect all histologic components, r/o areas of malignancy; immunohistochemistry (AFP, beta-HCG, placental alkaline phosphatase) may complement routine histology

DIFFERENTIAL DIAGNOSIS

- Sacrococcygeal, pelvic tumors:
  - external mass: lipoma, meningocele, lipomeningocele, hemangioma, bone malformation, abcess, pilonidal cyst, epidermal cyst, sarcomas of bone or soft tissues
  - internal mass: neuroblastoma, lymphoma, chordoma
- Gonadal tumors:
  - ovary: appendicitis, ovarian cyst, tubal pregnancy, pelvic abcess, epithelial carcinoma, sex cord–stromal tumors, pelvic sarcomas, lymphoma
  - testis: hydrocele, hematocele, hernia, torsion, sex cord–stromal tumors, paratesticular rhabdomyosarcoma, leukemia/lymphoma
- *Abdominal, retroperitoneal tumors:* renal anomalies, hydronephrosis, multicystic kidney disease, mesenteric cysts, intestinal duplications, Wilms tumor, neuroblastoma, rhabdomyosarcoma, lymphoma, liver tumors
- *Mediastinal tumors:* inflammatory adenopathy, bronchial or enteric cysts, thymic cysts, ectopic thyroid, lymphangioma, lymphoma, chest wall sarcomas, neuroblastoma, thymoma
- *Brain tumors (pineal, suprasellar):* pineoblastoma, pineocytoma, astrocytoma, craniopharyngioma

TREATMENT

- Tx largely defined by presence or absence of malignant histologic elements in tumor

- Teratoma (pure, benign histology):
  - *1° management:* complete surgical resection; sacrococcygeal tumors require coccygectomy to prevent recurrence; resect promptly to avoid risk of malignant transformation
  - *follow-up:* exam, serum AFP and beta-HCG, w/or w/o imaging q3–6 mos × 3 y
  - *outcome:* >90% recurrence free; some risk of benign local recurrence; some risk of malignant degeneration of unresected tumor
- Immature teratoma (pure histology or w/teratoma; *no malignant elements*):
  - *1° management:* complete surgical resection; sacrococcygeal tumors require coccygectomy to prevent recurrence; resect promptly to avoid risk of malignant transformation
  - *follow-up:* exam, serum AFP and beta-HCG, imaging q3–6 mos × 3 y
  - *outcome:* >90% recurrence free; small risk of local recurrence; small risk of malignant recurrence
- Malignant GCT:
  - tumors containing *any* yolk sac/endodermal sinus tumor, embryonal carcinoma, choriocarcinoma, or germinoma elements
  - testis, stage I:
    - *1° management:* complete surgical resection by radical inguinal orchiectomy; lymph node dissection not routinely used in children
    - *follow-up:* exam, serum AFP and beta-HCG, imaging q3–6 mos × 3 y
  - *outcome:* ~80% recurrence free; recurrences salvageable by platinum-based chemotherapy
  - testis, stages II–IV; all other sites, stages I–IV:
    - *1° management:* initial surgical resection or biopsy only, dependent on feasibility; multiagent chemotherapy including cisplatin or carboplatin; delayed resection of residual tumor
    - *follow-up:* exam, serum AFP and beta-HCG, imaging q3–6 mos × 3 y
    - *outcome:* ~85% recurrence free; some recurrences salvageable by high-dose chemotherapy, autologous marrow or stem cell transplant

COMPLICATIONS

- Surgery and chemotherapy-related side effects
- Death due to malignant tumor progression or recurrence (~10%)

WHEN TO REFER

- All cases require input from appropriate team of pediatric specialists experienced in evaluation, Dx, treatment, follow-up of this family of tumors—pediatric surgeon, pediatric radiologist, pediatric pathologist, pediatric oncologist
- Pts requiring chemotherapy should be cared for by pediatric oncologist

BACKGROUND

- *Definition/mechanism of injury:* due to abnormally mobile testis, which allows twisting of spermatic cord that represents vascular pedicle to testicle. Initially, venous congestion due to obstruction caused by this twisting occurs. Process then can progress to marked swelling, venous thrombosis, arterial thrombosis w/tissue ischemia, eventually testicular infarction, death. Tortion a true surgical emergency
- *Degree of injury depends on two factors:* degree of rotation (number of twists), duration of torsion
- *Incidence:* 1/~150 males; two-thirds of all cases occur in second decade of life, w/another peak in neonatal period
- Left side more commonly involved than right side
- Two types:
  – extravaginal: when testis and cord twist because of nonfixation of testis, cord, and processus vaginalis; almost exclusively occurs in neonatal period
  – intravaginal: torsion within tunica vaginalis due to bell-clapper deformity seen w/ abnormally high involvement of tunica on spermatic cord
- Etiology often obscure; trauma may be initiating factor (~20% of time). Most cases have no antecedent event

CLINICAL MANIFESTATIONS

- *Pain:* almost always first symptoms; may be gradual in onset or sudden; one-third pts have had similar previous episodes that resolved spontaneously
- Tenderness to palpation
- Swelling, erythema of scrotum; can be marked ↑ in size so palpation difficult
- Nausea, vomiting
- Loss of cremasteric reflex on affected side—not specific, but relatively sensitive
- Testicle may have transverse, high-riding lie
- Usually no dysuria or voiding symptoms

DIFFERENTIAL DIAGNOSIS

- Torsion of vestigial appendices: testis appendix, hydatid of Morgagni, testis epididymis
- Epididymitis, epididymo-orchitis
- Hydrocele, varicocele
- Inguinal hernia
- Trauma (eg, ruptured testicle)
- Tumors

DIAGNOSIS

- Radiographic examinations:
  – nuclear medicine scans: goal is to distinguish between ↑ flow to testicle oftentimes seen w/epididymitis vs. ↓ or absent flow to testicle seen w/torsion
  – color Doppler ultrasound: goal is to identify ↓ or absent arterial flow to affected testicle
  – both have sensitivity ranges 80–90% but can be misleading and do take time to perform, esp nuclear medicine scan
- Hx, physical exam keys to decision-making process regarding operative management. If any doubt, surgical exploration mandatory

TREATMENT

- When torsion suspected or cannot be ruled out, surgical exploration via scrotal incision should be undertaken
- If torsion found, fixation via scrotal orchidopexy required of affected side if still viable as well as fixation of contralateral side
- Orchiectomy may be necessary when testicle clearly nonviable, and often case w/extravaginal torsion in newborn setting
- Any child w/acute scrotal complaints requires immediate evaluation, attention

TETANUS

JANET E. SQUIRES

BACKGROUND

- Noncommunicable neurologic disease manifested by severe muscle spasms
- *Cause:* potent exotoxin from anaerobic bacteria *Clostridium tetani,* ubiquitous in soil/feces
- *Typical clinical situations:* wound w/deep puncture trauma/devitalized tissue, newborn w/unclean umbilical stump
- Major problem worldwide; rare in US
- *CDC statistics:* 1995–97 in US: 124 cases, 5% < age 20, one neonate; 87% of cases had not received primary series tetanus vaccine
- *Toxoid vaccine nearly "ideal":* highly effective, safe, inexpensive

CLINICAL MANIFESTATIONS

- Acute onset of hypertonia/painful muscular contractions, usually of muscles of jaw, neck (lockjaw)/generalized muscle spasms
- Symptoms exacerbated by external stimuli
- In partially immunized persons, muscle spasms may be mild, may be localized
- Incubation period 2 d–2 mos, most <2 wks; symptoms most intense in first 2 wks, gradually subside
- Death may occur from asphyxia during spasms
- Disease self-limited; in surviving pt, prognosis good unless hypoxic injuries occurred

LABORATORY FEATURES

- Diagnosis clinical
- Suspect wounds should be cultured, although *C. tetani* growth rare

DIFFERENTIAL DIAGNOSIS

- Hypocalcemic tetany
- Poisoning (eg, strychnine)
- Drug reaction (eg, phenothiazine)
- Hysteria, conversion reactions
- Seizures (esp in neonatal tetani)

TREATMENT

- Prevent further toxin from affecting CNS:
  - clean wounds, debride devitalized tissue, remove foreign bodies
  - tetanus immune globulin (TIG): 500 U for neonate/3,000–6,000 U for adult, using part of dose locally near wound, remainder IM
  - antibiotics: metronidazole, 30 mg/kg/d in 4 div doses IV/oral, penicillin G, 100,00 U/kg/d in 4 div doses IV
- Supportive care to control tetanic spasms:
  - airway management single most important care; ventilation if necessary
  - pharmacotherapy for spasms (wide range of Tx/doses): diazepam, 0.1–0.5 mg/kg/dose q2–8h; morphine, 0.1–0.15 mg/kg/dose q3–6h; pentobarbital, 2–4 mg/kg/dose q4–6h
  - avoidance of external stimuli
  - excellent nursing care: fluids, nutrition, care for urinary/stool retention
  - steroids controversial

COMPLICATIONS

- Aspiration pneumonia
- Death/hypoxic injury from respiratory compromise
- 2° bacterial infections
- Fractures
- Stress ulcers
- *Autonomic nervous system dysfunction:* hypertension, arrhythmias

PREVENTION

- 1° active immunization indicated for all persons:
  - age <7 yrs: series of 5 doses, per ACIP guidelines
  - age 7–12: series of 3 doses, per ACIP guidelines
  - age 12–16: Td booster after initial series, then Td booster q10y as adult
- Proper management of penetrating/contaminated wounds:
  - surgical debridement
  - use of tetanus immune globulin/vaccine (modified Red Book, American Academy of Pediatrics, 1997)

	Clean Minor Wound	Other Wounds
≥3 prior vaccine doses	vaccine if > 10 y	vaccine if > 5 y
uncertain, or <3 prior vaccine doses	vaccine, no TIG	vaccine, TIG

WHEN TO REFER

- Referral for hospital ICU indicated for suspected case, to support airway
- Tetanus reportable disease to public health

BACKGROUND

- Symptom of acute ↓ in serum calcium, not independent disease
- Symptoms result from rapid ↓ in serum calcium level/low ionized calcium (<3.5 mg/dL = 0.88 mMol/L)
- Neonatal forms usually transient/result from acute hormonal changes
- *Neonatal early prematurity:* calcitonin surge; delay PTH response (mother of IDDM); infant of mother w/hyperparathyroidism; perinatal anoxia
- *Neonatal late form (5–10 d of age):* results from parathyroid/vitamin D deficiency: maternal vitamin D deficiency; parathyroid agenesis; ↑ serum phosphate (dietary loading); hypomagnesemia
- In infant several weeks of age to adult, hypocalcemia most often prolonged, w/episodes of tetany that result from *vitamin D deficiency/resistance* (vitamin D deficiency, malbsorption, liver disease, chronic renal disease); *parathyroid resistance/deficiency* (parathyroid hypoplasia: DiGeorge syndrome, hypoparathyroidism, polyglandular autoimmune syndrome); *calcium redistribution/sequestration* (hyperventilation, massive transfusion citrated blood); ↑ *uptake of calcium by bone* ("hungry bone syndrome" in early treatment of rickets); *hypomagnesemia* resulting from chronic intestinal losses (enteric fistula, pancreatitis, malabsorption, short bowel syndrome); renal tubular wasting (aminoglycoside Tx, amphotericin, chemotherapy [cis platinum], cyclosporine; diuretic Tx, postobstuctive diuresis); endocrine disorders (diabetic ketoacidosis; hypoparathyroidism); rapid restoration of protein/calorie balance after malnutrition

CLINICAL MANIFESTATIONS

- Provoked by handling
- *Trousseau sign:* extension of fingers, w/thumb tightly adducted into palm/wrist flexed
- Chvostek sign (hyperexcitability of facial muscles) elicited by tapping over muscles
- *Carpopedal spasm:* paralytic state of hands/feet w/toes pointed down/↑ arching of foot
- Muscle fasiculation followed by focal/grand mal seizures
- Laryngospasm

LABORATORY FEATURES

- Low ionized calcium (<3.5 mg/dL [0.88 mMol/L])
- Low magnesium levels (<1.0 mg/dL)
- *EKG changes:* prolonged Q-T interval
- Low vitamin D level, low intact parathyroid hormone/↑ serum phosphorous

DIFFERENTIAL DIAGNOSIS

- Hyperkalemia
- Hypokalemia
- Hypomagnesemia
- Dystonic reaction

TREATMENT

- *Principal options:* calcium replacement, vitamin D supplements, magnesium replacement
- *Symptomatic treatment:* restore ionized calcium to normal by correcting underlying cause if possible
- Elemental calcium replacement, 10 mg/kg (0.5 mEq/kg) IV over 10–20 min under EKG monitoring; to stabilize, follow w/10 mg/kg over 4–6 h; repeat if necessary; aim to restore serum calcium to 7 mg/dL in premature infants/8 mg/dL in full-term infant; in older child, prolonged IV 20–40 mg elemental calcium/60–100 mg/kg oral supplementation required for restoration (advantage: rapid correction; disadvantage: dangerous bradycardia w/rapid infusion); tissue necrosis if extravasation outside of vein (use only well-functioning IV access/catheter for infusion; gastric irritation from calcium supplements may lead to pain/bleeding esp w/calcium chloride (avoid if possible)
- *Vitamin D supplements:* IV calcitriol, 0.01 µg/kg/1,25 dihydroxy cholecalciferol 0.125–0.25 µg may be required in older children after calcium restored to asymptomatic level/for prolonged periods in pts w/chronic renal failure, hypoparathyroidism, pseudo-hypoparathyroidism, Fanconi syndrome, liver disease; prophylactic use of vitamin D–supplemented milk 400 IU/qt, calcitriol supplementation early in renal failure/vitamin D–resistant rickets prevent hypocalcemia
- *Magnesium supplements:* magnesium sulfate, 20% (4 mEq/1mL) 0.4–0.8 mEq/kg (50–100 mg/kg) IV or IM indicated if serum magnesium <1 mEq/L; tetany not responsive to calcium replacement/if seizures occur; oral supplements: elemental magnesium, 3–6 mg/kg/d div 6–8 hourly as magnesium gluconate or magnesium oxide continued until stable serum magnesium levels occur; potential side effects of magnesium include abdominal cramping, diarrhea w/oral replacement, local irritation w/IM replacement, respiratory depression, sedation w/IV administration

COMPLICATIONS

- Muscle excitability
- Cramping/muscle stiffness
- Laryngeal closure w/tight adduction of vocal cords during intubation

WHEN TO REFER

- Referral indicated if cause not obvious/tetany prolonged
- If long-term Tx anticipated

BACKGROUND

- Most common cause of cyanotic congenital heart disease beyond infancy
- Most cases nonfamilial
- No known etiology; association w/22q-chromosomal abnormality noted

ANATOMY AND PATHOPHYSIOLOGY

- *Classic anatomic features of TOF:* large ventricular septal defect (VSD), pulmonic stenosis (PS), usually infundibular (but many variations), overriding aorta, right ventricular hypertrophy
- Large VSD allows for shunting between right/left ventricles. Severity of pulmonary stenosis determines direction/degree of shunting
- Natural Hx of PS is to progress

CLINICAL PRESENTATION

- Most severe cases diagnosed in neonatal period when newborn evaluated for cyanosis; typically more severe degree of PS may be ductus dependent for pulmonary blood flow
- Outpt Dx beyond newborn period typically occurs during evaluation of murmur and/or cyanosis
- Cyanosis may be absent to severe; desaturation may not be clinically apparent and discovered only w/pulse oximetry
- Clubbing may occur w/central cyanosis after age 6 mos
- *Murmurs:* S1 normal/S2 variable depending on degree of PS; w/↑ severity of PS, pulmonic component of S2 becomes softer/even inaudible; systolic click may/may not be present; most pts have systolic murmur along left mid to upper sternal border; murmur sometimes accompanied by thrill generated by PS; as PS ↑ in severity, murmur becomes shorter as less blood crosses right ventricular outflow tract/more shunted across VSD; diastolic murmurs uncommon in simple TOF; continuous murmur suggests PDA/collaterals
- Squatting may occur (↓ systemic venous return of desaturated blood/↑ systemic arterial resistance, which ↓ right-to-left shunt, thereby ↑ pulmonary blood flow/arterial saturation) Squatting not usually seen now because patients usually repaired earlier; infant might pull legs to chest
- CHF occurs in patients with TOF and pulmonary atresia w/large systemic aorto-pulmonary collaterals or surgical shunts; CHF not usually seen even in "pink tet"

LABORATORY EVALUATION

- *Echocardiogram:* definitive Dx made w/2D echo (cardiac catheterization still done in some centers prior to surgery)
- *Chest x ray:* heart size normal w/concave pulmonary artery segment; pulmonary vascularity normal to ↓ depending on degree of PS/presence of collaterals; classic description: boot-shaped heart ("coeur en sabot"); right aortic arch seen in 20–30% pts
- *EKG:* RVH (tall R wave in V1 w/abrupt change to biphasic R wave in V2), RAD (+90 to +180) expected findings in unoperated pt; after complete repair, RBBB present in most pts
- Pulse oximetry: desaturation to 85% may not be clinically apparent; pulse oximetry provides noninvasive assessment of oxygenation; mild desaturation detected by oximetry may be first indication that Dx TOF/not simple VSD; cyanosis may be aggravated by activity, fever; hypercyanotic spells (see below) require special mention
- Hgb/Hct: in response to desaturation, Hgb ↑ in effort to improve tissue oxygenation by ↑ O_2-carrying capacity; even if resting pulse oximetry normal, ↑ Hgb/Hct suggest pt chronically desaturated; imperative to check RBC indices and RDW in addition to Hgb/Hct in presence of iron deficiency, Hgb/Hct might be normal and relative anemia overlooked; can predispose to CVA and "tet" spell. Increasing Hgb/Hct suggests ↑ cyanosis

COMPLICATIONS

- *Hypercyanotic spells:* O_2 saturation variable in TOF (even infants clinically pink at rest at risk for episodes of severe desaturation); "tet" spells are characterized by ↑ cyanosis, hyperpnea, disappearance of the murmur, irritability, and metabolic acidosis; may occur at any time, esp. upon awakening or feeding; although frequently self-limiting, episodes can be life threatening; therapeutic maneuvers include knee chest position, morphine sulfate, 0.1–0.2 mg/kg IM/SubQ or slow IV, propranolol, 0.15–0.25 mg/kg slow IV, phenylephrine, NaHCO₃ (1 mEq/kg) volume expansion, O_2 (limited value); if these measures fail, ketamine and general anesthesia can be tried; hypercyanotic spells considered indication for surgical intervention (po propranolol also used to prevent recurrences)

- Cerebrovascular accidents:
  – hypoxia: CVA usually due to hypoxemia; risk further aggravated by iron deficiency anemia; infants should be on iron-fortified formulas/iron supplementation may be necessary; normal Hgb suggests relative anemia in cyanotic pt
  – polycythemia: Hct >65% poses risk for CVA 2° to hyperviscosity/resultant thrombosis; polycythemia may require cautious phlebotomy/volume replacement; dehydration esp dangerous in polycythemic pt; polycythemia can also cause coagulopathy
  – intracardiac right to left shunt predisposes to systemic arterial embolization from spontaneous intravascular thromboses and during catheterization
- Infection:
  – bacterial endocarditis: TOF high-risk lesion for bacterial endocarditis; most common organisms strep viridans/staph aureus; pts require SBE prophylaxis for dental procedures, etc
  – brain abscess: because most pts repaired by 2 yrs of age, rarely seen; should be considered in pts w/fever/changing neurologic status

LONG-TERM CONSIDERATIONS

- Most pts, following successful complete repair, function normally unless residual defects
- Special considerations include:
  – sports participation: level of participation depends on presence of residual defects; w/good results, no restrictions; recommendation should be made in consultation w/pediatric cardiologist
  – SBE prophylaxis: even w/o hemodynamically significant residual lesions, all pts continue to require SBE prophylaxis
  – arrhythmias: PVCs on routine EKG should prompt cardiac reevaluation; life-threatening arrhythmias can occur in postop pts, esp those w/residual defects

WHEN TO REFER

- All patients w/TOF should be under care of pediatric cardiologist; in consultation w/cardiac surgeon makes recommendation regarding timing of palliative surgery or complete repair; patient should also be followed by general pediatrician familiar w/certain features of TOF

THALASSEMIA MAJOR

BACKGROUND

- Most commonly occurs in following ethnic groups: Mediterranean Sea countries, Central Africa, India, China, Southeast Asia
- Anemia results from ↓/absent synthesis of alpha or beta globin chain of Hgb
- ↓ in alpha or beta globin chain synthesis has deleterious effects on erythrocyte production/survival; cells poorly hemoglobinized/destroyed in bone marrow; unbalanced chain synthesis leads to inclusion formation/hemolysis

CLINICAL MANIFESTATIONS

- Presents in infancy/early childhood w/pallor, failure to thrive, hepatosplenomegaly
- W/transfusion Tx pts have normal growth/development until ~10 yrs of age when growth retardation begins/puberty delayed

LABORATORY FEATURES

- Hgb very low
- *RBC indices:* mean corpuscular volume/mean corpuscular Hgb ↓
- *Peripheral blood smear:* marked hypochromia, microcytosis, anisocytosis, poikilocytosis, target cells, large numbers of normoblasts
- *Hgb electrophoresis:* Hgb F—no Hgb A detected
- Thalassemia minor detected in both parents
- *Bone marrow shows marked erythroid hyperplasia w/erythroid:* myeloid ratio ≥20:1
- Serum iron level ↑ w/slightly ↑ total iron-binding capacity
- Biosynthesis studies of blood reticulocytes/bone marrow cells show unbalanced globin chain synthesis

DIFFERENTIAL DIAGNOSIS

- Iron deficiency anemia
- Leukemia
- Viral syndrome

TREATMENT

- Regular blood transfusions given to maintain Hgb levels 10–14 g/dL; usually requires 10–15 cc/kg q3–5 wks
- Deferoxamine given daily by SubQ infusions to remove excess iron that results from blood transfusions
- Bone marrow transplantation using HLA-matched sibling donor successful in curing ~80% pts

COMPLICATIONS

- Possible transmission of viral infections from blood transfusions
- Iron overload may result in CHF/cardiac arrhythmias, growth retardation, delayed onset of puberty, diabetes mellitus, hypoparathyroidism, cirrhosis of the liver

PREVENTION

- Genetic counseling of population at risk to prevent marriage between carriers
- Antenatal Dx/abortion of affected fetuses

WHEN TO REFER

- Pts should be referred at presentation to confirm Dx/set treatment guidelines
- Monthly blood transfusion may be carried out by primary care physicians w/appropriate guidelines
- Pts should be evaluated q6 mos by pediatric hematologist to monitor treatment, identify complications

THALASSEMIA MINOR

CLINICAL MANIFESTATIONS

- Asymptomatic
- Mild anemia unresponsive to oral iron Tx

LABORATORY FEATURES

- *Hgb:* 8–10 g/dL
- *RBC indices:* mean cell volume ↓; mean cell corpuscular Hgb ↓
- *RBC count:* normal or mildly ↓
- *Peripheral blood smear:* mild hypochromia, microcytosis, occasional anisocytosis, poikilocytosis, target cells, basophilic stippling
- *Hgb electrophoresis:* ↑ Hgb A2 (4–7%); may have mild ↑ Hgb F

DIFFERENTIAL DIAGNOSIS

- Iron deficiency anemia
- Anemia of chronic disease

TREATMENT

- None necessary (chronic iron administration may lead to toxicity from iron overload/should be avoided)

COMPLICATIONS

- None

WHEN TO REFER

- Usually not necessary

THROMBOSIS, DEEP VEIN

ENRIQUE CRIADO AND MARK A. FARBER

BACKGROUND

- Venous stasis, hypercoagulability, intimal injury pathogenic basis of deep vein thrombosis (DVT); unusual in children
- *Risk factors:* previous DVT, indwelling venous catheter, older age, malignancy, prolonged bed rest or immobility, stroke, paralysis, pregnancy, obesity, multiple trauma, major surgery, hip/knee replacement, pelvic/lower extremity fractures, venous malformations, myeloproliferative disorders, hyperfibrinogenemia, 1° hypercoagulable states:
  - resistance to activated protein C (factor V Leiden mutation)
  - antithrombin III deficiency
  - protein C deficiency
  - protein S deficiency
- *Most common 1° hypercoagulability cause:* resistance to action of activated protein C (anticoagulant protein synthesized by liver, produced by presence of mutant factor V [factor V Leiden] preventing binding of activated protein C to factor V)
- *Major consequences of DVT:* pulmonary embolization (PE)/chronic venous insufficiency (CVI)
- PE can occur early w/DVT
- *CVI:* late sequela of DVT/caused by venous valvular incompetence/partial, complete venous obstruction; typically presents years after thrombotic event; major cause of long-term morbidity; treatment of DVT not only to prevent PE but to minimize sequela CVI

CLINICAL MANIFESTATIONS

- Limb pain, discomfort, tenderness, swelling; most often asymptomatic; Sx vague/nonspecific
- *Most common sign/best clinical predictor:* acute onset of unilateral limb swelling not caused by trauma/infection
- Pain on limb palpation/Homan sign little value in Dx; DVT cannot be palpated unlike some superficial VTs
- Fever rarely caused by DVT; clinical Dx DVT unreliable/inaccurate even in experienced hands

- Acute obstruction of iliac/common femoral vein can cause massive extremity swelling/severe limb pain/termed *phlegmasia alba dolens*
- Venous pressure at capillary level can compromise tissue perfusion; presents w/extreme limb swelling, pain, cyanosis, skin blistering, extensive skin necrosis *(phlegmasia cerulea dolens)*; limb threatening/may require emergency venous thrombectomy

LABORATORY FEATURES

- Duplex scanning test of choice for Dx (sensitivity/specificity >90%)
- Ascending venography rarely indicated; proximal iliac vein/caval thrombosis difficult to diagnose w/duplex scanning/can be diagnosed w/CT scan/MRI
- D-dimer serum levels have little clinical applicability (very low specificity)

DIFFERENTIAL DIAGNOSIS

- Bilateral lower extremity swelling more likely 2° to systemic illnesses (cardiogenic edema/hypoproteinemia); onset of swelling rarely acute
- Unilateral limb lymphedema/presents insidiously over months/years, nonpitting
- Limb swelling from infection/trauma (important to remember that DVT may occur in conjunction w/other problems)

TREATMENT

- *Best treatment:* prevention
- *Goals of Tx:* PE prevention/thrombus propagationn avoidance/maximal thrombus resolution
- Systemic heparinization/followed by chronic anticoagulation effective in preventing PE/does little to promote resolution of thrombus
- Catheter-directed thrombolytic Tx when thrombotic burden large/iliac, femoral veins occluded in symptomatic pts
- Venous thrombectomy indicated when acute venous hypertension jeopardizes limb

COMPLICATIONS

- PE most common complication; w/adequate treatment, unusual
- Limb-threatening ischemia
- *Heparin-induced thrombocytopenia:* platelet count should be monitored in any pt receiving heparin

PREVENTION

- Prophylaxis when at least 3 risk factors for DVT present
- *Optimal DVT prophylaxis:* SubQ heparin (low molecular weight heparin has advantage of single daily dose)
- If contraindications for SubQ heparin, pneumatic sequential compression devices applied to legs can provide adequate protection; compliance difficult
- Early ambulation following surgery, adequate hydration, avoidance of prolonged bed rest
- No data to support use of caval filters for prevention of PE in pediatric population

WHEN TO REFER

- Episode of DVT w/o identifiable cause referred to coagulation service for hypercoagulability evaluation
- DVT/known, suspected venous malformation to prevent recurrence/pulmonary embolization
- Severe swelling/acute skin changes from acute DVT referred to vascular surgeon for possible catheter-directed thrombolytic Tx/venous thrombectomy

THRUSH, CANDIDAL DIAPER RASH, AND OTHER SKIN INFECTIONS

MARTIN E. WEISSE

BACKGROUND

- Thrush most frequently found in first 2 mos of life, but rarely in first wk
- Candidal diaper dermatitis presents later, w/peak incidence at 3–4 mos of age
- Candidal paronychia usually occurs in age groups where sucking on fingers and thumbs common
- Colonization of mother risk factor for thrush; antibiotic use ↑ risk for both thrush and diaper dermatitis
- *Candida albicans* species that causes almost all cases of these infections
- Severe or recalcitrant disease, and infections occurring outside of usual age distribution should alert clinician to possible immunodeficiency

CLINICAL MANIFESTATIONS

- Thrush appears as white plaques on one or more of mucosal surfaces in oral pharynx: buccal, lingual, palatal, gingival, labial
- Diaper dermatitis usually appears in intertriginous areas as confluent papular eruption w/satellite papules. Diaper dermatitis due to other causes may become colonized w/*Candida* after ≥3 d, causing atypical features
- Candidal paronychia occurs on fingers, almost never on toes; may be differentiated from other causes of fungal onychomycosis by prominence of inflammation of surrounding skin

LABORATORY FEATURES

- Scrapings of plaques of thrush demonstrates yeast cells and pseudohyphae on KOH preparation or Gram stain. Culture on fungal media of scrapings of any of these infections reveals organism
- Other laboratory tests unnecessary, except in severe cases to investigate for immune deficiency

DIFFERENTIAL DIAGNOSIS

- *Thrush:* milk adherent to tongue after feeding
- *Candidal diaper dermatitis:* irritant diaper dermatitis, secondary staphylococcal dermatitis, seborrhea, psoriasis
- *Candidal paronychia:* bacterial paronychia, tinea onychomycosis

TREATMENT

- Thrush:
  – oral nystatin suspension usually first line of treatment
  – manual removal of plaques w/gauze aids resolution
  – clotrimazole troches (placing troche in nipple and allowing infant to suck) have been used
  – gentian violet applied topically may be useful for recalcitrant infections
  – miconazole oral gel probably most effective topical Tx but unavailable in US
  – for immune-compromised pts, topical amphotericin B or oral azole preparations may be necessary
- Candidal diaper dermatitis:
  – topical nystatin in either cream, ointment, or powder form usually effective
  – Clotrimazole 1% cream or miconazole 2% ointment also usually quite effective
  – combination preparations (antifungal + topical steroid) should be avoided, as steroid usually too potent for infant's skin. If topical steroid desired for symptomatic relief, hydrocortisone 1% usually sufficient
  – systemic treatment w/oral azoles almost never necessary
- Candidal paronychia:
  – keeping affected digit dry (not in mouth!) may be all that is necessary
  – topical therapy w/nystatin, clotrimazole, spectazole, others all effective

COMPLICATIONS

- All infections superficial; should not cause any scarring or other complications
- If more severe infections occur (candidal esophagitis, invasive disease, recalcitrant infection), immune deficiency should be suspected

PREVENTION

- Keeping infant's diaper area clean and dry, and avoiding unnecessary antibiotic exposure most important preventive measures

WHEN TO REFER

- No reason to refer for usual manifestations of these diseases. Recalcitrant or particularly severe disease may necessitate referral

BACKGROUND

- Identified in children 0–19 yrs of age, most 0–5 yrs
- Equal M:F ratio
- Arises from epithelial remnants of thyroglossal duct as developing thyroid gland descends from its origin at base of tongue to just above suprasternal notch

CLINICAL MANIFESTATIONS

- Mobile, soft, nontender, round, smooth swelling in neck
- Usually in midline (20% within 2 cm of midline)
- Moves w/swallowing/tongue protrusion most at level of hyoid bone; may present anywhere from base of tongue to just above suprasternal notch

LABORATORY AND IMAGING STUDIES

- T_3, T_4, TSH when Hx/physical findings suggestive of hypothyroidism
- Ultrasound of neck to identify presence of thyroid gland in normal location
- Radioisotope scan to confirm presence of functioning thyroid in normal location

DIFFERENTIAL DIAGNOSIS

- Dermoid cyst
- Branchial cleft cyst
- Ectopic thyroid gland
- Lymph node
- Hypertrophied pyramidal lobe of thyroid
- Thyroid nodule
- Lipoma
- Hemangioma

TREATMENT

- *Asymptomatic pt:* Sistrunk surgical procedure, which includes resection of cyst w/center of hyoid bone/duct to base of tongue
- *Infected cyst:* incision/drainage w/delayed resection following course of antibiotics/resolution of inflammation

COMPLICATIONS

- Untreated:
  - 50% become infected
  - 1% risk of malignancy
- Surgically excised w/Sistrunk procedure:
  - 4% risk of recurrence
  - 14% risk of recurrence if previously infected
  - 1% risk of removal of ectopic thyroid gland misdiagnosed as thyroglossal duct cyst

WHEN TO REFER

- Referral should occur at time of presentation

BACKGROUND

- Thyrotoxicosis refers to clinical syndrome that results from excessive levels of thyroid hormone in blood. Graves disease commonest cause of thyrotoxicosis in pediatric age group. Symptoms develop insidiously, often missed in early stages. Graves disease is organ-specific defect in suppressor T-cells allowing development of antibody to thyrotropin (TSH) receptor. Antibody stimulates thyroid gland, results in unregulated production, release of thyroid hormone. Form of thyrotoxicosis occurs in neonatal period due to transplacental passage of an antibody from mother who has or has had Graves disease

CLINICAL MANIFESTATIONS

- Nervousness, irritability, declining school performance, weight loss in spite of good appetite, heat intolerance, fatigability, palpitations
- Goiter, prominent eyes, exophthalmos, tremors, proximal muscle weakness, tachycardia, wide pulse pressure
- In neonatal period baby usually normal at birth but within a week becomes nervous, irritable, jittery, loses weight. Liver, spleen may be enlarged child may go into heart failure. Eyes may be prominent
- Some children present w/unilateral or bilateral exophthalmos w/no other Sx. This is called euthyroid Graves and requires treatment only if thyroid hormone levels ↑

LABORATORY FEATURES

- Serum thyrotropin (TSH) suppressed below normal values
- Serum thyroid hormones, free thyroxine (FT4), free triiodothyronine (FT3) ↑ above normal values for age
- Measurement of thyroid stimulating antibodies or radioactive iodine uptake not necessary. Ultrasound only required if gland irregular

DIFFERENTIAL DIAGNOSIS

- Anxiety
- Ingestion of thyroid hormone
- Subacute thyroiditis
- Iodine ingestion
- Pituitary resistance to thyroid hormone

TREATMENT

- Children tolerate excess thyroid hormone better than adults do. Relief for tremors, tachycardia can be achieved w/beta blockers. In newborn propanalol, 2 mg/kg/d; in older children, 10 mg/kg/d

Antithyroid Drugs

- Propylthiouracil (PTU) or methimazole (MZ) controls synthesis of thyroid hormone. PTU, 10 mg/kg/d or MZ, 0.5–1.0 mg/kg/d in div doses appear to be equally effective. MZ has longer half-life than PTU, may be given 2×/d
- Takes 6–12 wks to control disease w/antithyroid drugs. Dose may be ↑ if no improvement in thyroid hormone levels in 8 wks. Compliance w/medication routine should always be considered when thyroid hormone levels remain ↑. As thyroid hormone levels return to normal, dose of antithyroid medication should be reduced, adjusted to maintain thyroid hormone levels within normal range
- Side effects of antithyroid medications occur in 3–5% of children. Include rashes, suppressed WBC count, abnormal liver enzymes, jaundice, arthralgias. All usually reversible when medication stopped. Changes in WBC count unpredictable. WBC counts should be performed if unexplained fever, mouth ulcers develop. Liver enzymes should be measured at each visit, antithyroid drugs stopped if AST > 100 units
- Once thyroid hormone levels stabilized, treatment should continue 18–24 mos. Remission rate in children ~40–50% over that time. Children w/large goiters, very severe thyrotoxicosis more likely not to go into remission. At end of this time antithyroid drugs should be withdrawn, blood levels followed. Relapse usually occurs within 6 mos

Surgery

- If remission fails to occur while on antithyroid drug Tx, subtotal or total thyroidectomy an option. Total thyroidectomy favored by some because it reduces risk of recurrence of hyperthyroidism from remnant. Complications of surgery include recurrent laryngeal nerve damage, hypoparathyroidism
- Thyroid surgery infrequent in children now so surgeon w/experience should be selected

Radioactive Iodine

- Radioactive iodine use still controversial but treatment of choice in children who have completed pubertal growth. Some centers using radioactive iodine as initial treatment. After children have been rendered euthyroid w/antithyroid drugs, 5–15 mC usually effective. Dose may be repeated in 6 mos if children not made euthyroid
- Radioactive iodine should be used w/caution if ophthalmopathy severe, because it may become worse. Worsening usually transient, can be controlled w/corticosteroids
- Goal of surgery, radioactive iodine should be to make child hypothyroid. Hypothyroidism much easier to manage than thyrotoxicosis resistant to antithyroid drugs

WHEN TO REFER

- To an endocrinologist at Dx, if difficulty in controlling thyroid hormone levels or side effects develop that do not respond to withdrawal of antithyroid drugs
- Prior to surgery, if radioactive iodine being considered
- To ophthalmologist if eye disease severe

BACKGROUND

- Frequently encountered; most benign (resolves w/growth)
- Distinguish benign from poorer prognosis/bowing may require orthopedic evaluation; treatment
- Divided into deformities primarily involving coronal plane (common)/sagittal plane (infrequent)
- *Coronal deformities:* physiologic genu varum/Blount disease; *Sagittal deformities:* congenital posteromedial bow of tibia, congenital pseudoarthrosis of tibia, fibular hemimelia; most frequent: physiologic genu varum
- Infants normally have some varus leg bowing; spontaneous resolution expected by age 2 yrs; rebound genu valgum may occur 2–5 yrs of age

CLINICAL MANIFESTATIONS: CORONAL DEFORMITIES

- *Physiologic genu varum:* varus alignment of legs involve both femur/tibia; associated w/mild external rotation contractures of hips/internal tibial torsion
- *Blount disease:* appearance often indistinguishable from physiologic genu varum; does not occur <18–24 mos of age; time that physiologic genu varum should be resolving; unlike physiologic bowing, Blount disease varus deformity isolated to tibia; prominent medial beak located in tibia just below knee can often be palpated

SAGITTAL PLANE DEFORMITIES

- *Congenital posteromedial bow of tibia:* clinically apparent at birth; sharp angular deformity of lower leg just above ankle w/apex of angulation posterior; ≥30° angulation common; mild shortening of affected limb/foot normal in appearance
- *Congenital pseudoarthrosis of tibia:* apex anterior tibial bowing; associated w/neurofibromatosis (70% of cases); fracture of dysplastic bone may be present at birth/detected by motion of extremity at apex of deformity/frequently associated w/crepitance
- *Fibular hemimelia:* tibia demonstrates apex anterior bow/often associated w/shortening of tibia/femur; generally foot abnormal/frequent valgus alignment of ankle/foot; often absence of one/more rays of lateral foot

LABORATORY FEATURES

- Laboratory evaluation generally not indicated except if suspicion of nutritional rickets, other metabolic bone disease, x-linked hypophosphatemic rickets (serum calcium, phosphorus, vitamin D, urine phosphorus excretion)
- *Radiographic evaluation:* all sagittal plane deformities warrant radiographic evaluation; coronal plane deformities generally do not unless no resolution of deformity by age 2 (to r/o Blount disease); if suspicion of metabolic bone disease/nutritional rickets radiographs of involved extremities warranted

DIFFERENTIAL DIAGNOSIS

- Rickets, x-linked type of hypophosphatemic rickets, renal osteodystrophy, skeletal dysplasias

TREATMENT

- *Physiologic genu varum:* great majority resolve w/o treatment; in extreme cases orthotic management
- *Blount disease:* pts <3 yrs of age w/mild deformity treated w/long leg braces designed to provide varus correcting force at knee; in more advanced cases/>3 yrs, surgery to correct varus alignment
- *Congenital posteromedial bow of the tibia:* resolves spontaneously within first 5 yrs of life; often left w/residual limb length discrepancy (may require epiphysiodesis/tibial lengthening in adolescence)
- *Congenital pseudoarthrosis of the tibia:* bracing used to prevent fracture/to stabilize pseudoarthrosis already present; surgery required in most cases to achieve union
- *Fibular hemimelia:* depending on severity may require orthotics/surgical management; if severe shortening of extremity, amputation/prosthetic fitting recommended

COMPLICATIONS

- *Blount disease:* recurrence
- *Posteromedial bow of tibia:* limb length discrepancy
- *Congenital pseudoarthrosis of tibia:* failure to achieve surgical union/recurrent fractures (may lead to recommendation of amputation/prosthetic fitting)

WHEN TO REFER

- *Coronal deformities:* varus tibial deformities not resolving by age 2 yrs referred for evaluation of possible Blount disease
- *Sagittal deformities:* all sagittal deformities warrant evaluation by pediatric orthopedist

TIBIA TORSION, INTERNAL

JAMES T. BENNETT

BACKGROUND

- Most common cause of in-toeing gait in early ambulator (18 mos–2 yrs)
- Historically treated w/number of different orthotics including Dennis Brown Bar, corrective shoes and/or wedges
- Now considered normal finding in most pts, reflecting intrauterine confinement as well as normal torsion that follows dermatomes

CLINICAL MANIFESTATIONS

- W/knees forward feet assume turned-in appearance
- Sighting down alignment of thigh w/knee flexed, foot turned inward (in contrast to normal adult where there is slight toe-out, consequence of external tibial torsion)
- Can be demonstrated in newborn period if hips internally rotated
- Often associated w/physiologic genu varum

LABORATORY FEATURES

- Severe in-toeing w/internal tibial torsion should be differentiated from infantile Blount in which significant varus (bow) deformity concomitant w/internal tibial torsion
- Radiographs include AP of lower extremities of child (after walking age)/measuring metaphyseal diaphyseal angulation

- Beaking of proximal tibia (>11°) usually associated w/Blount disease
- For older pts in whom internal tibial torsion persists, absolute magnitude of torsion can be calculated by CT scan through hip, knee, ankles

DIFFERENTIAL DIAGNOSIS

- Other causes of in-toeing include deformity of foot (metatarsus adductus, talipes equino varus, clubfoot)/femoral anteversion

TREATMENT

- No treatment indicated for majority of pts w/natural Hx one of resolution of internal tibial torsion *almost* universally
- *Bracing:* occasionally Dennis Brown Bar used to alter pt's sleeping posture/can be used > age 18 mos, generally < age 2½; no alteration of actual torsion of tibia, rather improvement in gait comes from stretching soft tissues at hips, knees, ankles
- No role for corrective shoes in internal tibial torsion
- Surgery for persistently severe in-toeing gait/distal tibial (and sometimes fibular) osteotomy can be entertained; generally deferred until pt 8–10 yrs of age allowing normal physiologic remolding to occur; prior to correction, femoral anteversion as 1°/contributing cause of in-toeing should be excluded

COMPLICATIONS

- Internal tibial torsion normal phenomenon in most toddlers/young children; major complication: overtreatment for this benign process
- Complications can occur following surgery (rarely necessary/should be deferred until pt ~8–10 yrs of age)

WHEN TO REFER

- Most managed w/o referral w/reassurance that pt's exam physiologic
- Avoid guaranteeing parents that child will "outgrow" this; although most do, occasional child (esp if concomitant neuropathic process such as mild cerebral palsy/myelodysplasia) will not
- Equip your office w/pt education booklets in which these common physiologic variations can be demonstrated to parents

TIBIA VARA (TV), INFANTILE AND ADOLESCENT (LATE ONSET) (Blount Disease)

RICHARD C. HENDERSON

BACKGROUND

- Also called Blount disease
- Results from ↓ growth in medial portion of proximal tibial growth plate
- One/both legs may be affected
- Most frequently develops ages 18–36 mos (infantile TV)/at puberty w/boys ages 10–13 yrs; girls 1–2 yrs earlier (adolescent TV)
- *Infantile TV:* somewhat more common in blacks and females; likely to be heavy/early walker
- *Adolescent* (late onset) *TV:* most very obese black males w/prevalence 2–3% in this at-risk group; very rare in whites/those <95th percentile weight for age
- Mechanical factors implicated in etiology of growth plate dysfunction; endocrine abnormalities/metabolic bone disease not involved

CLINICAL MANIFESTATIONS

- Infantile TV:
  – most common presenting complaint: toddler w/persistent/worsening "bowed-leg" deformity; if neglected may present later w/severe deformity
  – internal tibia torsion usually present in addition to varus deformity; may be severe
- Adolescent TV:
  – presenting complaint may be progressive "bowed-leg" deformity, often developing rapidly during growth spurt, and/or knee pain
  – Dx often delayed due to lack of symptoms, very obese body habitus that obscures even severe deformity, hesitancy of typical pt (obese adolescent black male) to seek medical evaluation

LABORATORY FEATURES

- Lab results expected to be normal; may r/o metabolic bone diseases such as hypophosphatemic rickets as cause of bowing
- X ray after age 24–30 mos diagnostic; prior to that age, x rays helpful, but not totally reliable; x rays rarely necessary for evaluation of most "bowed legs"

DIFFERENTIAL DIAGNOSIS

- Internal tibial torsion (ITT):
  – common, benign, self-limited condition that may be quite marked, asymmetric, associated w/tripping
  – gives false appearance of varus at knees when child seen standing w/hips externally rotated/knees slightly flexed
  – *clinical exam:* w/child supine/limb rotated to position patella straight anteriorly shows bowing to be all distal to tibial tubercle; proximal tibia/knee joint not truly in varus
  – children <18–24 mos can be observed; ITT expected to improve; infantile TV worsens
  – x rays rarely needed to r/o ITT as cause of "bowed legs"
  – metabolic bone disease (most commonly hypophosphatemic rickets)
  – bone dysplasias (most commonly metaphyseal chondrodysplasia)
  – stature >25th percentile, negative family Hx for short stature or bowing in adults, and x rays showing no abnormalities other than at the knee help r/o uncommon causes of bowing

TREATMENT

- Most always surgical (bracing sometimes used in mild cases of infantile TV diagnosed early)
- Deformity often recurrent, particularly infantile TV treated after age 4–5 yrs; repeat surgery may be required

COMPLICATIONS

- In addition to varus deformity, shortening of ≥4 cm may occur if disease unilateral
- In severe cases of infantile TV, irreversible bone bridge may form as early as age 6–8 yrs/prevent further growth in medial portion of proximal tibial growth plate; severe shortening, angular deformity, distortion of knee joint surface result

WHEN TO REFER

- Condition may be subtle early in disease process; referral usually not necessary for Dx
- All cases of TV should be referred to orthopedic surgeon; progressive/almost always require surgical treatment
- When early Dx/treatment more surgical options; w/infantile TV, much greater likelihood that growth plate dysfunction will be reversible

BACKGROUND

- Most frequently found 3–10 yrs of age w/peak occurrence ~7 yrs; prevalence drops sharply > age 13
- Incidence of simple/chronic tics 1–13%; for Tourette 0.4%
- M:F ratio 2:1 for simple/chronic tics, 3–4:1 for Tourette
- Etiology unclear for simple/chronic tics but in families w/one tic disorder, individuals at higher risk for other tic disorders/obsessive compulsive disorder; for Tourette, genetic factors play an important role (strong association w/obsessive compulsive disorder/attention deficit hyperactivity disorder)

CLINICAL MANIFESTATIONS

- All tics stress sensitive; can be exacerbated/accentuated w/stress
- Simple twitching, nose movements, eye blinking, throat clearing, simple vocal noises
  – simple tics transient (come/go, often change)
  – chronic tics more persistent/enduring, do not generally change
- Tourette: chronic motor tics that can occur in any part of body/often complex; phonic tics begin 1–2 yrs after onset of motor tics/usually simple squeaking, grunting, coughing, throat clearing; coprolalia uncommon

LABORATORY FEATURES

- No specific tests used; EEG/neuroimaging noncontributory

DIFFERENTIAL DIAGNOSIS

- Myoclonus, chorea, akathesia, dystonia, tremors, athetosis
- Huntington chorea, Wilson disease, obsessive compulsive disorder

TREATMENT

- Simple/chronic tics:
  – reassurance for simple tics: vast majority disappear w/age
  – behavior Tx/hypnosis for chronic tics may help pt suppress tics in public
  – pt/family education regarding nonvolitional neuropsychiatric nature of tic disorders
  – anxiolytics *not* recommended except for short periods of extreme stress; psychotherapy may also be warranted in such cases
- Tourette
  – dopamine D_2 receptor antagonists (side effects: sedation, cognitive dulling, akathesia, dystonia, weight gain, tardive dyskinesia):
    ○ haloperidol, 0.25 µg gradually ↑ as needed up to 6 µg/d
  – pimozide, 1 µg gradually ↑ as needed up to 10 µg/d
  – alpha$_2$ adrenergic receptor agonist: (side effects: primarily sedation, potential hypotension/rebound hypertension w/sudden cessation of medication):
    ○ clonidine, 0.05 µg gradually ↑ as needed to 0.25 µg/d

COMPLICATIONS

- *Simple:* transient nature
- *Chronic:* rarely may interfere w/social function
- *Tourette:* often associated w/behavioral/emotional problems, obsessive compulsive disorder, ADHD, affective disorder

PROGNOSIS

- *Simple:* good; benign/transient
- *Chronic:* generally good; likely to diminish/disappear in adolescent
- *Tourette:* lifelong disorder; waxes/wanes; may improve in late adolescence/adulthood; symptomatic improvement up to 70% of cases w/haloperidol/pimozide; symptomatic improvement up to 30% of cases w/clonidine

WHEN TO REFER

- *Simple:* generally not necessary
- *Chronic:* generally not necessary unless tics significantly interfere w/social/school functioning
- *Tourette:* generally refer to child and adolescent psychiatrist/pediatric neurologist due to complex nature of illness, medication management

BACKGROUND

- *Dermatophytosis:* group of related fungi that live in soil, on animals, on humans/capable of infecting keratinized tissue such as stratum corneum, hair, nails; these infections, known as tineas, manifest in variety of disease patterns depending on involved site. Dermatophytic genera involved include Trichophyton, Microsporum, Epidermophyton

	Tinea capitis	Tinea corporis	Tinea cruris	Tinea pedis
Etiology	• T. tonsurans (90%) • M. canis	• E. floccosum • T. rubrum	• Trichophyton species • E. floccosum	• T. rubrum • T. mentagrophytes • E. floccosum
Population	• Prepubertal children • Blacks > whites	• All ages • Animal workers	• Postpubertal • Males > females	• Late childhood, adults • Males > females
Transmission	• Direct contact w/infected person, animal, or fomite	• Direct contact w/infected human, animal, or soil	• Most individuals have Tinea pedis, which is transferred from feet to crural area by hands	• Walking barefoot on contaminated floor
Predisposing conditions	• Asymptomatic carrier in family • Sharing combs, brushes, hats • Overcrowded conditions	• Autoinoculation from feet or scalp • Warm, humid climate	• Obesity • Tight clothing • Warm, humid climate • Sports participation	• Public pool or showers • Infected family member • Occlusive footwear • Hot, humid weather
Clinical manifestations	• Round patches of scale w/or w/o alopecia • Inflammatory pustules • Black dot sign: broken-off hairs near surface • Kerion: painful inflammatory tumor w/hair loss, draining pustules on surface	• Erythematous, scaly plaques w/sharply defined papulovesicular border, central clearing located on trunk, extremities, face • W/or w/o pruritus	• Well-marginated, erythematous scaly half-moon–shaped plaques in crural folds, upper thighs • W/or w/o pruritus	• Scaling, maceration, fissures of toe web spaces • Vesiculopustular eruption • Erythema, fine scaling, hyperkeratosis of plantar, lateral foot
Laboratory features	• KOH preparation • Fungal culture	• KOH preparation • Fungal culture	• KOH preparation • Fungal culture	• KOH preparation • Fungal culture
Differential diagnosis	• Seborrheic dermatitis • Psoriasis • Alopecia areata • Traction alopecia • Impetigo • Furunculosis • Histiocytosis	• Pityriasis rosea • Nummular eczema • Contact dermatitis • Erythema annulare • Psoriasis	• Intertrigo • Erythrasma • Psoriasis • Candidiasis • Irritant	• Erythrasma • Candida • Psoriasis • Eczema • Impetigo • Contact dermatitis
Treatment	• Oral antifungals • Kerion: prednisone 14 d tapering course w/or w/o oral antibiotics	• Topical antifungals • Oral antifungals for resistant/severe cases	• Topical antifungals • Oral antifungals for resistant/severe cases	• Topical antifungals • Oral antifungals if nail involvement
Prevention	• Examine all household contacts for asymptomatic carriers		• Loose cotton underwear • Bland absorbent powder	• Shower shoes • Open footwear • Antifungal foot powder

MEDICATIONS

- Topical antifungals:
  – imidazoles: clotrimazole (Lotrimin), miconazole (Micatin), ketaconazole (Nizoral)
  – allylamines: naftifine (Naftin), terbinafine (Lamisil), butenafine (Mentax)
  – treatment regimen: apply bid × 4 wks or until 3 wks after lesions cleared
- Oral antifungals:
  – griseofulvin:
    ○ children: microsize 15–20 mg/kg/d or ultramicrosize 7.5 mg/kg/d × 4–12 wks; adult: microsize 500–1,000 mg/d or ultramicrosize 330–750 mg/d × 4–12 wks; take w/fatty food to enhance absorption (ie, milk/ice cream); use sunblock during summer months
    ○ side effects: rare but include headache, nausea, vomiting, photosensivity, ↓ effect of warfarin/oral contraceptives
    ○ labs: obtain CBC/LFT's if on medication >6 wks
  – others: terbinafine, itraconazole, indicated for treatment of Tinea capitis in children allergic to/intolerant of griseofulvin; not yet FDA approved as first-line agent in pediatric population
    ○ ketoconazole: not recommended in view of rare but fatal hepatotoxicity

COMPLICATIONS

- 2° bacterial infection, scarring alopecia from kerion, "id" reaction

WHEN TO REFER

- Referral indicated when Dx in doubt, for development of serious complications/if disease fails to respond to adequate course of Tx despite good compliance

RICHARD J. MIER

BACKGROUND

- *Definition:* twisted neck, usually w/head laterally flexed/rotated on neck
- Causes may be congenital/acquired; include: congenital muscular torticollis; postnatal positioning; gastoesophageal reflux; strabismus; rotatory atlantoaxial subluxation; upper respiratory tract infections; tumors of posterior fossa/brainsteam; medications (phenothiazines); cervical disc calcification; occipitocervical malformations; trauma; CNS malformations; viral myositis; JRA; pseudotumor cerebri; dystonias; vertebral tumors (osteoid osteoma); myositis ossificans progressiva
- Muscular causes by far most common

CLINICAL MANIFESTATIONS

- Congenital muscular torticollis (CMT) draws head into lateral flexion on affected side/rotates chin to contralateral side
- W/CMT may be other positional deformities, including hip dysplasia, facial asymmetry, plagiocephaly
- Olive-shaped swelling in sternocleidomastoid (SCM) muscle appears early in postnatal period/regresses by 1 yr, even if torticollis persists
- W/congenital occipitocervical abnormalities, including vertebral fusion (Klippel-Feil), look for low hairline, short neck, webbing
- W/strabismus, resulting head tilt goes away/at least gets much better when child lies down, compared to sitting
- Painful acquired torticollis may be associated w/osteoid osteoma/osteoblastoma
- Gastroesophageal reflux may cause torticollislike positioning
- Any local inflammation (ie, pharyngitis) may cause self-limited torticollis directly/may occasionally lead to rotatory subluxation of C1–C2, w/persistent symptoms

DIFFERENTIAL DIAGNOSIS

- *Congenital:* radiographs of cervical spine should be performed on any infant w/congenital torticollis before physical Tx begun
- *Congenital:* ultrasonography/radiographs of hips because of association of torticollis w/developmental dysplasia of hip
- *Congenital:* CT scan should be performed for congenital torticollis if radiographic abnormality, webbing, short neck, low hairline, rigid deformity, neurologic abnormality, if no olive/shortening of SCM muscle
- *Acquired:* after radiographs, CT (for suspected bony lesion)/MRI (for soft tissue, cord lesion) for older child if symptoms severe/persistent, if cause not apparent
- *Acquired:* technetium bone scan for suspected bony vertebral tumor

TREATMENT

- *For congenital muscular torticollis:* physical Tx beginning w/therapist, continuing at home
- Lateral flexion of head away from tight side w/rotation toward affected side
- 10 gentle repetitions, holding at max range 3–4 ×/d
- Persistent tightness may require surgical correction w/postop Tx/splinting
- Early strabismus surgery may be indicated for ocular torticollis to prevent facial asymmetry

COMPLICATIONS

- Failure to discover congenital occipitocervical malformation before beginning Tx may result in cord injury
- Persistently ↓ ROM results in growth disturbances, facial/cranial asymmetry

WHEN TO REFER

- Most cases of congenital muscular torticollis improve w/time/many cases of acquired torticollis self-limited
- Refer for congenital muscular torticollis not improving by time infant is 6 mos
- Refer when Dx doubt/if initial Tx proves ineffective

TOURETTE SYNDROME (TS) AND RELATED DISORDERS
L. JARRETT BARNHILL

BACKGROUND

- *Tourette syndrome (TS):* nonprogressive, developmental movement disorder
- Like other movement disorders, tic disorders are:
  - exacerbated by fatigue, distress, intense affect
  - ↓ during relaxation/intense concentration
  - variably suppressed but w/sense of building pressure/explosion movements
  - once considered rare, TS may present in 1–6/1,000; if all tic disorders considered, incidence rises to 4–10% of school-aged children
  - M:F ratio 3–4:1
  - age of onset varies; mean onset of simple motor tics 6–7 yrs of age; mean age of onset of vocal tics 8–10 yrs of age
  - majority of pts w/tic disorders have mild forms of disorder
  - pts w/more severe movements have > incidence of associated coprolalia, echolalia, palilalia, copropraxia, echopraxia, significant behavior disturbances

CLINICAL MANIFESTATIONS

- *Simple motor tics:* rapid, involuntary, repetitive, nonrhythmic, meaningless movements
- *Complex motor tics:* series of movements, often preceded by sensory phenomena, overlap stereotypies/compulsive behaviors
- *Phonic tics:* vocalizations ranging from sniffing, coughing, throat clearing to barking/forced expiratory sounds
- Complex vocal tics may involve words/phrases
- Coprolalia uncommon (10–20% of severe ticquers); no longer included in diagnostic criteria
- Tourette syndrome:
  - presence of motor/phonic tics for at least 1 yr
  - age of onset < age 21
  - variable course, w/waxing/waning severity, as well as changing pattern of tic distribution
  - r/o other movement disorders
- Other tic disorders:
  - <1 yr in duration (transient tic disorder)
  - lack combined motor/phonic tics
  - unchanging distribution (chronic motor/phonic tic disorder)

DIFFERENTIAL DIAGNOSIS

- Pediatric autoimmune neurologic disorders associated w/streptococcal diseases (PANDAS) may account for up to 5% of new cases of tic disorders:
  - abrupt onset
  - negative family Hx
  - negative past Hx
  - exposure to/clinical infection w/group A beta-hemolytic strep
  - symptoms emerge wks after infection
  - persist for several mos
  - gradually abate
  - ↑ ASO, anti-streptococcal DNA-ASE B titers
  - treatment w/penicillin/plasmapheresis
- Wilson disease
- Drug-induced movement disorders may be caused by:
  - antihistaminics
  - anticonvulsants
  - tricyclic antidepressants
  - serotonin reuptake inhibitors
  - phenothiazine derivatives
  - caffeine
  - psychostimulants
  - myoclonic movements (nonsuppressible, associated w/movement initiation)
  - paroxysmal movement disorders (focal epileptiform discharges from basal ganglia)

COMPLICATIONS

- Waxing/waning of movements complicate treatment
- 40–60% may have obsessive-compulsive symptoms (OCS)/clinical obsessive-compulsive disorder (OCD)
  - OCD more common in females genetically vulnerable to TS
  - many pts display age-related transitions from tic disorder to obsessive-compulsive disorder (OCD)
  - emergence of tics in pts w/previous OCD
- 30–40% of pts w/TS have associated ADHD:
  - 1.5% of children treated w/stimulants develop tics
- Anxiety disorders, social phobic behaviors common
- Impulse control, oppositional defiant, conduct disorders lead to psychiatric referral
- Sleep disorders including parasomnias/sleep apneas have incidence of ~15%
- Migraine/vascular headaches frequently reported
- Tardive dyskinesia:
  - 20% treated w/neuroleptics
  - manifest as motor/phonic tics (tardive Tourette)
  - pts w/TS at ↑ risk for neuroleptic-induced movement disorders

TREATMENT

- Treatment criteria:
  - painful/socially disruptive tics
  - cause subjective distress, teasing
  - provoke self-consciousness/social avoidance, esp among adolescents
  - exacerbation of symptoms w/puberty
  - behavioral/emotional comorbidity
- Clonidine/guanfacine: alpha andrenergic agonists:
  - mild tic disorders
  - comorbid ADHD/conduct disorder
- Clonazepam: benzodiazepine:
  - axial/dystonic movements
  - comorbid anxiety disorders
  - sedation may limit usefulness
- Serotonin reuptake inhibitors (SSRIs):
  - fluoxetine (Prozac)
  - sertraline (Zoloft)
  - paroxetine (Paxil)
  - fluvoxamine (Luvox)
  - citalopram (Celexa)
  - venlafaxine (Effexor)
  - associated obsessive-compulsive disorder
  - presence of TS may limit response to SSRI monotherapy for OCD
- Neuroleptics should be reserved for:
  - severe tic disorders resistant to alternative
  - pts exquisitely sensitive to extrapyramidal side effects: akathisia, drug-induced dysphoria, tardive dyskinesias
  - commonly used: haloperidol (Haldol), pimozide (Orap), risperidone (Risperdal), olanzapine (Zyprexa), quetiapine (Seroquel)
- Stimulants often discontinued after onset of motor/phonic tics:
  - pts may require stimulants for persistent ADHD
  - unresponsive to antidepressant/alpha agonists
  - pts w/long-standing tic disorders, stimulants cautiously reintroduced, closely monitored

WHEN TO REFER

- Pts w/severe tic disorders resistant to standard treatments
- Severe comorbid psychopathology
- Atypical clinical course
- Use local Tourette Syndrome Association for support groups, information, clinical resources

BACKGROUND

- *Staphylococcus aureus* and *Streptococcus pyogenes* (group A beta-hemolytic streptococci) can both cause life-threatening shock syndromes w/abrupt onset, rapid progression leading to multiorgan dysfunction, potential for substantial risk of death
- In staphylococcal toxic shock, toxin (TSST-1) that triggers process absorbed from mucosal site colonized w/TSST-1 producing strain. TSST-1 is superantigen that causes systemic cytokine release by inducing polyclonal activation of T lymphocytes. Tissue-invasive staphylococcal infection or sepsis rarely demonstrated
- When menses-associated toxic shock accounted for >90% of cases, site of colonization was vagina, use of highly absorbent tampons implicated in promotion of localized replication of *Staphylococcus aureus*
- In prepubescent children, colonization of mucosa of upper respiratory tract most common, although minor skin lesions also implicated. Surgical wounds may also become colonized w/toxin-producing strains, but these lesions rarely show clinical evidence of localized inflammation
- Toxic shock syndrome associated w/*Streptococcus pyogenes* infection almost always occurs in association w/tissue-invasive infectious process. Blood culture positive in close to 60% of cases due to *S. pyogenes*. Marked propensity for development of rapidly progressive cellulitis that may evolve into necrotizing fasciitis or myositis
- Portal of entry for invasive streptococcal infection commonly skin lesion (or multiple skin lesions), w/antecedent varicella infection playing prominent role in childhood cases. Otherwise, infection usually initiated in respiratory tract or as 1° bacteremia

CLINICAL MANIFESTATIONS

- *Staphylococcal toxic shock syndrome* has abrupt onset w/high fever, headache, myalgia, vomiting, profuse diarrhea, altered sensorium
- Diffuse erythroderma, mucosal erythema, profound hypotension emerge within hours of onset of symptoms
- Leukocytosis, thrombocytopenia, evidence for impaired renal function, ↑ AST and ALT, ↑ CPK reflecting rhabdomyolysis are among common laboratory manifestations
- *Streptococcal toxic shock* usually presents as relentlessly progressive tissue-invasive infection (usually of skin) that evolves into toxic shock syndrome, usually by second or third day following onset of tissue invasion
- Necrotizing skin infections characterized by edema, erythema, intense pain. As soft tissue lesion evolves perfusion of skin impaired w/emergence of bluish or violaceous hue w/or w/o superficial vesicles. As illness progresses, hypotension, multiorgan system dysfunction develop, w/renal impairment, liver dysfunction, adult respiratory distress syndrome, cerebral dysfunction

---

Streptococcal Toxic Shock

Microbiologic

Isolation of *S. pyogenes* from normally sterile site (required for definite case). Blood culture positive in ~60% of cases.

Clinical

- Hypotension (systolic BP <5% ile age) and
- 2 or more of following:
  - renal impairment
  - coagulopathy
  - liver involvement
  - adult respiratory distress syndrome
  - generalized erythematous macular rash
  - soft tissue necrosis (fasciitis, myositis, or gangrene)

Staphylococcal Toxic Shock

Isolation of *S. aureus* from mucosal site or colonized (but usually not inflamed) wound.

Blood culture rarely positive

- Temperature ≥ 39°C, systolic hypotension
- Rash w/subsequent desquamation
- Involvement of 3 or more organ systems:
  - GI: vomiting, profuse diarrhea
  - muscle: myalgia, ↑ CPK
  - renal: BUN or creatinine > 2× normal
  - liver: ALT and/or AST > 2× normal
  - thrombocytopenia
  - disorientation
  - mucous membrane erythema

LABORATORY FEATURES

- Evidence for multiorgan system dysfunction typical of toxic shock mediated by both organisms. Renal, hepatic dysfunction commonly reflected by ↑ BUN, creatinine, ↑ serum concentrations of AST, ALT. Diffuse rhabdomyolysis reflected by ↑ serum CPK more common in staphylococcal TSS, but ↑ CPK may be observed w/localized necrotizing myositis in invasive streptococcal infection. Leucocytosis, immature neutrophils, thrombocytopenia typical of both syndromes

DIFFERENTIAL DIAGNOSIS

- Severity, rapidly progressive temporal evolution of these syndromes should distinguish them from illnesses commonly mentioned in differential Dx. Following disorders in differential Dx:
  - Rocky Mountain spotted fever
  - leptospirosis
  - measles
  - sepsis due to *N. meningitidis*, *S. pneumoniae*, enteric gram-negative bacteria, *P. aeruginosa*

TREATMENT

- Fluid, electrolyte (possibly w/colloid) resuscitation critical to stabilization of pts w/shock associated w/either infection
- In menstruating females, vagina must be examined, any tampon or foreign body removed, secretions obtained for culture
- For staphylococcal infection, provision of IV beta-lactamase stable antistaphylococcal penicillin (oxacillin, 200 mg/kg/d div q6h or nafcillin) required
- Invasive streptococcal infection can be treated initially w/penicillin G, third-generation cephalosporin, or antistaphylococcal penicillin. However, evidence that more rapid sterilization of necrotizing soft tissue infections can be achieved w/clindamycin; certain experts favor use of penicillin and clindamycin for these infections
- Clinical suspicion of necrotizing fasciitis followed by documentation of presence of necrosis by surgical biopsy, debridement of involved tissue important in controlling this form of invasive streptococcal infection
- IV immunoglobulin has been employed in streptococcal TSS w/anecdotal evidence suggesting possible benefit, but efficacy unproved. Whether such products contain toxin-specific neutralizing antibodies or interfere w/cytokine-mediated processes unknown

PREVENTION

- Recurrences of staphylococcal TSS, particularly menses-associated TSS, usually prevented by prohibiting, markedly limiting use of tampons. Highly absorbent tampons implicated in national outbreak of TSS have been removed from market
- If course of antistaphylococcal treatment used for initial episode of TSS effective in terminating vaginal colonization w/*S. aureus*, risk of recurrence should be low; however, limited tampon use still prudent
- Nearly 30% of childhood invasive streptococcal infections associated w/varicella infection. Therefore, varicella vaccine important in prevention of infections
- Strains of group A streptococci that cause invasive infection can be transmitted to close contacts in home or in child-care settings, including schools. Awareness of risk of invasive infection in close contacts can have implications for management of illnesses in these individuals

COMPLICATIONS

- Case fatality rate in typical menses-associated staphylococcal toxic shock syndrome <5%, when physicians were acutely aware of syndrome. Sporadic cases may or may not have as favorable an outcome
- Death-to-case ratio in streptococcal TSS can be as high as 30%. Identification, surgical management of necrotizing pyogenic tissue invasion (fasciitis, myositis, endometritis, empyema) can be important adjunct to effective clinical management

WHEN TO REFER

- Both of these syndromes require rapid, effective interventions to prevent fatal outcome. Evolution of staphylococcal TSS very rapid (over hrs). If effective control of shock can be accomplished w/fluids, electrolytes, colloid, syndrome and probable etiology recognized, appropriate antistaphylococcal antibiotic treatment initiated, most pts can be stabilized within 18–36 hrs. Early consultation w/infectious diseases, critical care consultants can help assure that early hrs of management optimized
- Invasive streptococcal infections, w/or w/o toxic shock syndrome, frequently require multidisciplinary team for effective management. Complex care of these pts can extend over several days. Referral to 3° center should be considered whenever aggressive, necrotizing tissue invasion occurs

BACKGROUND

- Etiologic agents are *Toxocara canis* (majority of cases) and *Toxocara cati*
- Worldwide distribution; seroprevalence 4–7% in US children w/estimated 10,000 cases of Toxocara infections per year in US
- Two major forms of disease: visceral larva migrans (VLM) and ocular larva migrans (OLM)
- VLM most frequently diagnosed in children <5 yrs of age, mean age 2 yrs; OLM most frequently diagnosed in children >5 yrs of age
- Identified risk factors include pica (geophagia) and exposure to puppies
- Pathogenesis: humans ingest Toxocara eggs (usually from soil), larvae hatch in GI tract, penetrate intestinal wall, are distributed to a variety of tissues (liver, lungs, heart, brain, muscle, eye), eliciting local immune response w/subsequent tissue damage
- Severity of symptoms depend on number of organisms ingested, degree of immune response

CLINICAL MANIFESTATIONS

- Hx pica, exposure to puppies common
- Majority of toxocara infections asymptomatic
- Sx VLM often varied, nonspecific: fever, malaise, anorexia, weight loss, abdominal complaints, hepatosplenomegaly, cough and/or wheeze, occasional rash or urticaria; rarely Sx of severe pneumonia, myocarditis, or meningoencephalitis
- Sx OLM more commonly include unilateral vision deficit occasionally w/strabismus; examination may reveal ≥1 posterior pole or peripheral pole granulomas, occasionally endophthalmitis or papillitis

LABORATORY FEATURES

- Humans do not excrete eggs or larvae; therefore stool examination can not be used to diagnose Toxocara infection
- Leukocytosis, hypereosinophilia, hypergammaglobulinemia more often present in VLM than OLM
- Tissue biopsies (eg, liver) not always positive, but may demonstrate granulomatous lesions w/eosinophils, neutrophils, rarely w/evidence of larvae
- Enzyme immunoassay (EIA) for Toxocara, available from CDC, some private laboratories, more useful in VLM than OLM (titer of ≥1:32 has sensitivity/specificity 78%/>90% in VLM and 73%/>90% in OLM). Positive titers do not prove current clinical infection w/organism
- Chest radiographs may demonstrate presence of infiltrates in VLM w/pulmonary involvement

DIFFERENTIAL DIAGNOSIS

- Sx VLM may be quite nonspecific, consistent w/variety of infectious diseases; added presence of marked eosinophilia, laboratory abnormalities noted may point toward Dx of migratory phase of a nematode, eosinophilic leukemia, or varied allergic disorders
- OLM must be differentiated from retinoblastoma as well as other infections producing retinal granulomas (eg, *Mycobacterium tuberculosis, Bartonella* spp., etc)

TREATMENT

- Efficacy of antihelmintic Tx variable, less effective in OLM
- Current drug of choice for symptomatic toxocariasis is diethylcarbamazine, 6 mg/kg/d in 3 doses × 7–10 d
- Alternative agents include albendazole (400 mg q12h × 3–5 d; 10 mg/kg/d in 2 doses × 5 d in one report) or mebendazole (100–200 mg bid × 5 d)
- Adjunctive Tx w/corticosteroids recommended in severe infections, esp in cases w/myocarditis/CNS involvement
- Severe retinal disease in OLM may require surgical management

COMPLICATIONS

- Recovery phase may be prolonged (up to 2 yrs) in significant infections
- Fatalities due to severe pulmonary, cardiac, or CNS disease are rare
- Permanent partial loss of vision may occur w/OLM

PREVENTION

- No vaccine available
- Address underlying etiologies of pica, if present
- Routine treatment of puppies, kittens w/antihelmintics to prevent Toxocara excretion
- Measures to ↓ contact w/animal feces (eg, proper disposal of cat, dog feces; cover sandboxes when not in use)
- Teach appropriate handwashing practices to young children

WHEN TO REFER

- Cases of suspected OLM should be referred to an ophthalmologist
- Referral indicated for other Toxocara infections if manifestations severe or Dx in doubt

BACKGROUND

- Parasitic infection by *toxoplasma gondii:*
  - worldwide distribution
  - definitive host: cat
- Infection of humans:
  - ingestion/inhalation of sporulated oocysts (ie, cleaning kitty litter box, eating unwashed fruits/vegetables contaminated by cysts, gardening in infected soil)
  - ingestion of infectious cysts in inadequately cooked meats
  - rarely by organ transplant, blood/leukocyte transfusion, laboratory accident
- congenital infection after 1° infection of immunocompetent pregnant woman/reactivation, 1° infection in immunocompromised pregnant woman
  - ○ risk of transmission across placenta by trimester: first < second < third
  - ○ if transmitted, risk of severe disease by trimester: first > second > third

CLINICAL MANIFESTATIONS

- Immunocompetent child/adult:
  - asymptomatic
  - lymphadenopathy w/or w/o fever/fatigue
  - rarely, organ involvement (heart, brain, eyes)
- Immunocompromised child/adult:
  - symptoms can be from 1° infection/reactivation
  - any organ can be involved: most commonly CNS/eyes
- Congenital infection:
  - asymptomatic (still at risk for later onset of chorioretinitis/developmental delay)
  - chorioretinitis, hydrocephalus, microcephalus, cranial calcifications, hepatosplenomegaly, jaundice, rash

LABORATORY DIAGNOSIS

- Specific studies:
  - *T. gondii* IgG specific: dye test, IFA, EIA, direct agglutination
  - *T. gondii* IgM specific: double-sandwiched IgM, ISAGA, EIA
  - other *T. gondii*–specific antibodies: IgA, EIA, IgE, EIA, ISAGA
  - PCR amplification/isolation of organism from blood, CSF, placenta, amniotic fluid
- Supporting studies:
  - hematologic abnormalities: thrombocytopenia, anemia, mild eosinophilia
  - liver abnormalities: direct hyperbilirubinemia
  - CSF: ↑ protein, pleocytosis, glucose either normal/low
  - chorioretinitis on ophthalmologic examination
  - cranial calcifications detected by head ultrasound, radiograph/CT

DIFFERENTIAL DIAGNOSIS

- Congenital toxoplasmosis:
  - congenital infections: CMV, rubella syndrome, syphilis, herpes simplex
  - neonatal bacterial sepsis
  - metabolic infections: galactosemia, tyrosinemia
  - hematologic diseases: immune thrombocytopenia, congenital leukemia
- Postnatal infections

TREATMENT

- Infection during pregnancy:
  - prevention of transmission across placenta: spiramycin (3 g/d po)
  - ↓ transmission across placenta by 50–60%/does not treat infected fetus
  - if fetal infection recognized; pyrimethamine (100 mg/d loading dose, then 50 mg/d po) *plus* sulfadiazine (100 mg/kg/d, max 4 g/d po), *plus* leucovorin (5–20 mg/d po), offsets leukopenia effects of treatment drugs
- Congenital infection:
  - optimal length of treatment not known; currently recommended to treat × 1 y
  - pyrimethamine (load: 2 mg/kg/d × 2 d [max 50 mg], then 1 mg/kg/d [max 25 mg]; after 2–6 mos can be switched to 3×/wk *plus* sulfadiazine (100 mg/kg/d div in 2 doses) *plus* leucovorin (5–20 mg 3×/wk)
- Immunocompetent w/o organ involvement: no treatment
- Immunocompromised/organ involvement:
  - pyrimethamine, sulfadiazine, leucovorin (doses as above)
  - treat 4–6 wks beyond resolution of symptoms

COMPLICATIONS

- 40–80% congenitally infected newborns who are asymptomatic at birth/untreated develop neurologic, ophthalmologic abnormalities over time

PREVENTION

- Avoid contact w/contaminated substances:
  - avoid cleaning cat's litter box during pregnancy; good hand washing if unavoidable
  - wear gloves while gardening; good hand washing after gardening/cleaning vegetables
  - cook meat thoroughly; good hand washing after handling raw meat

WHEN TO REFER

- If organ involvement present in any pt
- If congenital infection suspected
- If infection in immunocompromised host suspected

BACKGROUND

- Usually occurs when viral infection wanes w/abrupt worsening/onset of new fever, stridor
- Can follow laryngotracheitis (croup), influenza, measles/other less significant URIs
- More commonly seen in late fall/late spring but may occur anytime
- Peak incidence 2–4 yrs of age
- *Usual causes: S. aureus, S. pyogenes, S. pneumoniae*

CLINICAL MANIFESTATIONS

- Prodrome of viral respiratory illness
- Abrupt onset of stridor/toxicity w/associated brassy cough, anxiety
- Voice often hoarse, raspy
- Fever usually associated w/stridor/toxicity
- Does not respond to racemic epinephrine typically
- Pt unable to improve air flow by any positional maneuver

LABORATORY FEATURES

- *WBC count / differential:* neutrophilia, immature forms seen on white count
- *Microbiology:* Gram stain/culture of secretions in subglottic trachea usually confirm etiology; organism isolated from blood cultures in <50% pts; most common bacteria cultured from subglottic trachea include toxin-producing strains of *S. aureus / S. pyogenes*
- *Radiographs:* should *not* be obtained if Dx bacterial tracheitis suspected; if radiographs obtained after intubation/for other reasons, lateral neck radiographs may show subglottic narrowing, irregular trachea/possible intraluminal mass w/distended hypopharynx; chest radiograph may show patchy parenchymal peribronchial infiltrate
- *Bronchoscopy:* observation of pseudomembranes/purulent secretions in subglottic trachea w/erythematous, edematous, eroded trachea/bronchi

DIFFERENTIAL DIAGNOSIS

- Viral laryngotracheitis/croup syndrome
- Epiglottis
- Retropharyngeal abscess, peritonsillar abscess, lingual tonsillitis
- Foreign body aspiration
- Angioneurotic edema (allergic laryngeal edema)
- Diphtheria

TREATMENT

- Maintenance of adequate airway 1° concern/goal of management w/minimal stimulation/agitation of pt while arranging appropriate evaluation
- When Dx bacterial tracheitis suspected, pt should be transported to 3° setting where artificial airway maintained
- >75% of cases require artificial airway w/median intubation period 6 d
- Antimicrobial agents effective against *S. aureus, H. influenzae* type B, streptococci required (eg, nafcillin, 100 mg/kg/d w/ceftriaxone, 50–75 mg/kg/d)/should be initiated after appropriate cultures obtained
- Antibiotics usually continued 10–14 d w/oral administration after defervescence/extubation

COMPLICATIONS

- Endotracheal tube plugging/accidental extubation w/subsequent cardiorespiratory arrest most common causes of morbidity/mortality
- Other complications include pneumonia, atelectasis, pulmonary edema, septicemia, retropharyngeal cellulitis
- Subglottic stenosis infrequent sequela, occurring in <3%

WHEN TO REFER

- Pts w/presumed bacterial tracheitis should be expediently transported to facility capable of bronchoscopy to establish Dx/remove necrotic debris, inspissated secretions
- Pts always need to be w/clinician who can obtain/maintain airway once initial Dx bacterial tracheitis considered prior to bronchoscopy

BACKGROUND

- *Four major types:* esophageal atresia w/distal TEF (~85%); pure esophageal atresia w/o TEF (10%); H-type TEF w/o esophageal atresia (4%); esophageal atresia w/proximal TEF, proximal + distal TEF (1%)
- *Incidence:* 1:3,000–4,000; slight male predominance
- Occurs at 4–8 wks gestation; no inheritance pattern/teratogen established

CLINICAL MANIFESTATIONS

- *Antenatal period:* polyhydramnios in 30% EA + TEF cases/80% pure EA
- *Immediate neonatal period:* esophageal atresia w/or w/o TEF presents w/excessive salivation, coughing, choking, cyanosis w/feeds
- Scaphoid abdomen associated w/pure EA; gastric distension common w/EA + TEF
- Failure to pass NG tube beyond ~10 cm suggests EA
- *Late neonatal period/infancy:* H-type TEF presents w/chronic cough (esp w/feeding), atypical wheezing, recurrent pneumonitis

ASSOCIATED FEATURES

- *50% associated anomalies:* esp GI/cardiac (VSD, right-sided aortic arch)
- *10% VATER (VACTERL) association:* Vertebral, Anal, Cardiac, TE fistula, Renal, Limb anomalies

RADIOGRAPHIC FEATURES

- NG tube stops in proximal esophageal pouch w/EA
- Absence of bowel gas w/pure EA
- Pulmonary infiltrates (particularly right upper lobe) suggest aspiration pneumonia, esp with H-type TEF
- Contrast esophagogram detects majority of H-type TEF; bronchoscopy/esophagoscopy may be necessary if Dx equivocal

DIFFERENTIAL DIAGNOSIS

- Esophageal stenosis (congenital/acquired 2° to severe GE reflux)
- Congenital esophageal web
- Extrinsic esophageal compression due to vascular ring
- Traumatic fistula/perforation due to endotracheal/NG tube
- H-type TEF differential Dx:
  - severe GER w/aspiration
  - atypical reactive airways disease
  - direct aspiration 2° dysfunctional suck/swallow

TREATMENT

- Neonate w/suspected EA + TEF:
  - consult pediatric surgeon
  - elevate head of bed 30°
  - continuous suctioning of proximal esophageal pouch by 10 French NG/Replogle tube
  - O_2/respiratory support if necessary (caution: mechanical ventilation can lead to gastric perforation)
  - prophylactic antibiotics usually indicated for pneumonitis
  - echocardiogram to evaluate aortic arch position/determine surgical approach (caution: echocardiogram should not delay transfer to surgical center)
- Surgical repair in first 1–2 d in stable neonate >2 kg: 1° esophageal anastomosis/ligation/division of TEF via right thoracotomy
- *Staged repair in small (<2 kg)/sick neonate/long-gap atresia:* immediate gastrostomy, division of TEF, later esophageal anastomosis (less common options: esophagostomy "spit fistula," gastric/colonic interposition for long-gap atresias)
- H-type TEF may be repaired via cervical approach rather than thoracotomy

COMPLICATIONS

- Immediate postop:
  - anastomotic leak, mediastinitis
  - pneumothorax
- Medium term:
  - tracheomalacia w/stridor due to early compression of trachea by dilated esophageal pouch; improves w/time
  - esophageal stricture (usually due to severe GER)
  - recurrence of TEF (rare)
- Long term:
  - chronic cough (croupy/brassy) common
  - gastroesophageal reflux (common, chronic, often severe complication of EA due to esophageal dysmotility; may lead to gastric metaplasia of esophagus, "Barrett esophagus," precancerous condition)
  - achalasia

PREVENTION

- No prevention exists for congenital TEF/EA
- Long-term treatment of GER w/H_2 blockers/prokinetic agents indicated in most pts; fundoplication surgery avoided due to esophageal dysmotility

WHEN TO REFER

- Pediatric surgeon should be consulted for any neonate w/suspected EA and/or TEF
- When H-type TEF suspected, radiologic evaluation is indicated; if results inconclusive/Dx still suspected, surgical consultation should be obtained

TRACHEOMALACIA

BACKGROUND

- Abnormality of consistency/structure of tracheal rings
- Inspiratory (extrathoracic)/expiratory (intrathoracic) narrowing of trachea
- Pathophysiology:
  - 1° tracheomalacia: absence/hypoplasia of tracheal rings
  - 2° tracheomalacia: caused by compression of tracheal rings from vascular rings, slings, congenital heart disease (ie, tetralogy of Fallot), congenital tumors (ie, bronchogenic cyst, teratoma); congenital malformation of rings 2° to tracheoesophageal fistula; or inflammatory destruction of cartilage (ie, polychondritis)
- Generally presents during neonatal period (most by 6 wks of age)
- In 1° tracheomalacia, symptoms almost always improve by 1 yr of age/have resolved by 2–3 yrs old
- Prognosis in cases of isolated 1° tracheomalacia is excellent

CLINICAL MANIFESTATIONS

- *Generalized noisy breathing:* stridor, wheezing, barky cough
- May be asymptomatic w/quiet, shallow breathing
- Worsens w/crying, agitation, feeding, infections
- *Positional changes:* prone/upright better than supine
- In general, child in no distress, though "near deathlike" episodes/recurrent pneumonia have been reported
- Coarse breath sounds often heard
- Symmetric monophonic wheezing noted, best heard over central airways/becomes quieter as stethoscope moved distally
- Stridor may also be noted
- Suprasternal/intercostal retractions (if present) usually mild

LABORATORY FEATURES

- Bronchoscopy:
  - flexible fiberoptic bronchoscopy can visualize extent of tracheomalacia/degree of tracheal collapse (rigid bronchoscopy may stent open trachea, making tracheomalacia more difficult to visualize)
  - bronchoscopy should be done under conscious sedation (general anesthesia may alter airway dynamics)
  - useful to r/o other pathologies that can mimic tracheomalacia
- Chest radiograph:
  - usually normal in tracheomalacia
  - may show reduced/interrupted caliber of trachea
  - most useful for r/o other abnormalities that can cause pt's symptoms
- Lateral neck:
  - usually normal
- Fluoroscopy:
  - may be normal in tracheomalacia
  - expiratory narrowing or collapse may be seen
- Barium swallow:
  - may see compression of esophagus from vascular malformation (useful in evaluating for vascular rings or slings)
- MRI:
  - most useful for visualizing vascular anomalies

DIFFERENTIAL DIAGNOSIS

- Asthma
- Foreign body
- Laryngomalacia
- Tracheal stenosis (congenital vs. acquired)
- Gastroesophageal reflux
- Recurrent croup or pneumonia
- Psychogenic (habit) cough

TREATMENT

- In most cases (esp in 1° tracheomalacia), no definitive Tx required
- Observation/reassurance indicated
- Chest physiotherapy/humidification may make pt more comfortable, aid in clearing airway secretions
- CPAP can prove useful in stenting open trachea in severe cases
- Surgical repair via aortopexy/placement of tracheal stents used in children w/severe, localized tracheomalacia
- Tracheostomy may be needed in severe cases w/life-threatening problems

COMPLICATIONS

- Significant retractions at rest
- Worsening w/feeding/sleep
- Failure to thrive
- High-pitched/persistent stridor beyond first year
- Difficult extubation if being mechanically ventilated

PREVENTION

- In cases of 2° tracheomalacia, earlier treatment of causative lesion can be associated w/better prognosis, though results highly variable

WHEN TO REFER

- In cases of 1° tracheomalacia, referral rarely needed once Dx made if child thriving
- In cases of 2° tracheomalacia, otolaryngology/pulmonary input should be obtained in majority of cases

BACKGROUND

- *M:F ratio:* 1.3:1
- *Mean age:* 23 mos; 90% pts 1–3 yrs of age
- Often related to preceding viral infections (eg, parvovirus B19, echovirus 11, others)
- May be related to prior exposure to aspirin, piperazine, sulfanomides, valproic acid, phenytoin, phenobarbital
- Familial cases reported; rare
- Recurrent cases reported; rare
- Seasonal variation, w/apparent clusters usually from June–October/November–March in different series

CLINICAL MANIFESTATIONS

- Previously well child
- Usually gradual onset of anemia, pallor, fatigue
- May present w/hypovolemia/shock
- Commonly follows viral infection

LABORATORY MANIFESTATIONS

- Anemia
- Reticulocytopenia in early stage; ↑ reticulocyte count in recovery stage
- WBC count usually normal/may be low, high
- Platelet count usually high (2° to high erythropoietin), but may be low 2° to viral suppression of bone marrow
- Nonfetal characteristics of RBCs present (eg, MCV normal for age; i antigen, fetal hemoglobin usually not ↑ [different from Blackfan-Diamond anemia])
- Bone marrow aspirate shows erythroblastopenia/erythroid maturation arrest in early stage; erythroid hyperplasia in later, recovery stage
- Erythroid progenitor cell cultures indicate ↓ BFUs in 50% pts/↓ CFU-Es in 30% pts
- Serum/cellular inhibitors of normal progenitor cells identified in some pts
- Erythropoietin levels high

DIFFERENTIAL DIAGNOSIS

- Blackfan-Diamond anemia (these pts present younger, have fetal characteristics of their RBCs; see above)
- Viral diseases
- Aplastic anemia
- Leukemia
- Drug-induced anemia

TREATMENT

- Watchful waiting
- Transfuse only if anemia clinically significant
- Prednisone, anabolic steroids, other immunosuppressive Tx have no proven role

COMPLICATIONS

- Severe anemia may lead to cardiac failure

WHEN TO REFER

- If Dx in doubt
- If disease lasts >6 wks

BACKGROUND

- Possibly most common cause of acute hip pain/limp in children; responsible for 0.4–0.9% hospital admissions
- Most frequently occurs 3–8 yrs w/peak incidence at 6 ys
- Males > females (2:1); blacks infrequently affected
- Hypothesized related to current/antecedent infection, trauma/allergic hypersensitivity
- Etiology unknown/Dx by exclusion
- Biopsy specimens reveal nonspecific synovitis
- Duration of symptoms 1 wk to as long as 8 wks

CLINICAL MANIFESTATIONS

- Acute onset of hip, anterior thigh/knee pain; limp, refusal to bear weight in child not systemically ill
- May have associated low-grade fever
- Limitation of motion may be realized early from positive log roll test; affected extremity may be held in flexion/external rotation; abduction, internal rotation most limited
- Muscle atrophy suggests chronic disorder

LABORATORY FEATURES

- CBC/ESR required in presence of constitutional symptoms/prolonged cases
- White count may be mildly elevated as may be ESR (usually <20)
- X ray indicated only to r/o other diagnoses
- Log roll test (physical exam) as sensitive as ultrasound Dx hip effusion

DIFFERENTIAL DIAGNOSIS

- Septic hip
- Osteomyelitis of proximal femur/pelvis
- Legg-Calvé-Perthes
- Juvenile arthritis
- Acute rheumatic fever
- Slipped capital femoral epiphysis
- Tumor of proximal femur or pelvis
- Toddler fracture

TREATMENT

- Bed rest/nonweight bearing until pain resolves, ROM improves
- Aspiration of hip if symptoms more severe (pain, refusal to walk, concern over sepsis)/if slow to resolve
- Traction may help resolve symptoms/ helps enforce bed rest

- NSAIDs (avoid ASA)
- Pain-free interval prior to resumption of full activities

COMPLICATIONS

- Too early return to activities may lead to recurrence/delay in resolution of symptoms
- Recurrence reportedly 4–17% of cases
- Association w/Legg-Calvé-Perthes disease ~1% but direct causative association not documented

WHEN TO REFER

- If question of sepsis
- Failure to improve w/bed rest/NSAIDs after 48 hrs
- Severe pain, marked limitation of motion, inability (refusal) to walk
- Persistent limp (>5–7 d)/recurrent episodes

BACKGROUND

- Occurs in 2.7/10,000 births; M:F ratio: 2:1
- *Definition:* abnormal/discordant connection between ventricle/its great artery (ie, RV to aorta, LV to pulmonary artery)
- *Embryology:* abnormality in conotruncal rotation/development of subaortic infundibulum, resulting in persistent relationship of aorta to right ventricle
- Occurs as *"simple"* TGA (D-transposition w/only additional defects being PDA, patent foramen ovale, small VSD)/*"complex"* TGA (w/LV [pulmonary] outflow obstruction, large VSD, single ventricle)
- *Terminology alert: corrected transposition* can refer to *congenitally* corrected (L-transposition/ventricular inversion)/*surgically* corrected (eg, D-transposition, S/P arterial switch operation) conditions
- *Recurrence risk:* 3–4% for first-degree relatives
- Primary care provider most likely to encounter postop pts w/residual problems (see Complications)

CLINICAL MANIFESTATIONS

- Symptoms:
  – deep cyanosis in first 12–24 h of life (simple TGA)
  – heart failure/mild cyanosis at 2 wks–2 mos (some complex TGA)
- Signs:
  – cyanosis/hypoxemia w/o respiratory distress, occasionally w/acidosis/shock
  – often no audible murmur in simple TGA
  – usually heart murmur in complex TGA (due to associated defects)

DIAGNOSTIC TESTS

- *Arterial blood gases:* hypoxemia w/compensated respiratory alkalosis (eg, pH = 7.40, $pCO_2 = 28$, $pO_2 = 30$)
- *"Hyperoxia test":* pO_2 remains <100 torr (usually <80 torr) on 100% FiO_2
- *Pulse oximetry:* sometimes inverted pre-/postductal O_2 saturation difference (lower body > upper body) if right-to-left ductal shunt due to transient high pulmonary vascular resistance/associated coarctation
- *EKG:* often normal; may show right ventricular hypertrophy
- CXR:
  – narrow mediastinum w/oval cardiac contour ("egg on a string")
  – cardiac size often normal (simple TGA); may be enlarged (complex)
  – pulmonary vascular markings normal/↑
- Echocardiogram:
  – often provides definitive Dx/assessment of all important features (esp for simple TGA)
  – useful to guide bedside Rashkind balloon atrioseptostomy
- *Cardiac catheterization and angiography:* often unnecessary; can provide additional evaluation of coronary artery anatomy/possible associated defects (eg, coarctation)

DIFFERENTIAL DIAGNOSIS

- Most other forms of cyanotic congenital heart disease (ie, tetralogy of Fallot, pulmonary atresia, total anomalous pulmonary venous drainage, tricuspid atresia), persistent pulmonary hypertension of the newborn

TREATMENT

- For *stabilization* of critically ill newborn:
  – prostaglandin E_1 (Prostin VR): 0.05–1 µg/kg/min
  – sodium bicarbonate, 4.2% neonatal solution: 1 mEq/kg or 2 mL/kg
- *Rashkind balloon atrioseptostomy:* catheter procedure creates atrial septal defect to allow improved mixing of pulmonary/systemic venous blood, provides palliation until time of surgery; may be performed at bedside
- Surgical repair:
  – for most pts w/simple TGA, arterial switch (Jatene) operation preferred, requiring coronary artery translocation, but preserving left ventricle as systemic pump
  – many pts w/simple TGA encountered years after atrial switch (Senning or Mustard) repair w/residuae (see Complications)
  – complex TGA often requires initial palliation (eg, Blalock-Taussig shunt) followed by eventual Rastelli repair (LV blood baffled to aorta through VSD and RV w/RV to PA extracardiac conduit) or Fontan repair (single ventricle to aorta w/direct connection of systemic veins to pulmonary arteries)
- *Chronic postop antiarrhythmic/anticongestive Tx*

COMPLICATIONS AND PREVENTION (Long-term postop surveillance)

- After atrial switch repair (RV remains systemic pump):
  – systemic/pulmonary venous obstruction
  – brady/tachyarrhythmias (eg, sick sinus syndrome, atrial flutter)
  – late-onset right ventricular failure
- After arterial switch repair (LV remains systemic pump):
  – supravalvar pulmonary stenosis
  – "neo-aortic" valve insufficiency
  – late coronary artery occlusion/obstruction
- Exercise prescription:
  – exercise testing can assess postop arrhythmias, limited cardiac reserve, degree of exercise intolerance
  – limit participation in high-intensity competitive athletics (after Fontan, Senning, Mustard repairs); usually no restrictions after arterial switch repair
- Endocarditis prophylaxis

WHEN TO REFER

- All cyanotic newborns
- Postop pts w/Sx of change in cardiac status (eg, palpitations, syncope, exertional dyspnea/intolerance)

BACKGROUND

- Diarrheal diseases most common illnesses of travelers of all ages
- Susceptibility in travelers due to combination of ↑ exposure to diarrheagenic organisms from fecally contaminated food/water, immunologic naïveté of host, not having encountered these organisms previously
- Most frequent during first few wks of visiting, but may develop at any time, including immediate period after arriving home
- Risk particularly high for children from developed world who visit ancestral homes of their parents in developing countries
- Detailed etiologic studies of diarrheal pathogens in pediatric-aged travelers have not been done; extrapolation must be made from studies of adult travelers/from children w/diarrhea resident in developing countries

CLINICAL MANIFESTATIONS

- Usually abrupt onset/self-limited, usually lasting only several days; occasionally persistent (lasting >14 d)
- Most often watery/may contain mucus; it occurs >3 ×/24 hrs; may be as often as every few hrs at onset
- Diarrhea often accompanied by nausea, vomiting, anorexia
- Low-grade fever (<101°F)/abdominal pain unusual
- Dehydration may develop
- Symptoms of dysentery (blood/mucus in stool, fever, abdominal pain) less common (<10% of pts)
- In pts who develop persistent diarrhea, stool usually watery/dehydration may be important part of illness

LABORATORY FEATURES

- Laboratory usually not helpful in managing this illness; etiologic Dx not possible in most developing countries/nor necessary for successful clinical management in most cases
- Identification of pathogens (primarily protozoa) usually only important in children w/persistent diarrhea

DIFFERENTIAL DIAGNOSIS

- Dx usually obvious, but occasionally other causes of diarrhea should be considered:
  – food allergy
  – food poisoning (Ciguatera fish poisoning)
  – insecticide poisoning

TREATMENT

- Oral rehydration solutions (ORS):
  – rehydration most important aspect of treatment; usually done w/oral rehydration solutions (ORS) carried in packet form by travelers; effective in treating dehydration due to any diarrheal pathogen, in any age group
  – ORS purchased by travelers in US include packets of glucose-based ORS, cereal-based ORS; can also be purchased in most countries of world
  – mixed, according to instructions, w/clean water/given ad lib to child to maintain hydration as long as diarrhea persists; if vomiting is present ORS should initially be given frequently in small quantities
- Antimicrobials:
  – no uniformity of opinion about use of antimicrobials in pediatric travelers' diarrhea; ORS alone may be adequate
  – in adult travelers, antimicrobials significantly shorten disease/routinely prescribed
  – if antimicrobial used in young children, TMP/SMX (trimethoprim [8 mg/kg]/sulfamethoxazole [40 mg/kg]) bid × 3 d) effective treatment for most bacterial enteropathogens; in older children (>16 yrs) fluoroquinolone (ie, ciprofloxacin/norfloxacin) highly effective
  – in cases of dysentery, antibiotics 1° treatment (TMP/SMX effective in most cases); Shigella have become resistant to many antimicrobials
- Feeding:
  – should be continued, along w/ORS (breast-feeding should not be interrupted)
  – no need to withhold food
- Adjunctive Tx:
  – adjunctive symptomatic Tx w/bismuth subsalicylate/loperamide advocated by some
  – loperamide should not be used in children <2 yrs of age
  – kaolin/pectin mixtures not useful in treatment

PREVENTION

- Ingested water/ice should be free of microbial contamination; commercially bottled, boiled, chlorinated, or filtered
- Well-cooked foods/fruits that can be peeled safe; fresh, uncooked vegetable salads (lettuce, tomatoes)/unpeeled fruits (strawberries), however, particularly likely to be fecally contaminated
- All travelers to developing countries should be advised to take packets of ORS w/them/plus antimicrobial

WHEN TO REFER

- Management of acute illness primarily done by parents/guardians
- If high fever (>102°F)/does not respond quickly to treatment go to local physician (names can often be obtained from staff of U.S. Travel Clinic; U.S. embassy in any developing country has medical clinic that can also be used for referrals
- Persistent diarrhea may need to be evaluated by pediatric gastroenterologist

Enteric pathogens most likely to cause Travelers' Diarrhea in children*

Enterotoxigenic *E. coli*	40–60%
Enteropathogenic *E. coli* (in children <1 yr of age)	10–20%
Shigella	5–10%
Salmonella	<5%
Rotavirus (in children <2 yrs of age)	5–10%
Campylobacter jejuni	<5%
Protozoa (*Giardia lamblia, E. histolytica,* Cyclospora)	<5%
Others or unknown pathogens	30–50%

*As extrapolated primarily from studies in adults.

TRICHINELLOSIS (TRICHINOSIS)

ZBIGNIEW S. PAWLOWSKI

BACKGROUND

- Occurs worldwide, usually in epidemic outbreaks among those consuming raw meat (pork/wild boar, bear, horse, walrus meat) infected w/nematode *Trichinella spiralis*
- Children, any age/sex, most frequently part of outbreak; isolated cases exceptional
- Higher exposure risk in immigrants, hunter's families/in rural population
- Clinical course variable/depends mainly on intensity of infection. Asymptomatic infections common; incubation period 5–50 d (usually 8–15 d); an acute stage (trichinellosis syndrome, allergic vasculitis) followed by prolonged myositis, metabolic, cardiac disorders/some complications
- In children clinical course may be more severe; recovery quicker than in adults; chronic sequelae rare
- Mortality in treated cases low (<1%)

CLINICAL MANIFESTATIONS

- Occasionally early diarrhea, sometimes prolonged
- Acute trichinellosis syndrome (fever, muscle pains, malaise)
- Early allergic vasculitis syndrome (conjunctival and subungual hemorrhages, periorbital edema)
- Late metabolic disorders (hypoproteinemia, hypokalemia, hypoglycemia)/cardiac, pulmonary, neurologic complications, flexor muscle contractions
- Chronic trichinellotic myalgia rare in children

LABORATORY FEATURES

- Eosinophilia (0.5–5.0 × 10^9/l); lack of eosinophilia poor prognostic sign
- Leukocytosis (15–50 × 10^9/l); starts together w/eosinophilia/ends earlier
- Serum creatine phosphokinase (CPK) activity/creatine level ↑
- Immunoglobulins IgE, IgG, IgM ↑
- *Electromyographic examination:* signs of acute myositis
- Hypoalbuminemia, hypokalemia, hypoglycemia starting 3rd wk of disease
- Serologic tests positive starting 3rd wk of infection
- Definite Dx by finding Trichinella larvae in muscle biopsy specimen (usually in adult pt from same outbreak)

DIFFERENTIAL DIAGNOSIS

- Diarrhea w/alimentary intoxication, gastroenteritis, drug allergy
- Trichinellosis syndrome w/viral infections (influenza), typhoid fever, leptospirosis, rheumatic fever, septicemia
- Allergic vasculitis w/dermatomyositis, periarteritis nodosa, angioneurotic edema, serum sickness, drug allergy

TREATMENT

- *Any diagnosed/suspected case in any period of infection:* anthelmintic against intestinal worms (albendazole, 15 mg/kg/d po in 2 doses × 5 d or pyrantel pamoate, 10 mg/kg/d po in 2 doses × 5 d)
- *Severe trichinellosis:* life-saving high doses of corticosteroids parenterally followed by 40–60 mg prednisone until fever/signs of allergic vasculitis disappear; later correction of metabolic disorders/treatment of complications
- *Mild trichinellosis:* treatment w/antipyretic/analgesic drugs
- Bed rest
- *Asymptomatic trichinellosis:* no treatment

COMPLICATIONS

- Acute cardiovascular insufficiency in early stage of severe trichinellosis
- Metabolic disorders (hypoalbuminemia, hypokalemia, hypoglycemia) starting 3rd wk of disease
- Various cardiac, pulmonary, neurologic complications in later stage of disease

PREVENTION

- Avoid eating raw/semiraw meat, esp of unknown origin
- Cooking, freezing (except Arctic strain), low-level gamma irradiation kill Trichinella larvae
- Public education, proper management of animals, meat hygiene important

WHEN TO REFER

- *All cases symptomatic trichinellosis require hospitalization:* best in specialized unit/at least until consult by clinical parasitologist

TRICHINOSIS

BACKGROUND

- *Trichinella spiralis* of worldwide distribution
- Found in temperate areas of world, rarely in tropics
- Male worms 1.4–2.0 mm/females 3–4 mm; male dies after copulation
- Infection occurs by eating infected poorly cooked meat, 80% from pork; polar/black bears in Arctic, bush pig in Africa, deer containing encapsulated larvae
- Larvae freed in stomach, mature in intestine, reach organs through lymphatics/blood, encyst only in striated muscles
- Encysted larvae remain infective for many years

CLINICAL MANIFESTATIONS

- Symptoms appear 1 wk after ingestion of infected meat when invasion of muscles occur; last for several days/weeks
- Symptoms due to allergic/toxic products of parasite
- Pruritus, formications, petechial, maculopapular exanthem/urticaria, muscle pain
- Splinter hemorrhages of fingers/toes conjunctiva; edema of eyelids/face
- Severity of symptoms directly proportional to parasite load

DIAGNOSIS

- Eosinophilia, periorbital edema, severe headache, myositis suggest Dx
- Muscle biopsy/demonstration of serum antibodies/high serum IgE also helpful

TREATMENT

- Corticosteroids helpful in suppressing allergic reaction early in infection
- Thiabendazole 25 mg/kg 2×/d × 7 d; mebendazole also useful
- Treatment not useful in older infections

DIFFERENTIAL DIAGNOSIS

- Dematomyositis resembles acute stage of trichinosis
- Skin eruption may resemble cutaneous eruptions of other infections

PROGNOSIS

- 5% pts die if untreated
- Prognosis poor in heavy infections
- Prognosis good in almost all cases if treatment initiated early

PREVENTION

- Adequate cooking of meat (58°C)
- Freezing at –18°C for 24 hrs also adequate

GNATHOSTOMIASIS

BACKGROUND

- *Gnathostoma spinigerum,* intestinal nematode of carnivores, cause human infection
- Common in Far East, Thailand, Japan, China
- Infection occurs when eating uncooked fish, duck, chicken containing infectious larvae
- Human dead end host; parasite cannot complete its life cycle in human

CLINICAL MANIFESTATIONS

- Immature worms migrate through abdominal/thoracic organs producing inflammation, hemorrhage
- Fever, urticaria, pain; subside within month as worms reach SubQ tissue
- Continued migration in skin leads to serpiginous itchy tracts/abscesses
- If reaches epidermis, resembles cutanea larva migrans
- In eyes produces cellulitis, uveitis, iritis
- In CNS results in lethal eosinophilic meningitis

DIAGNOSIS

- High index of suspicion in endemic area w/clinical picture as described above
- Biopsy of suspected area of swelling demonstrates worm
- Eosinophilia in peripheral blood/CSF

TREATMENT

- Surgical removal when feasible only sure treatment
- Prevention by adequate cooking of fish, chicken, duck

ANGIOSTRONGYLIASIS CANTONENSIS

BACKGROUND

- Caused by *Angiostrongylus cantonensis,* rat lung worm
- Larvae passed in feces of rats/ingested by snails, slugs to develop into third-stage infectious larvae/may be carried by freshwater crabs/prawns
- When ingested by human, dead end host; dies after reaching CNS
- Found in Far East/several small Pacific islands

CLINICAL MANIFESTATIONS

- Severe headaches, visual impairment, paresthesias, paralysis of 6th/7th nerves in ~7%
- Meningeal irritation in ~15%
- Outcome usually favorable in contrast to gnathostomiasis

TREATMENT AND PREVENTION

- No known treatment; anthelminthic Tx should not be used, esp in heavy infections because of severe inflammatory reaction to killed parasites
- Proper cooking of infected snails, prawns, crabs
- Freezing of crustaceans/mollusks at –15° × 12 h kills infective larvae

DRACUNCULOSIS

BACKGROUND

- Caused by *Dracunculus medinensis* (guinea worm)
- Common in geographic dry areas (west, central, northeast africa, Middle East, Iran, Pakistan, India, Caribbean islands)
- *D. medinensis* large 1–2 mm wide; males rarely attain 12 cm, females 50–120 cm
- Humans get infected by drinking raw water containing copepods (cyclops), intermediate host containing infective larvae
- Females migrate to skin surface, usually extremities/release large numbers of larvae on contact w/water; larvae ingested by copepods

CLINICAL MANIFESTATIONS

- No symptoms of infection until female approaches skin
- Intense inflammation around protruding worm
- Severe symptoms of malaise, fever, urticaria/other erythematous rashes appear
- Worm dies after discharging larvae, become calcified/visible on x rays
- Possible to have >1 worm

DIAGNOSIS

- Clinical picture characteristic
- Wetting area results in release of larvae, which may be examined microscopically
- Fluorescent antibody test helps detection of infection earlier

TREATMENT

- Extraction of worm traditional treatment/should be done carefully, slowly over few days to avoid breakage of worm
- If worm broken severe cellulitis develops
- If worm is palpable, surgical removal possible
- Metronidazole, 250 mg tid × 7 d; thiabendazole, 25 mg/kg bid × 2 d; or niridazole (Ambilhar), 25 mg/kg tid × 7 d: topical/systemic antibodies for 2° infection
- Sanitary/public health measures prevent dissemination of infection

BACKGROUND

- Caused by flagellated protozoan *Trichomonas vaginalis;* spread primarily by sexual contact/from mother's birth canal to neonates
- *Incubation period:* 4–20 d

CLINICAL PRESENTATION (FEMALES)

- Asymptomatic (25–50%)
- Yellow to gray-green vaginal discharge (50–75%), frothy (8–50%), w/fishy odor (10%), exacerbated during/after menstrual period
- Vaginal itching (23–82%); can be severe
- Dyspareunia (10–50%)
- Dysuria (30–50%)/lower abdominal pain
- Punctate bleeding sites on cervix (1–2% by visual examination, 45% by colposcopy)
- Edematous vaginal walls (20–75%)

CLINICAL PRESENTATION (MALES)

- Urethral infection (100%), usually asymptomatic; if symptomatic, urethral discharge in 50%
- Prostatitis

LABORATORY EVALUATION

- Wet mount of vaginal/urethral discharge mixed in warm saline/motile protozoa w/4 anterior flagellates; slightly larger than polymorphonuclear cells; sensitivity 40–80%
- Protozoa may be seen in urine
- *Papanicolaou smear positive:* sensitivity 56–70%
- Other tests usually not done:
  - immunofluorescent antibody: sensitivity 80–90%
  - ELISA test: sensitivity 90%
  - latex agglutination: sensitivity 90%
  - culture: sensitivity 95%

DIFFERENTIAL DIAGNOSIS

- Other causes of vaginitis/urethritis:
  - *Neisseria gonorrhoea*
  - *Chlamydia trachomatis*
  - bacterial vaginosis
  - herpes simplex

TREATMENT

- Metronidazole:
  - adolescents/adults; 40 mg/kg po in single dose (max 2 g) (82–95% effective); if this fails, give 500 mg bid po × 7 d; if this fails, use 2 g 1×/d × 3 d
  - children: 15 mg/kg/d po div tid × 7 d (max dose 1/g)
  - no drinking alcohol for 48 h after start of treatment; causes nausea/flushing
  - do not use in first trimester of pregnancy; in first trimester, use gentle douching solution of 2 tbsp vinegar in qt of H_2O daily to 2×/wk

OTHER CONSIDERATIONS

- If found in children, do sexual abuse evaluation
- Evaluate/treat sexual partner(s)
- No sexual intercourse until cured/asymptomatic
- *Prevention:* abstinence/condoms

WHEN TO REFER

- Most pts managed w/o referral

BACKGROUND

- *Mycobacterium tuberculosis:* acid-fast bacillus. Bacilli are aerobic, nonspore forming, nonmotile, slightly curved or straight, w/length 1–10 μm
- ~1.3 million cases tuberculous disease, 400,000 tuberculous-related deaths occur annually among children <15 yrs of age worldwide
- Transmission usually person to person by mucous droplets that become airborne when individual w/pulmonary tuberculosis coughs, sneezes, laughs, or sings. Epidemiologic studies indicate children w/1° pulmonary tuberculosis rarely, if ever, infect other children or adults
- Droplets containing tubercle bacilli dry, become droplet nuclei, which may remain suspended in air for hours. Factor most closely correlated w/infectivity is positive acid-fast smear of sputum
- *Tuberculous infection:* asymptomatic tuberculin skin test convertor w/o evidence of pulmonary or extrapulmonary disease
- *Tuberculous disease:* pulmonary disease (pneumonia, hilar adenopathy) and/or manifestations of extrapulmonary disease
- Although reasons for ↑ in tuberculosis vary, important causes probably epidemic of HIV infection, immigration of people to US from countries w/high rates tuberculosis, poor performance of aspects of public health system
- Interval between initial tuberculous infection and onset of disease may be several weeks or many years
- Case rates of tuberculosis for all ages highest in urban, low-income areas, nonwhite racial, ethnic groups, among whom > two-thirds reported cases in US now occur. Foreign-born persons ~ one-third all new cases
- Although infected children of all ages at ↑ risk for developing tuberculous disease, infants, postpubertal adolescents highest risk. Other risk factors for progression of infection to disease include recent close contact w/infected person, recent skin test conversion, immunodeficiency (particularly HIV), IV drug use
- Incubation period from initial infection to development of positive reaction to tuberculin skin ~2–10 wks. Risk for developing disease highest in first 2 yrs after infection

CLINICAL MANIFESTATIONS

- Most infected children, adolescents symptomatic when tuberculin reaction found positive
- 1° complex of tuberculous infection usually not demonstrable on chest radiograph
- Early clinical manifestations occurring 1–6 mos after initial infection can include ≥1 of following: fever, weight loss, cough, night sweats, chills, lymphadenopathy of hilar, mediastinal, cervical, other nodes, pulmonary involvement of segmental lobe, occasionally w/consolidation, atelectasis, pleural effusion, miliary tuberculosis, tuberculous meningitis
- Extrapulmonary disease (miliary, meningeal, renal, bone, or joint) occurs ~25% children <15 yrs of age
- Clinical manifestations in pts w/drug-susceptible vs. drug-resistant tuberculosis indistinguishable

DIAGNOSTIC TESTS

- Isolation of tubercle bacilli by culture from early-morning gastric aspirates (usually 3), sputum, pleural fluid, CSF, urine, or other body fluids or biopsy material establishes Dx. In young child, best culture material for Dx pulmonary tuberculosis usually early-morning gastric aspirate
- *Mycobacterium tuberculosis:* slow-growing microorganism w/recovery taking as long as 10 wks by older culture methods, 2–3 wks by newer radiometric methods
- Even w/optimal culture techniques, organism isolated from <50% children, 75% infants w/pulmonary tuberculosis
- AFB-stained smears of sputum or body fluids using Ziehl-Neelsen method or auramine/rhodamine staining for fluorescent microscopy should be obtained
- Histologic examination in biopsy material should be obtained. *Mycobacterium tuberculosis* cannot be distinguished from other mycobacteria in AFB-stained smears or biopsy material
- Polymerase chain reaction for DNA identification or restriction fragment length polymorphism analysis (DNA fingerprinting) available, approved for smear-positive respiratory tract specimens. Currently available in limited reference laboratories, research laboratories
- Culture material should always be obtained when no source case isolate available, source case isolate drug resistant, child immunocompromised, or child has extrapulmonary disease
- *Tuberculin skin testing:* skin test is only practical tool for diagnosing tuberculous infection in asymptomatic individuals
- In most children, tuberculin reactivity first appears 2–10 wks, occasionally as long as 12 wks after initial infection
- Children w/positive tuberculin skin test, but no evidence of disease warrant family investigation; children w/positive tuberculin skin test and/or evidence of disease mandate identification of source case
- Proper determination of "positive reaction" must use specific guidelines
- Overall emphasis to control tuberculosis in US should be placed on access to health care; thorough Hx taking of exposure to infectious persons; timely, effective contact investigations; proper interpretation of Mantoux skin tests; appropriate use of Tx including directly observed Tx

- Previous BCG vaccination never contraindication to tuberculin testing
- Negative Mantoux tuberculin skin test never excludes tuberculous infection or disease
- Other strengths of PPD skin test antigens (1 or 250 TU) should not be used because of lack of standardization

Positive Mantoux Skin Test in Children

- *Reaction ≥5 mm:*
  – children in close contact w/known/suspected infectious cases of tuberculosis
  – children suspected to have tuberculosis
  – children receiving immunosuppressive Tx or w/immunosuppressive conditions, including HIV infection
  - *Reaction ≥10 mm:*
  – children at ↑ risk of dissemination:
  ° young age: <4 yrs of age
  ° other medical risk factors, including Hodgkin disease, lymphoma, diabetes mellitus, chronic renal failure, or malnutrition
  – children w/↑ environmental exposure:
  ° frequently exposed to adults who are HIV infected, homeless, users of illicit drugs, residents of nursing homes, incarcerated or institutionalized persons, migrant farm workers
  ° travel, exposure to high prevalence regions of the world
  - *Reaction ≥15 mm:*
  – children ≥4 yrs of age w/o any risk factors

Tuberculin Skin Test Recommendations

- Immediate skin testing:
  – contacts of persons w/confirmed or suspected infectious tuberculosis
  – children w/radiographic or clinical findings suggesting tuberculosis
  – children immigrating from endemic countries
  – children w/travel Hx to endemic countries
- Annual testing:
  – children infected with HIV
  – incarcerated adolescents
- Testing q2–3 yrs:
  – children exposed to HIV infected, homeless, residents of nursing homes, institutionalized adolescents or adults, users of illicit drugs, incarcerated adolescents or adults, migrant farm workers
- Considered testing at 4–6 and 11–16 yrs of age:
  – children whose parents immigrated (w/unknown tuberculin skin test status) from regions of the world w/high prevalence of tuberculosis
  – children w/o specific risk factors who reside in high-prevalence areas

Recommended treatment for drug-susceptible tuberculosis in infants, children, and adolescents

Infection or Disease Category	Regimen	Remarks
Asymptomatic infection (positive skin test, no disease):		
Isoniazid: susceptible	9 mos I/d	If daily Tx not possible, 2×/wk Tx may be used 9 mos
Isoniazid: resistant	6–9 mos R/d	Treat HIV-infected children × 12 mos
Isoniazid/rifampin: resistant	Consult a tuberculosis expert	
Pulmonary (including hilar adenopathy)	6 mo regimen (standard): 2 mos I, R, Z/d, followed by 4 mos I, R daily, *or* 2 mos I, R, Z/d followed by 4 mos I, R 2×/wk	If possible drug resistance a concern, add another drug (ethambutol or streptomycin) to initial 3 drug Tx until drug susceptibility determined. Do not use 2 drug 9 mo regimen
	9 mo regimen (alternative): 9 mos I, R/d, *or* 1 mo I, R/d, followed by 8 mos, I, R 2×/wk	Give drugs 2/3 ×/wk under direct observation in initial phase if nonadherence likely
		For hilar adenopathy, regimens consisting of 6 mos I, R/d, 1 mo I, R/d, followed by 5 mos I, R, 2×/wk, have been successful in areas where drug resistance rare
Meningitis, disseminated (miliary), bone/joint, HIV-infected children	2 mos I, R, Z, S/d, followed by 10 mos I, R/d, *or* 2 mos I, R, Z, S/d followed by 10 mos I, R 2×/wk	Streptomycin given in initial Tx until drug susceptibility is known
		For pts who may have acquired tuberculosis in geographic areas where resistance to streptomycin common, capreomycin (15–30 mg/kg/d) or kanamycin (15–30 mg/kg/d) may be used instead of streptomycin
Extrapulmonary other than meningitis, disseminated (miliary), or bone/joint	Same as for pulmonary disease	See "Pulmonary"

Key: I = isoniazid; R = rifampin; Z = pyrazinamide; S = streptomycin sulfate

PATIENTS AT INCREASED RISK FOR DRUG RESISTANCE

- Pts w/Hx treatment w/antituberculous medications (including source case for current contact)
- Contacts of pt with drug-resistant tuberculosis
- Foreign-born persons
- Residents of areas in US where prevalence of drug resistance documented (most experts include isoniazid resistance rates ≥4%)
- Pts (or source contact) whose smears/cultures remain positive after 2 mos antituberculous Tx

ADDITIONAL OBSERVATIONS

- Directly observed Tx means health-care worker/other responsible, mutually agreed upon individual (not family member) present when medications administered to pt; directly observed Tx recommended for treatment of tuberculosis in US
- Use corticosteroids in children w/tuberculous meningitis to reduce vasculitis inflammation as result of intracranial pressure; most experts consider 1–2 mg/kg/d prednisone equivalent for 6–8 wks appropriate
- Report all cases of tuberculosis to local public health authorities; collaborative efforts w/public health agencies should be undertaken w/all cases of tuberculosis, family investigations/Tx

COMPLICATIONS

- Nearly all children w/tuberculous infection adequately treated respond to treatment unless drug resistance present
- CNS infection carries w/it significant mortality/morbidity; delay in Dx/treatment significant predictor of poor outcome
- Pulmonary disease carries excellent prognosis when appropriate treatment utilized

WHEN TO REFER

- Most pts managed w/collaborative efforts of local public health authorities/tuberculosis experts
- Cases of extrapulmonary tuberculosis should be referred/managed by infectious disease specialist/tuberculosis expert
- Referral always indicated when tuberculosis in differential Dx, but no Dx made; in all children w/serious complications following Dx, referral/consultation should be performed
- Multidrug-resistant cases

TUBEROUS SCLEROSIS COMPLEX (TSC)

MANUEL R. GOMEZ

BACKGROUND

- *Definition:* autosomal dominant disease, involving virtually any organ, manifested by formation of well-circumscribed islands of tissue expressing excessive cellular proliferation (*hamartomas*), or impaired cellular migration and differentiation (*hamartias*) in the parenchyma. Less often, malignant tumor growth (*hamartoblastoma*), but only in kidney

Hamartomas

- Example: renal angiomyolipoma (AML), uncommon tumor that may exist as solitary tumor in non-TSC individuals but often multiple in TSC pts, particularly females. Accepted that ≥2 hamartomas in organ or hamartomas in ≥2 of following organs: skin, brain, eyes, heart, kidneys, lungs indicative of TSC. Less often hamartomas found on gums, nasal mucosa, liver, pancreas, pituitary gland, thyroid, adrenals, thymus, gonads, uterus, vagina, spleen, lymph nodes
- Hamartomas cause symptoms by compression and displacement of organ's parenchyma, by obstructing blood, CSF or alveolar air circulation, or by bleeding from tumor
- Development, growth of hamartomas age related. This chronology differs between organs.
- Severity of symptoms depends on size, number of lesions

Hamartias

- Examples: hypomelanotic skin macules or white spots, and cortical tubers
- First does not cause symptoms but cortical tubers often cause of seizures, mental subnormality
- Aorta and other large-caliber arteries may also express wall defects that lead to aneurysmal formation in thoracic or abdominal segment
- Lesions may appear as radiographic osteomatous thickening in long bones, calvarium, or vertebras as well as phalangeal cysts, dental enamel defects (pits)

Hamartoblastoma

- Only in kidney malignant tumor (renal cell carcinoma) may develop in pts w/TSC

Diagnostic Features of TSC (lesions in BOLD FONT are pathognomonic if two or more are present in an organ, or if more than one organ is affected, or if two direct relatives have the lesion)

Organs	Hamartias	Hamartomas
Brain	Cortical tuber	Subependymal nodes or SEGAs
Retina	Retinal depigmented areas	Astrocytic retinal hamartomas
Skin	Hypomelanotic macules	Facial angiofibromas
		Fibrous forehead plaques
		Ungual fibromas
		Shagreen plaques(s)
Heart		Rhabdomyomas
Kidney	Renal cysts	Angiomyolipomas; RCC
Liver		Angiomyolipoma(s)
Pancreas		Islet cell adenoma
Colon-rectum		Hamartomatous polyp
Adrenal		Angiomyolipoma
Thyroid		Fetal or papilliform thyroid adenoma
Gonads		Ovarian or testicular angiomyolipoma
Teeth		Enamel pits in 1° or deciduous teeth
Bones		Phalangeal cysts; calvarial thickenings
Large arteries		Wall defects: resulting in aneurysm of aorta, subclavian, carotid, cerebral, vertebral, renal

SEGA = Subependymal giant cell astrocytoma   RCC = Renal cell carcinoma

---

GENETICS

- Two gene loci mapped in families w/TSC mutations
- First gene locus to be detected, TSC1, in chromosome region 9q34
- Proposed protein product has been named *hamartin*
- Second gene, TSC2, in region 16p13 and protein product called *tuberin*. Both genes seem to function independently as tumor suppressors
- Birth incidence 1/7,000–1/9,000
- ~65% of affected individuals new mutants
- Each of two TSC genes involved in ~same number of cases

CLINICAL MANIFESTATIONS (DEPEND ON AFFECTED ORGAN)

- *Brain:* most often involved organ in TSC pts, presents three types of lesions
- Cortical tubers from which seizures emanate. Greater number of tubers, earlier seizure onset and more likely seizures generalized, frequent, long in duration, resistant to anticonvulsants. Seizures presenting complaint of 92% of pts of all ages, occur in 84% of individuals w/TSC. Except in newborn period seizures almost always presenting complaint of TSC pts. Seizures may be simple partial, complex partial or generalized, including infantile spasms. Infantile spasms usually begin ages 4–9 mos and are presenting sign of 65% of infants w/TSC. Mental handicap only occurs in ~45% of children, adults w/TSC: these are pts whose seizures began in first 4–5 yrs of life. Neurologic disabilities include, in addition to mental handicap, childhood autism, attention deficient hyperactivity disorder (ADHD), disruptive behavior
- Cerebral hamartomas result from unsuppressed cellular multiplication of periventricular germinal matrix. Begin as small lesion of little or no growth that may remain asymptomatic and calcify or start to grow faster. When growth continues, become subependymal giant cell astrocytomas (SEGA) and because of location near foramina of Monro, can block CSF circulation, causing intracranial hypertension, ventricular dilatation. Only ~6% of pts w/TSC will develop one or more intraventricular SEGA that lead to hydrocephaly. Cellular components have characteristics of both neurons and glia
- *Eyes:* retinal hamartomas present in ~50% of TSC pts (if examined by indirect ophthalmoscopy after pupils have been dilated). Usually asymptomatic. Histologically not different from SEGA. When >1 present, Dx of TSC confirmed.

- *Skin:* examining skin w/adequate illumination (sunlight or Wood lamp) may demonstrated hypomelanotic macules, very common sign that by itself not sufficient for definite Dx of TSC. Two or more white spots would be suggestive but not convincing. Conversely, absence of white spots does not mitigate against the Dx. Facial angiofibroma (FAF), also called adenoma sebaceum, present in ~50% of TSC pts who have reached puberty but uncommon <5 yrs of age. Can be mistaken w/angiofibroma of multiple endocrine neoplasia type 1 (MEN1). FAF is a hamartoma that may cause only cosmetic problems but can be of great concern with excessive growth
- *Heart:* >50% of fetuses, newborn infants w/TSC have cardiac rhabdomyoma(s) demonstrable w/echocardiography. Majority asymptomatic. Others present w/cardiac failure associated either w/Wolff-Parkinson-White (WPW) syndrome (of reentrant circuit) or from obstructive intracavitary tumor(s). Rhabdomyomas tend to regress gradually from birth or on after few years of no change. When echocardiogram reveals present of cardiac rhabdomyomas, close to 75% of time pt has TSC. Conversely 60% of infants w/TSC have cardiac rhabdomyomas. Surgical treatment of the obstructive tumor seldom necessary. More often medical treatment required for WPW syndrome
- *Kidneys:* infants w/TSC may be born w/polycystic kidneys. Association of TSC and adult polycystic kidney disease type 1 (APKD1), due to deletion or mutation of two contiguous genes TSC2 and adult polycystic kidney disease type 1, both located on chromosome 16p13. Infant should be recognized before signs of renal insufficiency w/uremia, abdominal distention, and ultrasound or CT scan evidence of multiple renal cysts appear. Renal angiomyolipomas (AML) are benign tumors that may bleed suddenly from ruptured aneurysmatic arteriole, cause hypovolemic shock. Rarely cause of renal failure. More common in females w/renal cell carcinoma, a malignant tumor that sends metasis to regional lymph nodes and the lungs, have similar presentation
- *Lungs:* pulmonary lymphangioleiomyomatsos (LALM) found almost exclusively in female pts after third decade of life. Symptoms include dyspnea, hemoptysis, recurrent spontaneous pneumothoracis or chylothorax, cystic changes in lung, resulting in lung hyperinflation, hypoxemia, hypercarbia, acidemia

LABORATORY FEATURES

- Imaging of brain w/CT and MRI essential. Unless SEGA threatening to block foramina of Monroe, no need to repeat CT more than yearly

- Echocardiography for detection of rhabdomyoma mandatory in all newborns at risk of having inherited TSC. If found, yearly exam will reveal shrinking of tumor
- Electrocardiography necessary to detect arrhythmia associated w/rhabdomyoma
- Angiomyolipomas (AML) and renal cysts best revealed by CT scan but ultrasound adequate for follow-up
- Microscopic UA may reveal unsuspected hematuria, ominous sign heralding possible catastrophic AML bleed
- Women w/TSC at risk of developing LALM; after reaching their twenties, should be aware of danger of pneumothorax and more serious progressive respiratory deficit

DIFFERENTIAL DIAGNOSIS

- Combination of seizures and mental retardation may be caused by focal cerebral dysplasia that not part of TSC

TREATMENT

- *Seizures:* epileptic seizures, partial or generalized, treated as soon as possible. Newborn infants have only partial motor seizures which may become generalized in form of infantile spasms at 4–9 mos. Seizures may not respond to usual antiepileptic drugs (AED). Vigabatrin more successful for infantile spasms than any other drug of choice. Other useful drugs include valproate, carbamazepine, lamotrigine, nitrozepam. Ketogenic diet may be effective. Partial and secondarily generalized seizures including infantile spasms not responding to AED could benefit from surgical removal of the cortical tuber or tubers causing them
- *Cardiac:* specific arrhythmias can be treated. Obstructive tumor rarely requires surgical treatment
- *Renal:* peritoneal dialysis available for pts in renal failure. Ultimately may need renal transplant. Hormonal Tx and O$_2$ supplement; when all fails, lung transplant only solution
- *Skin:* for cosmetic reasons FAF can be removed w/laser beam but necessary to obtain pt's cooperation. Very active youngsters may not be amenable for treatment unless placed under general anesthesia, an unnecessary step <10 yrs of age

WHEN TO REFER

- Infants w/TSC and infantile spasms should be referred to pediatric neurologist for Tx.

BACKGROUND

- Epizootic infection caused by *Francisella tularensis*
- Primarily disease of wild animals perpetuated in nature by contaminated environment, ectoparasites, acute/chronic carriers
- Common illness in certain geographic regions of southeastern/midwestern US
- Illness characterized by 7 clinical syndromes
- Commonly have Hx tick bite/rabbit exposure; more common in males than females, but occurs at all ages

ORGANISM/TRANSMISSION

- *Francisella tularensis:* small, gram-negative, pleomorphic, nonmotile, non-spore-forming coccobacillus
- Transmitted by dozens of biting/blood-sucking insects that serve as vectors; ticks/wild rabbits source for most of human cases in endemic areas
- Animal reservoirs include wild rabbits, squirrels, sheep, beavers, muskrats; animal bites, including those from cats/squirrels, have transmitted infection
- In US, disease carried by *Dermacentor andersonii* (Rocky Mountain wood tick), *Dermacentor variabilis* (American dog tick), *Dermacentor occidentalis* (Pacific Coast dog tick), *Amblyomma americanum* (Lone Star tick)
- Following inoculation into skin, organism multiplies locally, after 2–5 d (range 1–10 d), produces erythematous, tender/pruritic papule; papule rapidly enlarges/forms ulcer w/black base; bacteria spread to regional lymph nodes producing lymphadenopathy/may spread to distant organs w/bacteremia

CLINICAL MANIFESTATIONS

- Tularemia often starts w/sudden onset of fever, chills, headache, generalized myalgias, arthralgias

Clinical Presentation of Tularemia

	Children	Adults
Lymphadenopathy	96%	65%
Fever (≥38.3°C)	87%	21%
Ulcer/eschar/papule	45%	51%
Myalgias/arthralgias	39%	2%
Headache	9%	5%

- In adults, most common site inguinal/femoral; in children, cervical lymphadenopathy
- Clinical manifestations of tularemia have classically been divided into 7 clinical syndromes:

	Children	Adults
Ulceroglandular	45%	51%
Glandular	25%	12%
Pneumonia	14%	18%
Oropharyngeal	4%	
Oculoglandular	2%	
Typhoidal	2%	12%
Unclassified	6%	11%

- Ulceroglandular/glandular tularemia account for ~75–85% of human disease
- Nodes may become fluctuant/drain spontaneously; majority resolve w/effective treatment
- Late suppuration of lymph nodes described in up to 25% of pts w/ulceroglandular/glandular tularemia; material taken from these late fluctuant nodes following successful antimicrobial treatment have revealed sterile necrotic tissue
- Tularemia also has been associated w/meningitis, pericarditis, hepatitis, peritonitis, endocarditis, osteomyelitis, sepsis, rhabdomyolosis w/acute renal failure, meningitis

DIFFERENTIAL DIAGNOSIS

- In up to 40% of pts w/tularemia, no Hx of epidemiologic contact w/animal/arthropod vector can be elicited
- Papular skin lesion may resemble sporotrichosis, infection w/*Staphylococcus aureus, Streptococcus pyogenes,* syphilis, anthrax, rat bite fever (*Spirillium* species minus), *Rickettsia tsutsugamushi* (scrub typhus), *Mycobacterium marinum* infections
- Glandular tularemia must be differentiated from plague, lymphogranuloma venerum, cat scratch disease

DIAGNOSIS

- Culture/isolation difficult
- Tularemia most frequently confirmed by serology; in standard agglutination tests, titer <1:20 not diagnostic because of nonspecific cross reactions
- False-negative serologic responses found early in infection; up to 30% of tests negative after 3 wks of infection; single titer of 1:160 should be interpreted as presumptive positive test; fourfold ↑ in titers considered diagnostic

TREATMENT

- Gentamicin, 1.7 mg/kg/dose IV/IM q8h, recently, use of twice-daily (5 mg/kg/day)/once-daily gentamicin has been reported; no data using once-daily gentamicin for tularemia currently exists)
- Streptomycin, 7.5–10 mg/kg/dose q12h IM considered drug of choice in adults; streptomycin, 30–40 mg/kg/d div 2 daily IM doses considered drug of choice in children
- Following clinical response in 3–5 d, dose can be reduced to 10–15 mg/kg/d in 2 div doses; Tx typically continued for 7–10 d; however, in mild-to-moderate cases w/48–72 hrs of afebrile course, 5–7 d of Tx successful
- *Alternative drugs:* tetracyclines/chloramphenicol (higher relapse rates); fluoroquinolones in adolescents/adults
- If untreated, symptoms of tularemia usually last 1–4 wks, but may continue for mos
- Overall mortality for untreated tularemia <8%
- Mortality <1% w/appropriate treatment/often associated w/long delays in Dx/treatment

WHEN TO REFER

- Most pts managed w/o referral
- Complicated cases of unresponsive pneumonia, sepsis/disseminated disease may be difficult to diagnose
- Seronegative/undiagnosed pts, pts w/complicated disease should be considered for presumptive Tx w/positive epidemiologic exposure in endemic areas; consultation appropriate in complicated cases

BACKGROUND

- Girls w/abnormal/missing X chromosome *associated w/* short stature, gonadal dysgenesis, dysmorphic features, other problems
- One of most common chromosomal disorders in girls:
  - 1.5% of all conceptions, but 99.9% spontaneously aborted
  - 1/2,000 female live births
- Turner karyotypes include:
  - *monosomy* X (45,X) (50% pts)
  - *structural abnormalities* of X such as isochromosome (17%), partial deletion, ring
  - *mosaicism* such as 45,X/46,XX (14%) or 45,X/46,XY (4%)
- Clinical manifestations caused by absent/abnormal expression of gene(s) on X chromosome important for growth/lymphatic formation; failure of meiotic pairing in germ cells
- Many of somatic abnormalities appear to relate to:
  - abnormal lymphatic development (causing edema/cystic hygroma formation)
  - abnormal endochondral bone formation (causing skeletal/growth abnormalities)

CLINICAL MANIFESTATIONS

- Short stature: 100%
  - average adult height = 4'8"
- Dysmorphic features:
  - very common: 50–75%
    - high palate, retrognathia
  - common: 25–50%
    - ptosis; epicanthal folds
    - prominent ears
    - low hairline; short or web neck
    - cubitus valgus; flat feet
    - short 4th metacarpals
    - nail dysplasia; edema of hands, feet
- Others:
  very common: >75%
    - chronic otitis media
    - learning disability (normal IQ)
  - common: 25–50%
    - strabismus
    - cardiovascular anomalies (coarctation, bicuspid aortic valve)
    - renal anomalies
    - multiple nevi
    - glucose intolerance
  - less common: <25%
    - hypothyroidism
    - scoliosis
- Pubertal delay or amenorrhea: 95%

LABORATORY TESTING

- *Karyotype:* only way to make definitive Dx; obtain karyotype when following features present in girls:
  - *infancy:* lymphedema, excessive nuchal skin, low hairline, and/or left-sided cardiac anomalies (Dx often obvious)
  - *childhood:* unexplained short stature (Dx often difficult)
  - *adolescence:* delayed puberty (no breast development by age 14)/1° amenorrhea (no menses by age 16)
- *Other studies:* LH/FSH usually ↑ in girls <4 or >10 yrs of age w/gonadal dysgenesis

EVALUATIONS AND FOLLOW-UP THERAPIES

- Short stature:
  - measure, plot height each visit
    - growth hormone 0.05 mg/kg/d
    - consider anabolic steroids (eg, oxandrolone)
- Gonadal dysgenesis:
  - assess karyotype for Y chromosome material
    - refer for gonadectomies if Y material present
  - assess pubertal development; LH/FSH
    - estrogen and progestin; usually begin age 14–15
  - counsel about sexual development/ fertility
    - refer to reproductive endocrinologist
- Cardiac anomalies:
  - echocardiogram (or MRI) at Dx; BP/ pulses each visit
    - referral to cardiologist; prophylactic antibiotics
  - repeat echocardiograms to r/o aortic root dilatation
- Renal anomalies:
  - renal ultrasound at Dx
    - refer to nephrologist; routine UAs
- Psychosocial:
  - assess for possible learning disabilities
    - refer to psychologist; work w/school system
  - provide social support
    - link w/Turner Syndrome Society
- Hearing loss:
  - assess for otitis media, hearing loss (at risk for conductive and sensorineural losses)
    - aggressive antibiotic and surgical management
    - refer to audiology and ENT specialists

- Strabismus:
  - assess at each visit (esp preschool yrs)
    - refer to ophthalmologist
- Dental problems:
  - assess for crowding of teeth, malocclusion
    - refer to orthodontist
- Orthopedic problems:
  - assess for scoliosis at each visit (esp ages 5–15)
    - refer to orthopedist
  - assess for flat feet routinely
    - advise concerning proper shoes; refer for orthotics
  - assess for lymphedema
    - salt restriction, elastic stockings
- Skin lesions:
  - assess for dysplastic nevi, keloids, psoriasis
    - refer to dermatology
- Dysmorphic features:
  - assess for web neck, malformed ears
    - refer to plastic surgeon
- Thyroid dysfunction
  - yearly thyroid function tests
    - thyroid hormone replacement

DIFFERENTIAL DIAGNOSIS

- Familial short stature
- Constitutional growth delay
- Noonan syndrome
- Hypothyroidism

WHEN TO REFER

- Refer to pediatric endocrinologist at time of Dx. Consider referral to 3° care center using a multidisciplinary approach

BACKGROUND

- *Incidence:* 1–7/100,000 US population/year
- *Prevalence:* 50–75 cases/100,000 US population
- Age of presentation in pediatric population:
  - 50% pts 16–20 yrs of age
  - 33% pts 11–15 yrs of age
  - unusual <6 yrs of age
- More common in Caucasians/Jewish population
- Males/females equally effected
- ↑ prevalence in first-degree relatives

CLINICAL MANIFESTATIONS

- Presenting features:
  - diarrhea: 95%
  - rectal bleeding: 95%
  - weight loss: 40%
  - abdominal pain: 10%
  - arthritis: 5%
  - growth failure: 2%
- Extraintestinal manifestations:
  - joint symptoms: 15% (most often sacroiliac/large joints of lower extremity)
  - skin (erythema nodosum, pyoderma gangrenosum): 2–5%
  - eyes (episcleritis): 1%
  - liver (sclerosing cholangitis, hepatitis, hepatic steatosis): 1–3%

LABORATORY FEATURES

- ↑ sed rate: 80%
- Anemia: 70%
- Hypoalbuminemia: 60%
- Thrombocytosis: 60%
- Occult blood in stool: positive
- Stool cultures: negative
- Ova/parasites: negative

DIFFERENTIAL DIAGNOSIS

- *Crohn disease:* gross blood less frequent; differentiated by growth failure, perianal disease, small bowel involvement
- *Infectious colitis:* differentiated by sudden onset, identifiable source w/other cases
- *Amebic colitis:* travel to endemic area w/identification of ameba in stool

TREATMENT

- *Mild–moderate disease:* Tx initiated w/5-ASA compound; moderate–severe symptoms treated w/corticosteroids; remissions maintained w/5-ASA compounds
- 5-aminosalicylic acid:
  - carrier drugs:
    - 5-ASA-sulfapyridine (sulfasalazine; Azulfidine; 30–50 mg/kg/d; usual adult dose 1–2 g bid)
    - 5-ASA-ASA (olsalazine; Dipentum: usual adult dose 500 mg bid)
  - delayed-release drugs:
    - 5-ASA coated in acrylic resin released at pH >6 (mesalamine; Asacol; 30–50 mg/kg/d: usual adult dose 800 mg tid)
    - 5-ASA encapsulated in ethylcellulose microspheres (mesalamine; Pentasa; 30–50 mg/kg/d: usual adult dose 1 g tid–qid)
  - enemas/suppositories:
    - mesalamine (Rowasa): effective in proctitis, distal ulcerative colitis
- Corticosteroids:
  - oral: 1–2 mg/kg/d (max 40–60 mg):
    - once remission achieved, lower by 5 mg q1–2 wks
    - attempt to achieve qod schedule
    - parenteral administration in severe disease
  - enemas, foams and suppositories:
    - effective in proctitis

- Alternative Tx:
  - surgery w/total colectomy/ileo-pouch anal anastomosis curative/eliminates possibility of colon cancer; problems associated w/surgery include more frequent bowel movements/inflammation of pouch; chronic inflammation of pouch may occur in up to 5% pts

COMPLICATIONS

- *Hemorrhage:* massive in 1–3%; usually preceded by herald bleed
- *Toxic megacolon:* acute life-threatening dilation of colon; treated w/antibiotics, decompression/surgery if necessary; may be precipitated by agents that slow gut transit
- *Carcinoma:* risk ~8% after 25 yrs in pts w/pancolitis; dysplasia screening starting 7/8 yrs after onset of symptoms

WHEN TO REFER

- Most pts should be referred to gastroenterologist experienced in Dx, management of inflammatory bowel disease

UMBILICAL ABNORMALITIES

FREDERICK J. RESCORLA

BACKGROUND

- Umbilicus in early gestation contains umbilical vessels, allantois, extrocoelomic yolk stalk containing vitelline (omphalomesenteric) duct/vessels
- Persistence of structures that normally obliterate/failure of closure of umbilical ring account for most abnormalities
- Umbilical hernia, most common umbilical defect, occurs in up to 1/6 children; more common in black infants/prematures
- Umbilical granulomas represent proliferation of granulation tissue at base of umbilicus
- Infected umbilical vessels, omphalitis/periumbilical necrotizing fasciitis extremely rare but require prompt treatment/surgical excision

Embryonic Structure	Normal Development	Failure of Obliteration/Closure
Vitelline/ omphalomesenteric duct	Obliterates at 7–8th wk of gestation	Umbilical fistula/sinus Umbilical (mucosal) polyp Meckel diverticulum Enteric cyst
Allantois	Forms cordlike urachus at 4–5 mos gestation	Patent urachus (50%) Urachal cyst/abscess (30%) Urachal sinus (15%) Urachal diverticulum (5%)
Umbilical ring	Closes	Umbilical hernia Omphalocele Hernia of umbilical cord

CLINICAL MANIFESTATIONS

- Umbilical hernia; usually present as asymptomatic umbilical ring defect; incarceration extremely rare/along w/significant spontaneous closure rate basis for initial nonop management
- Omphalocele/hernia of umbilical cord (defect <4 cm) present as neonatal umbilical defect w/amnion/peritoneum covering underlying bowel
- Presence of urine/intestinal contents draining from umbilicus indicates patent urachus/umbilical fistula, respectively; rare to have both urinary/enteric drainage
- Urachal abnormalities often present as wet, edematous, enlarged umbilical cord that will not slough
- Urachal cysts often small/undetected until later when tender infraumbilical mass presents as urachal abscess; more common in older children/adults
- External urachal sinus presents w/intermittent periumbilical pain/tenderness
- Umbilical granulomas appear after cord separation as mass of pink granulation tissue at base of umbilicus

LABORATORY FEATURES

- If opening present catheter can be placed/radiographic contrast study obtained to identify urachal/omphalomesenteric remnants
- Urachal abnormalities can be further delineated by ultrasound, voiding cystourethrogram

TREATMENT

- *Umbilical hernia:* most undergo spontaneous closure; initial fascial defects <0.5 cm nearly always close; initial defects >1.5 cm less likely to close; recommendation: observation until 4–5 yrs of age, then surgical repair
- *Omphalocele/hernia of umbilical cord:* surgical repair in newborn period
- *Umbilical granuloma:* topical treatment w/silver nitrate sticks; most resolve after several treatments; persistence may indicate presence of umbilical polyp related to enteric involvement/should be excised
- *Umbilical fistula:* surgical excision
- *Urachal defects:* surgical excision. If urachal abscess involves multiple structures, initial treatment w/incision/drainage, antibiotics may be warranted
- *Infected umbilical vessels, omphalitis, periumbilical necrotizing fasciitis:* antibiotics/surgical excision

WHEN TO REFER

- *Umbilical hernia:* at 4–5 yrs of age when considering operative repair; presence/Hx incarceration (unusual)
- *Omphalocele/hernia of umbilical cord:* time of Dx
- *Urachal abnormalities:* time of Dx
- *Umbilical fistula, sinus/mucosal polyp:* time of Dx
- *Umbilical granuloma:* persistence after several treatments w/silver nitrate
- *Omphalitis, infected umbilical vessels, periumbilical necrotizing fasciitis:* time of Dx

BACKGROUND

- 1% boys, 3%, girls have symptomatic urinary tract infection (UTI) during first 10 yrs of life w/peak incidence during first year of life
- Except in first 8–12 wks of life when infection of urinary tract may be 2° to hematogenous source, UTI believed to arise by ascending route following entry of bacteria via urethra
- Enterobacteriaceae most common organisms isolated from infected urinary tract
- Risk factors for UTI include previous UTI, anatomic or functional abnormality of urinary tract, ABO-blood-group, nonsecretor phenotype, use of urinary catheter, recent sexual intercourse, possibly immunocompromising medical illness
- Renal growth occurring during first 5 yrs of life impaired when scarring present.

Risk factors for renal scarring include having first episode of pyelonephritis < age 3, grades IV, V vesicoureteral reflux in conjunction w/bacteriuria, delay in instituting Tx after establishment of pyelonephritis

CLINICAL MANIFESTATIONS

- Young children w/UTI often do not present w/specific urinary tract symptoms. After 5 yrs of age classic Sx infection (fever, dysuria, urgency, costovertebral angle tenderness) usually present
- Localization of infection to kidneys or bladder based on clinical presentation not sufficiently accurate to specifically direct management. Pts w/fever, costovertebral angle tenderness usually assumed to have pyelonephritis until proven otherwise, but as many as 25% children w/o symptoms of pyelonephritis have renal bacteriuria based on ureteral catheterization or bladder-washout test

LABORATORY FEATURES

- Generally required:
  – urine specimen for urine analysis (UA), culture. Specimens ideally obtained by suprapubic bladder aspiration or by urethral catheterization in non-toilet-trained child, by voided midstream technique in toilet-trained child. After collection urine should be refrigerated, processed within 24 h
  – UA analysis includes leukocyte esterase, nitrite components of "dipstick" biochemical tests along w/microscopic examination for WBCs, bacteria. In clinical practice dipstick and culture most accurate and cost effective tests for UTI. Microscopy adds little to diagnostic evaluation

Criteria for Dx UTIs

Method of Collection	Colony Count (Pure Culture)	Probability of Infection (%)
Suprapubic aspiration	Gram-negative bacilli: any number	> 99
	Gram-positive cocci: > few thousand	
Catheterization	> 10^5	95
	10^4–10^5	Infection likely
	10^3–10^4	Suspicious; repeat
	< 10^3	Infection unlikely
Clean-voided		
Boy	> 10^4	Infection likely
Girl	3 specimens: > 10^5	95
	2 specimens: > 10^5	90
	1 specimen: > 10^5	80
	5×10^4–10^5	Suspicious; repeat
	10^4–5×10^4	Symptomatic; suspicious; repeat
	10^4–5×10^4	Asymptomatic; infection unlikely
	< 10^4	Infection unlikely

Reprinted with permission from Hellerstein S. Recurrent urinary tract infections in children. Pediatr Infect Dis J. 1982;1:271–281. Copyright 1982.

DIFFERENTIAL DIAGNOSIS FOR POSITIVE URINE CULTURE

- Contaminated specimen
- Urethritis, vaginitis, cervicitis, prostatitis
- Foreign body including nephrolithiasis
- Renal (intrarenal or perinephric) abscess
- Entero- or vaginovesical fistula

TREATMENT

- Hospitalization considered for child <5 yrs of age suspected of having UTI, appearing systemically ill
- Broad antibiotic coverage for group B streptococcus and Enterobacteriaceae required during first 8 wks of life pending results of blood, CSF cultures. After newborn period, sulfonamides, aminopenicillins, nitrofurantoin, trimethoprim/sulfamethoxazole have established efficacy in treatment of uncomplicated UTI
- When fever has resolved, pts initially managed on parenteral Tx for UTI may then complete Tx w/oral antibiotic for total of 7–10 d
- Males, females <5 yrs of age should undergo radiologic evaluation of urinary tract following their first UTI. Prior to evaluation, child should have prophylactic antibiotic coverage (nitrofurantoin, sulfisoxazole, or trimethoprim/sulfamethoxazole)

COMPLICATIONS

- Recurrent infection most common complication
- Bacteremia and/or meningitis may accompany UTI in neonate
- Long-term complications occur as consequence of scarring; include growth failure, hypertension, renal failure

PREVENTION FOR RECURRENT UTI

- Prompt treatment of infection
- Prophylactic antibiotics
- Consider possible voiding dysfunction
- For sexually active pts, postcoital antimicrobial use or alternative method of contraception for diaphragm-using females
- Avoid use of indwelling catheters

WHEN TO REFER

- Most pts managed w/o referral
- Referral indicated for serious complications, when pt fails to respond to initial Tx, or when radiologic evaluation abnormal

BACKGROUND

- Urticaria, angioedema related conditions that often occur together (50% pts have both, 40% have only urticaria, 10% have only angioedema)
- Both disorders characterized by vasodilation; ↑ vascular permeability; extravasation of fluid, protein caused by mast cell–derived mediators or complement-derived activators. Urticaria involves superficial dermis, whereas angioedema takes place in submucosa, deep dermis, SubQ tissue
- Urticaria, angioedema have many causes:
  - *IgE-mediated:* foods (eg, shellfish, peanuts, eggs, wheat, milk, chocolate, strawberries), drugs (eg, penicillin, sulfonamides), infection (eg, viral, streptococcal), insect stings (eg, *Hymenoptera*), parasites, inhalants (animal dander, molds, pollen)
  - *circulating immune complexes:* serum sickness, hepatitis B infection, systemic lupus erythematosus, Epstein-Barr virus infection
  - *drug induced:* direct stimulant effect on mast cells (eg, codeine, radiocontrast media, hyperosmolar solutions, etc), abnormalities of arachidonic acid metabolism (symptoms worsen 20–40% pts w/urticaria who take NSAIDs)
  - physical stimuli (eg, cold, sunlight, pressure, vibration)
  - idiopathic
  - associated w/rare syndromes (eg, mastocytosis)
- Urticaria, angioedema classified as acute if process lasts <6 wks (most common form in children) or chronic if present for ≥6 wks (more likely in middle-aged pts)

CLINICAL MANIFESTATIONS

- Erythematous papules or plaques that may be round/oval/form rings or incomplete rings. In areas of confluence of lesions, polycyclic appearance may be observed
- Lesions may have pale halo and upon resolution may have dusky center
- Pruritus common
- In urticaria, individual lesions transient, last ≤24 h (usually 20 min–3 h)

- Systemic symptoms generally absent, but direct involvement of viscera may cause hoarseness, respiratory distress, vomiting, diarrhea, abdominal pain, arthralgias, headache, syncope, hypotension or shock
- If coexisting angioedema exists, pt exhibits diffuse, often well-demarcated, non-pitting swelling w/predilection for periorbital, perioral areas, where there is loose SubQ tissue, or hands and feet

DIFFERENTIAL DIAGNOSIS

- *Erythema multiforme:* lesions fixed (often lasting ≥ 7 d), manifest central change in color (eg, darker red, white, gray) or formation of bulla or crust. In addition, lesions of erythema multiforme annular and do not take on varied shapes often seen in urticaria
- Insect bites
- Mastocytosis
- *Urticarial vasculitis:* lesions persist >24 h

LABORATORY FEATURES

- *Acute urticaria (w/or w/o angioedema); no systemic symptoms:* in children, most such cases produced by acute infection (eg, viral, streptococcal), foods, or medications. Laboratory studies to determine etiology should be directed by Hx, physical examination
- *Chronic urticaria (w/or w/o angioedema); no systemic symptoms:* unusual presentation in children, adolescents; no etiology found in most cases (75–90%). Laboratory studies should be directed by Hx, physical examination. However, some authorities recommend performance of minimal laboratory evaluation, including CBC, sed rate, chemistry panel, UA

TREATMENT

- Remove or avoid identified precipitant
- Antihistamines first line of Tx:
  - begin w/first-generation H_1 antagonist (eg, hydroxyzine, 2–5 mg/kg/d, div qid [10–25 mg qid for adolescents]), ↑ dose as tolerated to control symptoms. Alternately, cetirizine (5–10 mg/d for children 6–11 yrs

of age, 10 mg for those ≥12 yrs of age) or second-generation, nonsedating H_1 antagonist (eg, loratidine [10 mg/d for pts ≥6 yrs of age] or others) may be selected, although these agents comparatively much more expensive
  - if pt experiences intolerable drowsiness w/first-generation H_1 antagonist, change to second-generation, nonsedating antihistamine. Bedtime dose of first-generation antihistamine may be used to provide additional control of symptoms while limiting daytime sedation
  - if response not optimal, consider one or more of following: (1) change to another class of first-generation H_1 antagonist, (2) add doxepin, which possesses potent H_1 antagonist effects [10–25 mg hs in pts ≥ 12 yrs of age], (3) use H_2 antagonist (eg, cimetidine or ranitidine) in conjunction w/H_1 antagonist because some pts benefit from combined Tx (H_2 antagonists should not be used alone in management of urticaria and angioedema)
- *Corticosteroids:* generally not required to manage acute urticaria and angioedema. However, short courses of agents (eg, prednisone, 1 mg/kg/d) may be of assistance in management of rare pts w/intractable symptoms not controlled by antihistamines. Corticosteroids should not be used to manage pts w/chronic urticaria
- *Special situations:* in general, evaluation, management of situations described below require consultation w/or referral to allergist/immunologist or dermatologist:
  - urticaria w/episodes of respiratory difficulty: provide pt w/injectable epinephrine (eg, EpiPen or EpiPen, Jr); refer
  - generalized urticaria or respiratory difficulty following insect sting: provide pt w/injectable epinephrine; refer for possible desensitization
  - chronic urticaria: consultation w/or referral to specialist indicated

WHEN TO REFER

- As described above

BACKGROUND

- Following menarche, adolescent female may have significant cycle-to-cycle variation until she begins to ovulate regularly
- Establishment of regular ovulatory menstrual cycle indication that hypothalamic-pituitary-ovarian (H-P-O axis) intact

Regular Uterine Bleeding

- FSH stimulates estrogen production, which creates endometrial growth (proliferative phase of menstrual cycle)
- After ovulation, corpus luteum develops, secreting progesterone, which stabilizes endometrium (luteal phase)
- If fertilization does not occur, regression starts. W/waning of progesterone and estrogen levels, endometrium undergoes necrotic changes that result in menstrual bleeding
- Ovulatory menstrual cycles usually occur at 21–35 d intervals
- Menstrual blood loss 40–80 ml; flow lasts 2–7 d

Dysfunctional Uterine Bleeding

- Defined as abnormal, excessive, irregular bleeding from endometrium unrelated to structural or systemic disease
- Blood loss may be >100 ml per menstrual period, amount that would result in iron deficiency anemia; flow may be >8–10 d
- Adolescent prone to anovulatory periods w/incomplete shedding of proliferative endometrium

CLINICAL MANIFESTATIONS

- Mild dysfunctional bleeding:
  - menses longer than normal, or cycle shortened ≥2 mos
  - flow slightly to moderately ↑
- Moderate dysfunctional bleeding:
  - menses moderately prolonged or cycle remains shortened w/frequent menses (q1–3 wks)
  - flow moderate to heavy
- Severe dysfunctional bleeding:
  - prolonged bleeding w/disruption of normal menstrual cycles
  - flow very heavy

DIFFERENTIAL DIAGNOSIS

- *Disorders of pregnancy:* threatened, incomplete, or missed abortion, molar pregnancy, ectopic pregnancy
- *Infectious causes:* pelvic inflammatory disease: salpingitis, endometritis, cervicitis
- *Blood dyscrasias:* thrombocytopenia (eg, idiopathic, leukemia, aplastic anemia, hypersplenism), clotting disorders, Von Willebrand disease/other disorders of platelet function, liver diseases
- *Endocrine disorders:* polycystic ovary syndrome, hypo- or hyperthyroidism, adrenal disease, diabetes mellitus, hyperprolactinemia
- *Vaginal abnormalities:* vaginitis, carcinoma
- *Cervical problems:* cervicitis, polyp, hemangioma, carcinoma
- *Uterine problems:* congenital anomalies, submucous myoma, polyp, carcinoma, use of intrauterine contraceptive device, tuberculosis, irregular bleeding associated w/use of hormonal contraceptives, ovulation bleeding, endometrial polyp
- *Ovarian problems:* cyst, abnormal corpus luteum function, steroid-secreting ovarian neoplasms, ovarian failure
- *Endometriosis*
- *Systemic diseases* (eg, liver diseases, renal diseases, cystic fibrosis)
- *Trauma*
- *Foreign body* (eg, retained tampon)
- *Arteriovenous malformation* at any site in female reproductive tract
- *Medication:* anticoagulants, platelet inhibitors, androgens, tricyclic antidepressants
- *Other disorders associated w/anovulation:* psychosocial problems, stress, eating disorders, obesity, athletic competition

PATIENT ASSESSMENT/EVALUATION

History

- Obtain complete Hx to determine likely Dx, as well urgency for immediate treatment because of profound or postural symptoms
- Date of menarche, menstrual pattern, duration, quantity/color of flow
- Use of tampons or other foreign objects
- Assess sexual activity, whether bleeding postcoital, use of contraceptives, previous sexually transmitted diseases (STD), recent exposure to new partner or partner w/STD
- General review of systems including recent stresses, weight changes, dietary practices, syncope, visual changes, headaches, GI symptoms, systemic disease, athletic competition, medication, illicit drugs
- Family hx polycystic ovarian syndrome (PCOS) and bleeding disorders

Physical Examination

- General assessment w/attention to height, weight, body type and fat distribution, BP (supine and standing)
- Evidence of androgen excess (acne, hirsutism, clitoromegaly)
- Thyroid palpation
- Other signs of bleeding such as petechiae or bruises
- Pelvic examination
  - pelvic exam in all sexually active teens to determine source of bleeding, to obtain cultures for STDs, to perform bimanual examination to assess ovarian masses, uterine fibroids, signs of PID, pregnancy
  - in virginal pt one-finger digital examination, often speculum examination, can be accomplished to check for foreign bodies within vagina, to palpate cervix, uterus, adnexae. If not, bimanual rectoabdominal examination or pelvic ultrasound can be helpful

Laboratory Tests

- Initial, all pts:
  - pregnancy test
  - CBC w/differential, platelets
  - in sexually active patients, tests for chlamydia and gonorrhea
- Menorrhagia at menarche, cyclic hemorrhage; severe bleeding:
  - coagulation studies (prothrombin time, partial thromboplastin time, bleeding time, Von Willebrand panel)
  - type, cross-match if acute severe hemorrhage or very low Hgb
- May be indicated:
  - a sed rate if pelvic infection a consideration
  - TSH
  - prolactin, endocrine tests for PCOS
  - pelvic ultrasound if examination cannot be accomplished, pt does not respond to treatment, abnormalities detected

TREATMENT

- *Objective:* to stop bleeding, prevent recurrence, provide long-term follow-up to pt. Estrogen heals over bleeding sites by causing further proliferation; progestins induce endometrial stability
- Mild dysfunctional bleeding:
  - Hgb level normal
  - observation, reassurance usually adequate
  - encourage pt to keep menstrual calendar so need for intervention in future can be assessed
  - iron supplement: to prevent anemia
  - antiprostaglandin medications, such as naproxen sodium, to reduce blood loss
- Moderate dysfunctional bleeding:
  - Hgb level often shows mild anemia
  - Tx consists of oral contraceptive pills (OCP) or oral medroxyprogesterone
  - course of oral iron should be prescribed to correct anemia
  - pt not bleeding at time of visit, pt or parent dislikes use of OCP, or there is medical contraindication to use of estrogen, oral medroxyprogesterone can be tried as initial Tx: 10 mg 1×/d × 10–14 d, started on day 14 of menstrual cycle (day 1 is first day of last period) or at time of visit. Pattern continued 3–6 mos
  - pts w/heavy or prolonged dysfunctional bleeding, initial use of an oral contraceptive, such as Lo/Ovral × 21 d. Useful regimen for heavy bleeding is Lo/Ovral 4×/d × 4 d, 3×/d × 3 d, and 2×/d × 2 wks. W/high doses of estrogen, antiemetics such as chlorpromazine, 5–10 mg, can be given 2 hrs before each dose of OCP. Normal withdrawal flow will follow 2–4 d after last hormone tablet. Treat for ≥3 mos before switching to cyclic oral medroxyprogesterone
- Severe dysfunctional bleeding:
  - Hgb level reduced, often <9 gm/dl. Clinical signs of blood loss may be present
  - pt should be admitted if:
    - initial Hgb <7 g
    - orthostatic signs present
    - bleeding heavy, Hgb <9 g/dl
  - transfusion should be considered if clinical signs of acute blood loss or Hgb extremely low
  - effective treatment is Ovral tablet q4h until bleeding slows or stops (usually 4–8 tablets), then q6h × 24 h, q8h × 48 h, then 2×/d to complete 21 d course of hormone. Alternatively, Lo/Ovral regimen can start w/q4h until bleeding controlled, then tapered to one tablet 4×/d × 4 d, 3×/d × 3 d, 2×/d × 2 wks
  - in acute severe hemorrhage, pt if NPO, conjugated estrogens, 25 mg IV q4h × 2–3 doses, sometimes used at same time that oral contraceptives initiated
  - if use of estrogen contraindicated, trial of progestin such as norethindrone acetate (Aygestin) or medroxyprogesterone, 10 mg can be given q4h, then tapered to regimen of 4×/d × 4 d, 3×/d × 3 d, 2×/d × 2 wks
  - if hormone regimen fails to control bleeding within 24–36 hrs, possibility of pelvic pathology should be excluded by ultrasound, anesthesia examination, dilation and curettage
  - iron Tx should be instituted along w/hormone Tx as soon as pt has stabilized (1–2 d)

FOLLOW-UP AND PROGNOSIS

- Pts w/thrombocytopenia (idiopathic, leukemia, or aplastic anemia) may require long-term management w/daily oral contraceptives or depoleuprolide (Depo-Lupron)
- Pts w/long Hx anovulatory cycles, dysfunctional uterine bleeding, PCOS have ↑ risk of later infertility, endometrial carcinoma. Regular withdrawal w/progestins (12–14 d/mo) or oral contraceptives should be prescribed

WHEN TO REFER

- Persistent bleeding
- Low hematocrit
- Chronic illness
- Clotting disorders (von Willebrand, thrombocytopenia)
- Anatomic abnormalities

VARICELLA-ZOSTER VIRUS INFECTIONS

ANNE A. GERSHON

BACKGROUND

- *Varicella:* most frequently occurs <10 yrs of age; *zoster:* unusual in otherwise healthy children; associated w/varicella in utero, immunosuppression including HIV infection; elderly age; has been reported rarely after immunization
- No sex predilection
- *Etiology of both:* varicella-zoster virus (VZV)
- Highly contagious to susceptibles (VZV antibody negative) as varicella; zoster due to reactivation of latent virus acquired during attack of varicella

CLINICAL MANIFESTATIONS

- Varicella:
  – evolving pruritic rash from maculopapules to vesicles to pustules to crusts
  – distribution of rash predominantly on trunk, face, head, including scalp
  – fever, malaise for several days
  – may be severe/even fatal in immunocompromised children (w/cancer, after transplantation, underlying AIDS)
- Zoster:
  – unilateral, often painful vesicular rash in dermatomal distribution

LABORATORY FEATURES

- Varicella:
  – routine laboratory values usually normal
  – occasionally followed by transient neutropenia, thrombocytopenia; WBC may be ↑ w/bacterial superinfection
  – Dx best made by viral antigen identification in skin lesions (smear stained w/fluorescein-labeled monoclonal antibody/viral culture of lesions)
  – fourfold rise in VZV antibody titer following disease diagnostic
- *Zoster:* as for varicella

DIFFERENTIAL DIAGNOSIS

- Varicella:
  – herpes simplex virus (HSV) infection
  – Stevens-Johnson syndrome
  – rickettsial pox
  – allergic skin reaction
  – scabies
- Zoster:
  – recurrent HSV infection

TREATMENT

- Varicella:
  – no specific treatment necessary for uncomplicated cases
  – acyclovir (30 mg/kg/d IV/1,500 mg/m^2/d, div tid) for those w/severe/potentially severe varicella; for oral Tx for adolescents, selected others (80 mg/kg/d div qid, po) × 5 d
- Zoster:
  – as for varicella; in addition, for adolescents w/zoster, famciclovir (500 mg tid po) × 7 d/valacyclovir (1 g tid po) × 7–14 d

COMPLICATIONS

- *Varicella:* major complication bacterial superinfection, particularly invasive group A beta hemolytic streptococci (w/possible sepsis, toxic shock, bone/soft tissue infection), also staphylococci
  – cerebellar ataxia (1/4,000), encephalitis (1/40,000)
  – 1° varicella pneumonia in immunocompromised pts, newborns whose mothers have active varicella at term, adults
- *Zoster:* particularly in elderly, postherpetic neuralgia (PHN); PHN very rare in children

PREVENTION

- Varicella:
  – most cases (90%) in otherwise healthy children prevented by active immunization w/licensed vaccine; 1 dose for children <13 yrs, 2 doses 4–8 wks apart used for adolescents >13 yrs
  – passive immunization w/varicella-zoster immune globulin (VZIG) for closely exposed susceptibles at high risk to develop severe varicella (immunocompromised pts, certain newborns, adults); dose: 1 vial q10 kg body weight; max 5 vials
- *Zoster:* no proven preventive

WHEN TO REFER

- Varicella:
  – if severe disease, including pneumonia, invasive streptococcal infection, prolonged (>7 d) formation of new lesions
  – if Dx unclear
  – if seemingly unusual complications develop after vaccination (severe rash, encephalitis, zoster)
  – if pt w/varicella thought to be immunosuppressed
- *Zoster:* PHN

GENERAL NOTE

- Vascular lesions common findings in newborns
- Distinction of benign, self-resolving types (eg, salmon patches) from persistent (eg, port-wine stains)/evolving lesions (eg, hemangiomas) usually made in nursery on clinical grounds; in some instances observation for few mos may be required

SALMON PATCH

BACKGROUND

- Also known as nevus simplex, erythema nuchae, angel's kiss, stork bite
- Most common vascular lesion in infancy
- Seen in 40% of newborns

CLINICAL MANIFESTATIONS

- Pink macule, w/or w/o telangiectasias, commonly located over nape of neck/glabella
- Also be seen on forehead, upper eyelids, nasolabial region
- Facial lesions fade in 1–2 yrs w/reappearance of erythema during episodes of crying, breath holding, straining
- Nuchal lesions commonly persist

PORT-WINE STAIN (PWS)

BACKGROUND

- Occurs in 0.3–0.5% of all newborns
- Also known as nevus flammeus
- M = F

CLINICAL MANIFESTATIONS

- Well-demarcated, pink to violaceous macule of any size, which at least partially blanches w/diascopy
- Usually unilateral/segmental
- Most commonly located on face/neck
- 5–8% of PWS in trigeminal distribution (V1 and/or V2) will have ocular/CNS involvement (Sturge-Weber syndrome)
- Port-wine stains persist/may become more violaceous, thicker/nodular w/advancing age

MANAGEMENT

- Pulsed tunable dye lasers can lighten color; multiple treatments are required
- Pts w/lesions in trigeminal distribution need ophthalmologic exams/careful clinical evaluation/follow-up for possible neurologic involvement
- Pts w/lesions on extremity/limb asymmetry should be evaluated for involvement of deeper vasculature/A-V fistulae (Klippel-Trenaunay/Parkes Weber syndromes, respectively)

VENOUS MALFORMATIONS

BACKGROUND

- Developmental venous anomalies

CLINICAL MANIFESTATIONS

- Usually present as soft, compressible, bluish SubQ nodules
- May also involve visceral structures
- Growth commensurate w/growth of child
- No involution occurs

COMPLICATIONS

- GI bleeding
- Pain from phleboliths

TREATMENT

- Symptomatic/cosmetically unacceptable lesions treated w/sclerosing agents, embolization, excision

CUTIS MARMORATA

BACKGROUND

- Physiologic response to cold temperatures accentuating cutaneous vascular network

CLINICAL MANIFESTATIONS

- Mottled, reticulated, bluish macules over trunk/extremities, vary in intensity
- Skin otherwise normal in appearance
- Color returns to normal w/warming

DIFFERENTIAL DIAGNOSIS

- Exaggerated cutis marmorata may be seen in Down syndrome, trisomy 18, Cornelia de Lange syndrome
- *Cutis marmorata telangiectatica congenita:* developmental anomaly in which vascular pattern typically coarser, asymmetrical, associated w/limb hemiatrophy/anomalies in other organs
- *Neonatal lupus erythematosus:* usually presents as erythematous macules/plaques in sun-exposed areas of skin after newborn period; rarely lesions congenital/telangiectatic

HEMANGIOMAS

BACKGROUND

- Most common benign tumors of childhood
- Occur in up to 2.5% of newborns/in 10–12% of Caucasian infants by 1 yr of age
- F:M ratio: 3:1
- ↑ incidence in premature infants <1,500 g, often multiple lesions

CLINICAL MANIFESTATIONS

- May have superficial ("strawberry") component, deep ("cavernous") component/both
- *Initial appearance of superficial lesions:* telangiectatic, red to violaceous macule/plaque often surrounded by zone of pallor
- Deeper lesions present as soft, SubQ mass
- Rapid growth over 4–6 mos, peaking at 10–12 mos before resolution begins
- 50–60% of lesions resolve by age 5, 70% by age 7, 97% by age 10–12 yrs
- Residual skin changes (eg, skin laxity, prominent vessels) remain in 40% of cases

DIFFERENTIAL DIAGNOSIS

- *Spider angioma:* central telangiectatic papule w/radiating vessels usually <1 cm; not congenital
- *Pyogenic granuloma:* usually an exophytic nodule of <1 cm that grows rapidly/tends to bleed spontaneously; not congenital
- *Lymphangiomas/venous malformations:* may be difficult to distinguish from SubQ hemangiomas by clinical examination; Hx of rapid growth during infancy points to hemangioma

COMPLICATIONS

- Interference w/vital functions (vision, airway)
- Ulceration
- *Platelet trapping:* true Kasabach-Merritt syndrome rare/may be primarily seen w/rare vascular tumor known as Kaposi hemangioendothelioma
- *Diffuse neonatal hemangiomatosis:* often too-numerous-to-count small hemangiomas in association w/visceral hemangiomas/intractable high output failure

MANAGEMENT

- Evaluate pts w/extensive hemangiomas of lower face/neck for subglottic involvement; may require urgent medical/surgical intervention
- Evaluate pts w/extensive facial hemangiomas for CNS/cardiac anomalies (PHACE syndrome)
- Evaluate infants w/numerous (>5) hemangiomas for visceral involvement
- Systemic/intralesional corticosteroids indicated for hemangiomas that interfere w/vital structures (eg, periorbital/subglottic lesions), visceral hemangiomatosis w/heart failure, those associated w/thrombocytopenia (Kasabach-Merritt syndrome), for extensive disfiguring hemangiomas
- Pulsed dye laser treatment of superficial hemangiomas under clinical trial
- Alpha-interferon may be needed for complicated lesions not responding to corticosteroids; monitor closely for neurological side effects (spasticity)

VENTRICULAR SEPTAL DEFECT

ROBERTA G. WILLIAMS

BACKGROUND

- Development of ventricular septum complex process involving invagination, compaction of ventricular cavity, wall, development/positioning of conal septum, and fusion of these structures at crux of heart where atrial septum, ventricular septum, two atrioventricular valves meet
- Example of failure of myocardial development is typical muscular ventricular septal defect (VSD)
- Positional abnormality of outflow septum as seen in tetralogy of Fallot results in malalignment type of VSD
- Failure of fusion may result in typical perimembraneous VSD or more serious atrioventricular septal (AKA A-V canal) defect
- Most VSDs isolated lesions in otherwise normal children, however, VSD most common cardiac lesion found in children w/chromosomal abnormalities and in fetal alcohol syndrome

PHYSIOLOGY

- Most defects small, cause no significant hemodynamic abnormality. Defects >2–3 mm diameter may allow enough left-to-right shunting to produce signs of left ventricular volume overload, pulmonary overcirculation
- Defects > one-half size of aorta associated w/transmission of high pressures to right ventricle, pulmonary artery (unless concomitant pulmonary outflow obstruction protects pulmonary artery)

CLINICAL FINDINGS

- Murmur of typical small VSD high pitched, begins w/first heart sound. Location, transmission depends on VSD location (perimembraneous defects: mid left, right sternal border; muscular: lower left, right sternal border or apex; subpulmonary: upper left, right sternal border
- If significant left-to-right shunt, hyperdynamic left ventricular apex palpable, diastolic rumble may be heard at apex, tachypnea, retractions may indicate pulmonary overcirculation. Infant may be pale, diaphoretic w/failure to thrive
- W/pulmonary hypertension, systolic murmur softer and shorter than typical VSD murmur or may disappear entirely

NATURAL HISTORY

- Both perimembraneous, muscular VSDs tend to close spontaneously or become smaller in first year of life. Closure of small defects may occur as late as adulthood, but usually complete by 4 yrs of age. Perimembraneous VSDs less likely to close in pts w/Down syndrome than those w/normal chromosomes
- Malalignment VSDs or those crossed by atrioventricular valve tissue virtually never close spontaneously

MANAGEMENT

- All pts w/VSD require endocarditis prophylaxis
- Small defects do not require closure unless associated w/endocarditis or aortic valve prolapse
- Defects large enough to produce symptoms of CHF usually closed surgically unless indication of progressive restriction in first 6–9 mos of life occurs
- Defects large enough to produce significant pulmonary artery hypertension should be closed before 9 mos of age; ideally, before 6 mos

WHEN TO REFER

- Most children w/pathologic cardiac findings should be referred directly to pediatric cardiologist
- Chest x ray, EKG, insensitive tests for small VSDs or in infants w/VSD and therefore ineffective screening tools
- Very localized, high-pitched, blowing systolic murmur at lower sternal border in infant w/no other abnormal findings may be safely observed for 1–2 mos before referral because murmur probably represents either transient tricuspid regurgitation or very small muscular VSD, which is likely to close early

VISCERAL LARVA MIGRANS

MICHAEL KATZ

BACKGROUND

• Causative agent most common form of condition, *Toxocara canis,* is roundworm parasite of dogs. Infects humans by same route as ascaris (ie, by ingestion of embryonated eggs from soil contaminated by dog feces). *Toxocara cati,* related ascarid of cats, can also cause syndrome, but far less common. Both species primarily resident in young animals (puppies, kittens). Roundworms of other animals can also cause syndrome, but do so only sporadically

• After eggs ingested, larvae hatch in small intestine, but—unlike larvae of ascaris—because they are in biologically foreign environment, begin an endless wandering, invading all organs. Degree of damage depends on number of larvae, tissue invaded. Most serious manifestation invasion of eye, wherein larva induces granuloma, which can resemble retinoblastoma when eye examined w/ophthalmoscope. (Eyes have been enucleated for that reason on mistaken belief they were affected by this tumor.) Systemic involvement, ocular disease do not occur simultaneously; now appears that strains of parasite may have different tropisms. Larvae of *Baylisascaris procyonis,* nematode parasite of raccoons, also can cause visceral larva migrans, but its incidence not known. Two reported cases of this infection in children ended in death due to meningoencephalitis, but virtually all organs involved, contained granulomas

• Source of infection soil contaminated by animal feces. Recreational sandboxes in which animals have defecated also frequent repositories of infected eggs. Eggs in soil must incubate ~2 wks before becoming infectious. Direct contact w/animal does not lead to infection

• Visceral infection affects primarily children 1–4 yrs of age, particularly those w/pica. Ocular disease tends to affect older children, 5–10 yrs of age

CLINICAL MANIFESTATIONS

• Lightly infected children—probably majority of those infected—asymptomatic. Those w/ocular disease have retinal granulomas, can present w/strabismus. Pts w/systemic disease febrile, tend to have protean symptoms, including malaise, cough, wheezing. In most severe cases can be patchy pneumonitis, myocarditis, encephalitis. Hypereosinophilia, hypergammaglobulinemia characteristic. Liver, spleen tend to be enlarged

LABORATORY FEATURES

• ↑ titers of isohemagglutinins to A, B blood groups strongly suggestive of Dx, if clinical symptoms compatible. Liver biopsy can reveal characteristic larvae, but negative specimen may simply reflect failure to hit right target. CDC offers ELISA test based on larval antigens. Test both sensitive, specific, positive in ~80% cases visceral disease; < sensitive in cases of ocular disease

DIFFERENTIAL DIAGNOSIS

• Condition needs to be differentiated from migratory stage of nematode infections in humans. Because of hypereosinophilia, hepatosplenomegaly, eosinophilic leukemia may need to be considered. It can be ruled out by examination of bone marrow. Retinal granulomas can give appearance of retinoblastoma

TREATMENT

• No drug specific or wholly effective. Following have been used in past: thiabendazole, 50 mg/kg/24 h daily [w/max 3 g/24 h] × 5 d. Diethylcarbamazine, 6 mg/kg/24 h in 3 div doses × 7 d. Effectiveness of either drug uncertain; both toxic. Benzimidazoles may be better choice, but still experimental in this condition. Albendazole, 10 mg/kg/24 h in 2 div doses × 5 d. Ivermectin, veterinary anthelmintic, recently introduced into human pharmacopeia as highly effective treatment of onchocerciasis, shows some promise in treatment of toxocariasis. Most children improve 2–3 wks, even if untreated. In cases of myocarditis or encephalitis, treatment w/corticosteroids appropriate

• Treatment of ocular disease must be carried out in consultation w/ophthalmologist. Drugs used as adjunct to surgical Tx. Systemic administration of corticosteroids reported to reduce inflammation. Thiabendazole po enters aqueous, vitreous humors. Most important component of treatment is surgical intervention, which may involve vitrectomy. Severely affected eyes, esp if pt blind may have to be enucleated

PREVENTION

• Treat puppies, kittens w/anthelmintics before purchase as pets. Keep recreational sandboxes covered when not in use

WHEN TO REFER

• Pediatricians need not refer children w/visceral larval migrans. Children w/ocular disease must be seen by ophthalmologist as soon as possible. However, often it is ophthalmologist who recognizes disease in child referred for problems w/vision, or w/strabismus

VITILIGO

BACKGROUND

- Most frequently begins between 10–30 yrs of age
- M:F ratio 1:1; both sexes affected equally; all races affected; 1% incidence
- Immunologic vs. neurotoxic self-destructive theories of causation
- Heritable disease; 30% pts w/affected family members; no distinct inheritance pattern
- Onset may be triggered by stressor (illness, crisis, life event)/trauma (physical injury, severe sunburn)

CLINICAL MANIFESTATIONS

- Chalk-white (depigmented), sharply defined macules, 5 mm–5 cm or larger
- Acquired. Progression by gradual enlargement of existing lesions/development of new depigmented macules; erythema may be observed at margins of macules
- Classification according to distribution; most common *generalized:* symmetrical distribution primarily involving pressure points of body/skin surrounding body orifices/intertriginous areas; progressive for years; *segmental:* linear, dermatomal distribution, more common in children, no family Hx, no associated disorders, rapidly progressive for 1 yr, then halts; *universalis:* total body involvement; may extend within sites of trauma (Koebner phenomenon)
- Perifollicular pigmentation may be present/represents repigmentation or residual pigmentation
- Premature graying; patchy white hairs within eyebrows, eyelashes, scalp hairs, halo nevi
- Partial repigmentation seen in roughly half of affected children; complete spontaneous repigmentation rare
- Ocular abnormalities such as iritis, chorioretinitis, retinal dilution observed

LABORATORY FEATURES

- Wood lamp examination: bright white macules
- Histopathology: normal epidermis w/absence of melanocytes in affected skin; Fontana-Masson/silver stains negative for melanin; DOPA reaction negative; mild lymphocytic infiltrate occasionally observed
- Potassium hydroxide examination: no fungi identified
- TSII, fasting blood glucose, CBC w/differential and/or ACTH stimulation test to r/o associated diseases
- Ophthalmologic examination to r/o iritis, chorioretinitis, retinal dilution

DIFFERENTIAL DIAGNOSIS

- Postinflammatory hyperpigmentation
- Pityriasis alba
- Tinea versicolor
- Piebaldism
- Hypomelanosis of Ito
- Waardenburg syndrome
- Tuberous sclerosis

TREATMENT

- *Sunscreen:* dual purposes: protection of involved skin from sunburn/limitation of tanning of normally pigmented skin; sunscreen with UVA, UVB, titanium dioxide (opaque), spf > 30 recommended
- *Camouflage:* Vitadye (ICN), Dy-o-Derm (Owen Laboratories), as well as self-tanning agents (Estée Lauder, Clinique) as temporary dyes; cover-up makeup such as Covermark (Lydia O'Leary), Dermablend (Flori Roberts) available for most skin hues
- *Topical corticosteroids:* initial treatment w/topical class I corticosteroid ointments applied daily recommended; if no response noted in 2 mos, unlikely to be effective; monitoring q2mos for signs of steroid atrophy required
- *Photochemotherapy:* not recommended for children <9 yrs of age; less than 20% body surface involvement can be treated w/topical psoralen w/ultraviolet A radiation (PUVA); more extensive disease requires oral PUVA; best employed by experienced dermatologist; therapy requires 6 mos of biweekly treatments to evaluate efficacy; if repigmentation noted, treatments continue for additional year; side effects include phototoxicity, nausea, photoaging, hyperpigmentation, increased risk of skin cancers, cataracts; ANA/ophthalmologic exam prior to initiation of PUVA
- *Minigrafting:* restricted to pts w/refractory segmental/limited vitiligo
- *Depigmentation:* restricted only to pts w/extensive vitiligo who have failed PUVA; treatment applied to normally pigmented skin; effect permanent, irreversible; side effects include sunburns, irreversibility of process

COMPLICATIONS

- May be associated w/Grave disease, Hashimoto thyroiditis, diabetes mellitus, hypoparathyroidism, pernicious anemia, alopecia areata, Addison disease, multiple endocrinopathy syndrome

PREVENTION

- Course highly variable; rapid onset followed by period of stability characteristic
- Treatment of associated diseases has no impact on course of vitiligo

WHEN TO REFER

- Referral to dermatologist indicated for confirmation of Dx/management

PITYRIASIS ALBA

BACKGROUND

- M:F ratio 1:1; both sexes equally affected; all races affected
- Most commonly presents between ages 3–16 yrs
- More commonly observed in pts w/personal/family Hx atopy
- Postulated to represent eczematous dermatitis w/resultant hypomelanosis due to postinflammatory hypopigmentation

CLINICAL MANIFESTATIONS

- Begin as pale pink to light brown macules w/indistinct borders; subtle erythema fades over weeks, w/residual off-white (hypopigmented) slightly scaly, ill-defined patches, 0.3–5 cm, persisting for years; may persist into adulthood
- Primarily affects face, in particular midforehead, cheeks, perioral/periorbital areas; neck, shoulders, back, limbs, trunk occasionally involved; generally limited to 1–5 lesions; rare generalized variant seen in adolescents/young adult with no Hx atopy
- Occasionally associated w/pruritus and/or burning

LABORATORY FEATURES

- Wood lamp examination: dull white to off-white macules, limited extent
- Potassium hydroxide examination: no fungi detected
- Histopathology: nonspecific; hyperkeratosis, parakeratosis, moderately dilated blood vessels in superficial dermis, slight perivascular infiltrate; papillary edema; melanocytes reduced in number

DIFFERENTIAL DIAGNOSIS

- Tinea versicolor
- Vitiligo
- Tuberous sclerosis

TREATMENT

- *No treatment:* generally self-limited in distribution/duration
- *Moisturizers:* frequent application (2–3 ×/d) of emollient (petroleum jelly) to affected areas to minimize scale/associated symptoms
- *Topical corticosteroids:* not recommended for facial lesions as only mildly effective. Conservative application of type VI/VII topical corticosteroids (hydrocortisone, alclomethasone dipropionate) may be employed for nonfacial lesions that are pruritic and/or scaly. Treatment limited to 10–14 d. Side effects include steroid atrophy

COMPLICATIONS

- None

PREVENTION

- Sunscreen use to limit increased pigmentation of adjacent normally pigmented skin

WHEN TO REFER

- Majority of pts managed w/o referral
- Referral to dermatologist if condition progressive in nature

BACKGROUND

- Refers to twisting of part or all of intestines or stomach resulting in obstruction, ischemia, or infarction
- Volvulus can be life threatening
- Most common cause malrotation of intestine
- Other causes in ambulatory pediatric setting include incomplete fixation of stomach, persistent omphalomesenteric remnant, and congenital adhesive band that may serve as points of volvulus
- Majority of pts presenting w/midgut volvulus are infants; 50% present within first month of life

CLINICAL MANIFESTATIONS

- Vomiting most common symptom (bilious vomiting in infant is malrotation w/volvulus until proven otherwise!)
- Intermittent crampy abdominal pain
- Abdominal distention; if obstruction proximal, abdominal girth may be normal
- ↓ frequency or cessation of stool or flatulence
- Bloody stools
- Dehydration

LABORATORY FEATURES

- Electrolytes: dehydration results in metabolic acidosis. May be particularly severe if bowel ischemia or infarction present
- Radiograph of abdomen: may reveal distended loops of bowel or conversely relatively gasless abdomen if obstruction from volvulus proximal
- Upper GI series: diagnostic for malrotation, volvulus. Malrotation present when ligament of Treitz in abnormal position. Ligament should normally be to left of spine, behind stomach. Volvulus results in either acutely obstructed point or, even more characteristically, obstructed point in shape of "beak"

DIFFERENTIAL DIAGNOSIS

- Gastroesophageal reflux
- Food allergy
- Gastroenteritis
- Incarcerated hernia
- Duodenal stenosis
- Pyloric stenosis
- Any other cause for abdominal pain and/or vomiting

TREATMENT

- When volvulus diagnosed, constitutes surgical emergency
- Fluid resuscitation w/antibiotic coverage for enteric organisms should be started
- Surgical procedure performed depends on source of volvulus
- Volvulus due to malrotation corrected by reducing volvulus by rotating mesentery in counterclockwise direction. Colon then mobilized to left side of abdomen while duodenum straightened, and small bowel mobilized to right side of abdomen. Appendix then removed. This constitutes Ladd procedure
- Volvulus of stomach corrected by reducing volvulus, then placing gastrostomy tube in order to pex stomach to abdominal wall
- Volvulus due to bowel wrapped around congenital omphalomesenteric remnant or adhesive band usually corrected by removing remnant or band, reducing volvulus
- Any frankly infarcted bowel must be removed. Depending on status of abdominal cavity, remaining bowel may be reconnected or brought to abdominal wall as stomas
- IV fluids, nasogastric suction, antibiotic coverages mainstays of postop treatment

COMPLICATIONS

- Most significant complication is short-gut syndrome resulting from significant loss of bowel due to infarction
- Sepsis may be component of volvulus if significant bowel injury has occurred
- Postop adhesions may cause bowel obstruction
- Recurrent volvulus may occur in 1–10% of cases
- Intestinal motility may be compromised for prolonged time after correction of volvulus

WHEN TO REFER

- Any infant w/bilious vomiting should be evaluated for potential volvulus
- Vomiting w/dehydration, or other signs of systemic instability

BACKGROUND

- Most common hereditary bleeding disorder, affecting at least 1% of population
- Quantitative/qualitative defects in von Willebrand factor (VWF) molecule, large multimeric glycoprotein synthesized in endothelial cell/megakaryocyte
- VWF involved in 1° hemostasis; essential for adhesion between platelets/vessel wall; carrier protein for factor VIII
- Most types of von Willebrand disease (VWD) inherited in autosomal dominant fashion/affect both sexes equally
- VWF acute-phase reactant; plasma levels ↑ by exercise, pregnancy, early infancy
- Current classification of VWD:
  - type 1: partial absence of normal functioning VWF
  - type 2A: loss of high molecular weight multimers, ↓ affinity for platelets
  - type 2B: ↑ affinity of VWF for platelets, loss of high molecular weight multimers
  - type 2M: loss of function (affinity for platelets) w/decreased normal multimers
  - type 2N: ↓ factor VIII binding ("Normandy variant")
  - type 3: total absence of VWF

CLINICAL MANIFESTATIONS

- Ecchymoses (large bruises >5 cm)
- Mucosal bleeding (epistaxis, gingival, menorrhagia, GI) variable (mild–severe)
- ↑ bleeding after trauma/surgical procedures (dental extractions, tonsillectomy)
- Deep hematomas/joint hemorrhage in type 3 pts

LABORATORY FEATURES

- Bleeding time/PTT abnormal ~60% pts; other screening tests (PT, fibrinogen, thrombin time, platelet count) normal except for low platelet count in rare pts w/type 2B VWD
- *Best single screening test for VWD:* VWF activity (plasma VWF ristocetin cofactor assay); normal values influenced by ABO blood groups (group O mean VWF activity = 0.89; lower limits = 0.53; groups A, B = 1.08; w/lower limit, 0.63 (U/mL)
- Factor VIII low ~50–60% of pts; if factor VIII only abnormal test, hemophilia A, female carriers of hemophilia A, type 2N VWD should be suspected
- Pts w/possible von Willebrand disease (positive bleeding Hx/family Hx, abnormal screening tests) should have confirmation/classification of Dx in reference laboratory; repeated testing frequently needed in mild/variant pts

DIFFERENTIAL DIAGNOSIS

- Hemophilia A
- Platelet function disorders
- Pseudo von Willebrand disease
- Antiphospholipid antibody syndrome

TREATMENT

- Select treatment option according to type of VWD
- For type 1/some type 2A pts use 1-deamino-8-D-arginine vasopressin (DDAVP):
  - IV: 0.3 µg/kg diluted in 10–20 mL saline injected over 10 min
  - intranasal: 150 µg w/precompression, metered spray pump (Ferring)
  - bleeding time shortened/factor VIII level ↑ 3–4 ×; doses may be repeated q12h
- Do not use DDAVP for type 2B/type 3 VWD; use replacement transfusion w/product containing intact VWF: Humate P (Centeon) 50 U/kg; repeat q12h for major surgery
- Plasma cryoprecipitates also effective, but may transmit blood-borne infectious agents

COMPLICATIONS

- Tachyphylaxis to repeated DDAVP doses
- Inadequate hemostasis
- Post-DDAVP hyponatremia in small children

WHEN TO REFER

- All pts w/new Dx/serious bleeding problem; refer to comprehensive hemophilia center/experienced hematologist

BACKGROUND

- Vulvovaginitis = vulvitis (vulvar inflammation) w/or w/o vaginitis (vaginal inflammation)
- Prepubertal child susceptible to vulvovaginitis due to:
  - hypoestrogenism, leading to atrophic vagina, thin hymen
  - poor hygiene; use of irritants (eg, bubble bath)
  - proximity of vagina and anus
  - lack of protective hair and labial fat pads
  - nonabsorbent clothing

CLINICAL MANIFESTATIONS

- Pruritus
- Vaginal discharge and/or odor
- Vaginal bleeding
- Dysuria
- Vulvar redness and irritation

DIFFERENTIAL DIAGNOSIS

- *Nonspecific vaginitis:* often associated w/alteration in vaginal flora, which may be due to change in aerobic flora or overpopulation w/fecal aerobes, anaerobes. Vaginal cultures consistent w/normal flora, including aerobic organisms such as *Staphylococcus epidermidis,* diphtheroids, *Streptococcus viridans,* enterococci, enterics
- Vulvovaginitis associated w/specific infectious agent:
  - bacterial infections: *Streptococcus pyogenes, Haemophilus influenzae, Staphylococcus aureus, Branhamella catarrhalis, Streptococcus pneumoniae, Neisseria meningitidis, Shigella*
  - sexually transmitted infections: *Neisseria gonorrhoeae, Chlamydia trachomatis,* herpes simplex virus, Trichomonas, human papilloma virus. These organisms may also be vertically transmitted at birth, and herpes may be transmitted by nonsexual contact
  - Candida: uncommon in prepubertal children in absence of antibiotic use, diabetes, immunosuppression, occlusive diapers
  - pinworms: esp if child has perineal or perianal pruritus

- Vaginal foreign body
- Vaginal/cervical polyp/tumor
- Urethral prolapse
- *Systemic illness:* measles, varicella, scarlet fever, Crohn disease, mononucleosis, Kawasaki disease
- *Vulvar skin disorders:* seborrhea, eczema, psoriasis, scabies, lichen sclerosus, autoimmune bullous diseases
- *Anomalies:* ectopic ureter, Mullerian/vaginal anomaly w/fistula
- *Physiologic leukorrhea:* common in neonates, postpubertal girls

EVALUATION

- All girls w/Sx of vulvovaginitis:
  - Hx: quality of discharge (color, odor, presence of blood), hygiene, medications, soaps, bubble bath, anal pruritus, enuresis, possibility of foreign body or sexual abuse (including behavioral changes), recent infections, Hx of eczema or other diseases
  - physical exam: general examination; inspect perineum, vulva, hymen, anterior vagina w/pt supine; visualize vagina, cervix w/pt prone in knee-chest position; rectoabdominal exam supine if indicated (girls w/persistent discharge, bleeding/pain)
- Girls w/persistent, purulent, or recurrent vaginal discharge or suspicion of sexual abuse:
  - laboratory specimens: obtain specimens for wet preparations, cultures w/nasopharyngeal Calgiswabs moistened w/saline, soft eyedropper, small feeding tube, or vaginal aspirator. Wet preparations include saline and 10% KOH. Cultures for *Neisseria gonorrhoeae, Chlamydia trachomatis,* and bacterial pathogens. Biggy agar culture for suspected Candida. Tape test for suspected pinworm

TREATMENT

- Nonspecific vaginitis:
  - good perineal hygiene, white cotton underpants, loose clothing, hand washing
  - sitz baths 10–15 min, 1–2×/d
  - avoid irritants such as bubble bath; use hypoallergenic soaps; no soap to vulva

  - A and D ointment, Desitin, or petroleum jelly to perineum
  - for persistent symptoms: review Dx, trial of antibiotics or estrogen cream
- Specific pathogen identified (in addition to above measures):
  - *Streptococcus pyogenes:* penicillin × 10 d
  - *Haemophilus influenzae:* amoxicillin, amoxicillin/calvulanate, cefixime, cefuroxime axetil, trimethoprim/sulfamethoxazole, erythromycin/sulfamethoxazole × 7 d
  - *Staphylococcus aureus:* cephalexin, dicloxacillin, amoxicillin-clavulanate, cefuroxime axetil × 7–10 d
  - *Streptococcus pneumoniae:* penicillin, erythromycin, trimethoprim/sulfamethoxazole, clindamycin
  - *Shigella:* trimethoprim/sulfamethoxazole, cefixime
  - *Chlamydia trachomatis:* erythromycin × 10–14 d, doxycycline (if ≥9 yrs) × 7 d
  - *Neisseria gonorrhoeae:* ceftriaxone IM or spectinomycin IM *plus* treatment for Chlamydia. Children >45 kg and ≥9 yrs can be treated w/adult regimens
  - *Candida:* topical nystatin, miconazole, clotrimazole or terconazole cream; fluconazole po in immunosuppressed
  - *Trichomonas:* metronidazole × 7–10 d
  - *pinworms (Enterobius vermicularis):* mebendazole
- Foreign body:
  - after removal, sitz baths × 2 wks

WHEN TO REFER

- Persistent vaginal discharge, bleeding/pain despite treatment
- Recurrent episodes of vaginitis
- Severe edematous vulvitis
- Suspicion of sexual abuse
- Vaginal bleeding
- Child does not tolerate office exam, may require exam under anesthesia

WILMS TUMOR

MARY JANE PETRUZZI AND DANIEL M. GREEN

BACKGROUND

- *Annual incidence <15 yrs:* age $8.9/10^6$ whites; $11.1/10^6$ African Americans
- *M:F ratio 1:1*
- Peak age 3–4 yrs of age (males, 36 mos unilateral/23 mos bilateral; females, 46 mos unilateral/30 mos bilateral)
- *Associated congenital anomalies:* aniridia, GU anomalies, hemihypertrophy, Beckwith-Wiedemann syndrome (BWS), Perlman syndrome, Denys-Drash syndrome (DDS), Simpson-Golabi-Behmel syndrome, WAGR (*W*ilms tumor, *A*niridia, *G*enitourinary malformations, mental *R*etardation) syndrome
- *Complex genetics:* >1 locus implicated: 11p13 (WT1 tumor suppressor gene), 11p15 (putative WT2 tumor suppressor gene), 16q (associated w/adverse outcome), 17q (linked to familial WT)
- Nephrogenic rests precursor lesions to Wilms tumor

CLINICAL MANIFESTATIONS

- *Most common presentation:* painless abdominal swelling
- 37% associated abdominal pain, 21% hematuria, 25% hypertension
- Ascites, hepatomegaly, superficial venous engorgement (2° to inferior vena cava obstruction) can occur
- Aniridia, facial/extremity asymmetry, abnormal genitalia sometimes found

LABORATORY EVALUATION

- CBC w/differential
- Liver function tests, renal function tests, serum calcium
- UA
- Blood (pt/parents) for molecular testing

- Bone marrow examination: clear cell sarcoma histology only

RADIOGRAPHIC EVALUATION

- *Abdominal ultrasound:* visualize kidneys, liver, IVC flow
- *Abdominal CAT scan:* opposite kidney, extent of mass, relationship to major vessels/other structures. CT does not preclude surgical inspection of opposite kidney
- *Abdominal MRI examination:* only if IVC patency/extent of thrombus not adequately documented by ultrasound
- Chest x ray to evaluate lung metastases (CT scan recommended by some)
- Bone scan not routinely required

DIFFERENTIAL DIAGNOSIS

- Neuroblastoma
- *Benign intrarenal lesions:* multicystic kidneys, renal carbuncles, hematomas
- *Other intrarenal neoplasms:* mesoblastic nephroma, renal cell carcinoma, rhabdoid tumor, malignant neurogenic tumor, non-Hodgkin lymphoma

NATIONAL WILMS TUMOR STUDY STAGING

- *Stage I:* tumor limited to kidney/completely excised; renal capsule intact; not ruptured before/during removal; no residual tumor apparent beyond margins of resection
- *Stage II:* tumor extends beyond kidney, but completely removed (ie, penetration through outer surface of renal capsule into perirenal soft tissues); vessels outside kidney substance infiltrated/contain tumor thrombus; tumor biopsied/local spillage confined to flank

- *Stage III:* residual nonhematogenous tumor confined to abdomen: hilar lymph/periaortic nodes involved, diffuse peritoneal contamination by tumor, spillage of tumor beyond flank before/during surgery, tumor penetrated through peritoneal surface, implants found on peritoneal surface, gross/microscopic spread beyond surgical margins, tumor not completely resectable because of local infiltration into vital structures
- *Stage IV:* hematogenous metastases (lung, liver, bone, brain)
- *Stage V:* bilateral renal involvement at Dx

TREATMENT

- *National Wilms Tumor Study (NWTS):* immediate nephrectomy/preop chemotherapy reserved for bilateral WT/extensive inferior vena cava thrombus; preop chemotherapy used by other cooperative Wilms tumor study groups

COMPLICATIONS

- *Treatment late effects:* radiation/anthracycline-related cardiac toxicity, radiation-associated pulmonary toxicity, renal/gonadal dysfunction, scoliosis, second malignancies

WHEN TO REFER

- Refer to center where multimodality treatment for pediatric malignant solid tumor possible; refer pts at ↑ risk for development of WT (hemihypertrophy, BWS, aniridia, WAGR syndrome, Denys-Drash syndrome, Perlman syndrome, Bloom syndrome, SGB syndrome) for appropriate screening/molecular evaluation

Histopathology	Treatment
Mesoblastic nephroma (90% diagnosed first year of life)	Surgery only
Favorable histology WT	Stage I and II (no radiation): vincristine, dactinomycin
	Stages III and IV: radiation, vincristine, dactinomycin, doxorubicin
Unfavorable histology WT	
Anaplasia	Radiation, vincristine, doxorubicin, cytoxan, etoposide
Clear Cell Sarcoma (bone/brain metastases)	Radiation, vincristine, doxorubicin, etoposide
Rhabdoid tumor (brain metastases or primary brain tumor)	Radiation, etoposide, carboplatin, cytoxan

BACKGROUND

- Usually presents w/signs of liver disease during adolescence
- Never seen <3 yrs of age
- *Incidence:* 1/30,000 overall
- *Inheritance:* autosomal recessive:
  - gene locus; chromosome 13 at 14q21
  - gene identification: copper-binding membrane-spanning protein w/P-type ATPase motifs that characterize metal transport proteins; bile canalicular membrane for transport of copper into bile; possible hepatocyte location

CLINICAL MANIFESTATIONS

- *Most common:* teenager w/hepatosplenomegaly/evidence of chronic liver disease
- Consider Dx in any pt w/unknown hepatocellular liver disease after 5 yrs of age (ie, ↑ transaminases)
- Coombs' negative hemolytic anemia, which may temporarily resolve
- Noninfectious hepatitis (hepatocellular enzyme elevation), which may temporarily resolve
- Acute fulminant liver failure:
  - clues: hemolytic anemia, extremely low alkaline phosphatase level, low uric acid level prior to renal failure
- *Neuropsychiatric:* predominantly in young adults but may be present in up to 50% of teenagers
- Neurologic: tremors/dysarthria
- Psychiatric: personality changes, irritability to psychosis/depression

DIAGNOSIS

- Kayser-Fleisher Ring: requires slit lamp examination by experienced ophthalmologist
  - may not be observed when only liver disease present
  - pathognomonic in children, not adults
- Ceruloplasmin <20 mg/dL 95% of pts; usually never >35 mg/dL by functional assay/may be higher by immune assay; great variability in normal ranges from laboratory to laboratory
- 24 h urine copper:
  - >100 µg/d sans chelator

- >1,000 µ/d after 750 mg/m^2/d penicillamine
- Liver copper >250 µ/g of liver (dry weight)
- *Liver pathology:* initially microscopic fat globules progressing to macroscopic fat globule accumulation in hepatocyte cytoplasm plus glycogenated nuclei; findings nonspecific; progress to cirrhosis; some cases show submassive necrosis/chronic active hepatitis

DIFFERENTIAL DIAGNOSIS

- Autoimmune hepatitis distinguished by positive FANA, smooth muscle antibody, liver-kidney microsomal antibody
- Alpha-1-antitrypsin (A1AT) deficiency distinguished by protease inhibitory phenotype, very low A1AT level
- *viral/drug-induced hepatitis:* acute/fulminant distinguished by appropriate studies
- Hepatic steatosis more commonly associated w/obesity
- *Indian childhood cirrhosis:* rarely documented in US

FAMILY STUDIES AFTER PROPOSITUS CARE

- AST/ceruloplasmin followed by liver biopsy in pts w/abnormal result
- Molecular techniques only in families w/defined gene defect (available only at research institutions) by haplotype analysis because most pts compound heterozygotes

TREATMENT

- *Diet:* avoid liver/shellfish; mushrooms, chocolate, nuts if possible
- *Medication:* penicillamine Tx of choice:
  - 250 mg qid/750 mg/m^2/div doses/25 mg/kg/d
  - ideally 30 min before or 2 hrs after meals
  - complications primarily immune-related; include most commonly rash/kidney damage detected by UA; controlled w/prednisone/reintroduction of penicillamine at very small dose w/gradual dose ↑

- late complications: renal, Goodpasture syndrome, lupus erythematosus, bone marrow suppression, pemphigus, myasthenia gravis
  - pyroxidine (25 mg/d) recommended by experts
- Alternatives to penicillamine chelators:
  - trientine (alternative chelator) 1.0–1.5 g/d in div doses/30 mg/kg/d; toxicity: bone marrow suppression, nephrotoxicity, skin, mucosal lesions, iron deficiency anemia
  - zinc acetate [Glazin, 25–50 mg tid]/zinc sulfate 50–220 mg, tid on empty stomach; toxicity includes gastric distress/mild pancreatic enzyme elevation

LIVER TRANSPLANTATION

- Indications:
  - fulminant liver failure
  - unresponsive to Tx within 3 mos
- *Success:* 75–80% 1 yr survival; even better results in Wilsonian fulminant hepatitis pts

EXPERIMENTAL THERAPIES

- Ammonium tetrathiolmolybdate when initial presentation neurologic
- Chelator plus zinc as acute Tx for liver disease
- Antioxidants

CONCERNS

- Adolescents (perhaps because they are asymptomatic) frequently do not take chelator; noncompliance more frequent in family members detected by screening before clinical evidence of liver disease
- *Pregnancy:* Tx should continue; if inadequate, zinc considered

WHEN TO REFER

- At time of tentative Dx to pediatric gastroeterologist experienced in Wilson pts
- Referral to liver transplant center when appropriate
- Routine follow-up w/primary physician reasonable w/yearly follow-up by specialist

BRENT W. WESTON

BACKGROUND

- Characterized by thrombocytopenia, susceptibility to infections, eczema
- Usually presents in first 2 yrs of life
- *Incidence:* $4/10^6$ male births
- Before bone marrow transplantation, median survival < 6 y, ~60% of death from infection, 25% bleeding, 5–10% malignancy (leukemia/lymphoma)
- Female carriers usually asymptomatic
- Related but milder disorder, X-linked thrombocytopenia, characterized by small platelets, normal immune function, no eczema, no propensity to develop malignancies
- Mutations in WAS gene characterized for WAS/X-linked thrombocytopenia
- Genetic testing provides pt Dx/carrier detection/prenatal Dx

CLINICAL MANIFESTATIONS

- *Bleeding:* usually mucosal/skin, not always related to thrombocytopenia severity (WAS platelets also dysfunctional)
- *Infections:* initially bacterial, followed by opportunistic as T cell number/function decline; recurrent otitis media, pneumonias, sinusitis, skin infections, sepsis common; draining ears, although classic, found in minority
- *Eczema:* often severe/infected w/staphylococci, other organisms; associated w/eosinophilia, moderately high IgE levels
- *Autoimmune features:* hemolytic anemia, vasculitis, renal disease, synovitis

LABORATORY FEATURES

- ↓ IgA/IgE, usually normal IgG, low IgM
- Lack of response to polysaccharide antigens (absent serum isohemagglutinins, poor response to *Haemophilus*/pneumococcal vaccines
- T cells develop progressive decline in number/function over several years; lymphopenia usually not apparent until 5/6 yrs of age
- Platelets small (half normal size)/turn over rapidly; ↓ thrombopoiesis; platelet counts 10,000–50,000; platelets function poorly; confirmation w/aggregation studies not necessary
- Hgb, RBC indices, neutrophils usually normal, unless associated autoimmune disorders present
- WAS genetic testing/HLA typing

DIFFERENTIAL DIAGNOSIS

- Immune thrombocytopenic purpura (ITP)
- Thrombotic thrombocytopenic purpura (TTP)
- Hemolytic uremic syndrome (HUS)
- Drug-induced thrombocytopenia
- Thrombocytopenia-absent radius syndrome (TAR)
- Malignancy
- Aplastic anemia
- Human immunodeficiency virus infection (HIV)
- 1° immunodeficiencies, including agammaglobulinemias, severe combined immunodeficiencies, ataxia telangiectasia, DiGeorge syndrome

TREATMENT

- Avoid salicylates/other inhibitors of platelet function
- Corticosteroids/IVIG sometimes used short term to treat episodes of worsening thrombocytopenia/various autoimmune disorders, w/variable results; IVIG also used as replacement Tx to prevent pyogenic infections
- Splenectomy often used early in course to control thrombocytopenia temporarily (should not delay definitive evaluation/treatment)
- Allogeneic bone marrow transplantation potentially curative

COMPLICATIONS

- Bleeding, infection, malignancies

WHEN TO REFER

- Refer to pediatric immunologist/hematologist if Dx suspected

Dyserythropoiesis, vs. folic acid deficiency, 145
Dysgenesis, complete gonadal, 372
    mixed gonadal, 372
    ovarian, 372
Dyskeratosis congenita, 23
Dyskinesia, 68
Dyslexia, 120
Dysmenorrhea, 121
    nonsteroidal anti-inflammatory drugs for, 121t
Dysplasia, bronchopulmonary, 55
    developmental, of hip, 197
    fibrous, 46
    multiple epiphyseal, in Legg-Calvé-Perthes disease, 241
    renal, 336, 336t
Dysrhythmias, 122, 122t

E

Ear, foreign body of, 148
    pain in, vs. otitis media, 293
Eccrine sweat duct, obstruction of, 264
Echinococcus, infestation with, 404
Echoviruses, 123
Eczema, in Wiskott-Aldrich syndrome, 456
Edema, cerebral, 67, 67t
    in submersion injury, 118
Education, in Down syndrome, 117
Educational achievement testing, for dyslexia, 120
Eickenella corrodens, in human bites, 39
Elapidae, 42
Elbow, fracture of, 153, 153t
    Little League, 247
    osteochondritis dissecans of, 290
    pulled (nursemaid), 332
Embryonal carcinoma, 406, 406t
Emery Deryfus muscular dystrophy, 269
Emphysema, in alpha-1-antitrypsin deficiency, 10
Enalapril, for cardiomyopathy, 61
    for hypertension, 211
Encephalitis, in rubella, 350
Encephalocele, 106t
Encephalopathy, 67, 182, 182t
Encephalotrigeminal angiomatosis, 97
Enchondroma, 46
Encopresis, 86, 124
Endocarditis, 125
    antibiotics for, 125t
    bacterial, in tetralogy of Fallot, 410
    prophylaxis for, 126t
Endocrine system, dysfunction of, hypertension associated with, 211
    vs. juvenile dermatomyositis, 105
    vs. uterine bleeding, 445
    in myelomeningocele, 272
Endodermal sinus tumor, 406, 406t
Endometriosis, vs. uterine bleeding, 445
Enema, for constipation, 86
    for encopresis, 124
Enigmatic diarrhea, 113, 113t
Entamoeba histolytica, in gastroenteritis, 165, 165t
Enteric fever, 352, 352t
Enteric pathogens, in travelers' diarrhea, 432t
Enteritis, vs. Crohn disease, 94
    vs. milk protein sensitivity, 265
Enterobacter, in folliculitis, 146

Enterobiasis, 25, 312, 349, 349t
Enterobius vermicularis, 312
Enterocolitis, 352t
    formula protein–induced, 265
    in Hirschsprung disease, 198
Enterocolitis syndrome, food-induced, 147
Enteropathy, gluten-sensitive, 65
Enterovirus, nonpolio human, 123
Enthesitis, 20
Enthesopathy-arthropathy, seronegative, 20
Enuresis, diurnal, 127
    nocturnal, 127
Enuresis alarms, 127
Environment, lead in, 240t
Eosinophilic granuloma, 46
Epidermal inclusion cyst, 263
Epidermolytic bullous ichthyosiform erythroderma, 219, 219t
Epidermolytic hyperkeratosis ichthyosiform erythroderma, 219, 219t
Epididymitis, 128
Epididymo-orchitis, 128
Epidural hematoma, 395, 395t
Epiglottitis, 129
    bacterial, 239
    vs. viral croup, 239
Epinephrine, for angioedema, 19
    for bronchiolitis, 54
    for complete heart block, 181
    for croup, 239
    for status asthmaticus asthma, 29
Epiphora, 130
Epiphysis, 151
    dysplasia of, in Legg-Calvé-Perthes disease, 241
    tumors of, 46
Epispadias, 216
Epistaxis, 131
Epsilon aminocaproic acid, for angioedema, 19
Epstein-Barr virus, in infectious mononucleosis, 224
Equinovarus, postural, vs. clubfoot, 76
Equinovarus congenita, 76
Erb engram, 49
Ergots, for migraine, 179t
Eruptions, from drugs, 119, 119t
    intertriginous, 228
Erythema, in molluscum contagiosum, 267
Erythema infectiosum, 141
Erythema marginatum, in rheumatic fever, 343, 343t
Erythema multiforme, 132
    vs. urticaria, 132t, 444
Erythema toxicum, 278
Erythrasma, 228
Erythroblastopenia, transient, 429
Erythroderma, epidermolytic bullous ichthyosiform, 219, 219t
    epidermolytic hyperkeratosis ichthyosiform, 219, 219t
    in atopic dermatitis, 31
    nonbullous congenital ichthyosiform, 219, 219t
Erythromycin, endocarditis prophylaxis with, 126t
    for acute otitis media with effusion, 293, 293t
    for afebrile pneumonia, 314
    for bacterial pneumonia, 315
    for chlamydial pneumonia, 315

Erythromycin (*cont.*)
    for diphtheria, 115
    for folliculitis, 146
    for furunculosis, 160
    for impetigo, 222
    for scarlet fever, 356
    for streptococcal infections, 308
Erythropoietin, recombinant, for anemia, 18
Escherichia coli, in breast abscess, 52
    in folliculitis, 146
    in gastroenteritis, 164, 164t
    in travelers diarrhea, 432t
Esophagitis, vs. gastroesophageal reflux, 167
Esophagus, burns of, 133
    foreign body of, 148
Esotropia, in strabismus, 391
Estrogen, for primary amenorrhea, 13
    for short stature, 375
    for uterine bleeding, 445
Ethosuximide, for absence seizures, 362
Ewing sarcoma, 134
Exanthem subitum, 347
Exotropia, in strabismus, 391
Extremity(ies), lower, overuse injuries of, 294
    stress fracture of, 294
    tendinitis of, 294
Eye(s), disorders of, 135
    foreign body of, 149
    hamartoma of, 438
    hemorrhage in, 212
    herpes simplex virus infection of, 196
    in Marfan syndrome, 253t
Eyelid(s), abnormal position of, 135

F

Facioscapulohumeral muscular dystrophy, 269, 269t
Factor IX concentrates, for hemophilia B, 188
Factor VIII concentrates, for hemophilia A, 187
Failure to thrive, in cystic fibrosis, 99
Famciclovir, for varicella, 446
Familial hypercholesterolemia, 209
Familial hypophosphatemic rickets, 345
Familial nephrogenic diabetes insipidus, 108
Fanconi anemia, 23
Farsightedness, 334
Fasciitis, necrotizing, periumbilical, 442, 442t
    streptococcal, 393
Fatty acids, free, in hypoglycemia, 213
Fecal soiling, 124
Femoral-neck shaft angle, in coxa vara, 90
Femur, anteversion of, 136
    capital epiphysis of, slipped, 380
    distal, fracture of, 156
        physis of, fracture of, 155
    retroversion of, 136
    shaft of, fracture of, 155, 155t
    torsion of, 136, 136t
Fetus, drug exposure in, 137
    hydronephrosis in, 207
Fever, enteric, 352, 352t
    in acute lymphocytic leukemia, 243
    in heat stroke, 182, 182t
    in neutropenia, 138, 284

Guaifenesin, for common cold, 80
Guanfacine, for Tourette syndrome, 422
Guillain-Barré syndrome, 176, 176t
Gynecologic disorders, vs. dysmenorrhea, 121

H

H1 antagonist, for angioedema, 19
Haemophilus influenzae, in cellulitis, 66t
  in conjunctivitis, 85
  in epiglottitis, 129
  in occult bacteremia, 140
Haemophilus influenzae vaccine, periorbital cellulitis and, 305
Hair loss, 9
Hallux valgus, 177
Haloperidol, for tics, 419
Hamartias, 438, 438t
Hamartoblastoma, 438
Hamartoma, 438, 438t
Hand, ganglia of, 163
Head injury, 82
  in femoral shaft fracture, 155, 155t
Head lice, 245
Headache, 180
  cluster, 178
  migraine, 178
    treatment of, 179, 179t
  muscle contraction, 180
  tension, 180
Hearing loss, in achondroplasia, 3
  otitis media and, 293
  vs. speech disorder, 382
Heart, in Kawasaki disease, 233
  in Noonan syndrome, 285
  tuberous sclerosis of, 438
Heart block, complete, 181
Heat stroke, 182, 182t
Helicobacter pylori, infection by, 183
Helminths, in gastroenteritis, 165, 165t
Hemangioma, 184, 447
  lobular capillary, 330, 330t
Hematochezia, asymptomatic, 324
Hematoma, epidural, 395, 395t
  subdural, 395, 395t
  subungual, 143
Hematopoietic growth factors, for aplastic anemia, 23
Hematuria, evaluation of, 185
Hemimelia, fibular, 416
Hemiplegia, in cerebral palsy, 68
Hemodialysis, for salicylate poisoning, 27
Hemolysis, in glucose-6-phosphate dehydrogenase anemia, 161
Hemolytic anemia, nonspherocytic, 161
Hemolytic-uremic syndrome, 186, 337, 338
Hemophilia A, 187
Hemophilia B, 188
Hemorrhage, in heat stroke, 182, 182t
  in Wiskott-Aldrich syndrome, 456
  subgaleal, 355t
Hemorrhagic reaction, in snake bite, 42, 42t
Hemorrhagic shock and encephalopathy syndrome, 182, 182t
Hemorrhoids, 189
Henoch-Schönlein purpura, 190
Hepatic ducts, cystic dilatation of, 73
Hepatic failure, inhalants and, 227
Hepatitis, vs. acetaminophen poisoning, 2
Hepatitis A, 191, 191t

Hepatitis A vaccine, 191
Hepatitis B, 192, 192t
Hepatitis B immunoglobulin, 192
Hepatitis B vaccine, 192
Hepatitis C, 193, 193t
Hepatitis E, 194
Hepatitis G, 194
Hepatomegaly, in heat stroke, 182, 182t
Hereditary angioedema, 19
Hereditary motor and sensory neuropathy, 69t
  type I, 64, 64t, 69, 69t
  type II, 64, 64t, 69, 69t
Hermaphroditism, true, 372
Hernia, inguinal, 195, 195t
  umbilical, 442, 442t
Heroin, fetal exposure to, 137
Herpes gladiatorum, 196
Herpes simplex virus, 196
  conjunctivitis from, 85
  in atopic dermatitis, 31
  type 1, 196
  type 2, 196
Herpetic whitlow, 196
Hilgenreiner-epiphyseal angle, in coxa vara, 90
Hip, developmental dysplasia of, 197
  fracture of, 155, 155t
  transient synovitis of, 430
Hirschsprung disease, 198
Histamine receptor antagonists, for gastritis, 183
  for ulcer disease, 183
Histiocytic disorders, malignant, 199
Histiocytosis, childhood, 199
Histoplasma capsulatum, 200
Histoplasmosis, 200, 200t
  vs. molluscum contagiosum, 267
Hobbies, lead in, 240t
Hodgkin disease, 201
Hookworms, 17, 349, 349t
Hot tubs, folliculitis from, 146
Human bites, 39
  clenched fist, 39
  occlusional, 39
Human chorionic gonadotropin, for cryptorchidism, 96
Human diploid cell vaccine, rabies prophylaxis with, 331
Human herpesvirus-6 infection, 347
Human herpesvirus-7 infection, 347
Human immunodeficiency virus (HIV) infection, 5, 5t, 176t
Human papillomavirus infection, genital, 202, 202t
  nongenital, 203, 203t
Human parvovirus B19, infection by, 141
Human rabies immune globulin, 331
Humerus, fracture of, 153
  proximal, fracture of, 157
Hydralazine, for cardiomyopathy, 61
  for hypertension, 211
Hydrocarbons, 204t
  halogenated, 204t
  ingestion of, 204
Hydrocele, 205
Hydrocephalus, 206
  shunt infection in, 377
Hydrochlorothiazide, for hypertension, 211
Hydronephrosis, fetal, 207

Hydroxychloroquine, for juvenile dermatomyositis, 105
  for polymyositis, 323
Hydroxyzine, for angioedema, 19
Hygroma, cystic, 100
Hymenolepiasis, 404
Hymenolepis nana, in gastroenteritis, 165, 165t
Hyperandrogenism, acne in, 4
Hypercalciuria, in renal stones, 208
  vs. hematuria, 185
Hypercholesterolemia, familial, 209
  familial combined, 209
Hypercoagulability, in deep vein thrombosis, 412
Hyperhomocystinemia, folic acid deficiency and, 145
Hyperkalemia, 338
Hyperlipidemia, 209, 209t
Hypernatremia, dehydration in, 103
Hyperopia, 334
Hyperosmolar agents, for cerebral edema, 67
Hyperphenylalaninemia, classification of, 309t
Hyperphosphatemia, 338
Hypertension, 210
  in renal failure, 338
  inhalants and, 227
  management of, 211
  portal, in alpha-1-antitrypsin deficiency, 10
Hyphema, 212
Hypoglycemia, 213
Hypogonadism, hypergonadotropic, vs. primary amenorrhea, 13
  hypogonadotropic, 215
    vs. primary amenorrhea, 13
Hypomagnesemia, tetany and, 409
Hypomelanosis of Ito, 214
Hyponatremia, in botulism, 47
Hypopigmentation, 214
Hypopituitarism, 215
Hypoproteinemia, in celiac disease, 65
Hypospadias, 216
Hypotension, in heat stroke, 182
Hypothermia, 217
  in submersion injury, 118
Hypothyroidism, acquired, 218, 218t
  congenital, 218, 218t
  short stature in, 375
Hysteria, 88

I

Ibuprofen, for common cold, 80
  for dysmenorrhea, 121t
  for migraine, 179t
  for pericarditis, 304
Ice water, submersion in, 118
Ichthyosis, 219
  lamellar, 219, 219t
  X-linked, 219, 219t
Ichthyosis vulgaris, 219, 219t
Idiopathic thrombocytopenic purpura, 220, 220t
Ileus, meconium, in cystic fibrosis, 99
Imipenem-cilastatin, for peritonitis, 306
Imipramine, for nocturnal enuresis, 127
Immune complexes, circulating, in angioedema, 19
  in urticaria, 444

Myopathy, 274
  inflammatory, in juvenile dermato-
    myositis, 105
Myopia, 334
Myositis, 275, 275t
Myotonic muscular dystrophy, 269, 269t
Myringitis, bullous, 276

N

Nadolol, for hypertension, 211
Nafcillin, for endocarditis, 125t
  for intervertebral disk infection, 229
  for osteomyelitis, 291t
  for sepsis, 369
  for septic arthritis, 370t
Nail, crush injury to, 143
  ingrown, 226
  injury to, 143
Nalidixic acid, for shigella infection, 374
Naproxen, for dysmenorrhea, 121t
Naratriptan, for migraine, 179t
Nasolacrimal duct, obstruction of, acquired,
    102
    congenital, 102
National Cholesterol Education Program,
    209
Navicular, accessory, 277
Nearsightedness, 334
Necrotizing fasciitis, periumbilical, 442,
    442t
Nectar americanus, 17
Neglect, 70
Neisseria gonorrhoeae, 172
Neisseria meningitidis, 259
  in occult bacteremia, 140
Neonates, acne in, 4
  cocaine effect on, 78
  listeriosis in, 246
  papules in, 278
  syphilis in, 400
Nephritis, 185
Nephronophthisis, juvenile, uremic
    medullary cystic kidney disease
    with, 336, 336t
Nephropathy, vs. hematuria, 185
Nephrotic syndrome, 279
  proteinuria with, 185
Nerve deafness, congenital, 280
Neural tube defect, 272
  folic acid deficiency and, 145
Neurobehavioral disorders, drugs and,
    137
Neuroblastoma, 281, 281t
Neurocutaneous melanosis, 282
Neurofibroma, 283
Neurofibromatosis 1, 283
Neurofibromatosis 2, 283
Neurogenic ptosis, 135
Neuroleptics, for Tourette syndrome, 422
Neurologic disorders, hypertension in,
    211
Neuroma, brachial plexus, 49
Neuromuscular degeneration, in kyphosis,
    236
Neuropathy, toxic, 176t
Neurotoxic reaction, in snake bite, 42, 42t
Neutropenia, autoimmune, 284, 284t
  congenital, 284, 284t
  cyclic, 284, 284t
  febrile, 138
  in acute lymphocytic leukemia, 243

Neutrophilic disorders, vs. gingivostomati-
    tis, 169
Neutrophils, 138
Nevic cells, 257
Nevus, congenital, 257
  congenital melanocytic, 311
Nevus achromicus, 214
Nevus anemicus, 214
Nevus depigmentosus, 214
Nevus of Ito, 311
Nevus of Ota, 311
Nevus spilus, 311
Niacin, 209
Niclosamide, for parasitic gastroenteritis,
    165t
Nifedipine, for hypertension, 211
  for migraine, 179t
Niridazole, for dracunculosis, 434
Nitroprusside, for hypertension, 211
  for myocarditis, 273
Non A-E hepatitis, 194
Nonbullous congenital ichthyosiform ery-
    throderma, 219, 219t
Nonpolio human enterovirus, 123
Nonsteroidal anti-inflammatory drugs, for
    asthma, 28
  for dysmenorrhea, 121t
  for juvenile ankylosing spondylitis, 20
  for juvenile rheumatoid arthritis, 232
  for Reiter syndrome, 335
Noonan syndrome, 285
Nose, foreign body of, 148
Nosebleeds, management of, 131
Nursemaid elbow, 332
Nutrition, in anorexia nervosa, 21
  in botulism, 47
  in bronchopulmonary dysplasia, 55
  in bulimia nervosa, 58
  in congestive heart failure, 84
  in Crohn disease, 94

O

Obesity, 286
  in myelomeningocele, 272
Obsessive-compulsive disorder, 22
Obstructive sleep apnea syndrome, 287
Occlusional bites, 39
Occupations, lead in, 240t
Ofloxacin, for gonorrhea, 172
  for pelvic inflammatory disease, 301
  for peritonitis, 306
Olecranon, fracture of, 153
Oligoarthritis, in juvenile rheumatoid
    arthritis, 232, 232t
Oligohydramnios, in hydronephrosis, 207
Omphalitis, 442, 442t
Omphalocele, umbilical cord, 442, 442t
Onchocerca volvulus, 142
Onchocerciasis, 142, 349, 349t
Oppositional defiant disorder, vs. conduct
    disorder, 83
Oral contraceptives, for uterine bleeding,
    445
Oral procedures, endocarditis prophylaxis
    in, 126t
Oral rehydration solution, for viral diar-
    rhea, 166
Orbit, cellulitis of, 305, 305t
  foreign body of, 149
Orchiectomy, 96
Orchitis, 128

Oropharynx, burns of, 133
Orthosis, for kyphosis, 236
Osgood-Schlatter disease, 289
Osteoarticular infection, streptococcal, 393
Osteoblastoma, 46
Osteochondritis dissecans, 234, 290
  of talus, 387
Osteochondroma, 46
Osteodystrophy, renal, 338
Osteoid osteoma, 46
Osteomyelitis, 291, 291t
Otitis externa, 292, 292t
Otitis media, acute, with effusion, 293, 293t
  adhesive, 293
  bacterial, common cold and, 80
  mastoiditis and, 256
Ototopic drops, for otitis externa, 292t
Ovary(ies), abnormalities of, vs. uterine
    bleeding, 445
  dysgenesis of, 372
Overuse injury, lower leg, 294
Oxacillin, for osteomyelitis, 291t
  for sepsis, 369
  for septic arthritis, 370t
Oxybutynin, for diurnal enuresis, 127
Oxycephaly, 93t
Oxycodone, for migraine, 179t
Oxygen therapy, for status asthmaticus
    asthma, 29
Oxygenation, in bronchopulmonary dyspla-
    sia, 55

P

p24 antigen, human immunodeficiency
    virus detection by, 5
Pacemaker, for complete heart block, 181
Pain, abdominal, 1
  growth and, 174
  in anterior knee, 234
  spinal, inflammatory, 20
  with menses, 121
Palate, cleft, 75
Pancreatitis, 295
Panic disorder, 22
Panner disease, vs. Little League elbow,
    247
Papular acrodermatitis, 296
Papular urticaria, 296
  arthropods and, 40
Papules, in molluscum contagiosum, 267
  neonatal, 278
Parainfluenza virus, in pneumonia, 319,
    319t
Parainfluenza virus infection, in laryngo-
    tracheobronchitis, 239
Paraphimosis, 302
Paraplegia, inherited spastic, 69t
Parasites, in cutaneous larva migrans, 392
  in gastroenteritis, 165, 165t
Parasitic infection, central nervous system,
    vs. meningoencephalitis, 260
  vs. sporotrichosis, 385
Parasympathetic nervous system, in scorpi-
    on sting, 41
Parathyroid gland, tetany and, 409
Paromomycin, for amebiasis, 12
Paronychia, candidal, 413
Paroxysmal atrial tachycardia, 122
Paroxysmal supraventricular tachycardia,
    122
Parvovirus infection, 141